NCC 国家癌症中心 NATIONAL CANCER CENTER 编

2020 中国肿瘤登记年报

CHINA CANCER REGISTRY ANNUAL REPORT

主　编　赫　捷　魏文强

副主编　张思维　郑荣寿

人民卫生出版社

·北　京·

图书在版编目（CIP）数据

2020 中国肿瘤登记年报：汉、英/国家癌症中心编
.—北京：人民卫生出版社，2022.2
ISBN 978-7-117-32453-3

Ⅰ.①2… Ⅱ.①国… Ⅲ.①肿瘤-卫生统计-中国
-2020-年报-汉、英 Ⅳ.①R73-54

中国版本图书馆 CIP 数据核字（2021）第 235552 号

人卫智网	www.ipmph.com	医学教育、学术、考试、健康，购书智慧智能综合服务平台
人卫官网	www.pmph.com	人卫官方资讯发布平台

2020 中国肿瘤登记年报
2020 Zhongguo Zhongliu Dengji Nianbao

编　　写：国家癌症中心
出版发行：人民卫生出版社（中继线 010-59780011）
地　　址：北京市朝阳区潘家园南里 19 号
邮　　编：100021
E - mail：pmph @ pmph.com
购书热线：010-59787592　010-59787584　010-65264830
印　　刷：北京顶佳世纪印刷有限公司
经　　销：新华书店
开　　本：889×1194　1/16　　印张：21
字　　数：607 千字
版　　次：2022 年 2 月第 1 版
印　　次：2022 年 7 月第 1 次印刷
标准书号：ISBN 978-7-117-32453-3
定　　价：178.00 元

编委会

张徐巾 张爱红 张竞丹 张海峰 张淑兰 张雅薇 张瑞欣 张源生 张韶凯 张慧玲 张增智
陆　艳 陆玉培 陆绍琦 陈　节 陈　茹 陈　萍 陈　琳 陈　琼 陈　静 陈　霞 陈小慧
陈仁忠 陈兰芬 陈伟强 陈冰霞 陈红艳 陈志虹 陈志萍 陈妙嫦 陈茂勇 陈建国 陈建顺
陈珍莲 陈顺平 陈艳芳 陈艳萍 陈晓红 陈燕芬 武　鸣 拉毛才让 苟丽萍 范　光 范　颖
范美霞 林　利 林　玲 林玉成 林鸿波 林超兰 欧阳乐 罗　源 罗　睿 罗文云 罗国良
罗艳丽 罗辉琴 和臣慧 和丽娜 季加孚 季洪兵 周　丽 周　林 周　衍 周　浩 周　婕
周　琦 周　慧 周　鑫 周义芬 周贤文 周昇杰 周金意 周建容 周建湘 周艳梅 周素霞
周晓梅 周敏茹 周婷婷 周锦涛 周新玉 郑小祥 郑冬柏 郑永萍 郑荣寿 郑裕明 单林涛
单保恩 宗　华 官文婷 陕国清 赵　丽 赵　培 赵　璨 赵小兰 赵会勇 赵海洲 赵彬茜
赵朝强 赵雅芳 郝士卿 郝庆华 荆国旗 胡　东 胡　池 胡　莹 胡　彪 胡　静 胡晓先
胡翠芳 茹夏丽 南　艳 柯　华 柯金练 查震球 柳以泽 哈艳茹 钞利娜 钟伟文 段乐永
段纪俊 段凯岚 保红莉 侯　亮 侯晓艳 俞　亮 俞　敏 独梅芝 施　燕 施长苗 姜　欣
姜方平 姜玉平 娄培安 洪　杰 宫舒萍 姚　霜 贺　玲 贺宇彤 贺绍琼 骆秀美 秦延锦
袁　帅 袁　湘 袁东娅 袁晓宇 耿文飞 莫兆波 莫桂琼 贾卫军 夏　冰 夏　亮 夏立环
夏丽莉 顾　凯 顾建芬 顾晓平 徐　红 徐　珏 徐　玲 徐　爽 徐　琴 徐　鹏 徐　薇
徐文超 徐玉銮 徐仙会 徐汉顺 徐红艳 徐贤雄 徐建强 徐绍和 徐海霞 徐媛锋 徐新红
凌海杰 高　从 高杨波 高秋生 高鸿敏 高瑞芳 郭　超 郭天骅 郭巧红 郭红革 郭启高
郭昌融 郭树岚 郭贵周 郭秋献 郭晓雷 郭颖贞 席云峰 唐　伟 唐士涛 涂波涌 陶小红
黄　丽 黄　静 黄一峰 黄飞平 黄永进 黄远田 黄国士 黄素勤 黄海浪 黄维娜 黄惠玲
曹　智 曹诗鹏 曹慷慷 龚建华 龚新洪 盛春宁 盛振海 盛根英 常　蓉 崔艳丽 符三乃
符为巨 符芳敏 庹吉妤 章　剑 章文华 章有建 淳志明 梁从凯 梁永春 梁志龙 梁伯衡
梁树军 梁鹏涛 梁翠敏 梁耀洁 彭　绩 彭　瑾 彭爱云 董　华 董　言 董　玲 董　洪
董建梅 蒋　丽 蒋　微 蒋素红 韩　奎 韩小玉 韩仁强 韩明明 韩湘意 覃忠书 景燕平
程立平 程向东 程志芳 程新和 鲁玲亚 曾　平 曾红梅 曾雄文 温之花 游宁静 谢　婧
谢威龙 谢淑雯 强德仁 靳万春 楚玉梅 赖永赣 雷芸华 雷宝琼 解　晔 赫　捷 蔡　伟
蔡红卫 管小琴 管元平 管丽娟 廖　顺 廖　倩 廖　涛 廖卓航 廖凌玲 漆苏洋 谯　宇
翟玉庭 熊　斌 熊　薇 熊晓世 熊润红 熊端萍 樊学琼 颜仕鹏 潘中伟 潘龙海 潘永富
潘定权 潘盛林 穆慧娟 戴　丹 戴　丽 戴　姮 戴招文 戴曙光 魏　丹 魏文强 魏矿荣
瞿　媛

Editorial Board

Wu Yanwei, Wu Haihong, Wu Yiping, Wu Xinhui, Qiu Hong, Qiu Lin, Qiu Yuqiong, He Fei, He Li, He Li, He Liu, He Jie, He Lei(Chaotian Qu), He Lei(Mouding Xian), He Liming, He Xiuling, He Daofeng, Yu Bin, Yu Jiahua, Gu Hanfeng, Zou Hong, Zou Yuewei, Ying Hongyan, Xin Jiakui, Wang Youku, Wang Yangjie, Shen Huan, Shen Feiqiong, Shen Chengfeng, Shen Jianxin, Shen Xiaowen, Song Guang, Song Yuhua, Song Lijun, Song Bingbing, Song Liangwen, Song Guohui, Zhang You, Zhang Long, Zhang Rong, Zhang Biao, Zhang Xing, Zhang Qiu, Zhang Li, Zhang Tao, Zhang Juan, Zhang Min, Zhang Yan, Zhang Ting, Zhang Xiaoling, Zhang Yijie, Zhang Yongzhen, Zhang Jizhi, Zhang Yaying, Zhang Quanshou, Zhang Yunqiu, Zhang Wuwu, Zhang Kunping, Zhang Yinan, Zhang Jianan, Zhang Jianlu, Zhang Siwei, Zhang Yanling, Zhang Yanyan, Zhang Xiaofeng, Zhang Xujin, Zhang Aihong, Zhang Jingdan, Zhang Haifeng, Zhang Shulan, Zhang Yawei, Zhang Ruixin, Zhang Yuansheng, Zhang Shaokai, Zhang Huiling, Zhang Zengzhi, Lu Yan, Lu Yupei, Lu Shaoqi, Chen Jie, Chen Ru, Chen Ping, Chen Lin ,Chen Qiong, Chen Jing, Chen Xia, Chen Xiaohui, Chen Renzhong, Chen Lanfen, Chen Weiqiang, Chen Bingxia, Chen Hongyan, Chen Zhihong, Chen Zhiping, Chen Miaochang, Chen Maoyong, Chen Jianguo, Chen Jianshun, Chen Zhenlian, Chen Shunping, Chen Yanfang, Chen Yanping, Chen Xiaohong, Chen Yanfen, Wu Ming, Lamao Cairang, Gou Liping, Fan Guang, Fan Ying, Fan Meixia, Lin Li, Lin Ling, Lin Yucheng, Lin Hongbo, Lin Chaolan, Ouyang Le, Luo Yuan, Luo Rui, Luo Wenyun, Luo Guoliang, Luo Yanli, Luo Huiqin, He Chenhui, He Lina, Ji Jiafu, Ji Hongbing, Zhou Li, Zhou Lin, Zhou Yan, Zhou Hao, Zhou Jie, Zhou Qi, Zhou Hui, Zhou Xin, Zhou Yifen, Zhou Xianwen, Zhou Shengjie, Zhou Jinyi, Zhou Jianrong, Zhou Jianxiang, Zhou Yanmei, Zhou Suxia, Zhou Xiaomei, Zhou Minru, Zhou Tingting, Zhou Jintao, Zhou Xinyu, Zheng Xiaoxiang, Zheng Dongbai, Zheng Yongping, Zheng Rongshou, Zheng Yuming, Shan Lintao, Shan Baoen, Zong Hua, Guan Wenting, Shan Guoqing, Zhao Li, Zhao Pei, Zhao Can, Zhao Xiaolan, Zhao Huiyong, Zhao Haizhou, Zhao Binqian, Zhao Zhaoqiang, Zhao Yafang, Hao Shiqing, Hao Qinghua, Jing Guoqi, Hu Dong, Hu Chi, Hu Ying, Hu Biao, Hu Jing, Hu Xiaoxian, Hu Cuifang, Ru Xiali, Nan Yan, Ke Hua, Ke Jinlian, Zha Zhenqiu, Liu Yize, Ha Yanru, Chao Lina, Zhong Weiwen, Duan Leyong, Duan Jijun, Duan Kailan, Bao Hongli, Hou Liang, Hou Xiaoyan, Yu Liang, Yu Min, Du Meizhi, Shi Yan, Shi Changmiao, Jiang Xin, Jiang Fangping, Jiang Yuping, Lou Peian, Hong Jie, Gong Shuping, Yao Shuang, He Ling, He Yutong, He Shaoqiong, Luo Xiumei, Qin Yanjin, Yuan Shuai, Yuan Xiang, Yuan Dongya, Yuan Xiaoyu, Geng Wenfei, Mo Zhaobo, Mo Guiqiong, Jia Weijun, Xia Bing, Xia Liang, Xia Lihuan, Xia Lili, Gu Kai, Gu Jianfen, Gu Xiaoping, Xu Hong, Xu Jue, Xu Ling, Xu Shuang, Xu Qin, Xu Peng, Xu Wei, Xu Wenchao, Xu Yuluan, Xu Xianhui, Xu Hanshun, Xu Hongyan, Xu Xianxiong, Xu Jianqiang, Xu Shaohe, Xu Haixia, Xu Yuanfeng, Xu Xinhong, Ling Haijie, Gao Cong, Gao Yangbo, Gao Qiusheng, Gao Hongmin, Gao Ruifang, Guo Chao, Guo Tianhua, Guo Qiaohong, Guo Hongge, Guo Qigao, Guo Changrong, Guo Shulan, Guo Guizhou, Guo Qiuxian, Guo Xiaolei, Guo Yingzhen, Xi Yunfeng, Tang Wei, Tang Shitao, Tu Boyong, Tao Xiaohong, Huang Li, Huang Jing, Huang Yifeng, Huang Feiping, Huang Yongjin, Huang Yuantian, Huang Guoshi, Huang Suqin, Huang Hailang, Huang Weina, Huang Huiling, Cao Zhi, Cao Shipeng, Cao Kangkang, Gong Jianhua, Gong Xinhong, Sheng Chunning, Sheng Zhenhai, Sheng Genying, Chang Rong, Cui Yanli, Fu Sannai, Fu Weiju, Fu Fangmin, Tuo Jiyu, Zhang Jian, Zhang Wenhua, Zhang Youjian, Chun Zhiming, Liang Congkai, Liang Yongchun, Liang Zhilong, Liang Boheng, Liang Shujun, Liang Pengtao, Liang Cuimin, Liang Yaojie, Peng Ji, Peng Jin, Peng Aiyun, Dong Hua, Dong Yan, Dong Ling, Dong Hong, Dong Jianmei, Jiang Li, Jiang Wei, Jiang Suhong, Han Kui, Han Xiaoyu, Han Renqiang, Han Mingming, Han Xiangyi, Qin Zhongshu, Jing Yanping, Cheng Liping, Cheng Xiangdong, Cheng Zhifang, Cheng Xinhe, Lu Lingya, Zeng Ping, Zeng Hongmei, Zeng Xiongwen, Wen Zhihua, You Ningjing, Xie Jing, Xie Weilong, Xie Shuwen, Qiang Deren, Jin Wanchun, Chu Yumei, Lai Yonggan, Lei Yunhua, Lei Baoqiong, Xie Ye, He Jie, Cai Wei, Cai Hongwei, Guan Xiaoqin, Guan Yuanping, Guan Lijuan, Liao Shun, Liao Qian, Liao Tao, Liao Zhuohang, Liao Lingling, Qi Suyang, Qiao Yu, Zhai Yuting, Xiong Bin, Xiong Wei, Xiong Xiaoshi, Xiong Runhong, Xiong Duanping, Fan Xueqiong, Yan Shipeng, Pan Zhongwei, Pan Longhai, Pan Yongfu, Pan Dingquan, Pan Shenglin, Mu Huijuan, Dai Dan, Dai Li, Dai Heng, Dai Zhaowen, Dai Shuguang, Wei Dan, Wei Wenqiang, Wei Kuangrong, Qu Yuan

前　言

肿瘤登记是对肿瘤流行情况、趋势变化和影响因素进行长期、连续、动态的系统性监测，是制定癌症预防控制策略、开展综合防控研究、评价防控效果的重要基础性工作。这项工作的标志性成果之一就是，每年以年报的形式及时发布全国肿瘤登记监测数据。中国肿瘤登记年报已成为我国癌症预防与控制不可或缺的宝贵资料，在不同历史时期均发挥了极其重要的作用。我国的肿瘤登记，自20世纪50年代起步至今，已走过60多年的发展历程，60年从无到有，从小到大，60年风雨兼程，愈挫弥坚，离不开几辈专业人士的拓荒与坚守，更离不开党和国家的引领与呵护，肿瘤登记工作已经探索出了符合我国实际的发展道路，成为我国癌症防控工作的重要组成部分。

目前，我国已建成覆盖全国的肿瘤登记随访监测系统，连续动态发布肿瘤登记年报，持续推进肿瘤生存随访。截至2020年底，肿瘤登记已覆盖全国1 152个县区，覆盖人口5.98亿，全国肿瘤登记中心也完成了《中国肿瘤登记数据集》团体标准立项及制定工作，完成了全国肿瘤登记信息平台建设工作，我国的肿瘤登记工作国际影响逐步扩大，国际评价我国为肿瘤登记数据质量一类地区，中国的肿瘤登记主动承担国际及区域肿瘤登记责任，不断为世界肿瘤登记工作贡献中国智慧。

肿瘤防控再出发，肿瘤登记要先行。随着肿瘤等慢性非传染性疾病在世界公共卫生问题中的比重逐步加重，癌症负担等慢病基础数据的必要性、连续性、重要性必将日益凸显，进一步提升肿瘤登记数据质量，促进登记数据与死因监测数据、临床诊疗信息数据以及人口数据、医保数据等其他信息的对接交换、互联互通，促进信息资源共享利用，是肿瘤登记工作的重中之重，也是大势所趋。

《2020中国肿瘤登记年报》是自2008年首次出版以来的第14卷。本年报汇总了2017年我国肿瘤登记地区癌症监测数据。国家癌症中心收到来自中国31个省（自治区、直辖市）及新疆生产建设兵团（未包括香港、澳门特别行政区和台湾省）821个肿瘤登记处上报数据。通过对数据审核和质量控制，有554个肿瘤登记处数据入选本年报。此次年报对所有癌症合计及22类癌症的发病和

Foreword

Cancer Registration is a long-term, continuous, dynamic and systematic monitoring system. It monitors the epidemic state, trend changes, and influence factors of cancer. Cancer Registration is the fundamental work of formulating cancer prevention and control strategies, launching comprehensive prevention and control research, and evaluating prevention and control results. One prominent achievement of cancer registration in China is to publish the *China Cancer Registry Annual Report*, which has been a great value for cancer prevention and control in different periods of the country. Since the primary stage in the 1950s, China cancer registration has gone through 60 years of development. In the past 60 years, it has developed from scratch, from small to large, and has experienced tremendous hardships. It is inseparable from the pioneering spirit and persistence of several generations of professionals, and also inseparable from the guidance and care of the Party and the State. China cancer registration has explored a way in line with the reality of our country, and has become an important part of cancer prevention and control in China.

At present, China has established a nationwide cancer registration and follow-up monitoring system, which can continuously and dynamically release Cancer Registry Annual Report, and constantly promotes follow-up of cancer survival. By the end of 2020, cancer registration has covered 1 152 counties and districts with population coverage of 598 million. The National Cancer Center has also completed the establishment and formulation of the association standard of *China Cancer Registration Data Set* and the construction of the National Cancer Registration Information Platform. The international influence of China cancer registration is gradually expanding. China has been evaluated as the first-class region in terms of the quality of cancer registration data. China actively takes the responsibility of international and regional cancer registration work, and constantly contributes China wisdom to the world.

Cancer prevention and control are having an unprecedented development opportunity, and cancer registration needs to start before the others to lead cancer prevention and control. With the increasing proportion of chronic non-infectious diseases such as cancer in the public health problem worldwide, the necessity, the continuity, and the importance of basic data of cancer and other chronic diseases will become increasingly prominent. Enhancing the quality of cancer registration data, promoting the exchange and interconnection of registration data and death causing data, the clinical diagnosis and treatment information data, population data, medical insurance data, and other information, and the sharing and utilization of information resources are the essential part and the general trend of cancer registration.

Since the first volume of *China Cancer Registry Annual Report* published in 2008, this book is the 14th Annual Report. In this volume, cancer surveillance data of China cancer registration areas in 2017 was

死亡数据进行了详细分析，并分地区、年龄别和性别比较了癌症分布差异。考虑到各省已经开始发布本地区的肿瘤负担数据，本次全国年报不再展示各省区县级的肿瘤登记数据。

60年转瞬即逝，肿瘤登记工作是中国人民防癌抗癌历程中浓墨重彩的一笔，但中国肿瘤登记的过去并未远去，我们仍在前辈开拓出的路上坚定前行。回顾中国肿瘤登记60年从小到大、从弱到强的发展历程，我们能够体会前辈的艰辛与坚守，我们更心存感激，我们更骄傲自豪，在建党100周年之际，我们几辈人薪火相传，已经探索出了符合中国实际的肿瘤登记道路！我们感恩前辈的筚路蓝缕，砥砺付出，最好的回报是传承和发展，我们深信，在党和国家健康中国战略的指引下，我国肿瘤登记工作必将会成绩斐然，再创辉煌！

在全国新冠肺炎疫情防控新常态环境下，肿瘤登记工作者在积极落实防控措施的前提下，不忘本职，无怨无悔地及时完成了年报数据上报清理、统计分析、编撰出版工作。《2020中国肿瘤登记年报》的顺利出版凝结着全国各肿瘤登记处全体工作人员的辛苦付出和50多位编写、审校人员的辛勤劳动，年报的出版也得到了国家疾病预防控制局、国家卫生健康委员会宣传司一如既往的具体指导和大力支持，我们在此表示衷心的感谢！

编者从登记点选择、数据清理、统计分析、图表呈现、文字描述等方面反复核实，力求做到数字真实、描述准确，竭力避免不必要的失误，然而由于水平和知识有限，加之入选年报的登记点数量剧增，数据体量巨大，工作中难免出现纰漏，敬请国内外同行和广大读者批评指正。

国家癌症中心

2021年6月

reported. A total of 821 cancer registries submitted data to National Cancer Center (NCC) in China, including 31 provinces (autonomous regions and municipalities) and Xinjiang Production and Construction Corps (not including Hong Kong, Macao Special Administrative Regions and Taiwan Province). After data quality control, a total of 554 cancer registries were included in the present *China Cancer Registry Annual Report*. In this volume, we summarized and analyzed data of the incidence and mortality for all cancers combined and 22 cancer sites by including overall analysis and analysis by age, sex and area. Considering that all provinces have begun to release the cancer burden data of their own regions, this national annual report will no longer show the cancer registration data at the county level.

Cancer registration is an important part of the anti-cancer process in China in the last 60 years. However, the history of China cancer registration has not passed away, and we are still proceeding on the way of our predecessors. We are grateful and proud of the hard work and persistence of our predecessors when looking back on the 60 years of development from small to large, from weak to strong of China cancer registration. Through the efforts of several generations, China cancer registration has explored a way in line with the reality of our country at the 100th anniversary of the founding of the Communist Party of China. We are grateful to the contribution of our predecessors and will continue the inheritance and development in return. We are convinced that China cancer registration will make brilliant achievements under the guidance of Healthy China Strategy of the Party and the State.

In the new period of regular prevention and control of COVID-19, all faculties of cancer registries did not forget their duties and complete the reporting, cleaning, analyzing and publishing works of the annual report without complaint while actively implementing epidemic prevention and control measures. The successful publication of *2020 China Cancer Registry Annual Report* embodies the hard work of all staff members in different cancer registries across the country. It also reflects the hard work of more than 50 editors and reviewers. National Administration of Disease Prevention and Control, Department of Publicity in National Health Commission of the People's Republic of China have also provided guidance and support in the publication of the *2020 China Cancer Registry Annual Report*. We acknowledge all staff working for the cancer registries and the editorial board who contributed to this publication.

In order to assure the data is real, objective, accurate and without unnecessary mistakes, the authors write carefully and verify repeatedly for choosing the cancer registries, cleaning data, doing statistical analysis, rendering charts and describing data. However, due to the knowledge limitation, and the intensively increased cancer registries, the vast data volume may lead to some mistakes in the work. Colleagues and readers are welcome to criticize and correct.

National Cancer Center

June 2021

目　　录

Contents

第一章 概 述

1 中国人群肿瘤登记系统

肿瘤登记是对癌症流行情况、趋势变化和影响因素进行长期、连续、动态的系统性监测，是制定癌症预防控制策略、开展综合防控研究、评价防控效果的重要基础性工作。我国的肿瘤登记工作已走过了60年发展历程，人群肿瘤登记工作在不同时期，都为国家癌症防控提供了科学翔实的肿瘤负担和流行情况，有力支撑了我国癌症防控政策策略制定和实施。

近几十年我国人群肿瘤登记工作进展迅速，成绩举世瞩目。2008年，原卫生部设立“肿瘤登记随访项目”并纳入“国家重大公共卫生专项中央财政转移支付项目”，在全国31个省（自治区、直辖市）及新疆生产建设兵团（未包括香港、澳门特别行政区和台湾省）逐步建立了覆盖全国的人群肿瘤登记和监测随访网络，逐步开展人群为基础的肿瘤发病、死亡和生存的信息收集工作。2015年原国家卫生和计划生育委员会、国家中医药管理局联合下发《肿瘤登记管理办法》，从制度上保证了全国肿瘤登记工作的顺利开展。多年来，在上级主管部门的领导和大力支持下，全国肿瘤登记处数量和质量逐年提升。截至2020年底，开展人群肿瘤登记工作的登记处为1 152个，覆盖5.98亿人口，目前收集到的肿瘤负担数据，能够较为全面地反映我国癌症发病、死亡、生存状况及变化趋势。

但我们也应看到，随着大数据时代的到来和现代网络信息技术的发展，传统登记监测手段的不足逐步显现，逐渐无法满足国家卫生决策、人民群众不断增长的健康需求及癌症预防、临床诊治、科学研究工作的及时高效服务需求。针对现阶段存在的肿瘤登记点数量不足和分布不均衡、肿瘤登记数据深度和广度不足、信息资源交互共享利用度低等问题，《健康中国行动——癌症防治实施方案（2019—2022年）》中，对肿瘤登记工作以制度标准、数据质量和资源共享为切入点，通过“扩面”“提质”“增效”三个方面的具体行动措施，全面推进肿瘤登记工作。“扩面”就是要通过修订

Chapter 1 Introduction

1 Population-based cancer registration system in China

Cancer Registration is a long-term, continuous, dynamic, systematic monitoring system. It monitors cancer's epidemic state, trend change and influence factor. Cancer Registration is the fundamental work of formulating cancer prevention and control strategies, launching comprehensive prevention and control research, and evaluating prevention and control results. After 60 years' development, the cancer registry provides scientific and detailed information about cancer burden and epidemic state for national cancer prevention and control, as well as supports the formulation and implementation of the cancer prevention and control policy in the different periods. In recent decades, our Cancer Registry has progressed rapidly, and its outstanding achievements have attracted worldwide attention.

Since 2008, the former Ministry of Health set up the "National Cancer Registration and Follow-up Program" to support the cancer registration in China with sustainable funding. All 31 provinces (autonomous regions, municipalities) and Xinjiang Production and Construction Corps in China (data of Hong Kong SAR, Macao SAR and Taiwan Province is not included) have gradually established a cancer registration framework. Population-based cancer incidence, mortality and survival information are collected through the cancer registration system. In 2015, the former National Health and Family Planning Commission and National Administration of Traditional Chinese Medicine co-published *Chinese Cancer Registration Management Regulation*, which provides a legal protection on cancer registration in China. Under the leadership of the Chinese government, there has been a steady increase in the numbers and quality of population-based cancer registries in China. Until the end of 2020, there are a total of 1 152 population-based cancer registries, with 598 million population coverage. Trends and updated statistics of cancer incidence, mortality and survival are comprehensively reported from the data the cancer registry collected.

However, with the advent of the big data era and the development of modern internet technology, the

《肿瘤登记管理办法(2015)》和《中国肿瘤登记工作指导手册(2016)》、发布肿瘤登记共识性政策文件和肿瘤登记工作实施方案、扩大登记年报覆盖面、落实省级责任制等工作进一步健全肿瘤登记报告制度。"提质"就是要通过推动国家肿瘤登记平台工程、建立多级肿瘤登记点专家团队、制定登记数据收集标准及随访监测数据质量标准等方面的工作,提升肿瘤登记数据质量。"增效"就是要通过加强肿瘤登记信息化建设、制定登记数据管理方法和数据信息安全管理方法、推进不同信息资源对接、开展大数据应用研究等,促进信息资源共享利用。

积极落实国家系列规划、计划等政策文件精神,国家癌症中心已基本完成了全国肿瘤登记信息平台的建设工作,今年年报的部分数据就是通过新的平台上报。相信在新的发展机遇下,中国的肿瘤登记工作必将实现肿瘤数据实时上报、动态监测和多维呈现,更为及时有效地为我国肿瘤防控的政策制定、工作实施、效果评估等提供坚实的科学依据,更好地服务健康中国战略。

deficiencies of traditional registration monitoring methods gradually emerged. It cannot fully support the national health decision making, satisfy the increasing demand of people's health concerns and fulfill the requirements of cancer prevention, clinical diagnosis, treatment and scientific research.

Due to the insufficient and unevenly distributed cancer registries, the insufficient data depth and breadth, and the low utilization of interactive sharing of information resources, *The Plan of Healthy China-The Implementation Plan of Cancer Prevention and Control (2019-2022)* develops three implementation strategies: "Coverage Expansion" "Quality Improvement" and "Efficiency Increment" to fully promote cancer registry from system standards, data quality and resource sharing aspects. "Coverage Expansion": by revising *Chinese Cancer Registration Management Regulation (2015)* and *Chinese Guideline for Cancer Registration (2016)*, releasing consensus policy of cancer registration and implementation proposal of cancer registration, expanding the coverage of the annual report and fulfilling provincial responsibility system to further improve the cancer registration system. "Quality Improvement": by promoting the "National Cancer Registration Platform Project", establishing a multi-level cancer registration expert team and developing the standards of registration data collection and data quality monitoring to improve the data quality of cancer registration. "Efficiency Increase": by strengthening the information construction of cancer registration, developing registration data management regulation and data security management regulation, promoting the integration of different resources, and conducting big data application research, to increase the efficiency of sharing and utilization of information resources.

National Cancer Center has mainly completed the construction of the National Cancer Registration Information Platform. Part of the data in this year's annual report was reported through the new platform. It is believed that under the new development opportunity, the cancer registration work of China will achieve real-time reporting, dynamic monitoring and multi-dimensional presentation. This work will provide solid scientific support for the policy formulation, work implementation, and effect evaluation of cancer prevention and control of China in a more timely and effective manner, so as to serve the "Healthy China" strategy better.

2 本年报数据

2.1 数据上报地区及范围

本年报数据收集截止时间为2020年12月31日，数据上报范围为2017年1月1日至2017年12月31日全年新发癌症发病和死亡个案数据（ICD-10编码范围：C00-96，D32-33，D42-43，D45-47），以及各肿瘤登记处2017年年中人口数据。上报2017年肿瘤登记数据的登记处分布在全国31个省（自治区、直辖市）及新疆生产建设兵团（未包括香港、澳门特别行政区和台湾省），合计登记处821个，覆盖人口563 934 185人，其中城市登记处298个，农村登记处523个。

2.2 数据质量控制及最终纳入数据

国家癌症中心根据《中国肿瘤登记工作指导手册（2016）》，参照国际癌症研究机构（IARC）/国际癌症登记协会（IACR）、《五大洲癌症发病率》第11卷对肿瘤登记质量的有关要求，从数据可比性、有效性和完整性等方面制定中国肿瘤登记年报数据纳入排除标准。依据标准对2017年肿瘤登记数据进行质量控制，同时充分考虑区域覆盖面，本年报最终纳入554个登记处数据。

全国554个肿瘤登记处2017年覆盖人口436 336 955人（男性221 134 960人，女性215 201 995人），占全国2017年年末人口数的31.39%。其中城市地区肿瘤登记处223个，覆盖人口213 246 283人，占入选年报中国肿瘤登记地区人口数的48.87%；农村地区肿瘤登记处331个，覆盖人口223 090 672人，占51.13%。

2 Data specification in this annual report

2.1 Data collection scope

NCC China required all population-based cancer registries to submit new diagnoses and deaths from cancer in 2017 (ICD-10: C00-96, D32-33, D42-43, D45-47), as well as the corresponding population data before December 31st, 2020. All those submitted data in 2017 are distributed in 31 provinces (autonomous regions, municipalities) and Xinjiang Production and Construction Corps (not including Hong Kong, Macao Special Administrative Regions and Taiwan Province). A total of 821 cancer registries submitted data to NCC China, covering a total of 563 934 185 population. Among the 821 cancer registries, 298 were urban cancer registries and 523 were rural cancer registries.

2.2 Data quality control and qualified data

According to *Chinese Guideline for Cancer Registration (2016)* and the standards of International Agency for Research on Cancer/International Association of Cancer Registries (IARC/IACR) on *Cancer Incidence in Five Continents, Vol. XI*, we have published a national criterion on data quality for Chinese cancer registration data from aspects of comparability, completeness and validity. We applied strict quality control on data and consider the wide coverage of different geographic areas in China. A total of 554 cancer registries were included in the present annual report.

The 554 cancer registries covered a total of 436 336 955 population (221 134 960 males, 215 201 995 females), accounting for 31.39% of the national population in 2017. Especially, there were 223 urban cancer registries covering 213 246 283 population (48.87%) and 331 rural cancer registries with population coverage of 223 090 672 (51.13%).

2.3 年报内容

本年报汇总了554个肿瘤登记处2017年癌症的发病、死亡及人口数据。详细描述了合计554个肿瘤登记处和各肿瘤登记处数据的质量控制指标,如死亡发病比例、病理诊断比例、仅有医学死亡证明书比例等。详细报道了合计癌症和22种癌症发病死亡数据指标包括:发病率、死亡率、中国人口标化率(2000年中国人口构成)、世界人口标化率(Segi's世界人口构成)、累积率、分年龄组发病率/死亡率、分性别发病率/死亡率等。部分癌症按亚部位和组织学分型进行了细化描述。分城市农村、东中西地区、七大区和各省(自治区、直辖市)及新疆生产建设兵团(未包括香港、澳门特别行政区和台湾省),比较了各地区癌症发病死亡差异。

2.3 Content of this annual report

The present annual report summarized data of the cancer incidence, mortality and demography through 554 cancer registration sites in 2017. We reported the quality control indicators including mortality incidence rate ratio (M/I), percentage of morphological verification (MV%), percentage of death certificate only (DCO%), et al, overall and by registration site. We reported data of new cases and deaths of all cancers and by site, including crude incidence, mortality, age-standardized rate (ASR) of China population in 2000, ASR of Segi's world population, cumulative rates, age and sex-specific rates. Moreover, we presented detailed distribution of subsite and morphology for some cancers. We compared cancer incidence and mortality rates by urban and rural areas, three geographic areas (eastern areas, central areas and western areas), the seven administrative districts (North China, Northeast China, East China, Central China, South China, Southwest China and Northwest China), and 31 provinces (autonomous regions, municipalities) and Xinjiang Production and Construction Corps (data of Hong Kong SAR, Macao SAR and Taiwan Province is not included).

第二章　方法和指标

肿瘤登记是系统性、经常性收集有关肿瘤及肿瘤病人信息的统计制度。目的是了解城乡居民癌症发病、死亡情况和生存状态，掌握癌症的疾病负担与变化趋势，以及在不同地区和人群中的分布特征，为国家和卫生行政部门制定癌症防治策略、规划与计划，为癌症基础研究及临床研究提供基本信息，为监测和评价癌症控制措施的效果提供基本依据。

1　建立肿瘤登记处

根据《肿瘤登记管理办法》要求：各级卫生计生行政部门、中医药管理部门应当加强肿瘤登记工作的组织和监督管理；各级各类医疗卫生机构要认真组织落实，做好肿瘤登记工作。经国务院批准，国家卫生健康委等 10 部委联合发布的《健康中国行动——癌症防治实施方案（2019—2022 年）》中明确要求实施癌症信息化行动，健全肿瘤登记报告制度，各级肿瘤登记中心负责辖区肿瘤登记工作的组织实施，各级各类医疗卫生机构履行肿瘤登记报告职责。到 2022 年，实现肿瘤登记工作在所有县区全覆盖，发布国家和省级肿瘤登记年报。提升肿瘤登记数据质量，建成肿瘤登记报告信息系统、质量控制标准和评价体系，提高报告效率及质量。到 2022 年，纳入国家肿瘤登记年报的登记处数量不少于 850 个。促进信息资源共享利用，加强肿瘤登记信息系统与死因监测、电子病历等数据库的对接交换，逐步实现资源信息部门间共享，推进大数据应用研究，提升生存分析与发病死亡趋势预测能力。规范信息管理，保护患者隐私和信息安全。

Chapter 2　Method and index

Cancer registration is a systematic and regular statistical system designed for collecting information on cancer and cancer patients. Cancer registration aims at understanding cancer incidence, mortality and survival in urban and rural areas, which helps to understand the current status and trends of cancer burden in different regions and populations. Cancer registration may provide accurate, up-to-date population-based cancer data which are vital for decision making on cancer prevention and control. The data may also provide basic information for cancer research and cancer surveillance.

1　Establishing a cancer registry

According to *Chinese Cancer Registration Management Regulation* published by the former National Health and Family Planning Commission and National Administration of Traditional Chinese Medicine, all medical institutions in different levels of China should conduct cancer registration.

With the approval of the State Council, *The Plan of Healthy China-The Implementation Plan of Cancer Prevention and Control (2019-2022)* issued by 10 ministries and commissions including the National Health Commission requires the implementation of cancer informatization actions and the improvement of the cancer registration reporting system. It also clearly states the responsibility of cancer registration centers for the organizing and implementing of the cancer registration work in their districts, and the responsibility of medical and health institutions at all levels for reporting the cancer registration situation.

By 2022, the cancer registration work should be fully covered in all districts and counties with national and provincial cancer registry annual report. The quality of cancer registration data will be improved. Also, the information system for the cancer registration report and the system for quality control standards and quality evaluation will be established. By

肿瘤登记处是连续性搜集、贮存、整理、统计分析、评价、阐述及报告肿瘤发病、死亡和生存信息资料的部门。肿瘤登记处所在区县，应建立完善的死因监测系统，同时能够获取准确的人口学资料。肿瘤登记处应覆盖全部市区或全县户籍人口。当地政府或卫生行政部门应制定和颁布实行肿瘤登记报告制度的法律法规或规范性文件，并配备相应的工作人员、经费及设备，同时制订肿瘤登记报告实施细则。

2022, the *China Cancer Registry Annual Report* should include no fewer than 850 registries. The sharing and utilization of information resources will be promoted; the docking and exchanging between cancer registration information system and death cause monitoring and electronic medical record and other databases will be strengthened; the sharing of resources and information among departments, and the promoting of the application of big data will be achieved; the ability of survival analysis and morbidity prediction will be improved; also, the information management and the protection of patients' privacy and information security will be standardized.

A cancer registry is a bureau for the collection, storage, management and analysis of data on persons with cancer. A cancer registry should be established based on the death surveillance system and accurate population statistics. The local governments or health bureaus should make regulations on cancer registration. They should also provide trained personnel, funding, equipment and cancer report regulations to support the establishment of cancer registries.

2 资料收集方法

肿瘤登记资料的收集分为被动和主动两种方法。被动是由各医疗机构定期报送肿瘤登记卡片到肿瘤登记处,或从死因监测部门获取肿瘤患者死亡信息。主动是登记员到各医疗单位、医疗保险机构查阅肿瘤新病例的诊疗病史,摘录肿瘤病历信息,或主动随访获取患者的生存信息。

为健全我国肿瘤登记信息系统、加强全国肿瘤登记工作规范化管理,获得及时、统一、准确的肿瘤发病、死亡和生存信息,使肿瘤登记工作满足当前癌症防治工作需要,国家癌症中心于 2019 年新开发了“中国肿瘤登记平台”。并于当年 7 月 1 日正式上线运行。中国肿瘤登记平台覆盖全国全部省份和区县,平台按照国家行政区划,采取国家-省-市-县-乡 5 级设立管理机构、登记处和上报机构,平台包括系统管理、登记、审核、随访、人口与寿命表、基线信息、导入导出、统计分析、实时呈现、在线培训模块等基本功能。

2 Methods of data collection

Case reporting methods are classified as active or passive. Cancer registries may passively receive the cancer registration cards from health-related institutions or vital statistics bureaus. Meanwhile, cancer registry personnel may actively retrieve the cancer data from health-related institutions, insurance bureaus and public security bureaus. Cancer registrars may actively follow up the cancer patients for their vital status.

The National Cancer Center newly developed the “China Cancer Registration Platform” in 2019, which was officially launched on 1st July of that year. The new platform is there to improve the national cancer registration information system and strengthen the standardized management of the national cancer registration work. Also, it is launched to obtain timely, unified and accurate information on the incidence, death and survival of cancers, so that the needs of current cancer prevention and treatment works can be met by the cancer registration works. The China Cancer Registration Platform covers all provinces, districts and counties throughout the country. According to the national administrative divisions, the platform uses the 5 levels divisions (national-provincial-municipal-county-township) to establish management agencies, registries and reporting agencies. The platform includes system management, registration, audit, follow-up, population and life expectancy table, baseline information, import and export, statistical analysis, real-time presentation, online training module and other fundamental functions.

2.1 信息收集渠道

肿瘤登记地区从相关部门收集辖区内肿瘤新发病例、死亡病例、生存信息和相关人口资料。病例资料的收集渠道包括登记地区各级医疗机构、医疗保险数据库、死因监测数据库、新型农村合作医疗数据库等。人口资料的来源包括人口普查资料和公安、统计部门有关资料等。

2.2 病例核实工作

肿瘤登记地区负责肿瘤病例的建卡和分类编码,并以身份证号作为标识。通过核对死因监测数据库,对遗漏病例进行补充建卡,对重复病例进行剔除。

2.3 随访工作

随访工作的开展采用被动随访和主动随访相结合的方式进行。肿瘤登记处首先将肿瘤发病库与全死因登记库进行被动匹配。未匹配上者通过定期访视、电话、书信、电子邮件等方式进行联系,并通过社区居委会、基层医疗卫生机构开展主动随访,以获取病例的生存情况(图 2-1)。

2.1 Data collecting channels

Cancer registries should collect cancer statistics including cancer incidence, cancer death, cancer survival and population data from all kinds of channels. The cancer registries may collect cancer statistics from clinics, hospitals, health insurance databases, death surveillance database and cooperative health insurance database in rural areas.

2.2 Cancer case certification

The cancer registries are responsible for making cancer case report forms, using identification card number as personal identification code. The cancer death records should also be matched with incidence database. The missing incidence cases should be supplemented and the duplicated cases should be deleted.

2.3 Follow-up practice

Both passive follow-up and active follow-up are used to collect the survival information of cancer cases. Staff of local registries linked the cancer records and death records based on identifiable information. Patients who were not linked to the death surveillance system were followed by regular visit, telephone, letter and e-mails etc. And obtain the survival status of those cases through community committees and primary medical and health institutions(Figure 2-1).

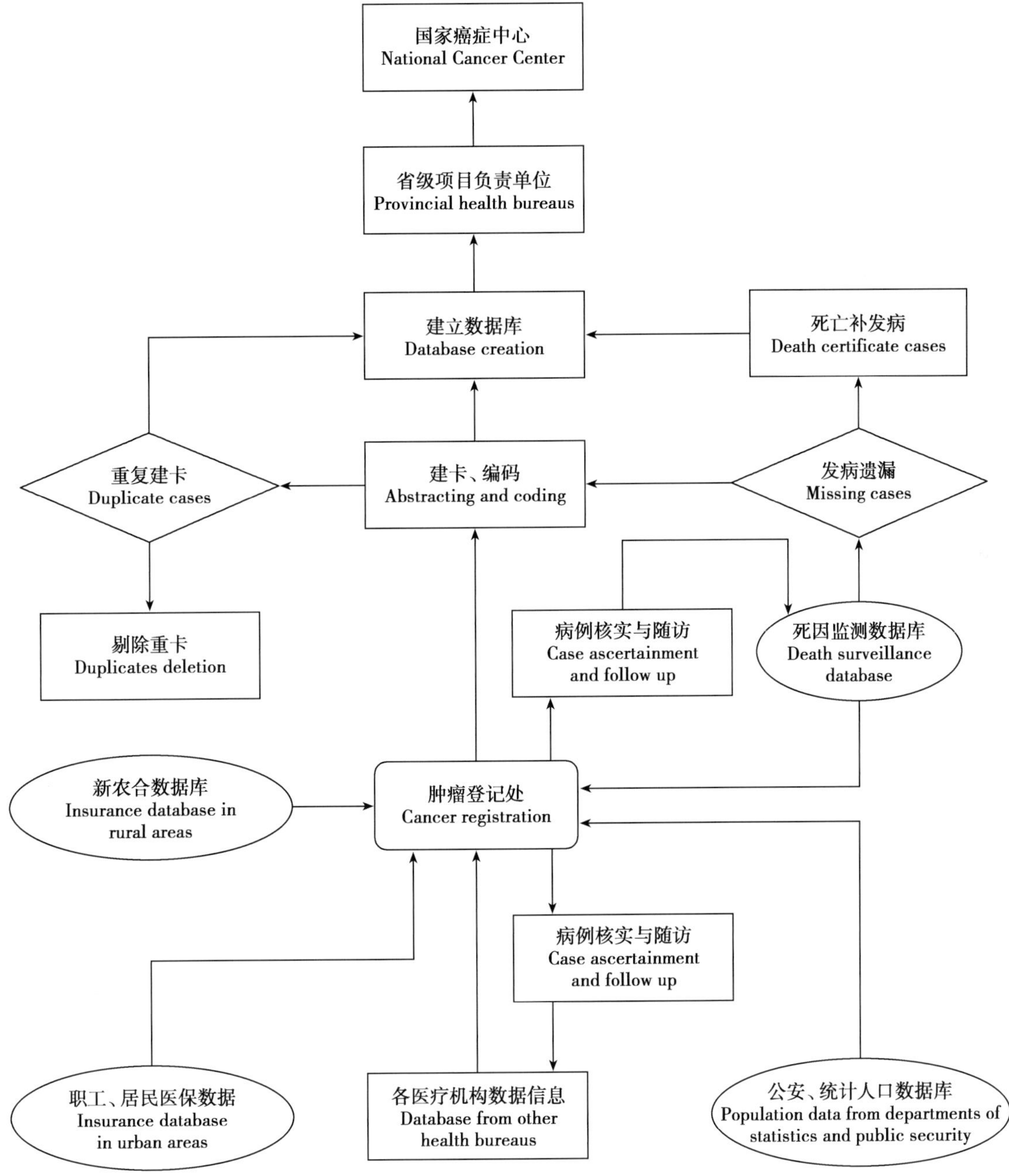

图 2-1　肿瘤登记工作流程图

Figure 2-1　Flow diagram of the cancer registration system

3 数据收集

肿瘤登记主要收集登记覆盖范围内全部癌症和中枢神经系统良性肿瘤及动态未定或未知肿瘤病例的发病、死亡和生存状态,以及登记覆盖人群的相关人口资料。为评估早诊早治效果,现已开始要求各登记处收集原位癌病例信息。

3.1 新发病例数据

个人信息包括姓名、性别、出生日期、年龄、身份证号码、住址、出生地、民族、婚姻状况、职业等;肿瘤信息包括发病日期、解剖学部位(亚部位)、组织学类型、诊断依据、病理和临床分期、治疗方法等;报告单位信息包括报告日期、诊断单位、报告单位、报告医生等。

3.2 死亡数据

肿瘤死亡资料来源于全人口死因登记报告,包括根本死因为非肿瘤原因的肿瘤病例的死亡资料。除发病信息外,还应包括死亡日期、实足年龄、死亡原因主要诊断、诊断级别和依据、死亡地点等。

3.3 生存随访数据

肿瘤病例随访资料包括最后接触时间、生存状态、是否失访、失访原因等。

3.4 人口数据

人口资料来源于我国人口普查资料和公安、统计部门逐年提供的人口资料。人口资料包括居民人口总数及其性别、年龄别人口数或构成。年龄组按0~岁、1~4岁、5~9岁、10~14岁……80~84岁、85岁及以上分组。为计算肿瘤相对生存率,需提供相应年份的寿命表。

3 Data collection

Cancer registries are required to collect data on all cancers' incidence, mortality and survival, including tumors of central nerve systems with benign or uncertain behaviors. The data of population coverage should also be collected. In order to evaluate the effect of early diagnosis and treatment, each registry was required to collect the information of cancer in situ cases.

3.1 Incidence data

We collect personal information of incident cases including age, sex, date of birth, age of diagnosis, identification number, address, place of birth, race, marital status and career. The detailed cancer information including date of diagnosis, anatomical site and sub-site, pathological, histological as well as cytological results, diagnosis basis, pathological and clinical stages, and treatment methods. The reporting date, clinics of diagnosis, reporting bureau and reporting doctors should be collected.

3.2 Mortality data

The cancer mortality data are from population-based all causes of death surveillance database. Besides personal information of cancer incidence, the mortality data should contain date of death, age of death, cause of death, place of death and diagnostic basis for death cause.

3.3 Survival data

The cancer survival statistics are from the follow-up data of the cancer patients. The detailed cancer survival information includes: last time of contact, vital status, causes of lost-to-follow up.

3.4 Population data

The population data originate from census data, departments of statistics or public security. The detailed population data covered the number of residents, sex, age-specific population or composition. The age group was divided into 0, 1-4, 5-9, 10-14, . . . 80-84, 85+. For relative survival calculation, the cancer registries should also provide life tables.

4 质量控制

质量控制贯穿肿瘤登记工作的全过程。肿瘤登记地区应在各个环节制定工作规范和质量控制程序,并严格执行。质量控制主要包括四个方面:可比性、完整性、有效性和时效性。

4.1 可比性

数据结果真实可比的基本先决条件是采用通用的标准或定义。通常而言,可比性是指发病率间的不同不是因各登记地区之间的数据质量和标准不同而产生。可比性涉及以下几个指标:对"发病"的定义,对原发、复发和转移的诊断标准、分类与编码,死亡证明等。

4.2 完整性

完整性是指在登记地区资料库的目标人群中发现所有发病病例的程度。常用的评价指标有死亡/发病比(M/I)、只有死亡证明书比例(DCO%)、形态学诊断确认比例(MV%)、病例的来源数与报告单数、不同时间发病率的稳定性、不同人群发病率的比较、年龄别发病率曲线、儿童癌症评价等等。俘获/再俘获方法也用来评价登记报告资料的完整性。

4.3 有效性

有效性是指登记病例中具有给定特征属性(例如肿瘤部位、年龄)的病例所占的比例。再摘录与再编码方法是评价有效性的最客观方法,一般由另一个观察者完成对登记地区记录与相关病例文件间仔细比较。常用的评价指标有形态学诊断确认比例(MV%),只有死亡证明书比例(DCO%)、部位不明百分比,年龄不明百分比等。癌症登记地区至少进行诸如年龄/出生日期、性别/部位、部位/组织学以及部位/组织学/年龄、基本变量有无遗漏信息等基本核对。

4 Quality control

The value of cancer registration relies on the data quality. This procedure aims at providing qualified cancer registration data with comparability, completeness, validity, and timeliness.

4.1 Comparability

Comparability is the extent to which coding and classification at a registry, together with the definitions of recording and reporting specific data items, adhere to standardized international guidelines. In the evaluation of the comparability of registration data, the following standards should be identical: the identification for tumor classification and coding, the definition of incidence, the identification of primary cancer and cancer recurrence or metastasis of an existing one, the criteria of death certification.

4.2 Completeness

The completeness of cancer registry data refers to the extent of all the incident cancers occurring in the population included in the cancer registration database. It is an extremely important attribute of a cancer registry's data. The methods which provide indication of the completeness include the following: Mortality/Incidence(M/I) ratios, percentage of death certificate only(DCO%), percentage of morphological verification of diagnosis(MV%), reporting avenues, stability of incidence rates over time, comparison of incidence rates in different populations, shape of age-specific curves and incidence rates of childhood cancers. The capture-recapture methods are also used to evaluate the completeness of registration data.

4.3 Validity

Validity is defined as the proportion of cases in a dataset with a given characteristic which truly have the attribute. Re-abstracting and re-coding are the principal methods which permit comparisons with respect to specified subsets of cases. Using diagnostic criteria (MV% and DCO%), missing information analysis and internal consistency methods, the validity of the cancer registration information can be verified.

4.4 时效性

时效性一般指从发病日期(诊断日期)到数据被利用时(年报、研究报告、论文)的间隔。登记地区应及时报告和获取癌症信息。目前对时效性的要求无统一的国际标准。为平衡与完整性和准确性的关系,国家癌症中心要求各登记地区于诊断年份后的30个月内提交数据。

4.4 Timeliness

Timeliness relates to the rapidity at which a registry can collect, process and report reliable and complete cancer data. It indicates the time to availability as the interval between date of diagnosis and the date the case was available in the registry for further use. The cancer registries should timely collect and report cancer statistics. Whilst there are no international guidelines for the timeliness of cancer registry data, NCC China requires the cancer registries should report cancer statistics in 30 months.

5 资料质量控制流程

国家癌症中心收到各肿瘤登记处上报资料后,首先检查资料的完整性。在确认资料完整后,使用IARC/IACR工具软件中的Check程序逐一检查所有记录的变量是否完整和有效,同时对不同变量之间是否合乎逻辑的一致性进行检查。然后使用数据分析软件及数据库软件生成统一表格,对登记数据的完整性和可靠性做出评估。各登记地区根据评估结果,对登记资料进行核实、补充与修改,将修改后的资料再次上报国家癌症中心,国家癌症中心将全国各登记地区数据进行汇总分析,并撰写年度报告(图2-2)。

5 Flow diagram of data quality control

After receiving the cancer registration data, NCC will first check the completeness of the cancer data. After that, IARC/IACR-check software would be used to check whether all the variables are complete and valid. The internal consistency of the dataset would also be checked. NCC would further publish specific data evaluation report to each registry. The local registries would follow the evaluation report to check and revise the cancer datasets once again. Qualified cancer dataset will be pooled and analyzed for annual national cancer report(Figure 2-2).

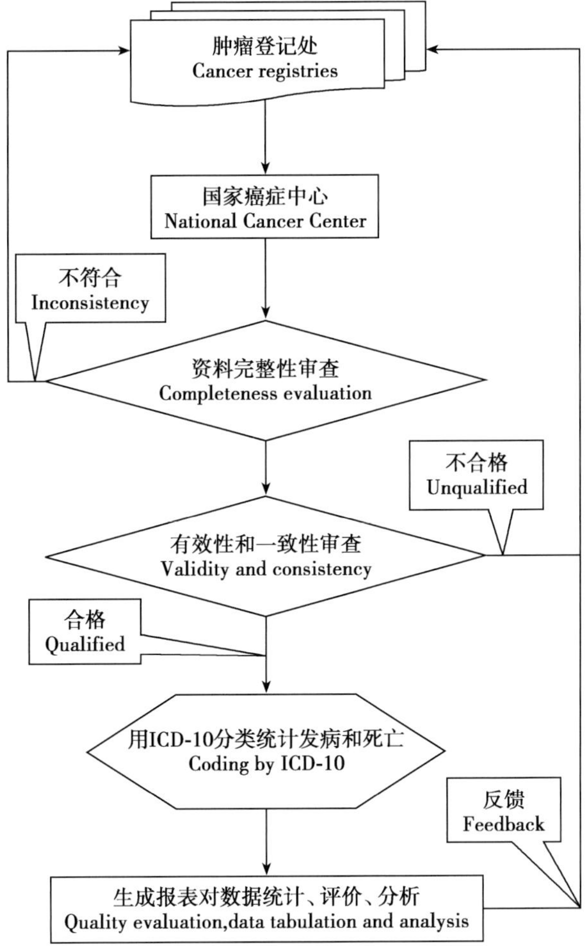

图 2-2　登记资料审核流程

Figure 2-2　Flow diagram of data quality

6 统计分类

6.1 癌症分类

参照国际上常用的癌症 ICD-10 分类统计表，根据 ICD-10 前三位“C”类编码，将癌症细分类为 59 部位、25 个大类，其中脑和神经系统包括良性及良恶性未定肿瘤（D32-33，D42-43）。真性红细胞增多症（D45）、骨髓增生异常综合征为（D46）、淋巴造血和有关组织动态未定肿瘤（D47）归入髓样白血病（C92）。原位癌暂未纳入统计分析。详见表 2-1、表 2-2。

6 Classification and coding

6.1 Cancer classification

Taken from the WHO cancer classification publications of ICD-10 version, Cancers were classified into 59 types and 25 categories with different anatomic sites. The neoplasms of cerebral and central nervous system(D32-33, D42-43) are included in the ICD-10 cancer dictionary. For myeloproliferative disease(D46) and myelodysplastic syndromes(D47), they are coded as myeloid leukemia (C92). Caricinoma in situ was not included in the analyses(Table 2-1, Table 2-2).

表 2-1 癌症统计分类表(ICD-10)

Table 2-1 classification used in statistic (bu ICD-10)

部位 **Site**	**ICD-10**
唇 Lip	C00
舌 Tongue	C01-02
口 Mouth	C03-06
唾液腺 Salivary glands	C07-08
扁桃腺 Tonsil	C09
其他口咽 Other oropharynx	C10
鼻咽 Nasopharynx	C11
下咽 Hypopharynx	C12-13
咽，部位不明 Pharynx, unspecified	C14
食管 Esophagus	C15
胃 Stomach	C16
小肠 Small intestine	C17
结肠 Colon	C18
直肠 Rectum	C19-20
肛门 Anus	C21
肝脏 Liver	C22
胆囊及其他 Gallbladder etc.	C23-24
胰腺 Pancreas	C25
鼻、鼻窦及其他 Nose, sinuses etc.	C30-31
喉 Larynx	C32
气管、支气管、肺 Trachea, bronchus & lung	C33-34
其他胸腔器官 Other thoracic organs	C37-38
骨 Bone	C40-41
皮肤黑色素瘤 Melanoma of skin	C43

续表

部位 Site	ICD-10
皮肤其他 Other skin	C44
间皮瘤 Mesothelioma	C45
卡波氏肉瘤 Kaposi sarcoma	C46
周围神经、其他结缔组织、软组织 Connective & soft tissue	C47,C49
乳腺 Breast	C50
外阴 Vulva	C51
阴道 Vagina	C52
子宫颈 Cervix uteri	C53
子宫体 Corpus uteri	C54
子宫,部位不明 Uterus,unspecified	C55
卵巢 Ovary	C56
其他女性生殖器 Other female genital organs	C57
胎盘 Placenta	C58
阴茎 Penis	C60
前列腺 Prostate	C61
睾丸 Testis	C62
其他男性生殖器 Other male genital organs	C63
肾 Kidney	C64
肾盂 Renal pelvis	C65
输尿管 Ureter	C66
膀胱 Bladder	C67
其他泌尿器官 Other urinary organs	C68
眼 Eye	C69
脑、神经系统 Brain,nervous system	C70-72,D32-33,D42-43
甲状腺 Thyroid	C73
肾上腺 Adrenal gland	C74
其他内分泌腺 Other endocrine	C75
霍奇金淋巴瘤 Hodgkin lymphoma	C81
非霍奇金淋巴瘤 Non-Hodgkin lymphoma	C82-86,C96
免疫增生性疾病 Immunoproliferative diseases	C88
多发性骨髓瘤 Multiple myeloma	C90
淋巴样白血病 Lymphoid leukemia	C91
髓样白血病 Myeloid leukemia	C92-94,D45-47
白血病,未特指 Leukemia,unspecified	C95
其他或未指明部位 Other and unspecified	O&U
所有部位合计 All sites	C00-96,D32-33,D42-43,D45-47
所有部位除外 C44 All sites except C44	C00-96,D32-33,D42-43,D45-47exc. C44

表 2-2　常用癌症分类统计表(大分类)

Table 2-2　Broad cancer classification of ICD-10

部位全称 **Full title of site**	部位缩写 **Short title of site**	**ICD-10**
口腔和咽喉(除外鼻咽) Oral cavity & pharynx except nasopharynx	口腔 Oral cavity & pharynx	C00-10,C12-14
鼻咽 Nasopharynx	鼻咽 Nasopharynx	C11
食管 Esophagus	食管 Esophagus	C15
胃 Stomach	胃 Stomach	C16
结直肠肛门 Colon,rectum & anus	结直肠 Colon-rectum	C18-21
肝脏 Liver	肝 Liver	C22
胆囊及其他 Gallbladder etc.	胆囊 Gallbladder	C23-24
胰腺 Pancreas	胰腺 Pancreas	C25
喉 Larynx	喉 Larynx	C32
气管、支气管、肺 Trachea,bronchus & lung	肺 Lung	C33-34
其他胸腔器官 Other thoracic organs	其他胸腔器官 Other thoracic organs	C37-38
骨 Bone	骨 Bone	C40-41
皮肤黑色素瘤 Melanoma of skin	皮肤黑色素瘤 Melanoma of skin	C43
乳房 Breast	乳房 Breast	C50
子宫颈 Cervix uteri	子宫颈 Cervix	C53
子宫体及子宫部位不明 Uterus & unspecified	子宫体 Uterus	C54-55
卵巢 Ovary	卵巢 Ovary	C56
前列腺 Prostate	前列腺 Prostate	C61
睾丸 Testis	睾丸 Testis	C62
肾及泌尿系统不明 Kidney & unspecified urinary organs	肾 Kidney	C64-66,C68
膀胱 Bladder	膀胱 Bladder	C67
脑、神经系统 Brain,nervous system	脑 Brain	C70-C72,D32-33,D42-43
甲状腺 Thyroid	甲状腺 Thyroid	C73
淋巴瘤 Lymphoma	淋巴瘤 Lymphoma	C81-86,C88,C90,C96
白血病 Leukemia	白血病 Leukemia	C91-95,D45-47
其他或未指明部位 Other and unspecified	其他 Other	Other
所有部位合计 All sites	合计 All sites	C00-96, D32-33, D42-43, D45-47

6.2 自然地区分类

城、乡分类根据国家标准 GB 2260—2019，将地级以上城市归于城市地区，县及县级市归于农村地区，同时综合考虑地区经济及生活方式等因素。

东、中、西部地区的划分采用国家统计局标准。

东部地区包括：北京市、天津市、河北省、辽宁省、上海市、江苏省、浙江省、福建省、山东省、广东省、海南省、香港特别行政区、澳门特别行政区、台湾省。

中部地区包括：黑龙江省、吉林省、山西省、安徽省、江西省、河南省、湖北省、湖南省。

西部地区包括：内蒙古自治区、广西壮族自治区、重庆市、四川省、贵州省、云南省、西藏自治区、陕西省、甘肃省、青海省、宁夏回族自治区、新疆维吾尔自治区。

七大区划分根据民政部区划分类（未包括香港、澳门特别行政区和台湾省）。

华北地区：北京市、天津市、河北省、山西省、内蒙古自治区。

东北地区：辽宁省、吉林省、黑龙江省。

华东地区：上海市、江苏省、浙江省、安徽省、福建省、江西省、山东省。

华中地区：河南省、湖北省、湖南省。

华南地区：广东省、广西壮族自治区、海南省。

西南地区：重庆市、四川省、贵州省、云南省、西藏自治区。

西北地区：陕西省、甘肃省、青海省、宁夏回族自治区、新疆维吾尔自治区。

6.2 Area classification

According to GB2260-2019 national standard, prefecture-level cities are classified into urban areas, whereas counties and county-level cities are classified into rural areas. And the socio-economic status of the areas are considered.

The classification of eastern areas, central areas and western areas is based on the standard of National Statistics Bureau. The eastern areas consists of provinces of Beijing, Tianjin, Hebei, Liaoning, Shanghai, Jiangsu, Zhejiang, Fujian, Shandong, Guangdong, Hainan, Hong Kong, Macao, Taiwan. The central areas consists of provinces of Heilongjiang, Jilin, Shanxi, Anhui, Jiangxi, Henan, Hubei and Hunan. The western areas consist of provinces of Inner Mongolia, Guangxi, Chongqing, Sichuan, Guizhou, Yunnan, Tibet, Shaanxi, Gansu, Qinghai, Ningxia and Xinjiang.

According to the standard from Ministry of Civil Affairs, the classification of these seven areas is shown as following (not including Hong Kong, Macao Special Administrative Regions and Taiwan Province):

North China: Beijing, Tianjin, Hebei, Shanxi, Inner Mongolia.

Northeast China: Liaoning, Jilin, Heilongjiang.

East China: Shanghai, Jiangsu, Zhejiang, Anhui, Fujian, Jiangxi, Shandong.

Central China: Henan, Hubei, Hunan.

South China: Guangdong, Guangxi, Hainan.

Southwest China: Chongqing, Sichuan, Guizhou, Yunnan, Tibet.

Northwest China: Shaanxi, Gansu, Qinghai, Ningxia, Xinjiang.

7 常用统计指标

7.1 年平均人口数

年平均人口数是计算发病(死亡)率指标的分母,精确算法是一年内每一天暴露于发病(死亡)危险的生存人数之和除以年内天数,但实际上很难掌握每一天的生存人数,因而常用年初和年末人口数的算术平均数作为年平均人口数的近似值。

$$\text{年平均人口数(人)}=\frac{\text{年初(上年末)人口数}+\text{年末人口数}}{2}$$

年中人口数指 7 月 1 日零时人口数,如果人口数变化均匀,年中人口数等于年平均人口数,可以用年中人口数代替年平均人口数。

7.2 性别、年龄别人口数

性别、年龄别人口数是指按男、女性别和不同年龄分组的人口数,建议用“内插法”推算。年龄的分组,规定以 5 岁划分年龄别:0~岁、1~4 岁、5~9 岁、10~14 岁……80~84 岁、85 岁及以上。

7.3 发病(死亡)率

发病(死亡)率又称为粗发病(死亡)率,是反映人口发病(死亡)情况最基本的指标,是指某年该地登记的每 10 万人口癌症新病例(死亡)数,反映人口发病(死亡)水平。

$$\text{发病(死亡)率(1/10 万)}=\frac{\text{某时期恶性肿瘤新病例(死亡)数}}{\text{某时期年平均人口数}}\times 100\,000$$

7.4 年龄别发病(死亡)率

人口的年龄结构是影响癌症发病(死亡)水平的重要因素,年龄别发病(死亡)率是统计研究的重要指标。

$$\text{某年龄组发病(死亡)率(1/10 万)}=\frac{\text{某年龄组发病(死亡)人数}}{\text{同年龄组人口数}}\times 100\,000$$

7 Statistical indicators

7.1 Average annual population

Average annual population is the denominator of the incidence(mortality) rates. The exact method to calculate is the average of persons at risk of incidence (mortality) each day in a specific year. Considering the complexity of the calculation, we often use the estimated calculation to quantify the population effectively. The formula is:

$$\text{Average annual population}=\frac{\text{population at the end of the year+population in the early of the year}}{2}$$

The mid-year population is the number of populations in 1st July at 0AM. If the population is relatively stable, the mid-year population can be used to represent average annual population.

7.2 Sex- and age-specific population

Sex-specific population is the population by sex. Age-specific population is the population by different age groups and it is can be calculated by interpolation. The ages may be grouped into classes of up to five years, for example, 0, 1-4, 5-9, 10-14... 80-84, 85+.

7.3 Incidence(mortality) rate

The incidence(mortality) rate is a measure of the frequency with which an event, such as a new case of cancer(cancer death) occurs in a population over a period.

$$\text{Incidence(mortality) rate per 100 000}=\frac{\text{new cases(new cancer death) ocurring during a given time period}}{\text{population at risk during the same time period}}\times 100\,000$$

7.4 Age-specific incidence(mortality) rate

Age is an important factor influencing the cancer incidence and mortality. Age-specific rate is important statistical indicator.

$$\text{Age-specific incidence(mortality) rate per 100 000}=\frac{\text{cases(cancer death) in a specific age group}}{\text{population in the age group}}\times 100\,000$$

7.5 年龄调整率(标准化率)

由于粗发病(死亡)率受人口年龄构成的影响较大,因此在对比分析不同地区的发病(死亡)率或同一地区人群不同时期的发病(死亡)水平时,为消除人口年龄结构对发病(死亡)水平的影响,需要计算按年龄标准化的发病(死亡)率,即指按照某一标准人口的年龄结构所计算的发病(死亡)率。本年报使用中国标准人口是 2000 年全国第五次人口普查的人口构成(简称:中标率),世界标准人口采用 Segi's 标准人口构成(简称:世标率)。表 2-3 为中国人口和世界人口年龄构成,可供计算年龄标准化率时选用。

年龄调整发病(死亡)率的计算(直接法):

(1) 计算年龄组发病(死亡)率。

(2) 以各年龄组发病(死亡)率乘以相应的标准人口年龄构成百分比,得到相应的理论发病(死亡)率。

(3) 将各年龄组的理论发病(死亡)率相加之和,即年龄标准化发病(死亡)率。

$$\text{年龄标准化发病(死亡)率(1/10万)} = \frac{\sum \text{标准人口年龄构成} \times \text{年龄别发病(死亡)率}}{\sum \text{标准人口年龄构成}}$$

7.5 Age-standardized rate (ASR)

Standardization is necessary when comparing populations with different age structures because age has such a powerful influence on cancer incidence and mortality. ASR is a summary measure of a rate that a population would have if it had a standard age structure.

In this annual cancer report, the population standards we used are the Segi's population and the fifth Chinese national census of 2000. Table 2-3 are the details of the population standards.

Direct method calculating incidence (mortality) rate:

(1) calculating the rates for subjects in a specific age category in a study population.

(2) calculating the weighted age-specific rates. The weights applied represent the relative age distribution of the standard population.

(3) adding up each weighted age-specific rate. The summary rates reflect the adjusted rates.

$$\text{ASR per 100 000} = \frac{\sum \text{standard population in corresponding age group} \times \text{age-specific rate}}{\sum \text{standard population}}$$

表 2-3 标准人口构成

Table 2-3 Standard Populations

年龄组/岁 Age group/ years	中国人口构成 2000 年 China standard population(2000)	世界人口构成 Segi's population	年龄组/岁 Age group/ years	中国人口构成 2000 年 China standard population(2000)	世界人口构成 Segi's population
0~	13 793 799	2 400	45~	85 521 045	6 000
1~	55 184 575	9 600	50~	63 304 200	5 000
5~	90 152 587	10 000	55~	46 370 375	4 000
10~	125 396 633	9 000	60~	41 703 848	4 000
15~	103 031 165	9 000	65~	34 780 460	3 000
20~	94 573 174	8 000	70~	25 574 149	2 000
25~	117 602 265	8 000	75~	15 928 330	1 000
30~	127 314 298	6 000	80~	7 989 158	500
35~	109 147 295	6 000	85+	4 001 925	500
40~	81 242 945	6 000	合计	1 242 612 226	100 000

7.6 分类构成

各类癌症发病(死亡)构成比可以反映各类癌症对居民健康危害的情况。癌症发病(死亡)分类构成比的计算公式如下:

$$\text{某癌症构成比}(\%)=\frac{\text{某癌症发病(死亡)人数}}{\text{总发病(死亡)人数}}\times 100$$

7.7 累积发病(死亡)率

累积发病(死亡)率是指某病在某一年龄阶段内的按年龄(岁)的发病(死亡)率进行累积的总指标。累积发病(死亡)率消除了年龄构成不同的影响,故不需要标准化便可以用于不同地区直接进行比较。癌症一般是计算 0~74 岁的累积发病(死亡)率。

$$\text{累积发病(死亡)率}(\%)=\{\sum[\text{年龄组发病(死亡)率}\times\text{年龄组距}]\}\times 100$$

7.8 截缩发病(死亡)率

通常对癌症是截取 35~64 岁这一易发年龄段计算,其标准人口构成是世界人口。

$$\text{截缩发病(死亡)率}(1/10\text{万})=\frac{\sum\text{截缩段各年龄组发病(死亡)率}\times\text{各段标准年龄构成}}{\sum\text{各段标准年龄构成}}$$

因为癌症在 35 岁以前是少发的,而在 65 岁以后其他疾病较多,干扰较大,所以采用 35~64 岁这一阶段的截缩发病(死亡)率比较确切,便于比较。

7.6 Relative frequency

The relative frequency indicates the proportion of new site-specific cancer cases in all cancers combined. The formular is:

$$\text{Relative frequency of a certain type of cancer }(\%)=\frac{\text{No. of cases of a particular cancer}}{\text{No. of cases of all cancers}}\times 100$$

7.7 Cumulative incidence (mortality) rate

A cumulative incidence (mortality) rate expresses the probability of the onset of cancer between birth and a specific age. The rate can be compared without age standardization as it is not affected by age structures. This is often expressed for population between 0 and 74 years.

$$\text{Cumulative incidence(mortality) rate }(\%)=\left[\sum(\text{age-specific incidence(mortality) rate}\times\text{width of the agegroup})\right]\times 100$$

7.8 Truncated incidence (mortality) rate

Truncated incidence rate is the calculation of rate over the truncated age-range 35-64, using WHO world standard population. The data are presented as truncated rates mainly because the accuracy of age-specific rates in the elderly may be much less certain and the rates in the young age groups may be rare.

$$\text{Truncated incidence (mortality) rate per 100 000}=\frac{\sum\text{trancated rate in a specific age group}\times\text{standard proportion of the age group}}{\sum\text{standard population}}$$

8 生存率

生存率是评价癌症治疗是否有效的关键指标。以人群为基础的肿瘤登记工作收集患者的生存资料，计算生存率以反映肿瘤人群的生存状况。某时间生存率，是指某一批随访对象中，生存期大于等于该时间的研究对象的比例，如五年生存率等。常用的生存率指标有观察生存率、净生存率和相对生存率。生存率实质是累积生存概率。

8.1 观察生存率

观察生存率分析中，以患者死亡为观察终点，包括死于肿瘤和其他原因。肿瘤登记资料常用寿命表法估计观察生存率。寿命表法应用定群寿命表的基本原理计算生存率，可利用截尾数据的不完全信息。

8.2 调整生存率/净生存率

观察生存率反映的是肿瘤患者的整体死亡状况。在很多情况下，人们关注于肿瘤患者死于肿瘤的信息。此时，常常需要计算调整生存率/净生存率。净生存率的关键是必须依据完整、准确的死因信息。在比较不同年龄、性别、社会经济学状况下癌症患者的生存率时，使用净生存率显得尤为重要，因为肿瘤外其他死因会影响癌症患者的生存状况。

净生存率可通过计算疾病特异性生存率(disease-specific survival rate)获得，即以患者死于该肿瘤为观察终点。若肿瘤患者死于肿瘤之外的其他原因，将与存活状态同等处理。

8 Survival rate

Survival rate is an overall index for measuring the effectiveness of cancer care. The survival rates calculated based on data from population-based cancer registries will therefore represent the average prognosis in the population. Survival rate can be expressed in terms of the percentage of those cases who were still alive after a specified interval (i. e. 5 years). The measures for survival rate calculation include observed survival rate, net survival rate, and relative survival rate, which are the cumulative probability of survival from diagnosis to the end of each time interval.

8.1 Observed survival rate

The observed or crude survival rate is simply the estimated probability of survival at the end of the specified period. It takes no account of the cause of death. Actuarial or life-table method provides a means for using all the follow-up information to calculate survival rate, which is often applied in population-based cancer survival analysis.

8.2 Adjusted survival/net survival rate

The observed survival rate can be interpreted as the probability of survival from cancer and all other causes of deaths combined. While this is a true reflection of total mortality in the patient group, the main interest is usually in describing mortality attributable to cancer. The concept of net (or adjusted) survival rate is the survival probability in the hypothesis that the patients only die from their cancer. It is a crucial measure for survival rate comparisons among patients with different age, sex and socio-economic status.

Net survival rate can be achieved through calculating cancer-specific survival rate, which relies on reliable individual cause of death. If the cancer patients die from causes other than cancer, it will be treated as alive.

8.3 相对生存率

当缺乏完整、准确的全死因信息时，净生存率指标往往较难通过疾病特异性生存率获取。此时，净生存率可以通过相对生存率来估计。相对生存率即为特定人群的观察生存率与该人群的期望生存率比值。根据全死因寿命表的死亡概率，可以求得一般人群的期望生存率。

$$相对生存率=\frac{观察生存率}{期望生存率}$$

如前所述，肿瘤登记资料中观察生存率常采用寿命表法。而期望生存率的计算常常分区间估计。估计方法有 Ederer Ⅰ、Ederer Ⅱ、Hakulinen 方法等。

8.3 Relative survival rate

Where death certificate is not publicly available, or certification of the cause of death is not sufficiently reliable, net survival rate is hardly achieved through cancer-specific survival rate, which needs the exact cause of death for cancer patients. Relative survival rate does not require information on the cause of death in the cancer patients. Relative survival rates are usually expressed as a ratio of the crude survival rate in the group of cancer patients and the corresponding expected survival rate in the general population. Observed survival rate can be achieved by life-table/actual methods, while expected survival rate can be estimated with methods of Ederer Ⅰ, Ederer Ⅱ and Hakulinen.

$$\text{Relative survival rate}=\frac{\text{observed survival rate}}{\text{expected survival rate}}$$

第三章 数据质量评价

Chapter 3 Evaluation of data quality

1 数据来源

2020年国家癌症中心收到全国821个登记处提交的2017年肿瘤登记资料，登记覆盖的区县约有980个。登记处分布在全国31个省（自治区、直辖市）及新疆生产建设兵团（未包括香港、澳门特别行政区和台湾省），其中地级以上城市298个，县和县级市523个。四川省上报资料登记处数量最多为131个，其次为云南省77个、江苏省和河南省各47个。北京市、天津市、广州市、石家庄市登记地区覆盖了全部区县，在本年报分城乡按2个登记处计（表3-1）。

1 Data sources

A total of 821 cancer registries submitted cancer registration data of 2017 to NCC China in 2020, covering about 980 districts and counties. A total of 31 provinces (autonomous regions, municipalities) and Xinjiang Production and Construction Corps (not including Hong Kong, Macao Special Administrative Regions and Taiwan Province) were covered by these registries, with a total of 298 prefecture-level cities and 523 counties (county-level cities). Sichuan province submitted data from most cancer registries (131), followed by Yunnan (77), Jiangsu and Henan (47). The data from Beijing, Tianjin, Shijiazhuang and Guangzhou covered all districts and counties. They were classified as urban and rural areas separately in this report (Table 3-1).

表3-1 2017年全国提交肿瘤登记资料的地区

Table 3-1 The cancer registries which submitted cancer statistics of 2017

省（自治区、直辖市） Province (autonomous region, municipality)	登记处数 No. of cancer registries	登记处名单 List of cancer registries
北京 Beijing	2	北京市 Beijing Shi、北京市郊区 Rural areas of Beijing Shi
天津 Tianjin	2	天津市 Tianjin Shi、天津市郊区 Rural areas of Tianjin Shi
河北 Hebei	28	石家庄市 Shijiazhuang Shi、石家庄市郊区 Rural areas of Shijiazhuang Shi、赞皇县 Zanhuang Xian、迁西县 Qianxi Xian、迁安市 Qian'an Shi、秦皇岛市 Qinhuangdao Shi、邯郸市邯山区 Hanshan Qu, Handan Shi、大名县 Daming Xian、涉县 She Xian、磁县 Ci Xian、武安市 Wu'an Shi、邢台市 Xingtai Shi、邢台县 Xingtai Xian、临城县 Lincheng Xian、内丘县 Neiqiu Xian、任县 Ren Xian、保定市 Baoding Shi、望都县 Wangdu Xian、安国市 Anguo Shi、张家口市宣化区 Xuanhuan Qu, Zhangjiakou Shi、张北县 Zhangbei Xian、承德市双桥区 Shuangqiao Qu, Chengde Shi、丰宁满族自治县 Fengning Manzu Zizhixian、沧州市 Cangzhou Shi、海兴县 Haixing Xian、盐山县 Yanshan Xian、衡水市冀州区 Jizhou Qu, Hengshui Shi、辛集市 Xinji Shi
山西 Shanxi	17	太原市杏花岭区 Xinghualing Qu, Taiyuan Shi、阳泉市 Yangquan Shi、平定县 Pingding Xian、盂县 Yu Xian、平顺县 Pingshun Xian、沁源县 Qinyuan Xian、阳城县 Yangcheng Xian、晋中市榆次区 Yuci Qu, Jinzhong Shi、昔阳县 Xiyang Xian、寿阳县 Shouyang Xian、稷山县 Jishan Xian、绛县 Jiang Xian、垣曲县 Yuanqu Xian、芮城县 Ruicheng Xian、洪洞县 Hongtong Xian、临县 Lin Xian、孝义市 Xiaoyi Shi

省(自治区、直辖市) Province (autonomous region, municipality)	登记处数 No. of cancer registries	登记处名单 List of cancer registries
内蒙古 Inner Mongolia	26	武川县 Wuchuan Xian、土默特右旗 Tumd Youqi、赤峰市红山区 Hongshan Qu, Chifeng Shi、赤峰市元宝山区 Yuanbaoshan Qu, Chifeng Shi、赤峰市松山区 Songshan Qu, Chifeng Shi、巴林左旗 Bairin Zuoqi、敖汉旗 Aohan Qi、通辽市科尔沁区 Horqin Qu, Tongliao Shi、科尔沁左翼中旗 Horqin Zuoyi Zhongqi、开鲁县 Kailu Xian、库伦旗 Hure Qi、奈曼旗 Naiman Qi、扎鲁特旗 Jarud Qi、呼伦贝尔市海拉尔区 Hailar Qu, Hulun Buir Shi、呼伦贝尔市扎赉诺尔区 Dalai Nur Qu, Hulun Buir Shi、阿荣旗 Arun Qi、莫力达瓦达斡尔族自治旗 Morin Dawa Daurzu Zizhiqi、鄂温克族自治旗 Ewenkizu Zizhiqi、陈巴尔虎旗 Chen Barag Qi、满洲里市 Manzhouli Shi、牙克石市 Yakeshi Shi、扎兰屯市 Zalantun Shi、额尔古纳市 Ergun Shi、根河市 Genhe Shi、巴彦淖尔市临河区 Linhe Qu, Bayannur Shi、锡林浩特市 Xilin Hot Shi
辽宁 Liaoning	15	沈阳市 Shenyang Shi、康平县 Kangping Xian、法库县 Faku Xian、大连市 Dalian Shi、庄河市 Zhuanghe Shi、鞍山市 Anshan Shi、本溪市 Benxi Shi、丹东市 Dandong Shi、东港市 Donggang Shi、营口市 Yingkou Shi、阜新市 Fuxin Shi、彰武县 Zhangwu Xian、辽阳县 Liaoyang Xian、盘锦市大洼区 Dawa Qu, Panjin Shi、建平县 Jianping Xian
吉林 Jilin	22	德惠市 Dehui Shi、吉林市 Jilin Shi、吉林市昌邑区 Changyi Qu, Jilin Shi、吉林市龙潭区 Longtan Qu, Jilin Shi、吉林市船营区 Chuanying Qu, Jilin Shi、吉林市丰满区 Fengman Qu, Jilin Shi、永吉县 Yongji Xian、蛟河市 Jiaohe Shi、桦甸市 Huadian Shi、磐石市 Panshi Shi、通化市 Tonghua Shi、柳河县 Liuhe Xian、梅河口市 Meihekou Shi、大安市 Da'an Shi、延吉市 Yanji Shi、图们市 Tumen Shi、敦化市 Dunhua Shi、珲春市 HunChun Shi、龙井市 Longjing Shi、和龙市 Helong Shi、汪清县 Wangqing Xian、安图县 Antu Xian
黑龙江 Heilongjiang	11	哈尔滨市道里区 Daoli Qu, Harbin Shi、哈尔滨市南岗区 Nangang Qu, Harbin Shi、哈尔滨市香坊区 Xiangfang Qu, Harbin Shi、尚志市 Shangzhi Shi、五常市 Wuchang Shi、勃利县 Boli Xian、牡丹江市东安区 Dong'an Qu, Mudanjiang Shi、牡丹江市阳明区 Yangming Qu, Mudanjiang Shi、牡丹江市爱民区 Aimin Qu, Mudanjiang Shi、牡丹江市西安区 Xi'an Qu, Mudanjiang Shi、海林市 Hailin Shi
上海 Shanghai	1	上海市 Shanghai Shi
江苏 Jiangsu	47	无锡市 Wuxi Shi、江阴市 Jiangyin Shi、宜兴市 Yixing Shi、徐州市 Xuzhou Shi、徐州市鼓楼区 Gulou Qu, Xuzhou Shi、常州市 Changzhou Shi、溧阳市 Liyang Shi、常州市金坛区 Jintan Qu, Changzhou Shi、苏州市 Suzhou Shi、常熟市 Changshu Shi、张家港市 Zhangjiagang Shi、昆山市 Kunshan Shi、太仓市 Taicang Shi、南通市 Nantong Shi、海安市 Hai'an Shi、如东县 Rudong Xian、启东市 Qidong Shi、如皋市 Rugao Shi、海门市 Haimen Shi、连云港市 Lianyungang Shi、连云港市赣榆区 Ganyu Qu, Lianyungang Shi、东海县 Donghai Xian、灌云县 Guanyun Xian、灌南县 Guannan Xian、淮安市淮安区 Huai'an Qu, Huai'an Shi、淮安市淮阴区 Huaiyin Qu, Huai'an Shi、淮安市清江浦区 Qingjiangpu Qu, Huai'an Shi、涟水县 Lianshui Xian、淮安市洪泽区 Hongze Qu, Huai'an Shi、盱眙县 Xuyi Xian、金湖县 Jinhu Xian、盐城市亭湖区 Tinghu Qu, Yancheng Shi、盐城市盐都区 Yandu Qu, Yancheng Shi、响水县 Xiangshui Xian、滨海县 Binhai Xian、阜宁县 Funing Xian、射阳县 Sheyang Xian、建湖县 Jianhu Xian、东台市 Dongtai Shi、盐城市大丰区 Dafeng Qu, Yancheng Shi、宝应县 Baoying Xian、丹阳市 Danyang Shi、扬中市 Yangzhong Shi、泰兴市 Taixing Shi、宿迁市宿城区 Sucheng Qu, Suqian Shi、宿迁市宿豫区 Suyu Qu, Suqian Shi、泗阳县 Siyang Xian

省(自治区、直辖市) Province (autonomous region, municipality)	登记处数 No. of cancer registries	登记处名单 List of cancer registries
浙江 Zhejiang	14	杭州市 Hangzhou Shi、宁波市鄞州区 YinzhouQu, Ningbo Shi、慈溪市 Cixi Shi、温州市鹿城区 Lucheng Qu, Wenzhou Shi、嘉兴市 Jiaxing Shi、嘉善县 Jiashan Xian、海宁市 Haining Shi、长兴县 Changxing Xian、绍兴市上虞区 Shangyu Qu, Shaoxing Shi、永康市 Yongkang Shi、开化县 Kaihua Xian、岱山县 Daishan Xian、仙居县 Xianju Xian、龙泉市 Longquan Shi
安徽 Anhui	38	合肥市 Hefei Shi、长丰县 Changfeng Xian、肥东县 Feidong Xian、肥西县 Feixi Xian、庐江县 Lujiang Xian、巢湖市 Chaohu Shi、芜湖市 Wuhu Shi、蚌埠市 Bengbu Shi、五河县 Wuhe Xian、淮南市大通区 Datong Qu, Huainan Shi、淮南市田家庵区 Tianjia'an Qu, Huainan Shi、淮南市谢家集区 Xiejiaji Qu, Huainan Shi、淮南市八公山区 Bagongshan Qu, Huainan Shi、淮南市潘集区 Panji Qu, Huainan Shi、凤台县 Fengtai Xian、马鞍山市 Ma'anshan Shi、当涂县 Dangtu Xian、濉溪县 Suixi Xian、铜陵市 Tongling Shi、铜陵市义安区 Yi'an Qu, Tongling Shi、安庆市宜秀区 Yixiu Qu, Anqing Shi、岳西县 Yuexi Xian、黄山市屯溪区 Tunxi Qu, Huangshan Shi、天长市 Tianchang Shi、阜阳市颍州区 Yingzhou Qu, Fuyang Shi、阜阳市颍东区 Yingdong Qu, Fuyang Shi、太和县 Taihe Xian、阜南县 Funan Xian、颍上县 Yingshang Xian、宿州市埇桥区 Yongqiao Qu, Suzhou Shi、灵璧县 Lingbi Xian、寿县 Shou Xian、霍邱县 Huoqiu Xian、金寨县 Jinzhai Xian、蒙城县 Mengcheng Xian、东至县 Dongzhi Xian、泾县 Jing Xian、宁国市 Ningguo Shi
福建 Fujian	12	福清市 Fuqing Shi、福州市长乐区 Changle Qu, Fuzhou Shi、厦门市 Xiamen Shi、厦门市同安区 Tong'an Qu, Xiamen Shi、厦门市翔安区 Xiang'an Qu, Xiamen Shi、莆田市涵江区 Hanjiang Qu, Putian Shi、永安市 Yong'an Shi、惠安县 Hui'an Xian、漳州市长泰区 Changtai Qu, Zhangzhou Shi、建瓯市 Jian'ou Shi、龙岩市新罗区 Xinluo Qu, Longyan Shi、龙岩市永定区 Yongding Qu, Longyan Shi
江西 Jiangxi	34	南昌市青云谱区 Qingyunpu Qu, Nanchang Shi、南昌市青山湖区 Qingshanhu Qu, Nanchang Shi、南昌市湾里区 Wanli Qu, Nanchang Shi、芦溪县 Luxi Xian、九江市浔阳区 Xunyang Qu, Jiujiang Shi、武宁县 Wuning Xian、新余市渝水区 Yushui Qu, Xinyu Shi、余江县 Yujiang Xian、赣州市章贡区 Zhanggong Qu, Ganzhou Shi、赣州市赣县区 Ganxian Qu, Ganzhou Shi、信丰县 Xinfeng Xian、大余县 Dayu Xian、上犹县 Shangyou Xian、崇义县 Chongyi Xian、龙南县 Longnan Xian、于都县 Yudu Xian、吉安市吉州区 Jizhou Qu, Ji'an Shi、峡江县 Xiajiang Xian、安福县 Anfu Xian、万载县 Wanzai Xian、上高县 Shanggao Xian、靖安县 Jing'an Xian、乐安县 Le'an Xian、宜黄县 Yihuang Xian、抚州市东乡区 Dongxiang Qu, Fuzhou Shi、上饶市信州区 Xinzhou Qu, Shangrao Shi、上饶市广丰区 Guangfeng Qu, Shangrao Shi、铅山县 Yanshan Xian、横峰县 Hengfeng Xian、弋阳县 Yiyang Xian、余干县 Yugan Xian、万年县 Wannian Xian、婺源县 Wuyuan Xian、德兴市 Dexing Shi
山东 Shandong	31	济南市 Jinan Shi、济南市章丘区 Zhangqiu Qu, Jinan Shi、济南市莱芜区 Laiwu Qu, Jinan Shi、青岛市 Qingdao Shi、青岛市黄岛区 Huangdao Qu, Qingdao Shi、淄博市临淄区 Linzi Qu, Zibo Shi、沂源县 Yiyuan Xian、滕州市 Tengzhou Shi、广饶县 Guangrao Xian、烟台市 Yantai Shi、招远市 Zhaoyuan Shi、临朐县 Linqu Xian、高密市 Gaomi Shi、济宁市任城区 Rencheng Qu, Jining Shi、汶上县 Wenshang Xian、梁山县 Liangshan Xian、曲阜市 Qufu Shi、邹城市 Zoucheng Shi、宁阳县 Ningyang Xian、肥城市 Feicheng Shi、乳山市 Rushan Shi、日照市东港区 Donggang Qu, Rizhao Shi、沂南县 Yinan Xian、沂水县 Yishui Xian、莒南县 Junan Xian、德州市德城区 Decheng Qu, Dezhou Shi、高唐县 Gaotang Xian、滨州市滨城区 Bincheng Qu, Binzhou Shi、菏泽市牡丹区 Mudan Qu, Heze Shi、单县 Shan Xian、巨野县 Juye Xian

续表

省(自治区、直辖市) Province (autonomous region, municipality)	登记处数 No. of cancer registries	登记处名单 List of cancer registries
河南 Henan	47	郑州市 Zhengzhou Shi、巩义市 Gongyi Shi、开封市祥符区 Xiangfu Qu, Kaifeng Shi、洛阳市 Luoyang Shi、孟津县 Mengjin Xian、新安县 Xin'an Xian、栾川县 Luanchuan Xian、嵩县 Song Xian、汝阳县 Ruyang Xian、宜阳县 Yiyang Xian、洛宁县 Luoning Xian、伊川县 Yichuan Xian、偃师市 Yanshi Shi、平顶山市 Pingdingshan Shi、鲁山县 Lushan Xian、郏县 Jia Xian、舞钢市 Wugang Shi、安阳市 Anyang Shi、林州市 Linzhou Shi、鹤壁市 Hebi Shi、新乡市 Xinxiang Shi、辉县市 Huixian Shi、焦作市 Jiaozuo Shi、孟州市 Mengzhou Shi、濮阳市华龙区 Hualong Qu, Puyang Shi、范县 Fan Xian、濮阳县 Puyang Xian、禹州市 Yuzhou Shi、漯河市 Luohe Shi、漯河市郾城区 Yancheng Qu, Luohe Shi、舞阳县 Wuyang Xian、临颍县 Linying Xian、三门峡市湖滨区 Hubin Qu, Sanmenxia Shi、南阳市卧龙区 Wolong Qu, Nanyang Shi、南召县 Nanzhao Xian、方城县 Fangcheng Xian、内乡县 Neixiang Xian、睢县 Sui Xian、虞城县 Yucheng Xian、信阳市浉河区 Shihe Qu, Xinyang Shi、罗山县 Luoshan Xian、固始县 Gushi Xian、沈丘县 Shenqiu Xian、郸城县 Dancheng Xian、太康县 Taikang Xian、西平县 Xiping Xian、济源市 Jiyuan Shi
湖北 Hubei	18	武汉市 Wuhan Shi、大冶市 Daye Shi、十堰市郧阳区 Yunyang Qu, Shiyan Shi、宜昌市 Yichang Shi、五峰土家族自治县 Wufeng Tujiazu Zizhixian、襄阳市 Xiangyang Shi、宜城市 Yicheng Shi、京山县 Jingshan Xian、钟祥市 Zhongxiang Shi、云梦县 Yunmeng Xian、荆州市 Jingzhou Shi、公安县 Gong'an Xian、洪湖市 Honghu Shi、麻城市 Macheng Shi、嘉鱼县 Jiayu Xian、通城县 Tongcheng Xian、恩施市 Enshi Shi、天门市 Tianmen Shi
湖南 Hunan	30	长沙市芙蓉区 Furong Qu, Changsha Shi、长沙市天心区 Tianxin Qu, Changsha Shi、长沙市岳麓区 Yuelu Qu, Changsha Shi、长沙市开福区 Kaifu Qu, Changsha Shi、长沙市雨花区 Yuhua Qu, Changsha Shi、长沙市望城区 Wangcheng Qu, Changsha Shi、长沙县 Changsha Xian、浏阳市 Liuyang Shi、株洲市芦淞区 Lusong Qu, Zhuzhou Shi、株洲市石峰区 Shifeng Qu, Zhuzhou Shi、攸县 You Xian、湘潭市雨湖区 Yuhu Qu, Xiangtan Shi、衡东县 Hengdong Xian、常宁市 Changning Shi、邵东县 Shaodong Xian、新宁县 Xinning Xian、岳阳市岳阳楼区 Yueyanglou Qu, Yueyang Shi、常德市武陵区 Wuling Qu, Changde Shi、慈利县 Cili Xian、益阳市资阳区 Ziyang Qu, Yiyang Shi、桃江县 Taojiang Xian、临武县 Linwu Xian、资兴市 Zixing Shi、道县 Dao Xian、宁远县 Ningyuan Xian、新田县 Xintian Xian、麻阳苗族自治县 Mayang Miaozu Zizhixian、洪江市 Hongjiang Shi、冷水江市 Lengshuijiang Shi、涟源市 Lianyuan Shi
广东 Guangdong	19	广州市 Guangzhou Shi、广州市郊区 Rural areas of Guangzhou Shi、南雄市 Nanxiong Shi、深圳市 Shenzhen Shi、珠海市 Zhuhai Shi、佛山市南海区 Nanhai Qu, Foshan Shi、佛山市顺德区 Shunde Qu, Foshan Shi、江门市 Jiangmen Shi、肇庆市端州区 Duanzhou Qu, Zhaoqing Shi、四会市 Sihui Shi、惠州市惠阳区 Huiyang Qu, Huizhou Shi、梅州市梅江区 Meijiang Qu, Meizhou Shi、梅州市梅县区 Meixian Qu, Meizhou Shi、阳江市阳东区 Yangdong Qu, Yangjiang Shi、阳山县 Yangshan Xian、东莞市 Dongguan Shi、中山市 Zhongshan Shi、揭西县 Jiexi Xian、罗定市 Luoding Shi

省(自治区、直辖市) Province (autonomous region, municipality)	登记处数 No. of cancer registries	登记处名单 List of cancer registries
广西 Guangxi	28	南宁市兴宁区 Xingning Qu,Nanning Shi、南宁市青秀区 Qingxiu Qu,Nanning Shi、南宁市江南区 Jiangnan Qu,Nanning Shi、南宁经济技术开发区 Nanning economic and technological development zone、南宁市西乡塘区 Xixiangtang Qu,Nanning Shi、南宁市良庆区 Liangqing Qu,Nanning Shi、南宁市东盟经济开发区 ASEAN Economic Development Zone,Nanning Shi、隆安县 Long'an Xian、宾阳县 Binyang Xian、柳州市 Liuzhou Shi、桂林市 Guilin Shi、梧州市 Wuzhou Shi、苍梧县 Cangwu Xian、北海市 Beihai Shi、合浦县 Hepu Xian、钦州市钦南区 Qinnan Qu,Qinzhou Shi、贵港市港北区 Gangbei Qu,Guigang Shi、贵港市港南区 Gangnan Qu,Guigang Shi、贵港市覃塘区 Qintang Qu,Guigang Shi、平南县 Pingnan Xian、玉林市 Yulin Shi、陆川县 Luchuan Xian、北流市 Beiliu Shi、百色市右江区 Youjiang Qu,Baise Shi、田阳县 Tianyang Xian、罗城仫佬族自治县 Luocheng Mulaozu Zizhixian、合山市 Heshan Shi、扶绥县 Fusui Xian
海南 Hainan	6	三亚市 Sanya Shi、五指山市 Wuzhishan Shi、琼海市 Qionghai Shi、定安县 Ding'an Xian、昌江黎族自治县 Changjiang Lizu Zizhixian、陵水黎族自治县 Lingshui Lizu Zizhixian
重庆 Chongqing	38	重庆市万州区 Wanzhou Qu,Chongqing Shi、重庆市涪陵区 Fuling Qu、重庆市渝中区 Yuzhong Qu,Chongqing Shi、重庆市大渡口区 Dadukou Qu,Chongqing Shi、重庆市江北区 Jiangbei Qu,Chongqing Shi、重庆市沙坪坝区 Shapingba Qu,Chongqing Shi、重庆市九龙坡区 Jiulongpo Qu,Chongqing Shi、重庆市南岸区 Nan'an Qu,Chongqing Shi、重庆市北碚区 Beibei Qu,Chongqing Shi、重庆市綦江区 Qijiang Qu,Chongqing Shi、重庆市大足区 Dazu Qu,Chongqing Shi、重庆市渝北区 Yubei Qu,Chongqing Shi、重庆市巴南区 Banan Qu,Chongqing Shi、重庆市黔江区 Qianjiang Qu,Chongqing Shi、重庆市长寿区 Changshou Qu,Chongqing Shi、重庆市江津区 Jiangjin Qu,Chongqing Shi、重庆市合川区 Hechuan Qu,Chongqing Shi、重庆市永川区 Yongchuan Qu,Chongqing Shi、重庆市南川区 Nanchuan Qu,Chongqing Shi、重庆市万盛经济技术开发区 Wansheng Economic and Technological Development Zone,Chongqing Shi、重庆市潼南区 Tongnan Qu,Chongqing Shi、重庆市铜梁区 Tongliang Qu,Chongqing Shi、重庆市荣昌区 Rongchang Qu,Chongqong Shi、重庆市璧山区 Bishan Qu,Chongqing Shi、重庆市梁平区 Liangping Qu,Chongqing Shi、丰都县 Fengdu Xian、垫江县 Dianjiang Xian、重庆市武隆区 Wulong Qu,Chongqing Shi、忠县 Zhong Xian、重庆市开州区 Kaizhou Qu,Chongqing Shi、云阳县 Yunyang Xian、奉节县 Fengjie Xian、巫山县 Wushan Xian、巫溪县 Wuxi Xian、石柱土家族自治县 Shizhu Tujiazu Zizhixian、秀山土家族苗族自治县 Xiushan Tujia Miaozu Zizhixian、酉阳土家族苗族自治县 Youyang Tujiazu Miaozu Zizhixian、彭水苗族土家族自治县 Pengshui Miaozu Tujiazu Zizhixian

省(自治区、直辖市) Province (autonomous region, municipality)	登记处数 No. of cancer registries	登记处名单 List of cancer registries
四川 Sichuan	131	成都市青羊区 Qingyang Qu,Chengdu Shi、成都市成华区 Chenghua Qu,Chengdu Shi、成都市龙泉驿区 Longquanyi Qu, Chengdu Shi、成都市新都区 Xindu Qu, Chengdu Shi、金堂县 Jintang Xian、成都市双流区 Shuangliu Qu,Chengdu Shi、成都市天府新区 Tianfu New Area,Chengdu Shi、成都市郫都区 Pidu Qu,Chengdu Shi、新津县 Xinjin Xian、彭州市 Pengzhou Shi、自贡市自流井区 Ziliujing Qu,Zigong Shi、自贡市贡井区 Gongjing Qu,Zigong Shi、自贡市大安区 Da'an Qu,Zigong Shi、自贡市沿滩区 Yantan Qu,Zigong Shi、荣县 Rong Xian、富顺县 Fushun Xian、攀枝花市东区 Dong Qu,Panzhihua Shi、攀枝花市西区 Xi Qu,Panzhihua Shi、攀枝花市仁和区 Renhe Qu,Panzhihua Shi、米易县 Miyi Xian、盐边县 Yanbian Xian、泸州市江阳区 Jiangyang Qu, Luzhou Shi、泸州市纳溪区 Naxi Qu, Luzhou Shi、泸州市龙马潭区 Longmatan Qu, Luzhou Shi、泸县 Lu Xian、合江县 Hejiang Xian、叙永县 Xuyong Xian、古蔺县 Gulin Xian、德阳市旌阳区 Jingyang Qu,Deyang Shi、中江县 Zhongjiang Xian、德阳市罗江区 Luojiang Qu,DeyangShi、广汉市 Guanghan Shi、什邡市 Shifang Shi、绵竹市 Mianzhu Shi、绵阳市涪城区 Fucheng Qu,Mianyang Shi、绵阳市游仙区 Youxian Qu,Mianyang Shi、绵阳市安州区 Anzhou Qu, Mianyang Shi、三台县 Santai Xian、盐亭县 Yanting Xian、梓潼县 Zitong Xian、北川羌族自治县 Beichuan Qiangzu Zizhixian、平武县 Pingwu Xian、江油市 Jiangyou Shi、广元市利州区 Lizhou Qu,Guangyuan Shi、广元市昭化区 Zhaohua Qu,Guangyuan Shi、广元市朝天区 Chaotian Qu,Guangyuan Shi、旺苍县 Wangcang Xian、青川县 Qingchuan Xian、剑阁县 Jiange Xian、苍溪县 Cangxi Xian、遂宁市船山区 Chuanshan Qu,Suining Shi、遂宁市安居区 Anju Qu,Suining Shi、蓬溪县 Pengxi Xian、射洪县 Shehong Xian、大英县 Daying Xian、内江市市中区 Shizhong Qu,Neijiang Shi、内江市东兴区 Dongxing Qu,Neijiang Shi、威远县 Weiyuan Xian、资中县 Zizhong Xian、隆昌市 Longchang Shi、乐山市市中区 Shizhong Qu,Leshan Shi、乐山市沙湾区 Shawan Qu,Leshan Shi、乐山市五通桥区 Wutongqiao Qu,Leshan Shi、乐山市金口河区 Jinkouhe Qu, Leshan Shi、犍为县 Jianwei Xian、井研县 Jingyan Xian、夹江县 Jiajiang Xian、沐川县 Muchuan Xian、峨边彝族自治县 Ebian Yizu Zizhixian、马边彝族自治县 Mabian Yizu Zizhixian、峨眉山市 Emeishan Shi、南充市顺庆区 Shunqing Qu, Nanchong Shi、南充市高坪区 Gaoping Qu, Nanchong Shi、南充市嘉陵区 Jialing Qu,Nanchong Shi、南部县 Nanbu Xian、营山县 Yingshan Xian、蓬安县 Peng'an Xian、仪陇县 Yilong Xian、西充县 Xichong Xian、阆中市 Langzhong Shi、眉山市东坡区 Dongpo Qu, Meishan Shi、眉山市彭山区 Pengshan Qu, Meishan Shi、仁寿县 Renshou Xian、洪雅县 Hongya Xian、丹棱县 Danleng Xian、青神县 Qingshen Xian、宜宾市翠屏区 Cuiping Qu, Yibin Shi、宜宾市叙州区 Xuzhou Qu, Yibin Shi、江安县 Jiang'an Xian、长宁县 Changning Xian、高县 Gao Xian、筠连县 Yunlian Xian、屏山县 Pingshan Xian、广安市广安区 Guang'an Qu,Guang'an Shi、广安市前锋区 Qianfeng Qu,Guang'an Shi、岳池县 Yuechi Xian、武胜县 Wusheng Xian、邻水县 Linshui Xian、华蓥市 Huaying Shi、达州市达川区 Dachuan Qu, Dazhou Shi、宣汉县 Xuanhan Xian、开江县 Kaijiang Xian、大竹县 Dazhu Xian、渠县 Qu Xian、万源市 Wanyuan Shi、雅安市雨城区 Yucheng Qu, Ya'an Shi、雅安市名山区 Mingshan Qu, Ya'an Shi、荥经县 Yingjing Xian、汉源县 Hanyuan Xian、石棉县 Shimian Xian、天全县 Tianquan Xian、芦山县 Lushan Xian、宝兴县 Baoxing Xian、巴中市巴州区 Bazhou Qu,Bazhong Shi、巴中市恩阳区 Enyang Qu,Bazhong Shi、通江县 Tongjiang Xian、南江县 Nanjiang Xian、平昌县 Pingchang Xian、资阳市雁江区 Yanjiang Qu,Ziyang Shi、安岳县 Anyue Xian、乐至县 Lezhi Xian、马尔康县 Barkam Xian、汶川县 Wenchuan Xian、理县 Li Xian、茂县 Mao Xian、松潘县 Songpan Xian、金川县 Jinchuan Xian、小金县 Xiaojin Xian、黑水县 Heishui Xian、若尔盖县 Zoigê Xian、红原县 Hongyuan Xian

省(自治区、直辖市) Province (autonomous region, municipality)	登记处数 No. of cancer registries	登记处名单 List of cancer registries
贵州 Guizhou	31	贵阳市花溪区 Huaxi Qu, Guiyang Shi、开阳县 Kaiyang Xian、息烽县 Xifeng Xian、清镇市 Qingzhen Shi、六盘水市钟山区 Zhongshan Qu, Liupanshui Shi、六盘水市六枝特区 Liuzhi Tequ, Liupanshui Shi、水城县 Shuicheng Xian、盘州市 Panzhou Shi、遵义市红花岗区 Honghuagang Qu, Zunyi Shi、遵义市汇川区 Huichuan Qu, Zunyi Shi、习水县 Xishui Xian、赤水市 Chishui Shi、安顺市西秀区 Xixiu Qu, Anshun Shi、镇宁布依族苗族自治县 Zhenning Buyizu Miaozu Zizhixian、毕节市七星关区 Qixingguan Qu, Bijie Shi、金沙县 Jinsha Xian、铜仁市碧江区 Bijiang Qu, Tongren Shi、玉屏侗族自治县 Yuping Dongzu Zizhixian、思南县 Sinan Xian、普安县 Pu'an Xian、册亨县 Ceheng Xian、黄平县 Huangping Xian、镇远县 Zhenyuan Xian、榕江县 Rongjiang Xian、雷山县 Leishan Xian、麻江县 Majiang Xian、都匀市 Duyun Shi、福泉市 Fuquan Shi、荔波县 Libo Xian、独山县 Dushan Xian、龙里县 Longli Xian
云南 Yunnan	77	昆明市五华区 Wuhua Qu, Kunming Shi、昆明市盘龙区 Panlong Qu, Kunming Shi、昆明市官渡区 Guandu Qu, Kunming Shi、昆明市西山区 Xishan Qu, Kunming Shi、昆明市东川区 Dongchuan Qu, Kunming Shi、昆明市晋宁区 Jinning Qu, Kunming Shi、昆明市呈贡区 Chenggong Qu, Kunming Shi、富民县 Fumin Xian、嵩明县 Songming Xian、禄劝彝族苗族自治县 Luquan Yizu Miaozu Zizhixian、安宁市 Anning Shi、曲靖市麒麟区 Qilin Qu, Qujing Shi、曲靖市沾益区 Zhanyi Qu, Qujing Shi、马龙县 Malong Xian、陆良县 Luliang Xian、富源县 Fuyuan Xian、宣威市 Xuanwei Shi、玉溪市红塔区 Hongta Qu, Yuxi Shi、玉溪市江川区 Jiangchuan Qu, Yuxi Shi、澄江县 Chengjiang Xian、通海县 Tonghai Xian、华宁县 Huaning Xian、易门县 Yimen Xian、峨山彝族自治县 Eshan Yizu Zizhixian、新平彝族傣族自治县 Xinping Yizu Daizu Zizhixian、元江哈尼族彝族傣族自治县 Yuanjiang Hanizu Yizu Daizu Zizhixian、保山市隆阳区 Longyang Qu, Baoshan Shi、施甸县 Shidian Xian、腾冲市 Tengchong Shi、龙陵县 Longling Xian、昌宁县 Changning Xian、昭通市昭阳区 Zhaoyang Qu, Zhaotong Shi、巧家县 Qiaojia Xian、绥江县 Suijiang Xian、水富县 Shuifu Xian、丽江市古城区 Gucheng Qu, Lijiang Shi、玉龙纳西族自治县 Yulong Naxizu Zizhixian、华坪县 Huaping Xian、景东彝族自治县 Jingdong Yizu Zizhixian、景谷傣族彝族自治县 Jinggu Daizu Yizu Zizhixian、镇沅彝族哈尼族拉祜族自治县 Zhenyuan Yizu Hanizu Lahuzu Zizhixian、江城哈尼族彝族自治县 Jiangcheng Hanizu Yizu Zizhixian、临沧市临翔区 Linxiang Qu, Lincang Shi、镇康县 Zhenkang Xian、沧源佤族自治县 Cangyuan Wazu Zizhixian、楚雄市 Chuxiong Shi、双柏县 Shuangbai Xian、牟定县 Mouding Xian、南华县 Nanhua Xian、姚安县 Yao'an Xian、大姚县 Dayao Xian、永仁县 Yongren Xian、元谋县 Yuanmou Xian、武定县 Wuding Xian、禄丰县 Lufeng Xian、个旧市 Gejiu Shi、开远市 Kaiyuan Shi、蒙自市 Mengzi Shi、弥勒市 Mile Shi、屏边苗族自治县 Pingbian Miaozu Zizhixian、建水县 Jianshui Xian、石屏县 Shiping Xian、泸西县 Luxi Xian、河口瑶族自治县 Hekou Yaozu Zizhixian、砚山县 Yanshan Xian、西畴县 Xichou Xian、丘北县 Qiubei Xian、富宁县 Funing Xian、景洪市 Jinghong Shi、大理市 Dali Shi、祥云县 Xiangyun Xian、弥渡县 Midu Xian、永平县 Yongping Xian、鹤庆县 Heqing Xian、梁河县 Lianghe Xian、盈江县 Yingjiang Xian、兰坪白族普米族自治县 Lanping Baizu Pumizu Zizhixian
西藏 Tibet	3	拉萨市城关区 Chengguan Qu, Lasa Shi、林芝市巴宜区 Bayi Qu, Linzhi Shi、山南市乃东区 Nedong Qu, Shannan Shi

省(自治区、直辖市) Province (autonomous region, municipality)	登记处数 No. of cancer registries	登记处名单 List of cancer registries
陕西 Shaanxi	42	西安市碑林区 Beilin Qu,Xi'an Shi、西安市莲湖区 Lianhu Qu,Xi'an Shi、西安市未央区 Weiyang Qu,Xi'an Shi、西安市雁塔区 Yanta Qu,Xi'an Shi、西安市高陵区 Gaoling Qu,Xi'an Shi、西安市鄠邑区 Huyi Qu,Xi'an Shi、铜川市王益区 Wangyi Qu,Tongchuan Shi、铜川市耀州区 Yaozhou Qu,Tongchuan Shi、宝鸡市金台区 Jintai Qu,Baoji Shi、宝鸡市陈仓区 Chencang Qu,Baoji Shi、凤翔县 Fengxiang Xian、岐山县 Qishan Xian、眉县 Mei Xian、陇县 Long Xian、千阳县 Qianyang Xian、麟游县 Linyou Xian、泾阳县 Jingyang Xian、渭南市临渭区 Linwei Qu,Weinan Shi、渭南市华州区 Huazhou Qu,Weinan Shi、潼关县 Tongguan Xian、大荔县 Dali Xian、合阳县 Heyang Xian、澄城县 Chengcheng Xian、蒲城县 Pucheng Xian、富平县 Fuping Xian、华阴市 Huayin Shi、延安市宝塔区 Baota Qu,Yan'an Shi、富县 Fu Xian、黄陵县 Huangling Xian、汉中市汉台区 Hantai Qu,Hanzhong Shi、城固县 Chenggu Xian、宁强县 Ningqiang Xian、绥德县 Suide Xian、安康市汉滨区 Hanbin Qu,Ankang Shi、汉阴县 Hanyin Xian、石泉县 Shiquan Xian、宁陕县 Ningshan Xian、紫阳县 Ziyang Xian、镇坪县 Zhenping Xian、旬阳县 Xunyang Xian、商洛市商州区 Shangzhou Qu,Shangluo Shi、镇安县 Zhen'an Xian
甘肃 Gansu	22	兰州市城关区 Chengguan Qu,Lanzhou Shi、兰州市七里河区 Qilihe Qu,Lanzhou Qu、兰州市西固区 Xigu Qu,Lanzhou Shi、兰州市安宁区 Anning Qu,Lanzhou Shi、兰州市红古区 Honggu Qu,Lanzhou Shi、白银市白银区 Baiyin Qu,Baiyin Shi、白银市平川区 Pingchuan Qu,Baiyin Shi、靖远县 Jingyuan Xian、景泰县 Jingtai Xian、天水市秦州区 Qinzhou Qu,Tianshui Shi、天水市麦积区 Maiji Qu,Tianshui Shi、武威市凉州区 Liangzhou Qu,Wuwei Shi、民勤县 Minqin Xian、古浪县 Gulang Xian、天祝藏族自治县 Tianzhu Zangzu Zizhixian、张掖市甘州区 Ganzhou Qu,Zhangye Shi、高台县 Gaotai Xian、静宁县 Jingning Xian、敦煌市 Dunhuang Shi、庆城县 Qingcheng Xian、临洮县 Lintao Xian、临潭县 Lintan Xian
青海 Qinghai	8	西宁市 Xining Shi、大通回族土族自治县 Datong Huizu Tuzu Zizhixian、西宁市湟中县 Huangzhong Xian,Xining Shi、海东市乐都区 Ledu Qu,Haidong Shi、民和回族土族自治县 Minhe Huizu Tuzu Zizhixian、互助土族自治县 Huzhu Tuzu Zizhixian、循化撒拉族自治县 Xunhua Salarzu Zizhixian、海南藏族自治州 Hainan Zangzu Zizhizhou
宁夏 Ningxia	11	银川市兴庆区 Xingqing Qu,Yinchuan Shi、银川市西夏区 Xixia Qu,Yinchuan Shi、银川市金凤区 Jinfeng Qu,Yinchuan Shi、贺兰县 Helan Xian、石嘴山市大武口区 Dawukou Qu,Shizuishan Shi、石嘴山市惠农区 Huinong Qu,Shizuishan Shi、平罗县 Pingluo Xian、青铜峡市 Qingtongxia Shi、固原市原州区 Yuanzhou Qu,Guyuan Shi、中卫市沙坡头区 Shapotou Qu,Zhongwei Shi、中宁县 Zhongning Xian
新疆 Xinjiang	7	乌鲁木齐市天山区 Tianshan Qu,Urumqi Shi、乌鲁木齐市米东区 Midong Qu,Urumqi Shi、克拉玛依市 Karamay Shi、库尔勒市 Korla Shi、和田市 Hotan Shi、和田县 Hotan Xian、新源县 Xinyuan Xian
兵团 Corps	3	第二师 Di'ershi、第七师 Diqishi、第八师 Dibashi

2 数据纳入标准

国家癌症中心成立肿瘤登记专家委员会和《中国肿瘤登记年报》编委会。在继往《中国肿瘤登记年报》数据入选原则基础上，根据《肿瘤随访登记技术方案》（卫生部疾病预防控制局 2009）、《中国肿瘤登记工作指导手册（2016）》中的数据质量要求，参照国际癌症研究机构（IARC）/国际癌症登记协会（IACR）对肿瘤登记数据的质量控制规则，经充分研究与讨论，制定了《2020 中国肿瘤登记年报》纳入排除标准。

本年报入选标准，注重肿瘤登记数据的真实性、稳定性和均衡性，根据登记地区的特点，综合评估该肿瘤登记处数据质量。重点考核指标要求发病率大于 175/10 万，死亡率水平基本不低于 100/10 万，MV%、DCO%、M/I 合理。并兼顾地区差异，综合考虑肿瘤登记处各个指标在本地区的合理范围。对于新建立第一次上报数据的登记处，在上述规则的原则上，考虑社会经济发展水平，工作基础、少数民族地区等因素综合评估后择优录取，MV%标准适当放宽。对于曾经被收录的登记处，在行政区划没有变化的情况下，一般粗率变化幅度不能超过 20%。对于曾经上报过数据，但未曾被收录的登记处，变化幅度如果不在上述范围内的，根据实际情况进一步核实评估。对于连续 5 年及以上被纳入年报的登记处数据，若个别指标不符合要求，但为保持连续性适当保留。

2 Data inclusion criteria

NCC has established a panel of cancer registry experts and the editorial committee of *China Cancer Registry Annual Report*. According to the principle of selecting the previous annual report data and based on *Technical Protocols of Cancer Registration and Follow up* by Ministry of Health 2009, *Chinese Guideline for Cancer Registration*(*2016*) and the quality control rules of cancer registration by the International Agency for Research on Cancer(IARC)/the International Agency for Cancer Registry (IACR), the editorial committee has established a comprehensive data inclusion and exclusion criteria of *2020 Chinese Cancer Registry Annual Report* after thorough investigation and discussion.

The data inclusion criteria were focused on the authenticity, stability, and comparability of cancer registry data quality. The quality of data was evaluated based on considering the characteristics of the corresponding regions. To pass the data inclusion criteria, one registry the data should have an incidence of more than 175 per 100 000, while the morality of the data should be greater or equal to 100 per 100 000. The MV%, DCO%, and M/I should be reasonable. Taking regional disparity into account, the proper ranges of quality control indexes of registration data differed by areas. For registries which submitted data for the first time, the quality control index MV% could be flexible. And registries were enrolled with due consideration of their social economic development level, working foundation and ethnic minority conditions. For registries which data have already been included in the report before, changes of crude rates should be less than 20% if the administrative divisions of the registries remained the same. For registries which have submitted data but have never been included in the report before, over 20% changes of crude rates should be evaluated according to the actual situation of registries. For registries which have been consecutively included in the report over 5 years, their data were included in this report even if individual indexes were not qualified, in order to guarantee data continuity.

3 肿瘤登记资料评价

3.1 覆盖人口、发病数和死亡数

提交数据的 821 个肿瘤登记地区 2017 年登记覆盖人口 563 934 185 人,其中城市地区为 256 986 805 人,占全部覆盖人口的 45.57 %,农村地区为 306 947 380 人,占 54.43%。全国登记地区覆盖人口占 2017 年全国年末人口数的 40.57%。2017 年报告癌症新发病例数合计 1 529 672 例,其中城市地区占 50.55%,农村地区占 49.45%。共计报告癌症死亡病例男女合计 898 693 例,城市地区占 47.82%,农村地区占 52.18%(表 3-2)。

3.2 数据质量评价

在提交 2017 年资料的 821 个登记处中,病理诊断比例(MV%)在 55%~95%的登记处有 618 个(75.27%),病理诊断比例(MV%)小于 55%和大于 95%的分别为 189 个和 14 个,占 24.73%。只有死亡医学证明书比例(DCO%)在 0~5%的登记处有 553 个(67.36%),DCO%为 0 的登记处有 194 个(23.63%),大于 5%的登记处有 74 个(9.01%)。死亡/发病比(M/I)为 0.55~0.85 的登记处有 583 个(71.01%),M/I 小于 0.55 和大于 0.85 的登记处分别为 221 个和 17 个,占 28.99%。

2017 年第一次提交数据的登记处有 216 个,占 26.31%。在与提交过 2016 年数据的 605 个登记处癌症发病率相比,变化幅度在 10%以内的登记处有 434 个,占提交过数据登记处总数的 71.74%。

3 Evaluation of cancer registration data

3.1 Population coverage, new cancer cases and cancer deaths

Among 821 cancer registries which submitted cancer statistics, the population coverage was 563 934 185, with 256 986 805 in urban areas (45.57%) and 306 947 380 in rural areas (54.43%). The covering population accounted for 40.57% of the overall national population of 2017. A total of 1 529 672 new cancer cases were reported in 2017. Among them, 50.55% were from urban areas and 49.45% were from rural areas. There were 898 693 new cancer deaths in 2017. The urban cancer deaths accounted for 47.82% of overall cancer deaths and rural cancer deaths accounted for 52.18% (Table 3-2).

3.2 Evaluation of data quality

Among the 821 registries which submitted the data of 2017, 618 registries (75.27%) had MV% between 55% and 95%. A total of 189 registries had MV% less than 55%, and 14 had MV% more than 95%, accounting for 24.73% of all registries. There were 553 registries having DCO% between 0 and 5%, accounting for 67.36% of all registries. A total of 194 registries (23.63%) reported no DCO cases, and 74 registries (9.01%) reported more than 5% of DCO cases. Among all registries, there were 583 registries (71.01%) having M/I between 0.55 and 0.85. 221 registries had M/I less than 0.55, 17 registries had M/I more than 0.85, accounting for 28.99%.

There were 216 registries (26.31%) submitted data to NCC for the first time. Compared with all cancer incidence rates in 2016, 434 registries reported a change of rate in 2017 less than 10%, accounting for 71.74% of all registries.

表 3-2 2017 年全国肿瘤登记地区覆盖人口、发病数、死亡数及主要质控指标

Table 3-2 The population coverage, new cancer cases, cancer deaths and major indicators for data quality of 2017 in cancer registration areas

序号 No.	肿瘤登记处 Cancer registries	人口数 Population	发病数 New cases	死亡数 Deaths	MV%	DCO%	M/I	发病率变化 Change for CR %	接受 Accepted
1	北京市 Beijing Shi	8 440 225	33 447	17 057	78. 93	0. 10	0. 51	3. 35	Y
2	北京市郊区 Rural areas of Beijing Shi	5 170 063	17 343	9 101	76. 69	0. 05	0. 52	2. 94	Y
3	天津市 Tianjin Shi	5 232 151	21 597	12 521	46. 77	0. 38	0. 58	-2. 48	Y
4	天津市郊区 Rural areas of Tianjin Shi	5 267 758	15 378	8 400	51. 59	0. 26	0. 55	4. 13	Y
5	石家庄市 Shijiazhuang Shi	2 280 772	6 342	3 375	81. 80	0. 09	0. 53	3. 30	Y
6	石家庄市郊区 Rural areas of Shijiazhuang Shi	2 388 370	5 423	3 397	79. 61	0. 98	0. 63	-2. 71	Y
7	赞皇县 Zanhuang Xian	271 277	628	470	67. 68	0. 16	0. 75	0. 62	Y
8	迁西县 Qianxi Xian	405 204	918	640	78. 43	1. 09	0. 70	4. 87	Y
9	迁安市 Qian'an Shi	762 246	1 519	1 239	68. 73	1. 32	0. 82	-11. 21	Y
10	秦皇岛市 Qinhuangdao Shi	1 439 381	3 280	2 048	82. 07	7. 38	0. 62	-2. 48	Y
11	邯郸市邯山区 Hanshan Qu, Handan Shi	520 540	1 025	696	74. 44	1. 95	0. 68	—	Y
12	大名县 Daming Xian	794 078	1 637	995	69. 70	2. 38	0. 61	3. 23	Y
13	涉县 She Xian	431 146	1 380	977	76. 59	0. 36	0. 71	4. 37	Y
14	磁县 Ci Xian	649 188	1 932	1 366	85. 04	0. 67	0. 71	4. 19	Y
15	武安市 Wu'an Shi	839 087	1 707	1 126	67. 60	0. 88	0. 66	-1. 84	Y
16	邢台市 Xingtai Shi	854 685	1 574	1 139	72. 94	0. 13	0. 72	-3. 48	Y
17	邢台县 Xingtai Xian	358 141	741	589	78. 41	0. 13	0. 79	-0. 35	Y
18	临城县 Lincheng Xian	213 989	434	303	70. 05	0. 92	0. 70	5. 34	Y
19	内丘县 Neiqiu Xian	274 907	613	431	70. 31	0. 33	0. 70	-2. 43	Y
20	任县 Ren Xian	338 738	744	606	84. 14	1. 61	0. 81	-7. 55	Y
21	保定市 Baoding Shi	1 174 481	2 608	2 103	69. 94	5. 10	0. 81	1. 01	Y
22	望都县 Wangdu Xian	259 070	520	308	71. 73	1. 92	0. 59	-1. 41	Y
23	安国市 Anguo Shi	384 613	951	642	72. 66	3. 58	0. 68	1. 04	Y
24	张家口市宣化区 Xuanhua Qu, Zhangjiakou Shi	265 276	577	374	76. 95	2. 08	0. 65	-6. 50	Y
25	张北县 Zhangbei Xian	364 410	1 235	784	74. 33	0. 73	0. 63	7. 68	Y
26	承德市双桥区 Shuangqiao Qu, Chengde Shi	314 082	643	392	69. 52	0. 16	0. 61	-6. 81	Y
27	丰宁满族自治县 Fengning Manzu Zizhixian	407 151	847	534	76. 86	0. 12	0. 63	-2. 15	Y

序号 No.	肿瘤登记处 Cancer registries	人口数 Population	发病数 New cases	死亡数 Deaths	MV%	DCO%	M/I	发病率变化 Change for CR %	接受 Accepted
28	沧州市 Cangzhou Shi	523 440	1 220	754	80. 49	0. 66	0. 62	3. 83	Y
29	海兴县 Haixing Xian	211 787	460	276	85. 43	2. 39	0. 60	0. 41	Y
30	盐山县 Yanshan Xian	441 126	883	592	80. 07	0. 23	0. 67	1. 32	Y
31	衡水市冀州区 Jizhou Qu, Hengshui Shi	344 796	793	596	67. 97	2. 65	0. 75	13. 82	Y
32	辛集市 Xinji Shi	634 569	1 444	905	81. 93	0. 83	0. 63	2. 76	Y
33	太原市杏花岭区 Xinghualing Qu, Taiyuan Shi	665 324	1 829	996	51. 61	8. 15	0. 54	18. 91	Y
34	阳泉市 Yangquan Shi	683 232	1 647	1 132	67. 58	5. 89	0. 69	4. 25	Y
35	平定县 Pingding Xian	316 322	732	426	7. 24	0. 14	0. 58	0. 60	
36	盂县 Yu Xian	307 011	600	418	98. 83	0. 00	0. 70	19. 05	
37	平顺县 Pingshun Xian	152 565	309	245	80. 91	9. 39	0. 79	3. 59	
38	沁源县 Qinyuan Xian	163 506	191	170	75. 39	0. 00	0. 89	-8. 13	
39	阳城县 Yangcheng Xian	383 416	1 480	905	78. 11	1. 82	0. 61	9. 33	Y
40	晋中市榆次区 Yuci Qu, Jinzhong Shi	611 747	1 436	802	56. 55	5. 29	0. 56	8. 54	Y
41	昔阳县 Xiyang Xian	235 745	464	282	100. 00	0. 00	0. 61	-13. 34	
42	寿阳县 Shouyang Xian	212 803	610	405	60. 98	1. 15	0. 66	7. 60	Y
43	稷山县 Jishan Xian	359 740	640	370	66. 88	0. 00	0. 58	18. 01	
44	绛县 Jiang Xian	286 234	304	181	42. 76	9. 21	0. 60	—	
45	垣曲县 Yuanqu Xian	223 981	470	317	95. 74	0. 00	0. 67	52. 97	
46	芮城县 Ruicheng Xian	406 065	476	353	99. 58	0. 00	0. 74	16. 29	
47	洪洞县 Hongtong Xian	717 236	1 649	833	59. 73	0. 00	0. 51	49. 23	Y
48	临县 Lin Xian	656 513	687	930	38. 72	0. 44	1. 35	39. 07	
49	孝义市 Xiaoyi Shi	393 815	405	259	17. 78	0. 00	0. 64	—	
50	武川县 Wuchuan Xian	175 985	271	121	100. 00	0. 00	0. 45	197. 51	
51	土默特右旗 Tumd Youqi	279 368	547	330	83. 00	5. 48	0. 60	-3. 81	Y
52	赤峰市红山区 Hongshan Qu, Chifeng Shi	429 471	986	501	64. 00	0. 00	0. 51	—	Y
53	赤峰市元宝山区 Yuanbaoshan Qu, Chifeng Shi	322 589	1 085	580	43. 78	0. 28	0. 53	—	Y
54	赤峰市松山区 Songshan Qu, Chifeng Shi	569 103	1 604	779	61. 10	0. 00	0. 49	—	Y
55	巴林左旗 Bairin Zuoqi	325 146	935	469	38. 50	0. 00	0. 50	—	Y
56	敖汉旗 Aohan Qi	542 754	1 204	746	63. 37	0. 00	0. 62	-3. 27	Y

续表

序号 No.	肿瘤登记处 Cancer registries	人口数 Population	发病数 New cases	死亡数 Deaths	MV%	DCO%	M/I	发病率变化 Change for CR %	接受 Accepted
57	通辽市科尔沁区 Horqin Qu, Tongliao Shi	785 368	1 835	939	60. 76	3. 43	0. 51	—	Y
58	科尔沁左翼中旗 Horqin Zuoyi Zhongqi	449 212	1 125	612	65. 16	0. 00	0. 54	2. 68	Y
59	开鲁县 Kailu Xian	385 809	1 094	606	49. 36	0. 09	0. 55	15. 28	Y
60	库伦旗 Hure Qi	174 296	429	228	59. 91	0. 00	0. 53	11. 14	Y
61	奈曼旗 Naiman Qi	399 730	936	630	70. 83	0. 11	0. 67	9. 46	Y
62	扎鲁特旗 Jarud Qi	302 815	719	323	77. 19	0. 00	0. 45	-0. 06	Y
63	呼伦贝尔市海拉尔区 Hailar Qu, Hulun Buir Shi	274 137	1 028	627	63. 23	0. 68	0. 61	5. 39	Y
64	呼伦贝尔市扎赉诺尔区 Dalai Nur Qu, Hulun Buir Shi	105 954	202	98	55. 94	0. 00	0. 49	—	
65	阿荣旗 Arun Qi	276 299	815	476	66. 87	1. 72	0. 58	2. 73	Y
66	莫力达瓦达斡尔族自治旗 Morin Dawa Daurzu Zizhiqi	274 462	347	204	40. 06	0. 00	0. 59	—	
67	鄂温克族自治旗 Ewenkizu Zizhiqi	133 812	450	278	74. 44	2. 22	0. 62	6. 84	Y
68	陈巴尔虎旗 Chen Barag Qi	57 737	115	96	0. 00	0. 00	0. 83	—	
69	满洲里市 Manzhouli Shi	85 311	228	146	63. 16	9. 21	0. 64	25. 44	Y
70	牙克石市 Yakeshi Shi	349 070	1 314	890	66. 82	4. 49	0. 68	0. 65	Y
71	扎兰屯市 Zalantun Shi	363 074	534	309	49. 06	5. 43	0. 58	—	
72	额尔古纳市 Ergun Shi	76 005	100	166	31. 00	7. 00	1. 66	—	
73	根河市 Genhe Shi	109 463	338	268	37. 57	18. 34	0. 79	3. 00	Y
74	巴彦淖尔市临河区 Linhe Qu, Bayannur Shi	441 518	1 155	727	82. 86	2. 94	0. 63	7. 13	Y
75	锡林浩特市 Xilin Hot Shi	246 610	932	388	85. 52	0. 00	0. 42	3. 68	Y
76	沈阳市 Shenyang Shi	3 806 854	15 889	9 741	57. 56	1. 76	0. 61	3. 89	Y
77	康平县 Kangping Xian	346 648	787	558	48. 92	3. 94	0. 71	-23. 20	
78	法库县 Faku Xian	444 054	1 443	1 005	65. 70	2. 29	0. 70	3. 90	Y
79	大连市 Dalian Shi	2 383 025	12 251	6 399	79. 47	0. 94	0. 52	6. 02	Y
80	庄河市 Zhuanghe Shi	897 072	3 808	2 320	75. 26	0. 21	0. 61	10. 32	Y
81	鞍山市 Anshan Shi	1 479 544	7 021	4 166	75. 19	1. 94	0. 59	9. 46	Y
82	本溪市 Benxi Shi	908 036	2 969	2 023	64. 70	0. 40	0. 68	-1. 39	Y
83	丹东市 Dandong Shi	778 268	2 650	1 664	72. 68	0. 45	0. 63	7. 55	Y
84	东港市 Donggang Shi	600 961	2 177	1 333	47. 86	0. 14	0. 61	3. 44	Y

续表

序号 No.	肿瘤登记处 Cancer registries	人口数 Population	发病数 New cases	死亡数 Deaths	MV%	DCO%	M/I	发病率变化 Change for CR %	接受 Accepted
85	营口市 Yingkou Shi	445 461	1 859	1 131	75. 20	2. 58	0. 61	16. 91	Y
86	阜新市 Fuxin Shi	622 036	2 360	1 736	57. 37	2. 92	0. 74	-3. 04	Y
87	彰武县 Zhangwu Xian	400 295	1 063	783	46. 10	0. 56	0. 74	27. 00	Y
88	辽阳县 Liaoyang Xian	469 468	1 223	968	64. 84	1. 88	0. 79	2. 46	Y
89	盘锦市大洼区 Dawa Qu, Panjin Shi	318 914	1 016	686	52. 76	0. 79	0. 68	3. 86	Y
90	建平县 Jianping Xian	581 990	1 717	1 306	53. 64	1. 34	0. 76	-7. 00	Y
91	德惠市 Dehui Shi	899 523	2 184	1 499	70. 79	2. 11	0. 69	7. 93	Y
92	吉林市 Jilin Shi	1 977 294	7 307	3 492	68. 55	4. 16	0. 48	-1. 37	
93	吉林市昌邑区 Changyi Qu, Jilin Shi	659 720	1 173	561	79. 62	0. 09	0. 48	—	
94	吉林市龙潭区 Longtan Qu, Jilin Shi	527 977	1 109	312	41. 39	45. 54	0. 28	—	
95	吉林市船营区 Chuanying Qu, Jilin Shi	492 529	250	151	71. 20	0. 00	0. 60	—	
96	吉林市丰满区 Fengman Qu, Jilin Shi	297 068	372	115	40. 86	17. 74	0. 31	—	
97	永吉县 Yongji Xian	397 508	555	317	43. 78	4. 50	0. 57	-29. 89	
98	蛟河市 Jiaohe Shi	432 211	1 239	412	72. 80	0. 16	0. 33	10. 71	
99	桦甸市 Huadian Shi	445 254	928	470	16. 59	1. 40	0. 51	21. 53	
100	磐石市 Panshi Shi	508 720	731	457	55. 95	0. 27	0. 63	-18. 32	
101	通化市 Tonghua Shi	443 051	1 210	816	67. 93	1. 24	0. 67	-17. 74	Y
102	柳河县 Liuhe Xian	363 836	1 167	474	91. 52	0. 77	0. 41	89. 45	
103	梅河口市 Meihekou Shi	620 322	1 696	800	64. 62	0. 53	0. 47	14. 56	Y
104	大安市 Da'an Shi	384 677	1 241	320	55. 92	0. 00	0. 26	34. 47	
105	延吉市 Yanji Shi	550 177	1 501	1 126	57. 83	2. 93	0. 75	6. 41	Y
106	图们市 Tumen Shi	112 771	361	254	41. 83	3. 32	0. 70	28. 37	Y
107	敦化市 Dunhua Shi	460 162	1 273	960	42. 42	2. 28	0. 75	2. 68	Y
108	珲春市 HunChun Shi	239 229	736	422	26. 77	19. 43	0. 57	18. 84	
109	龙井市 Longjing Shi	156 781	455	227	47. 03	1. 54	0. 50	20. 93	Y
110	和龙市 Helong Shi	175 700	457	363	25. 82	10. 50	0. 79	-22. 66	
111	汪清县 Wangqing Xian	221 124	813	669	28. 78	5. 41	0. 82	-0. 85	
112	安图县 Antu Xian	223 605	371	400	40. 16	0. 00	1. 08	-37. 91	
113	哈尔滨市道里区 Daoli Qu, Harbin Shi	755 331	2 486	1 593	73. 37	1. 17	0. 64	7. 92	Y

续表

序号 No.	肿瘤登记处 Cancer registries	人口数 Population	发病数 New cases	死亡数 Deaths	MV%	DCO%	M/I	发病率变化 Change for CR %	接受 Accepted
114	哈尔滨市南岗区 Nangang Qu, Harbin Shi	1 020 802	3 368	2 078	71. 73	1. 01	0. 62	4. 01	Y
115	哈尔滨市香坊区 Xiangfang Qu, Harbin Shi	763 423	2 735	1 649	89. 21	0. 51	0. 60	13. 99	Y
116	尚志市 Shangzhi Shi	592 301	1 365	811	83. 08	0. 88	0. 59	33. 64	Y
117	五常市 Wuchang Shi	977 500	2 313	1 033	67. 32	3. 42	0. 45	754. 85	
118	勃利县 Boli Xian	307 249	806	493	87. 84	0. 37	0. 61	277. 33	Y
119	牡丹江市东安区 Dong'an Qu, Mudanjiang Shi	193 587	639	364	85. 60	0. 16	0. 57	12. 18	Y
120	牡丹江市阳明区 Yangming Qu, Mudanjiang Shi	233 087	549	368	81. 42	0. 55	0. 67	-14. 64	
121	牡丹江市爱民区 Aimin Qu, Mudanjiang Shi	267 121	982	654	85. 44	1. 43	0. 67	10. 95	Y
122	牡丹江市西安区 Xi'an Qu, Mudanjiang Shi	242 092	717	446	85. 91	0. 84	0. 62	-16. 01	Y
123	海林市 Hailin Shi	377 859	1 027	714	73. 22	0. 10	0. 70	13. 17	Y
124	上海市 Shanghai Shi	6 027 423	34 810	16 467	73. 63	0. 47	0. 47	7. 34	Y
125	无锡市 Wuxi Shi	2 563 044	9 856	5 746	73. 36	0. 48	0. 58	3. 00	Y
126	江阴市 Jiangyin Shi	1 251 788	4 749	2 851	76. 21	0. 04	0. 60	0. 01	Y
127	宜兴市 Yixing Shi	1 081 818	3 503	2 800	69. 00	0. 77	0. 80	9. 97	Y
128	徐州市 Xuzhou Shi	2 062 454	6 519	3 270	68. 03	6. 26	0. 50	-0. 61	Y
129	徐州市鼓楼区 Gulou Qu, Xuzhou Shi	8 349 630	19 872	11 747	67. 02	2. 50	0. 59	—	Y
130	常州市 Changzhou Shi	2 461 967	10 056	5 641	76. 42	0. 18	0. 56	5. 76	Y
131	溧阳市 Liyang Shi	791 174	2 561	1 550	73. 96	0. 08	0. 61	4. 50	Y
132	常州市金坛区 Jintan Qu, Changzhou Shi	549 958	2 279	1 445	67. 75	0. 18	0. 63	0. 93	Y
133	苏州市 Suzhou Shi	3 521 559	13 778	7 320	78. 87	3. 59	0. 53	7. 47	Y
134	常熟市 Changshu Shi	1 068 873	3 750	2 552	58. 40	2. 24	0. 68	-5. 17	Y
135	张家港市 Zhangjiagang Shi	927 805	4 362	2 256	67. 81	0. 00	0. 52	8. 11	Y
136	昆山市 Kunshan Shi	843 128	3 479	1 728	78. 47	0. 43	0. 50	6. 81	Y
137	太仓市 Taicang Shi	484 882	1 915	1 158	69. 61	0. 00	0. 60	-6. 00	Y
138	南通市 Nantong Shi	1 949 572	7 963	5 382	63. 43	0. 88	0. 68	-5. 01	Y
139	海安市 Hai'an Shi	932 019	3 926	2 729	68. 36	0. 33	0. 70	12. 73	Y
140	如东县 Rudong Xian	1 027 265	3 929	2 854	63. 27	0. 08	0. 73	-3. 96	Y
141	启东市 Qidong Shi	1 117 674	5 714	3 491	63. 18	0. 04	0. 61	5. 12	Y

续表

序号 No.	肿瘤登记处 Cancer registries	人口数 Population	发病数 New cases	死亡数 Deaths	MV%	DCO%	M/I	发病率变化 Change for CR %	接受 Accepted
142	如皋市 Rugao Shi	1 424 867	5 522	3 921	72. 00	0. 09	0. 71	3. 50	Y
143	海门市 Haimen Shi	998 425	4 301	2 862	65. 57	0. 14	0. 67	0. 54	Y
144	连云港市 Lianyungang Shi	1 035 611	2 475	1 536	69. 29	1. 82	0. 62	4. 04	Y
145	连云港市赣榆区 Ganyu Qu, Lianyungang Shi	1 195 775	2 814	1 752	56. 22	0. 82	0. 62	11. 60	Y
146	东海县 Donghai Xian	1 239 118	2 653	1 980	66. 42	1. 28	0. 75	5. 13	Y
147	灌云县 Guanyun Xian	1 040 972	2 194	1 676	61. 62	0. 77	0. 76	2. 05	Y
148	灌南县 Guannan Xian	819 099	1 590	1 135	52. 58	0. 31	0. 71	-1. 65	Y
149	淮安市淮安区 Huai'an Qu, Huai'an Shi	1 168 558	3 721	2 624	67. 40	0. 16	0. 71	2. 68	Y
150	淮安市淮阴区 Huaiyin Qu, Huai'an Shi	925 442	2 445	1 721	70. 31	1. 39	0. 70	0. 02	Y
151	淮安市清江浦区 Qingjiangpu Qu, Huai'an Shi	568 208	1 263	833	67. 30	3. 72	0. 66	9. 98	Y
152	涟水县 Lianshui Xian	1 144 516	2 670	2 122	77. 68	0. 71	0. 79	-4. 73	Y
153	淮安市洪泽区 Hongze Qu, Huai'an Shi	381 793	1 072	786	70. 62	1. 21	0. 73	1. 47	Y
154	盱眙县 Xuyi Xian	799 257	2 043	1 467	69. 60	0. 39	0. 72	5. 79	Y
155	金湖县 Jinhu Xian	351 330	1 124	736	78. 20	0. 98	0. 65	-0. 78	Y
156	盐城市亭湖区 Tinghu Qu, Yancheng Shi	699 700	2 254	1 396	62. 95	0. 18	0. 62	1. 85	Y
157	盐城市盐都区 Yandu Qu, Yancheng Shi	706 535	2 798	1 907	75. 38	0. 00	0. 68	2. 14	Y
158	响水县 Xiangshui Xian	623 993	1 632	1 119	60. 54	0. 92	0. 69	—	Y
159	滨海县 Binhai Xian	1 229 953	2 991	1 933	66. 97	0. 00	0. 65	1. 70	Y
160	阜宁县 Funing Xian	1 127 246	3 193	2 217	66. 11	0. 03	0. 69	9. 42	Y
161	射阳县 Sheyang Xian	958 932	3 206	2 327	62. 69	0. 06	0. 73	2. 37	Y
162	建湖县 Jianhu Xian	787 678	2 592	1 786	75. 96	0. 12	0. 69	-1. 21	Y
163	东台市 Dongtai Shi	1 117 921	4 031	2 989	74. 80	0. 07	0. 74	0. 76	Y
164	盐城市大丰区 Dafeng Qu, Yancheng Shi	714 462	3 074	2 034	68. 51	0. 10	0. 66	1. 98	Y
165	宝应县 Baoying Xian	912 480	2 379	1 911	63. 56	3. 66	0. 80	13. 84	Y
166	丹阳市 Danyang Shi	808 297	3 719	2 608	63. 70	0. 05	0. 70	-0. 41	Y
167	扬中市 Yangzhong Shi	281 972	1 065	877	74. 08	0. 00	0. 82	4. 44	Y
168	泰兴市 Taixing Shi	1 193 122	4 299	2 682	84. 55	1. 84	0. 62	9. 74	Y
169	宿迁市宿城区 Sucheng Qu, Suqian Shi	737 101	1 526	841	76. 67	0. 98	0. 55	—	Y

续表

序号 No.	肿瘤登记处 Cancer registries	人口数 Population	发病数 New cases	死亡数 Deaths	MV%	DCO%	M/I	发病率变化 Change for CR %	接受 Accepted
170	宿迁市宿豫区 Suyu Qu, Suqian Shi	501 395	925	484	52. 54	4. 32	0. 52	—	
171	泗阳县 Siyang Xian	1 068 314	2 874	2 211	66. 84	3. 58	0. 77	—	Y
172	杭州市 Hangzhou Shi	7 424 858	30 540	13 300	82. 15	0. 26	0. 44	5. 16	Y
173	宁波市鄞州区 Yinzhou Qu, Ningbo Shi	266 922	1 123	544	81. 66	0. 18	0. 48	—	Y
174	慈溪市 Cixi Shi	1 051 059	4 151	2 318	69. 36	2. 22	0. 56	7. 14	Y
175	温州市鹿城区 Lucheng Qu, Wenzhou Shi	765 657	3 162	1 404	76. 63	0. 03	0. 44	16. 70	Y
176	嘉兴市 Jiaxing Shi	549 422	2 653	1 186	74. 22	0. 08	0. 45	7. 40	Y
177	嘉善县 Jiashan Xian	391 087	2 219	1 091	74. 27	0. 18	0. 49	5. 63	Y
178	海宁市 Haining Shi	690 323	2 652	1 291	76. 66	0. 04	0. 49	7. 90	Y
179	长兴县 Changxing Xian	632 382	2 460	1 201	80. 53	0. 00	0. 49	11. 86	Y
180	绍兴市上虞区 Shangyu Qu, Shaoxing Shi	722 563	3 707	1 616	82. 03	1. 83	0. 44	4. 52	Y
181	永康市 Yongkang Shi	610 034	2 472	1 131	77. 18	6. 19	0. 46	19. 99	Y
182	开化县 Kaihua Xian	360 826	1 068	582	72. 66	0. 09	0. 54	2. 35	Y
183	岱山县 Daishan Xian	183 539	1 213	604	73. 87	0. 25	0. 50	10. 64	Y
184	仙居县 Xianju Xian	515 413	2 142	1 049	67. 23	0. 05	0. 49	9. 06	Y
185	龙泉市 Longquan Shi	290 795	1 074	529	72. 25	0. 00	0. 49	13. 67	Y
186	合肥市 Hefei Shi	2 646 361	7 861	4 446	65. 34	1. 84	0. 57	3. 15	Y
187	长丰县 Changfeng Xian	769 755	2 179	1 277	51. 40	0. 23	0. 59	11. 77	Y
188	肥东县 Feidong Xian	1 064 353	3 557	2 147	61. 15	0. 06	0. 60	6. 95	Y
189	肥西县 Feixi Xian	824 326	3 784	2 223	53. 91	1. 80	0. 59	7. 16	Y
190	庐江县 Lujiang Xian	1 206 276	4 705	3 107	58. 47	1. 28	0. 66	1. 18	Y
191	巢湖市 Chaohu Shi	858 200	2 778	1 665	42. 87	0. 00	0. 60	-0. 68	Y
192	芜湖市 Wuhu Shi	1 481 986	4 553	2 492	66. 57	0. 00	0. 55	1. 25	Y
193	蚌埠市 Bengbu Shi	1 148 839	2 220	994	73. 78	0. 09	0. 45	0. 48	
194	五河县 Wuhe Xian	688 499	1 641	1 020	63. 38	0. 67	0. 62	10. 95	Y
195	淮南市大通区 Datong Qu, Huainan Shi	185 581	387	99	99. 22	0. 00	0. 26	—	
196	淮南市田家庵区 Tianjia'an Qu, Huainan Shi	525 299	1 439	354	73. 94	0. 35	0. 25	—	
197	淮南市谢家集区 Xiejiaji Qu, Huainan Shi	291 975	920	510	72. 61	4. 46	0. 55	—	Y

续表

序号 No.	肿瘤登记处 Cancer registries	人口数 Population	发病数 New cases	死亡数 Deaths	MV%	DCO%	M/I	发病率变化 Change for CR %	接受 Accepted
198	淮南市八公山区 Bagongshan Qu, Huainan Shi	155 539	332	62	52.71	0.30	0.19	—	
199	淮南市潘集区 Panji Qu, Huainan Shi	404 490	1 099	428	58.96	0.00	0.39	—	
200	凤台县 Fengtai Xian	618 041	1 240	551	59.35	0.00	0.44	—	
201	马鞍山市 Ma'anshan Shi	638 317	2 269	1 253	80.26	0.18	0.55	5.53	Y
202	当涂县 Dangtu Xian	476 922	1 617	949	67.84	1.42	0.59	12.64	Y
203	濉溪县 Suixi Xian	1 175 821	1 621	1 023	36.58	1.17	0.63	—	
204	铜陵市 Tongling Shi	446 701	1 346	952	64.71	3.49	0.71	-0.79	Y
205	铜陵市义安区 Yi'an Qu, Tongling Shi	292 940	920	622	68.37	0.00	0.68	-4.49	Y
206	安庆市宜秀区 Yixiu Qu, Anqing Shi	168 915	319	137	52.98	0.00	0.43	—	
207	岳西县 Yuexi Xian	417 061	788	52	62.31	0.38	0.07	—	
208	黄山市屯溪区 Tunxi Qu, Huangshan Shi	233 875	227	141	72.69	14.54	0.62	—	
209	天长市 Tianchang Shi	617 285	1 436	993	87.26	7.87	0.69	-8.50	Y
210	阜阳市颍州区 Yingzhou Qu, Fuyang Shi	767 000	1 828	973	39.11	0.00	0.53	-2.90	Y
211	阜阳市颍东区 Yingdong Qu, Fuyang Shi	660 770	1 500	947	52.07	0.33	0.63	0.49	Y
212	太和县 Taihe Xian	1 755 330	4 911	2 950	69.64	0.69	0.60	1.93	Y
213	阜南县 Funan Xian	1 723 076	3 722	2 287	52.36	2.36	0.61	—	Y
214	颍上县 Yingshang Xian	1 779 080	3 829	1 817	75.58	0.00	0.47	—	
215	宿州市埇桥区 Yongqiao Qu, Suzhou Shi	1 724 950	4 261	2 725	56.11	1.74	0.64	12.53	Y
216	灵璧县 Lingbi Xian	1 032 800	2 941	1 743	64.67	0.24	0.59	10.16	Y
217	寿县 Shou Xian	1 196 255	3 013	1 996	81.81	3.12	0.66	1.36	Y
218	霍邱县 Huoqiu Xian	1 634 235	2 847	684	54.37	0.00	0.24	—	
219	金寨县 Jinzhai Xian	682 982	1 441	864	67.45	0.69	0.60	-2.89	Y
220	蒙城县 Mengcheng Xian	1 107 270	2 292	1 387	26.31	0.00	0.61	-19.07	
221	东至县 Dongzhi Xian	479 084	1 202	736	53.00	0.00	0.61	29.67	Y
222	泾县 Jing Xian	305 066	775	462	79.10	1.55	0.60	-1.87	Y
223	宁国市 Ningguo Shi	1 146 146	455	290	64.18	2.64	0.64	—	
224	福清市 Fuqing Shi	1 362 996	3 670	2 213	73.38	5.29	0.60	-10.99	Y

序号 No.	肿瘤登记处 Cancer registries	人口数 Population	发病数 New cases	死亡数 Deaths	MV%	DCO%	M/I	发病率变化 Change for CR %	接受 Accepted
225	福州市长乐区 Changle Qu, Fuzhou Shi	731 291	1 892	1 111	60. 47	0. 42	0. 59	-0. 19	Y
226	厦门市 Xiamen Shi	1 566 576	4 217	2 800	79. 91	0. 00	0. 66	-14. 52	Y
227	厦门市同安区 Tong' an Qu, Xiamen Shi	348 058	901	667	62. 60	0. 22	0. 74	0. 22	Y
228	厦门市翔安区 Xiang' an Qu, Xiamen Shi	350 411	968	611	53. 31	0. 00	0. 63	9. 56	Y
229	莆田市涵江区 Hanjiang Qu, Putian Shi	445 872	1 412	901	78. 40	1. 20	0. 64	1. 78	Y
230	永安市 Yong' an Shi	332 150	890	545	69. 66	0. 56	0. 61	5. 17	Y
231	惠安县 Hui' an Xian	799 735	2 057	1 237	71. 90	0. 00	0. 60	32. 06	Y
232	漳州市长泰区 Changtai Qu, Zhangzhou Shi	209 616	431	357	82. 83	0. 00	0. 83	-0. 92	Y
233	建瓯市 Jian' ou Shi	553 571	1 409	1 020	54. 15	0. 28	0. 72	2. 55	Y
234	龙岩市新罗区 Xinluo Qu, Longyan Shi	528 847	1 574	788	56. 04	0. 00	0. 50	-3. 26	Y
235	龙岩市永定区 Yongding Qu, Longyan Shi	507 629	1 240	814	68. 23	0. 16	0. 66	-0. 26	Y
236	南昌市青云谱区 Qingyunpu Qu, Nanchang Shi	269 523	551	411	64. 25	3. 27	0. 75	—	Y
237	南昌市青山湖区 Qingshanhu Qu, Nanchang Shi	412 800	894	511	67. 67	0. 45	0. 57	—	Y
238	南昌市湾里区 Wanli Qu, Nanchang Shi	668 071	1 313	944	67. 02	0. 91	0. 72	0. 45	Y
239	芦溪县 Luxi Xian	268 500	538	295	81. 04	2. 79	0. 55	-2. 14	Y
240	九江市浔阳区 Xunyang Qu, Jiujiang Shi	287 077	657	402	71. 23	2. 13	0. 61	8. 51	Y
241	武宁县 Wuning Xian	392 922	846	575	72. 93	0. 24	0. 68	2. 36	Y
242	新余市渝水区 Yushui Qu, Xinyu Shi	862 987	1 627	946	62. 20	4. 49	0. 58	0. 70	Y
243	余江县 Yujiang Xian	368 767	825	386	62. 18	1. 33	0. 47	39. 59	
244	赣州市章贡区 Zhanggong Qu, Ganzhou Shi	486 298	1 167	746	72. 32	0. 43	0. 64	-0. 47	Y
245	赣州市赣县区 Ganxian Qu, Ganzhou Shi	564 403	1 107	670	59. 71	1. 90	0. 61	9. 07	Y
246	信丰县 Xinfeng Xian	685 815	1 314	751	77. 63	0. 46	0. 57	—	Y
247	大余县 Dayu Xian	296 961	568	359	63. 20	2. 82	0. 63	4. 87	Y

续表

序号 No.	肿瘤登记处 Cancer registries	人口数 Population	发病数 New cases	死亡数 Deaths	MV%	DCO%	M/I	发病率变化 Change for CR %	接受 Accepted
248	上犹县 Shangyou Xian	265 761	512	318	63.87	2.73	0.62	6.81	Y
249	崇义县 Chongyi Xian	193 692	348	211	67.24	2.59	0.61	-2.72	Y
250	龙南县 Longnan Xian	312 831	646	385	62.54	0.93	0.60	2.04	Y
251	于都县 Yudu Xian	865 811	1 938	1 181	60.78	1.34	0.61	29.18	Y
252	吉安市吉州区 Jizhou Qu, Ji'an Shi	359 712	753	486	74.50	0.40	0.65	—	Y
253	峡江县 Xiajiang Xian	188 883	335	192	78.21	0.00	0.57	10.14	Y
254	安福县 Anfu Xian	396 220	818	475	62.47	0.37	0.58	2.76	Y
255	万载县 Wanzai Xian	488 423	1 047	663	61.32	1.91	0.63	6.46	Y
256	上高县 Shanggao Xian	336 526	651	413	64.21	2.30	0.63	2.95	Y
257	靖安县 Jing'an Xian	152 543	293	224	63.48	3.41	0.76	2.94	Y
258	乐安县 Le'an Xian	355 370	631	393	70.68	2.85	0.62	4.87	Y
259	宜黄县 Yihuang Xian	229 646	414	241	73.43	2.90	0.58	6.22	Y
260	抚州市东乡区 Dongxiang Qu, Fuzhou Shi	451 376	797	481	76.54	3.01	0.60	0.16	Y
261	上饶市信州区 Xinzhou Qu, Shangrao Shi	426 190	1 111	680	72.46	1.71	0.61	5.54	Y
262	上饶市广丰区 Guangfeng Qu, Shangrao Shi	793 415	1 443	877	66.74	0.97	0.61	7.56	Y
263	铅山县 Yanshan Xian	438 125	769	571	62.29	0.26	0.74	-4.27	Y
264	横峰县 Hengfeng Xian	189 794	419	285	65.39	3.10	0.68	1.64	Y
265	弋阳县 Yiyang Xian	362 794	657	485	64.54	0.00	0.74	—	Y
266	余干县 Yugan Xian	923 670	1 711	1 031	60.32	3.97	0.60	-1.12	Y
267	万年县 Wannian Xian	368 564	707	430	63.65	1.70	0.61	-3.82	Y
268	婺源县 Wuyuan Xian	344 017	703	445	62.87	1.14	0.63	8.50	Y
269	德兴市 Dexing Shi	300 697	539	325	61.41	0.56	0.60	6.81	Y
270	济南市 Jinan Shi	3 750 268	12 447	6 508	74.71	1.31	0.52	0.24	Y
271	济南市章丘区 Zhangqiu Qu, Jinan Shi	1 040 671	3 999	2 306	72.62	2.08	0.58	—	Y
272	济南市莱芜区 Laiwu Qu, Jinan Shi	987 219	3 654	1 896	37.06	0.11	0.52	—	Y
273	青岛市 Qingdao Shi	1 816 159	5 190	3 121	77.55	2.49	0.60	-11.73	Y
274	青岛市黄岛区 Huangdao Qu, Qingdao Shi	1 248 093	4 376	2 868	55.85	11.38	0.66	8.47	Y
275	淄博市临淄区 Linzi Qu, Zibo Shi	617 110	2 160	1 242	70.97	3.84	0.58	3.20	Y

续表

序号 No.	肿瘤登记处 Cancer registries	人口数 Population	发病数 New cases	死亡数 Deaths	MV%	DCO%	M/I	发病率变化 Change for CR %	接受 Accepted
276	沂源县 Yiyuan Xian	572 676	1 886	1 198	70. 04	1. 22	0. 64	2. 55	Y
277	滕州市 Tengzhou Shi	1 725 390	4 775	2 824	77. 47	1. 49	0. 59	1. 41	Y
278	广饶县 Guangrao Xian	524 735	1 649	1 079	80. 96	0. 67	0. 65	32. 03	Y
279	烟台市 Yantai Shi	1 849 554	7 066	4 074	66. 74	4. 09	0. 58	15. 57	Y
280	招远市 Zhaoyuan Shi	565 364	2 409	1 635	57. 45	0. 66	0. 68	24. 64	Y
281	临朐县 Linqu Xian	924 630	2 878	1 899	74. 84	0. 66	0. 66	-4. 49	Y
282	高密市 Gaomi Shi	903 879	2 855	2 118	68. 27	1. 40	0. 74	7. 52	Y
283	济宁市任城区 Rencheng Qu, Jining Shi	1 267 527	2 776	1 181	85. 41	0. 22	0. 43	-7. 89	
284	汶上县 Wenshang Xian	816 972	2 338	1 469	75. 71	4. 53	0. 63	-0. 80	Y
285	梁山县 Liangshan Xian	820 826	2 382	1 218	81. 65	0. 92	0. 51	6. 29	Y
286	曲阜市 Qufu Shi	655 813	1 928	1 131	59. 60	0. 10	0. 59	22. 51	Y
287	邹城市 Zoucheng Shi	1 198 965	3 742	2 222	75. 76	0. 29	0. 59	18. 87	Y
288	宁阳县 Ningyang Xian	836 736	2 684	1 769	78. 32	1. 38	0. 66	-4. 61	Y
289	肥城市 Feicheng Shi	991 680	3 829	2 524	72. 00	0. 42	0. 66	20. 61	Y
290	乳山市 Rushan Shi	551 263	2 272	1 401	57. 97	5. 50	0. 62	9. 66	Y
291	日照市东港区 Donggang Qu, Rizhao Shi	936 492	2 588	963	81. 88	3. 75	0. 37	-3. 74	
292	沂南县 Yinan Xian	962 780	2 576	1 635	74. 30	0. 12	0. 63	7. 48	Y
293	沂水县 Yishui Xian	1 163 369	3 113	2 043	75. 68	4. 50	0. 66	27. 13	Y
294	莒南县 Junan Xian	853 733	2 720	1 724	49. 23	0. 40	0. 63	25. 04	Y
295	德州市德城区 Decheng Qu, Dezhou Shi	641 330	1 217	609	45. 77	0. 00	0. 50	-38. 90	
296	高唐县 Gaotang Xian	512 634	1 510	952	74. 77	3. 25	0. 63	25. 13	Y
297	滨州市滨城区 Bincheng Qu, Binzhou Shi	689 106	2 087	1 132	72. 07	0. 00	0. 54	3. 93	Y
298	菏泽市牡丹区 Mudan Qu, Heze Shi	1 615 732	3 792	2 530	29. 88	0. 34	0. 67	-17. 05	
299	单县 Shan Xian	1 270 491	3 550	1 779	61. 66	0. 39	0. 50	1. 11	Y
300	巨野县 Juye Xian	1 088 512	2 935	2 090	38. 53	1. 70	0. 71	2. 37	Y
301	郑州市 Zhengzhou Shi	3 075 125	7 890	2 877	68. 76	1. 89	0. 36	-3. 86	
302	巩义市 Gongyi Shi	842 520	1 939	1 074	57. 92	5. 72	0. 55	-31. 75	
303	开封市祥符区 Xiangfu Qu, Kaifeng Shi	729 265	1 718	1 032	76. 14	0. 29	0. 60	-1. 57	Y
304	洛阳市 Luoyang Shi	1 618 677	4 703	2 903	76. 23	1. 70	0. 62	2. 23	Y

序号 No.	肿瘤登记处 Cancer registries	人口数 Population	发病数 New cases	死亡数 Deaths	MV%	DCO%	M/I	发病率变化 Change for CR %	接受 Accepted
305	孟津县 Mengjin Xian	465 988	1 361	818	73. 62	1. 47	0. 60	-0. 78	Y
306	新安县 Xin'an Xian	541 654	1 389	880	72. 35	1. 37	0. 63	0. 19	Y
307	栾川县 Luanchuan Xian	354 077	880	566	76. 48	0. 23	0. 64	5. 52	Y
308	嵩县 Song Xian	620 654	1 572	1 079	71. 82	0. 25	0. 69	-5. 44	Y
309	汝阳县 Ruyang Xian	525 235	1 274	776	74. 88	2. 59	0. 61	5. 11	Y
310	宜阳县 Yiyang Xian	709 954	1 920	1 220	74. 27	1. 15	0. 64	79. 80	Y
311	洛宁县 Luoning Xian	503 215	1 282	768	72. 85	0. 31	0. 60	10. 30	Y
312	伊川县 Yichuan Xian	917 634	2 086	1 345	73. 78	0. 05	0. 64	8. 47	Y
313	偃师市 Yanshi Shi	632 334	1 823	1 044	75. 70	2. 91	0. 57	8. 68	Y
314	平顶山市 Pingdingshan Shi	923 747	2 143	1 287	73. 87	0. 14	0. 60	-1. 80	Y
315	鲁山县 Lushan Xian	945 756	2 377	1 891	71. 14	1. 39	0. 80	7. 08	Y
316	郏县 Jia Xian	634 148	1 518	897	69. 10	0. 72	0. 59	—	Y
317	舞钢市 Wugang Shi	315 750	816	403	36. 03	7. 11	0. 49	—	
318	安阳市 Anyang Shi	1 172 385	3 091	1 443	71. 14	18. 70	0. 47	23. 94	
319	林州市 Linzhou Shi	1 125 386	3 489	2 250	84. 35	1. 23	0. 64	1. 14	Y
320	鹤壁市 Hebi Shi	652 145	1 810	1 154	68. 40	2. 82	0. 64	-0. 89	Y
321	新乡市 Xinxiang Shi	907 105	2 367	795	89. 48	0. 04	0. 34	—	
322	辉县市 Huixian Shi	879 390	2 406	1 620	75. 52	0. 33	0. 67	2. 06	Y
323	焦作市 Jiaozuo Shi	803 415	2 301	752	81. 75	3. 13	0. 33	—	
324	孟州市 Mengzhou Shi	382 809	843	481	98. 58	0. 00	0. 57	—	
325	濮阳市华龙区 Hualong Qu, Puyang Shi	465 799	1 440	683	76. 39	1. 81	0. 47	-11. 59	Y
326	范县 Fan Xian	545 567	1 222	605	51. 55	0. 00	0. 50	—	Y
327	濮阳县 Puyang Xian	1 125 250	3 103	1 847	61. 97	0. 00	0. 60	3. 47	Y
328	禹州市 Yuzhou Shi	1 288 374	3 239	2 596	77. 37	1. 02	0. 80	7. 15	Y
329	漯河市 Luohe Shi	808 882	2 169	1 385	68. 97	2. 12	0. 64	—	Y
330	漯河市郾城区 Yancheng Qu, Luohe Shi	497 556	1 297	862	66. 08	2. 54	0. 66	5. 30	Y
331	舞阳县 Wuyang Xian	540 479	1 425	912	57. 68	4. 98	0. 64	—	Y
332	临颍县 Linying Xian	686 677	1 350	636	66. 74	3. 48	0. 47	—	
333	三门峡市湖滨区 Hubin Qu, Sanmenxia Shi	294 274	905	548	72. 93	0. 22	0. 61	9. 40	Y
334	南阳市卧龙区 Wolong Qu, Nanyang Shi	928 511	2 391	1 510	68. 38	2. 22	0. 63	-7. 75	Y
335	南召县 Nanzhao Xian	550 750	1 464	891	77. 53	1. 71	0. 61	—	Y

续表

序号 No.	肿瘤登记处 Cancer registries	人口数 Population	发病数 New cases	死亡数 Deaths	MV%	DCO%	M/I	发病率变化 Change for CR %	接受 Accepted
336	方城县 Fangcheng Xian	1 158 727	2 875	1 738	82. 19	0. 21	0. 60	-8. 29	Y
337	内乡县 Neixiang Xian	733 247	1 977	1 343	72. 08	1. 37	0. 68	-0. 04	Y
338	睢县 Sui Xian	855 819	2 095	1 308	65. 25	0. 00	0. 62	-1. 20	Y
339	虞城县 Yucheng Xian	1 128 144	2 742	1 613	74. 29	0. 00	0. 59	-15. 63	
340	信阳市浉河区 Shihe Qu, Xinyang Shi	646 610	1 464	852	76. 78	3. 21	0. 58	-1. 19	Y
341	罗山县 Luoshan Xian	757 784	2 106	1 318	71. 56	0. 24	0. 63	17. 52	Y
342	固始县 Gushi Xian	1 845 804	6 560	2 587	82. 56	0. 63	0. 39	8. 20	
343	沈丘县 Shenqiu Xian	1 198 162	3 357	2 052	64. 73	4. 77	0. 61	1. 15	Y
344	郸城县 Dancheng Xian	1 393 534	3 647	2 462	66. 16	0. 96	0. 68	11. 15	Y
345	太康县 Taikang Xian	1 621 143	5 022	2 917	70. 39	0. 00	0. 58	—	Y
346	西平县 Xiping Xian	885 442	2 299	1 460	70. 90	2. 91	0. 64	4. 52	Y
347	济源市 Jiyuan Shi	721 704	1 946	1 206	72. 35	0. 26	0. 62	-5. 22	Y
348	武汉市 Wuhan Shi	4 845 055	18 687	10 116	88. 11	0. 47	0. 54	1. 43	Y
349	大冶市 Daye Shi	885 702	2 289	1 414	77. 68	2. 14	0. 62	-2. 30	Y
350	十堰市郧阳区 Yunyang Qu, Shiyan Shi	563 600	1 247	885	72. 98	0. 00	0. 71	-4. 59	Y
351	宜昌市 Yichang Shi	1 277 449	3 770	2 247	69. 79	2. 60	0. 60	6. 90	Y
352	五峰土家族自治县 Wufeng Tujiazu Zizhixian	199 120	494	357	76. 92	1. 82	0. 72	8. 35	Y
353	襄阳市 Xiangyang Shi	1 470 792	3 460	2 238	48. 44	9. 51	0. 65	9. 54	Y
354	宜城市 Yicheng Shi	52 5401	1 253	889	44. 05	0. 48	0. 71	3. 95	Y
355	京山县 Jingshan Xian	633 603	1 448	875	70. 51	0. 28	0. 60	0. 42	Y
356	钟祥市 Zhongxiang Shi	1 015 600	2 284	1 442	82. 05	0. 18	0. 63	1. 26	Y
357	云梦县 Yunmeng Xian	539 886	1 541	795	59. 70	0. 06	0. 52	-2. 96	Y
358	荆州市 Jingzhou Shi	1 207 805	2 697	1 748	85. 09	0. 00	0. 65	—	Y
359	公安县 Gong'an Xian	878 867	2 664	1 761	76. 73	0. 49	0. 66	-0. 42	Y
360	洪湖市 Honghu Shi	847 808	1 907	1 383	69. 59	0. 10	0. 73	2. 95	Y
361	麻城市 Macheng Shi	1 169 512	3 056	2 022	73. 95	0. 56	0. 66	5. 45	Y
362	嘉鱼县 Jiayu Xian	372 198	789	479	65. 40	3. 93	0. 61	-3. 60	Y
363	通城县 Tongcheng Xian	407 286	920	514	76. 85	1. 52	0. 56	64. 93	Y
364	恩施市 Enshi Shi	806 495	2 047	1 233	81. 78	0. 20	0. 60	8. 86	Y
365	天门市 Tianmen Shi	1 354 123	3 510	2 247	69. 83	0. 00	0. 64	7. 76	Y
366	长沙市芙蓉区 Furong Qu, Changsha Shi	395 903	1 525	1 004	75. 87	3. 15	0. 66	17. 06	Y

续表

序号 No.	肿瘤登记处 Cancer registries	人口数 Population	发病数 New cases	死亡数 Deaths	MV%	DCO%	M/I	发病率变化 Change for CR %	接受 Accepted
367	长沙市天心区 Tianxin Qu, Changsha Shi	467 753	1 707	995	76. 86	0. 06	0. 58	15. 43	Y
368	长沙市岳麓区 Yuelu Qu, Changsha Shi	697 672	1 356	1 005	77. 65	4. 42	0. 74	-14. 01	Y
369	长沙市开福区 Kaifu Qu, Changsha Shi	481 900	1 804	1 180	76. 77	1. 77	0. 65	22. 40	Y
370	长沙市雨花区 Yuhua Qu, Changsha Shi	679 686	1 718	1 234	76. 89	0. 29	0. 72	9. 53	Y
371	长沙市望城区 Wangcheng Qu, Changsha Shi	562 953	1 331	1 039	75. 51	0. 15	0. 78	19. 33	Y
372	长沙县 Changsha Xian	775 500	2 258	1 353	73. 25	1. 90	0. 60	—	Y
373	浏阳市 Liuyang Shi	1 487 452	3 096	2 302	73. 90	0. 03	0. 74	—	Y
374	株洲市芦淞区 Lusong Qu, Zhuzhou Shi	240 662	682	409	73. 17	4. 69	0. 60	37. 99	Y
375	株洲市石峰区 Shifeng Qu, Zhuzhou Shi	247 638	609	418	71. 92	3. 94	0. 69	-15. 13	Y
376	攸县 You Xian	821 078	1 644	1 155	71. 35	0. 06	0. 70	6. 92	Y
377	湘潭市雨湖区 Yuhu Qu, Xiangtan Shi	517 809	1 546	735	73. 93	0. 52	0. 48	-1. 23	Y
378	衡东县 Hengdong Xian	761 598	1 482	1 099	71. 05	2. 83	0. 74	0. 22	Y
379	常宁市 Changning Shi	965 700	1 738	1 363	65. 07	0. 29	0. 78	—	Y
380	邵东县 Shaodong Xian	1 342 863	3 165	2 131	75. 20	5. 12	0. 67	1. 79	Y
381	新宁县 Xinning Xian	653 550	1 137	830	66. 31	0. 53	0. 73	9. 13	
382	岳阳市岳阳楼区 Yueyanglou Qu, Yueyang Shi	517 949	1 335	738	76. 55	2. 70	0. 55	7. 66	Y
383	常德市武陵区 Wuling Qu, Changde Shi	429 095	1 157	861	71. 39	5. 70	0. 74	38. 18	Y
384	慈利县 Cili Xian	702 623	1 559	914	73. 89	1. 35	0. 59	6. 65	Y
385	益阳市资阳区 Ziyang Qu, Yiyang Shi	433 297	1 008	728	74. 80	2. 38	0. 72	8. 28	Y
386	桃江县 Taojiang Xian	892 899	1 982	1 164	78. 51	1. 51	0. 59	18. 48	Y
387	临武县 Linwu Xian	385 100	833	510	79. 23	1. 92	0. 61	8. 10	Y
388	资兴市 Zixing Shi	380 499	845	567	78. 58	1. 18	0. 67	19. 84	Y
389	道县 Dao Xian	808 266	1 770	1 016	70. 62	3. 84	0. 57	27. 64	Y
390	宁远县 Ningyuan Xian	889 799	1 867	1 176	72. 63	4. 02	0. 63	—	Y
391	新田县 Xintian Xian	446 250	781	567	67. 73	2. 94	0. 73	-1. 37	Y

序号 No.	肿瘤登记处 Cancer registries	人口数 Population	发病数 New cases	死亡数 Deaths	MV%	DCO%	M/I	发病率变化 Change for CR %	接受 Accepted
392	麻阳苗族自治县 Mayang Miaozu Zizhixian	398 807	759	494	67. 06	3. 29	0. 65	8. 13	Y
393	洪江市 Hongjiang Shi	429 777	760	530	71. 71	0. 92	0. 70	1. 23	Y
394	冷水江市 Lengshuijiang Shi	371 500	931	569	67. 78	9. 02	0. 61	—	Y
395	涟源市 Lianyuan Shi	1 144 000	2 374	1 494	77. 00	5. 01	0. 63	-3. 19	Y
396	广州市 Guangzhou Shi	4 432 956	17 144	8 331	77. 61	0. 78	0. 49	5. 21	Y
397	广州市郊区 Rural areas of Guangzhou Shi	4 545 761	12 151	6 341	77. 33	0. 42	0. 52	1. 66	Y
398	南雄市 Nanxiong Shi	509 564	1 138	792	60. 19	3. 34	0. 70	-5. 23	Y
399	深圳市 Shenzhen Shi	4 096 196	9 406	3 745	72. 00	6. 86	0. 40	9. 68	Y
400	珠海市 Zhuhai Shi	1 173 270	3 390	1 381	60. 27	0. 86	0. 41	2. 29	Y
401	佛山市南海区 Nanhai Qu, Foshan Shi	1 413 684	4 082	2 209	68. 01	0. 00	0. 54	-5. 29	Y
402	佛山市顺德区 Shunde Qu, Foshan Shi	1 401 290	4 718	2 642	66. 89	0. 04	0. 56	19. 84	Y
403	江门市 Jiangmen Shi	676 685	2 223	1 273	77. 64	0. 76	0. 57	4. 49	Y
404	肇庆市端州区 Duanzhou Qu, Zhaoqing Shi	402 587	1 204	666	72. 34	0. 50	0. 55	-11. 74	Y
405	四会市 Sihui Shi	427 036	950	690	52. 00	0. 00	0. 73	-17. 70	Y
406	惠州市惠阳区 Huiyang Qu, Huizhou Shi	384 119	1 138	675	57. 82	11. 69	0. 59	—	Y
407	梅州市梅江区 Meijiang Qu, Meizhou Shi	356 591	1 056	587	78. 60	2. 84	0. 56	—	Y
408	梅州市梅县区 Meixian Qu, Meizhou Shi	612 499	1 708	1 115	74. 59	0. 00	0. 65	8. 23	Y
409	阳江市阳东区 Yangdong Qu, Yangjiang Shi	505 586	1 068	216	64. 14	0. 00	0. 20	—	
410	阳山县 Yangshan Xian	569 466	1 199	471	53. 04	9. 84	0. 39	65. 60	
411	东莞市 Dongguan Shi	2 113 081	5 887	2 900	72. 79	0. 32	0. 49	-5. 99	Y
412	中山市 Zhongshan Shi	1 611 596	5 155	2 716	83. 67	0. 00	0. 53	13. 35	Y
413	揭西县 Jiexi Xian	850 790	2 512	1 180	65. 61	0. 00	0. 47	16. 98	Y
414	罗定市 Luoding Shi	1 290 108	2 348	1 740	54. 94	3. 58	0. 74	-2. 02	Y
415	南宁市兴宁区 Xingning Qu, Nanning Shi	334 134	892	512	60. 20	2. 47	0. 57	-11. 18	Y
416	南宁市青秀区 Qingxiu Qu, Nanning Shi	733 504	1 518	846	79. 12	0. 33	0. 56	7. 31	Y

续表

序号 No.	肿瘤登记处 Cancer registries	人口数 Population	发病数 New cases	死亡数 Deaths	MV%	DCO%	M/I	发病率变化 Change for CR %	接受 Accepted
417	南宁市江南区 Jiangnan Qu, Nanning Shi	373 365	746	588	40.08	0.13	0.79	-6.23	Y
418	南宁经济技术开发区 Nanning economic and technological development zone	150 921	252	171	48.41	3.97	0.68	—	
419	南宁市西乡塘区 Xixiangtang Qu, Nanning Shi	796 000	2 149	1 090	48.21	14.15	0.51	-6.14	Y
420	南宁市良庆区 Liangqing Qu, Nanning Shi	288 470	704	317	65.34	0.00	0.45	—	
421	南宁市东盟经济开发区 ASEAN Economic Development Zone, Nanning Shi	38 064	89	67	52.81	1.12	0.75	—	Y
422	隆安县 Long'an Xian	422 396	890	511	56.63	0.11	0.57	31.94	Y
423	宾阳县 Binyang Xian	1 057 876	2 719	1 608	71.64	0.00	0.59	1.31	Y
424	柳州市 Liuzhou Shi	1 796 801	4 596	2 745	69.84	0.07	0.60	-7.12	Y
425	桂林市 Guilin Shi	783 166	2 300	1 328	75.00	0.22	0.58	3.83	Y
426	梧州市 Wuzhou Shi	794 633	1 932	1 248	65.42	0.98	0.65	0.21	Y
427	苍梧县 Cangwu Xian	407 192	936	641	53.85	1.18	0.68	-1.27	Y
428	北海市 Beihai Shi	710 402	2 085	1 122	65.08	0.62	0.54	2.89	Y
429	合浦县 Hepu Xian	933 297	2 409	1 804	51.18	2.57	0.75	-1.97	Y
430	钦州市钦南区 Qinnan Qu, Qinzhou Shi	515 499	1 058	548	59.07	0.00	0.52	—	Y
431	贵港市港北区 Gangbei Qu, Guigang Shi	724 600	1 379	901	70.49	7.40	0.65	16.62	Y
432	贵港市港南区 Gangnan Qu, Guigang Shi	704 498	1 374	826	70.96	0.00	0.60	-8.41	Y
433	贵港市覃塘区 Qintang Qu, Guigang Shi	606 098	1 100	746	38.45	0.00	0.68	-10.86	
434	平南县 Pingnan Xian	1 524 724	4 009	2 242	64.83	0.00	0.56	41.00	Y
435	玉林市 Yulin Shi	667 478	1 472	795	17.60	0.00	0.54	—	
436	陆川县 Luchuan Xian	794 267	1 463	977	0.00	0.00	0.67	—	
437	北流市 Beiliu Shi	1 515 002	2 055	1 836	44.33	0.00	0.89	-10.72	
438	百色市右江区 Youjiang Qu, Baise Shi	380 028	750	426	53.60	0.00	0.57	-6.06	Y
439	田阳县 Tianyang Xian	355 567	676	427	31.95	19.67	0.63	—	
440	罗城仫佬族自治县 Luocheng Mulaozu Zizhixian	386 902	746	451	78.55	0.00	0.60	12.71	Y

序号 No.	肿瘤登记处 Cancer registries	人口数 Population	发病数 New cases	死亡数 Deaths	MV%	DCO%	M/I	发病率变化 Change for CR %	接受 Accepted
441	合山市 Heshan Shi	119 106	343	268	66. 47	0. 00	0. 78	10. 08	Y
442	扶绥县 Fusui Xian	460 012	1 186	937	37. 44	2. 28	0. 79	1. 57	Y
443	三亚市 Sanya Shi	615 867	1 650	664	34. 48	0. 00	0. 40	-9. 89	
444	五指山市 Wuzhishan Shi	105 600	262	103	48. 47	1. 15	0. 39	-14. 14	
445	琼海市 Qionghai Shi	499 311	1 202	761	83. 94	0. 25	0. 63	-5. 65	Y
446	定安县 Ding'an Xian	288 237	708	357	37. 85	0. 56	0. 50	2. 95	Y
447	昌江黎族自治县 Changjiang Lizu Zizhixian	232 000	567	325	37. 74	0. 00	0. 57	2. 10	Y
448	陵水黎族自治县 Lingshui Lizu Zizhixian	370 141	1 032	371	26. 07	0. 00	0. 36	-5. 41	
449	重庆市万州区 Wanzhou Qu, Chongqing Shi	1 624 387	4 900	3 732	70. 35	0. 92	0. 76	-2. 69	Y
450	重庆市涪陵区 Fuling Qu, Chongqing Shi	1 162 063	3 052	1 665	62. 42	1. 70	0. 55	-3. 75	Y
451	重庆市渝中区 Yuzhong Qu, Chongqing Shi	656 363	2 100	1 178	63. 10	1. 95	0. 56	-0. 52	Y
452	重庆市大渡口区 Dadukou Qu, Chongqing Shi	332 700	1 094	574	79. 62	0. 00	0. 52	—	Y
453	重庆市江北区 Jiangbei Qu, Chongqing Shi	849 800	1 665	656	63. 24	0. 66	0. 39	-33. 72	
454	重庆市沙坪坝区 Shapingba Qu, Chongqing Shi	1 120 013	2 846	2 071	75. 30	0. 35	0. 73	-7. 63	Y
455	重庆市九龙坡区 Jiulongpo Qu, Chongqing Shi	932 463	2 662	1 627	64. 73	0. 11	0. 61	-0. 22	Y
456	重庆市南岸区 Nan'an Qu, Chongqing Shi	858 100	3 452	1 325	57. 65	0. 09	0. 38	12. 30	
457	重庆市北碚区 Beibei Qu, Chongqing Shi	794 509	2 644	1 576	66. 07	0. 87	0. 60	-9. 22	Y
458	重庆市綦江区 Qijiang Qu, Chongqing Shi	817 346	1 957	662	76. 44	0. 46	0. 34	—	
459	重庆市大足区 Dazu Qu, Chongqing Shi	763 900	2 608	1 752	34. 43	2. 88	0. 67	60. 30	Y
460	重庆市渝北区 Yubei Qu, Chongqing Shi	1 470 900	4 835	2 944	81. 43	0. 02	0. 61	8. 68	Y
461	重庆市巴南区 Banan Qu, Chongqing Shi	1 005 800	2 686	1 697	69. 14	0. 97	0. 63	5. 54	Y
462	重庆市黔江区 Qianjiang Qu, Chongqing Shi	462 000	1 241	680	63. 82	0. 40	0. 55	22. 99	Y

续表

序号 No.	肿瘤登记处 Cancer registries	人口数 Population	发病数 New cases	死亡数 Deaths	MV%	DCO%	M/I	发病率变化 Change for CR %	接受 Accepted
463	重庆市长寿区 Changshou Qu, Chongqing Shi	833 012	2 318	1 649	88. 52	0. 47	0. 71	-15. 48	Y
464	重庆市江津区 Jiangjin Qu, Chongqing Shi	1 331 900	3 722	2 384	64. 99	0. 00	0. 64	2. 39	Y
465	重庆市合川区 Hechuan Qu, Chongqing Shi	1 374 979	3 529	2 121	94. 05	0. 00	0. 60	-3. 96	Y
466	重庆市永川区 Yongchuan Qu, Chongqing Shi	1 096 100	3 587	2 450	70. 70	0. 47	0. 68	—	Y
467	重庆市南川区 Nanchuan Qu, Chongqing Shi	564 300	276	401	82. 25	0. 00	1. 45	-84. 73	
468	重庆市万盛经济技术开发区 Wansheng economic and technological development zone, Chongqing Shi	272 451	631	379	67. 19	0. 00	0. 60	-8. 31	Y
469	重庆市潼南区 Tongnan Qu, Chongqing Shi	682 300	1 936	1 094	66. 27	0. 57	0. 57	-1. 22	Y
470	重庆市铜梁区 Tongliang Qu, Chongqing Shi	684 357	2 181	1 479	62. 31	8. 76	0. 68	-4. 21	Y
471	重庆市荣昌区 Rongchang Qu, Chongqing Shi	701 000	846	968	40. 78	0. 35	1. 14	—	
472	重庆市璧山区 Bishan Qu, Chongqing Shi	695 200	1 673	1 408	86. 19	0. 00	0. 84	—	Y
473	重庆市梁平区 Liangping Qu, Chongqing Shi	674 000	950	561	34. 53	0. 42	0. 59	-36. 79	
474	丰都县 Fengdu Xian	625 600	1 482	779	60. 05	0. 13	0. 53	5. 56	Y
475	垫江县 Dianjiang Xian	693 958	1 466	1 165	21. 96	0. 95	0. 79	—	
476	重庆市武隆区 Wulong Qu, Chongqing Shi	346 700	892	564	22. 42	57. 74	0. 63	14. 21	
477	忠县 Zhong Xian	788 834	2 314	1 507	70. 66	0. 91	0. 65	2. 03	Y
478	重庆市开州区 Kaizhou Qu, Chongqing Shi	1 183 074	4 061	2 775	61. 81	0. 07	0. 68	3. 97	Y
479	云阳县 Yunyang Xian	896 600	2 362	1 770	86. 33	0. 00	0. 75	-12. 49	Y
480	奉节县 Fengjie Xian	803 300	2 334	1 549	64. 70	8. 53	0. 66	—	Y
481	巫山县 Wushan Xian	462 300	984	297	56. 10	0. 00	0. 30	—	
482	巫溪县 Wuxi Xian	397 868	976	521	34. 02	0. 10	0. 53	—	Y
483	石柱土家族自治县 Shizhu Tujiazu Zizhixian	386 500	944	692	77. 22	0. 00	0. 73	—	Y

续表

序号 No.	肿瘤登记处 Cancer registries	人口数 Population	发病数 New cases	死亡数 Deaths	MV%	DCO%	M/I	发病率变化 Change for CR %	接受 Accepted
484	秀山土家族苗族自治县 Xiushan Tujiazu Miaozu Zizhixian	491 300	503	683	59. 84	0. 60	1. 36	—	
485	酉阳土家族苗族自治县 Youyang Tujiazu Miaozu Zizhixian	556 500	738	722	74. 12	0. 00	0. 98	-51. 09	
486	彭水苗族土家族自治县 Pengshui Miaozu Tujiazu Zizhixian	516 400	1 032	766	67. 64	0. 00	0. 74	—	Y
487	成都市青羊区 Qingyang Qu, Chengdu Shi	681 411	2 497	1 498	67. 96	4. 57	0. 60	18. 47	Y
488	成都市成华区 Chenghua Qu, Chengdu Shi	738 166	2 489	1 531	67. 58	0. 76	0. 62	—	Y
489	成都市龙泉驿区 Longquanyi Qu, Chengdu Shi	672 292	1 922	1 287	68. 21	5. 67	0. 67	2. 58	Y
490	成都市新都区 Xindu Qu, Chengdu Shi	782 870	1 899	1 322	71. 88	1. 11	0. 70	—	Y
491	金堂县 Jintang Xian	901 403	2 966	1 778	68. 88	7. 72	0. 60	—	Y
492	成都市双流区 Shuangliu Qu, Chengdu Shi	582 093	1 690	1 020	81. 95	0. 18	0. 60	—	Y
493	天府新区 Tianfu New Area, Chengdu Shi	589 218	1 535	947	80. 33	8. 73	0. 62	—	Y
494	成都市郫都区 Pidu Qu, Chengdu Shi	588 034	1 441	1 054	75. 09	4. 86	0. 73	—	Y
495	新津县 Xinjin Xian	317 154	1 219	735	70. 55	3. 28	0. 60	—	Y
496	彭州市 Pengzhou Shi	803 997	2 891	1 846	68. 73	0. 93	0. 64	0. 82	Y
497	自贡市自流井区 Ziliujing Qu, Zigong Shi	393 420	1 360	880	84. 85	0. 00	0. 65	8. 38	Y
498	自贡市贡井区 Gongjing Qu, Zigong Shi	287 531	867	593	43. 60	1. 50	0. 68	5. 23	Y
499	自贡市大安区 Da'an Qu, Zigong Shi	446 694	1 155	768	48. 05	0. 00	0. 66	—	Y
500	自贡市沿滩区 Yantan Qu, Zigong Shi	355 206	755	515	17. 88	0. 00	0. 68	0. 40	
501	荣县 Rong Xian	685 004	1 317	907	28. 85	1. 52	0. 69	—	
502	富顺县 Fushun Xian	1 075 595	2 606	1 733	69. 26	0. 00	0. 67	—	Y
503	攀枝花市东区 Dong Qu, Panzhihua Shi	287 086	825	253	84. 97	2. 42	0. 31	—	

续表

序号 No.	肿瘤登记处 Cancer registries	人口数 Population	发病数 New cases	死亡数 Deaths	MV%	DCO%	M/I	发病率变化 Change for CR %	接受 Accepted
504	攀枝花市西区 Xi Qu, Panzhihua Shi	133 352	521	303	76. 97	0. 38	0. 58	—	Y
505	攀枝花市仁和区 Renhe Qu, Panzhihua Shi	233 420	526	323	70. 34	1. 71	0. 61	19. 05	Y
506	米易县 Miyi Xian	221 725	456	241	75. 22	0. 88	0. 53	34. 63	Y
507	盐边县 Yanbian Xian	208 864	256	67	67. 58	5. 47	0. 26	—	
508	泸州市江阳区 Jiangyang Qu, Luzhou Shi	676 329	2 001	1 337	34. 53	0. 05	0. 67	—	
509	泸州市纳溪区 Naxi Qu, Luzhou Shi	465 720	881	511	71. 06	4. 77	0. 58	—	Y
510	泸州市龙马潭区 Longmatan Qu, Luzhou Shi	370 424	1 145	750	63. 67	0. 35	0. 66	-7. 06	Y
511	泸县 Lu Xian	1 072 035	3 188	2 057	32. 21	0. 09	0. 65	20. 63	Y
512	合江县 Hejiang Xian	900 869	2 205	1 264	72. 65	0. 50	0. 57	3. 87	Y
513	叙永县 Xuyong Xian	725 070	1 335	704	62. 70	1. 57	0. 53	—	
514	古蔺县 Gulin Xian	876 241	1 527	882	31. 04	0. 20	0. 58	—	
515	德阳市旌阳区 Jingyang Qu, Deyang Shi	697 353	2 166	1 448	71. 93	0. 74	0. 67	13. 83	Y
516	中江县 Zhongjiang Xian	1 399 224	2 656	1 968	55. 65	3. 69	0. 74	14. 53	Y
517	德阳市罗江区 Luojiang Qu, Deyang Shi	247 532	636	498	68. 08	0. 47	0. 78	6. 42	Y
518	广汉市 Guanghan Shi	603 706	1 747	1 205	77. 79	0. 46	0. 69	-5. 28	Y
519	什邡市 Shifang Shi	432 636	1 320	970	70. 23	0. 08	0. 73	-1. 91	Y
520	绵竹市 Mianzhu Shi	501 082	1 595	1 189	60. 25	1. 19	0. 75	-2. 83	Y
521	绵阳市涪城区 Fucheng Qu, Mianyang Shi	523 646	1 767	1 098	70. 12	6. 79	0. 62	126. 29	Y
522	绵阳市游仙区 Youxian Qu, Mianyang Shi	480 631	1 389	861	76. 24	0. 22	0. 62	14. 32	Y
523	绵阳市安州区 Anzhou Qu, Mianyang Shi	449 172	963	693	69. 37	1. 14	0. 72	-7. 56	Y
524	三台县 Santai Xian	1 422 783	3 898	2 386	55. 90	0. 62	0. 61	20. 53	Y
525	盐亭县 Yanting Xian	596 770	2 279	1 798	71. 13	0. 13	0. 79	-1. 42	Y
526	梓潼县 Zitong Xian	384 490	773	282	35. 71	26. 78	0. 36	—	
527	北川羌族自治县 Beichuan Qiangzu Zizhixian	237 601	502	344	39. 04	0. 20	0. 69	21. 06	Y
528	平武县 Pingwu Xian	178 840	115	26	66. 96	0. 00	0. 23	—	

续表

序号 No.	肿瘤登记处 Cancer registries	人口数 Population	发病数 New cases	死亡数 Deaths	MV%	DCO%	M/I	发病率变化 Change for CR %	接受 Accepted
529	江油市 Jiangyou Shi	878 551	2 405	1 470	81. 16	0. 12	0. 61	—	Y
530	广元市利州区 Lizhou Qu, Guangyuan Shi	492 066	1 334	940	75. 34	0. 52	0. 70	—	Y
531	广元市昭化区 Zhaohua Qu, Guangyuan Shi	232 559	638	354	66. 77	0. 31	0. 55	—	Y
532	广元市朝天区 Chaotian Qu, Guangyuan Shi	188 381	609	300	82. 59	0. 00	0. 49	80. 20	Y
533	旺苍县 Wangcang Xian	450 954	998	544	68. 04	1. 00	0. 55	-12. 48	Y
534	青川县 Qingchuan Xian	230 867	518	331	68. 73	0. 39	0. 64	4. 82	Y
535	剑阁县 Jiange Xian	657 662	1 790	1 299	48. 77	0. 45	0. 73	0. 32	Y
536	苍溪县 Cangxi Xian	758 097	1 686	1 127	42. 35	0. 06	0. 67	—	Y
537	遂宁市船山区 Chuanshan Qu, Suining Shi	666 039	1 571	1 149	77. 91	0. 19	0. 73	20. 02	Y
538	遂宁市安居区 Anju Qu, Suining Shi	782 701	1 668	1 244	67. 03	0. 48	0. 75	32. 45	Y
539	蓬溪县 Pengxi Xian	718 241	1 644	1 144	57. 66	0. 79	0. 70	—	Y
540	射洪县 Shehong Xian	972 379	2 179	1 493	69. 25	0. 05	0. 69	-4. 17	Y
541	大英县 Daying Xian	553 902	1 183	837	71. 01	0. 08	0. 71	—	Y
542	内江市市中区 Shizhong Qu, Neijiang Shi	513 199	972	568	81. 38	1. 13	0. 58	—	
543	内江市东兴区 Dongxing Qu, Neijiang Shi	884 110	1 617	995	48. 98	0. 62	0. 62	2. 08	
544	威远县 Weiyuan Xian	677 699	1 060	596	25. 28	0. 19	0. 56	—	
545	资中县 Zizhong Xian	1 278 141	2 925	2 353	48. 00	0. 62	0. 80	-21. 76	
546	隆昌市 Longchang Shi	773 544	1 645	1 171	80. 97	0. 85	0. 71	—	Y
547	乐山市市中区 Shizhong Qu, Leshan Shi	630 693	1 908	1 186	86. 90	0. 00	0. 62	18. 93	Y
548	乐山市沙湾区 Shawan Qu, Leshan Shi	178 354	326	228	65. 03	3. 68	0. 70	-5. 87	
549	乐山市五通桥区 Wutongqiao Qu, Leshan Shi	301 658	627	507	92. 98	2. 07	0. 81	—	Y
550	乐山市金口河区 Jinkouhe Qu, Leshan Shi	49 268	44	48	59. 09	0. 00	1. 09	—	
551	犍为县 Jianwei Xian	559 530	1 100	724	32. 27	0. 09	0. 66	—	Y
552	井研县 Jingyan Xian	401 694	777	644	27. 41	0. 00	0. 83	—	
553	夹江县 Jiajiang Xian	346 427	555	424	74. 59	0. 00	0. 76	-12. 67	

续表

序号 No.	肿瘤登记处 Cancer registries	人口数 Population	发病数 New cases	死亡数 Deaths	MV%	DCO%	M/I	发病率变化 Change for CR %	接受 Accepted
554	沐川县 Muchuan Xian	252 726	119	103	39. 50	1. 68	0. 87	—	
555	峨边彝族自治县 Ebian Yizu Zizhixian	158 721	102	75	37. 25	6. 86	0. 74	—	
556	马边彝族自治县 Mabian Yizu Zizhixian	220 385	113	61	36. 28	1. 77	0. 54	—	
557	峨眉山市 Emeishan Shi	432 848	1 000	690	69. 70	0. 20	0. 69	—	Y
558	南充市顺庆区 Shunqing Qu, Nanchong Shi	665 727	3 431	1 090	50. 31	0. 64	0. 32	—	
559	南充市高坪区 Gaoping Qu, Nanchong Shi	596 843	1 524	1 070	72. 77	0. 00	0. 70	-11. 54	Y
560	南充市嘉陵区 Jialing Qu, Nanchong Shi	702 499	1 839	879	32. 30	0. 38	0. 48	—	
561	南部县 Nanbu Xian	1 257 296	2 614	789	56. 54	0. 46	0. 30	—	
562	营山县 Yingshan Xian	912 440	2 274	1 145	33. 38	0. 13	0. 50	—	
563	蓬安县 Peng'an Xian	681 819	1 629	942	21. 06	0. 43	0. 58	—	
564	仪陇县 Yilong Xian	1 082 014	2 355	1 465	62. 80	2. 51	0. 62	24. 88	
565	西充县 Xichong Xian	603 738	1 644	681	45. 32	0. 18	0. 41	—	
566	阆中市 Langzhong Shi	844 683	2 958	1 835	66. 73	0. 41	0. 62	6. 73	Y
567	眉山市东坡区 Dongpo Qu, Meishan Shi	884 862	2 118	1 329	79. 23	1. 04	0. 63	17. 85	Y
568	眉山市彭山区 Pengshan Qu, Meishan Shi	331 992	716	519	67. 18	0. 14	0. 72	23. 21	Y
569	仁寿县 Renshou Xian	1 531 443	3 527	2 918	56. 59	1. 22	0. 83	10. 17	Y
570	洪雅县 Hongya Xian	350 800	215	71	74. 88	0. 47	0. 33	—	
571	丹棱县 Danleng Xian	145 949	294	200	35. 71	5. 44	0. 68	—	Y
572	青神县 Qingshen Xian	194 093	404	317	72. 03	0. 00	0. 78	14. 37	Y
573	宜宾市翠屏区 Cuiping Qu, Yibin Shi	845 478	2 159	1 313	50. 35	0. 05	0. 61	4. 90	Y
574	宜宾市叙州区 Xuzhou Qu, Yibin Shi	1 023 976	1 993	912	68. 09	0. 50	0. 46	15. 81	
575	江安县 Jiang'an Xian	564 056	889	525	54. 78	0. 00	0. 59	—	
576	长宁县 Changning Xian	465 193	1 045	714	71. 29	0. 29	0. 68	2. 45	Y
577	高县 Gao Xian	534 148	719	283	41. 03	0. 00	0. 39	—	
578	筠连县 Yunlian Xian	444 389	592	227	73. 82	1. 35	0. 38	—	
579	屏山县 Pingshan Xian	312 780	291	232	24. 05	7. 22	0. 80	—	
580	广安市广安区 Guang'an Qu, Guang'an Shi	897 156	2 519	1 799	71. 73	2. 98	0. 71	7. 27	Y

续表

序号 No.	肿瘤登记处 Cancer registries	人口数 Population	发病数 New cases	死亡数 Deaths	MV%	DCO%	M/I	发病率变化 Change for CR %	接受 Accepted
581	广安市前锋区 Qianfeng Qu, Guang'an Shi	369 787	928	441	36. 96	0. 22	0. 48	—	
582	岳池县 Yuechi Xian	1 170 827	2 157	1 057	79. 14	0. 97	0. 49	—	
583	武胜县 Wusheng Xian	836 823	1 749	490	38. 02	0. 69	0. 28	—	
584	邻水县 Linshui Xian	1 026 874	1 379	629	36. 04	2. 76	0. 46	—	
585	华蓥市 Huaying Shi	362 490	493	346	76. 67	1. 01	0. 70	—	
586	达州市达川区 Dachuan Qu, Dazhou Shi	1 158 342	2 192	1 165	54. 01	0. 73	0. 53	—	Y
587	宣汉县 Xuanhan Xian	1 323 382	2 373	1 519	81. 50	0. 67	0. 64	35. 53	
588	开江县 Kaijiang Xian	59 0261	931	637	51. 45	4. 73	0. 68	—	
589	大竹县 Dazhu Xian	1 114 182	2 599	1 571	70. 87	0. 77	0. 60	-1. 05	Y
590	渠县 Qu Xian	1 365 468	2 565	2 004	44. 76	0. 86	0. 78	—	Y
591	万源市 Wanyuan Shi	550 130	650	482	52. 46	0. 00	0. 74	-2. 52	
592	雅安市雨城区 Yucheng Qu, Ya'an Shi	346 113	874	537	60. 41	3. 32	0. 61	2. 57	Y
593	雅安市名山区 Mingshan Qu, Ya'an Shi	279 847	632	401	65. 66	2. 06	0. 63	4. 26	Y
594	荥经县 Yingjing Xian	147 386	397	250	80. 35	0. 00	0. 63	-0. 37	Y
595	汉源县 Hanyuan Xian	322 310	732	489	58. 47	0. 41	0. 67	-1. 73	Y
596	石棉县 Shimian Xian	122 054	312	219	66. 03	2. 56	0. 70	0. 12	Y
597	天全县 Tianquan Xian	152 215	423	253	66. 67	0. 47	0. 60	23. 48	Y
598	芦山县 Lushan Xian	121 008	325	195	76. 92	0. 92	0. 60	11. 28	Y
599	宝兴县 Baoxing Xian	58 456	143	88	66. 43	0. 70	0. 62	4. 50	Y
600	巴中市巴州区 Bazhou Qu, Bazhong Shi	676 551	1 085	765	45. 44	3. 13	0. 71	—	
601	巴中市恩阳区 Enyang Qu, Bazhong Shi	571 062	669	260	49. 33	1. 79	0. 39	—	
602	通江县 Tongjiang Xian	746 161	1 135	656	82. 38	0. 00	0. 58	—	
603	南江县 Nanjiang Xian	664 283	1 097	726	79. 49	0. 36	0. 66	10. 36	
604	平昌县 Pingchang Xian	799 280	1 222	535	49. 35	0. 82	0. 44	—	
605	资阳市雁江区 Yanjiang Qu, Ziyang Shi	1 081 171	2 847	1 774	47. 14	0. 07	0. 62	13. 57	Y
606	安岳县 Anyue Xian	1 607 930	2 149	1 150	63. 24	0. 19	0. 54	—	
607	乐至县 Lezhi Xian	825 863	2 071	1 520	68. 13	0. 10	0. 73	25. 47	Y
608	马尔康县 Barkam Xian	55 663	44	17	95. 45	0. 00	0. 39	—	
609	汶川县 Wenchuan Xian	94 552	140	104	80. 71	0. 71	0. 74	17. 51	

续表

序号 No.	肿瘤登记处 Cancer registries	人口数 Population	发病数 New cases	死亡数 Deaths	MV%	DCO%	M/I	发病率变化 Change for CR %	接受 Accepted
610	理县 Li Xian	44 250	96	88	95. 83	2. 08	0. 92	—	
611	茂县 Mao Xian	112 484	171	113	58. 48	25. 15	0. 66	—	
612	松潘县 Songpan Xian	74 066	70	28	87. 14	0. 00	0. 40	—	
613	金川县 Jinchuan Xian	72 434	45	19	35. 56	0. 00	0. 42	—	
614	小金县 Xiaojin Xian	80 586	62	61	27. 42	24. 19	0. 98	—	
615	黑水县 Heishui Xian	63 183	38	13	31. 58	0. 00	0. 34	—	
616	若尔盖县 Zoigê Xian	79 934	27	8	62. 96	0. 00	0. 30	—	
617	红原县 Hongyuan Xian	48 878	41	19	36. 59	24. 39	0. 46	—	
618	贵阳市花溪区 Huaxi Qu, Guiyang Shi	602 716	734	454	68. 39	0. 14	0. 62	-41. 26	
619	开阳县 Kaiyang Xian	369 516	935	704	74. 22	0. 86	0. 75	-14. 51	
620	息烽县 Xifeng Xian	222 137	263	181	33. 84	7. 98	0. 69	—	
621	清镇市 Qingzhen Shi	464 615	991	611	77. 40	1. 41	0. 62	11. 94	Y
622	六盘水市钟山区 Zhongshan Qu, Liupanshui Shi	527 809	878	433	27. 22	2. 28	0. 49	-22. 82	
623	六盘水市六枝特区 Liuzhi Tequ, Liupanshui Shi	508 472	1 324	827	41. 84	0. 08	0. 62	1. 88	Y
624	水城县 Shuicheng Xian	671 142	564	313	29. 61	5. 85	0. 55	—	
625	盘州市 Panzhou Shi	1 045 712	2 364	1 737	46. 66	1. 61	0. 73	—	Y
626	遵义市红花岗区 Honghuagang Qu, Zunyi Shi	865 349	313	119	70. 93	9. 27	0. 38	—	
627	遵义市汇川区 Huichuan Qu, Zunyi Shi	567 401	736	324	65. 22	0. 68	0. 44	-33. 00	
628	习水县 Xishui Xian	519 600	676	346	37. 13	9. 76	0. 51	—	
629	赤水市 Chishui Shi	242 402	489	513	54. 40	1. 64	1. 05	4. 71	
630	安顺市西秀区 Xixiu Qu, Anshun Shi	617 043	1 665	914	91. 41	0. 54	0. 55	15. 59	Y
631	镇宁布依族苗族自治县 Zhenning Buyizu Miaozu Zizhixian	268 379	855	624	79. 53	0. 00	0. 73	27. 61	Y
632	毕节市七星关区 Qixingguan Qu, Bijie Shi	1 151 393	1 737	754	77. 20	1. 38	0. 43	5. 00	
633	金沙县 Jinsha Xian	573 280	1 036	727	94. 79	0. 48	0. 70	-14. 82	
634	铜仁市碧江区 Bijiang Qu, Tongren Shi	281 956	698	315	84. 53	0. 72	0. 45	28. 24	Y
635	玉屏侗族自治县 Yuping Dongzu Zizhixian	120 181	256	81	42. 97	1. 17	0. 32	—	

序号 No.	肿瘤登记处 Cancer registries	人口数 Population	发病数 New cases	死亡数 Deaths	MV%	DCO%	M/I	发病率变化 Change for CR %	接受 Accepted
636	思南县 Sinan Xian	500 681	896	237	27. 90	4. 58	0. 26	—	
637	普安县 Pu'an Xian	258 861	412	66	89. 81	9. 71	0. 16	—	
638	册亨县 Ceheng Xian	182 179	461	464	68. 11	1. 30	1. 01	47. 90	
639	黄平县 Huangping Xian	265 220	418	177	31. 82	0. 00	0. 42	—	
640	镇远县 Zhenyuan Xian	210 744	272	152	85. 66	8. 82	0. 56	—	
641	榕江县 Rongjiang Xian	288 864	370	263	26. 49	1. 62	0. 71	—	
642	雷山县 Leishan Xian	119 776	214	101	76. 17	0. 00	0. 47	11. 14	
643	麻江县 Majiang Xian	123 263	196	156	36. 22	1. 02	0. 80	—	
644	都匀市 Duyun Shi	425 156	1 373	483	70. 87	0. 07	0. 35	37. 30	
645	福泉市 Fuquan Shi	295 168	489	379	56. 65	0. 61	0. 78	13. 09	
646	荔波县 Libo Xian	128 479	191	102	26. 70	6. 28	0. 53	—	
647	独山县 Dushan Xian	272 222	263	128	15. 97	0. 00	0. 49	—	
648	龙里县 Longli Xian	161 628	457	308	43. 54	10. 94	0. 67	—	Y
649	昆明市五华区 Wuhua Qu, Kunming Shi	583 144	1 842	1 007	80. 67	0. 81	0. 55	—	Y
650	昆明市盘龙区 Panlong Qu, Kunming Shi	553 732	1 516	1 063	51. 98	14. 12	0. 70	12. 15	Y
651	昆明市官渡区 Guandu Qu, Kunming Shi	525 229	1 207	836	60. 89	0. 08	0. 69	-2. 46	Y
652	昆明市西山区 Xishan Qu, Kunming Shi	546 072	1 460	965	70. 68	0. 00	0. 66	-2. 36	Y
653	昆明市东川区 Dongchuan Qu, Kunming Shi	312 511	353	65	29. 46	0. 85	0. 18	-39. 58	
654	昆明市晋宁区 Jinning Qu, Kunming Shi	284 246	569	242	63. 62	0. 00	0. 43	—	
655	昆明市呈贡区 Chenggong Qu, Kunming Shi	116 766	245	110	79. 18	0. 00	0. 45	—	
656	富民县 Fumin Xian	149 613	259	163	3. 47	0. 00	0. 63	—	
657	嵩明县 Songming Xian	306 948	567	434	52. 73	0. 00	0. 77	—	Y
658	禄劝彝族苗族自治县 Luquan Yizu Miaozu Zizhixian	420 374	718	430	67. 13	0. 00	0. 60	14. 53	
659	安宁市 Anning Shi	276 288	776	276	90. 08	0. 00	0. 36	—	
660	曲靖市麒麟区 Qilin Qu, Qujing Shi	715 900	1 446	847	45. 37	2. 77	0. 59	10. 28	Y
661	曲靖市沾益区 Zhanyi Qu, Qujing Shi	444 831	817	533	52. 63	0. 00	0. 65	-6. 82	Y
662	马龙县 Malong Xian	209 562	343	201	30. 90	3. 21	0. 59	—	

续表

序号 No.	肿瘤登记处 Cancer registries	人口数 Population	发病数 New cases	死亡数 Deaths	MV%	DCO%	M/I	发病率变化 Change for CR %	接受 Accepted
663	陆良县 Luliang Xian	652 302	2 244	279	23. 62	0. 36	0. 12	—	
664	富源县 Fuyuan Xian	749 219	1 717	813	38. 26	5. 07	0. 47	13. 39	
665	宣威市 Xuanwei Shi	1 551 701	3 292	2 146	41. 40	0. 00	0. 65	—	Y
666	玉溪市红塔区 Hongta Qu, Yuxi Shi	450 322	1 031	602	73. 62	1. 16	0. 58	1. 02	Y
667	玉溪市江川区 Jiangchuan Qu, Yuxi Shi	282 923	522	286	67. 82	0. 57	0. 55	—	Y
668	澄江县 Chengjiang Xian	145 809	331	172	68. 28	2. 11	0. 52	-0. 53	Y
669	通海县 Tonghai Xian	289 488	571	323	70. 75	0. 00	0. 57	37. 73	Y
670	华宁县 Huaning Xian	212 830	360	247	51. 39	0. 00	0. 69	0. 01	
671	易门县 Yimen Xian	165 734	394	252	75. 38	0. 00	0. 64	14. 87	Y
672	峨山彝族自治县 Eshan Yizu Zizhixian	155 614	391	249	58. 31	3. 32	0. 64	4. 15	Y
673	新平彝族傣族自治县 Xinping Yizu Daizu Zizhixian	278 464	514	286	76. 07	0. 00	0. 56	-11. 90	
674	元江哈尼族彝族傣族自治县 Yuanjiang Hanizu Yizu Daizu Zizhixian	210 441	483	285	73. 91	0. 00	0. 59	52. 63	Y
675	保山市隆阳区 Longyang Qu, Baoshan Shi	940 860	1 846	1 195	72. 86	0. 00	0. 65	-1. 07	Y
676	施甸县 Shidian Xian	347 168	625	402	65. 12	0. 00	0. 64	-4. 38	Y
677	腾冲市 Tengchong Shi	665 127	1 312	745	75. 84	0. 00	0. 57	2. 91	Y
678	龙陵县 Longling Xian	286 099	400	214	43. 75	5. 25	0. 54	—	
679	昌宁县 Changning Xian	353 913	632	368	65. 35	0. 00	0. 58	37. 15	
680	昭通市昭阳区 Zhaoyang Qu, Zhaotong Shi	825 089	977	800	22. 72	0. 00	0. 82	—	
681	巧家县 Qiaojia Xian	443 960	678	341	38. 35	0. 00	0. 50	—	
682	绥江县 Suijiang Xian	169 892	304	171	25. 00	0. 00	0. 56	—	
683	水富县 Shuifu Xian	105 738	199	120	14. 07	0. 00	0. 60	12. 78	
684	丽江市古城区 Gucheng Qu, Lijiang Shi	157 397	389	236	62. 72	1. 54	0. 61	22. 19	Y
685	玉龙纳西族自治县 Yulong Naxizu Zizhixian	220 671	417	237	80. 34	5. 04	0. 57	7. 27	Y
686	华坪县 Huaping Xian	161 825	271	191	51. 29	38. 38	0. 70	18. 99	
687	景东彝族自治县 Jingdong Yizu Zizhixian	366 337	538	242	29. 37	0. 00	0. 45	—	

序号 No.	肿瘤登记处 Cancer registries	人口数 Population	发病数 New cases	死亡数 Deaths	MV%	DCO%	M/I	发病率变化 Change for CR %	接受 Accepted
688	景谷傣族彝族自治县 Jinggu Daizu Yizu Zizhixian	301 230	536	391	69. 78	0. 00	0. 73	—	Y
689	镇沅彝族哈尼族拉祜族自治县 Zhenyuan Yizu Hanizu Lahuzu Zizhixian	213 803	356	113	25. 84	0. 00	0. 32	—	
690	江城哈尼族彝族自治县 Jiangcheng Hanizu Yizu Zizhixian	117 302	279	121	10. 39	0. 00	0. 43	—	
691	临沧市临翔区 Linxiang Qu, Lincang Shi	325 915	597	327	75. 38	0. 00	0. 55	-4. 00	
692	镇康县 Zhenkang Xian	182 187	249	149	15. 66	0. 00	0. 60	—	
693	沧源佤族自治县 Cangyuan Wazu Zizhixian	185 151	299	190	78. 26	0. 33	0. 64	21. 07	
694	楚雄市 Chuxiong Shi	530 491	1 181	618	82. 64	1. 10	0. 52	18. 79	Y
695	双柏县 Shuangbai Xian	163 824	306	174	83. 33	0. 00	0. 57	22. 39	Y
696	牟定县 Mouding Xian	215 653	449	232	83. 52	0. 00	0. 52	49. 05	Y
697	南华县 Nanhua Xian	243 690	411	249	34. 06	0. 24	0. 61	22. 55	
698	姚安县 Yao'an Xian	203 652	356	219	80. 62	0. 00	0. 62	5. 67	
699	大姚县 Dayao Xian	278 292	487	321	26. 08	0. 21	0. 66	96. 36	
700	永仁县 Yongren Xian	111 284	191	120	80. 10	0. 00	0. 63	—	
701	元谋县 Yuanmou Xian	220 286	392	231	75. 51	0. 00	0. 59	3. 28	Y
702	武定县 Wuding Xian	278 847	408	316	74. 51	0. 74	0. 77	—	
703	禄丰县 Lufeng Xian	434 138	1 026	467	60. 92	0. 00	0. 46	—	
704	个旧市 Gejiu Shi	384 363	990	676	62. 63	3. 13	0. 68	12. 97	Y
705	开远市 Kaiyuan Shi	286 251	606	334	42. 08	10. 73	0. 55	-10. 86	Y
706	蒙自市 Mengzi Shi	415 612	730	433	74. 25	0. 00	0. 59	-8. 40	Y
707	弥勒市 Mile Shi	541 785	764	542	70. 29	0. 13	0. 71	-0. 35	
708	屏边苗族自治县 Pingbian Miaozu Zizhixian	160 045	354	266	74. 01	0. 00	0. 75	5. 81	Y
709	建水县 Jianshui Xian	543 441	953	619	69. 67	0. 73	0. 65	4. 45	Y
710	石屏县 Shiping Xian	316 785	593	360	57. 00	0. 00	0. 61	6. 46	Y
711	泸西县 Luxi Xian	444 305	825	465	50. 42	0. 00	0. 56	-9. 55	Y
712	河口瑶族自治县 Hekou Yaozu Zizhixian	92 795	139	71	38. 85	0. 00	0. 51	—	
713	砚山县 Yanshan Xian	481 011	793	425	93. 82	0. 00	0. 54	—	
714	西畴县 Xichou Xian	261 364	433	240	23. 56	0. 00	0. 55	—	

续表

序号 No.	肿瘤登记处 Cancer registries	人口数 Population	发病数 New cases	死亡数 Deaths	MV%	DCO%	M/I	发病率变化 Change for CR %	接受 Accepted
715	丘北县 Qiubei Xian	491 243	886	536	2. 71	0. 00	0. 60	55. 07	
716	富宁县 Funing Xian	418 535	441	339	83. 45	0. 00	0. 77	—	
717	景洪市 Jinghong Shi	425 821	1 052	702	44. 96	0. 19	0. 67	-0. 10	Y
718	大理市 Dali Shi	630 467	1 020	483	76. 76	1. 27	0. 47	-21. 69	
719	祥云县 Xiangyun Xian	477 968	701	391	93. 15	0. 00	0. 56	-11. 59	
720	弥渡县 Midu Xian	323 126	474	273	50. 84	4. 64	0. 58	—	
721	永平县 Yongping Xian	185 685	182	61	71. 43	0. 00	0. 34	—	
722	鹤庆县 Heqing Xian	280 483	211	65	72. 99	0. 00	0. 31	—	
723	梁河县 Lianghe Xian	172 163	228	100	82. 46	0. 00	0. 44	—	
724	盈江县 Yingjiang Xian	316 104	384	173	72. 92	1. 56	0. 45	—	
725	兰坪白族普米族自治县 Lanping Baizu Pumizu Zizhixian	223 190	290	206	80. 00	1. 03	0. 71	-33. 31	
726	拉萨市城关区 Chengguan Qu, Lasa Shi	210 410	123	79	35. 77	4. 07	0. 64	—	
727	林芝市巴宜区 Bayi Qu, Linzhi Shi	44 176	58	15	29. 31	31. 03	0. 26	-10. 77	
728	山南市乃东区 Naidong Qu, Shannan Shi	64 169	110	9	9. 09	0. 00	0. 08	—	
729	西安市碑林区 Beilin Qu, Xi'an Shi	679 588	1 675	1 029	89. 67	4. 12	0. 61	5. 32	Y
730	西安市莲湖区 Lianhu Qu, Xi'an Shi	669 708	3 968	3 034	74. 14	1. 21	0. 76	96. 29	Y
731	西安市未央区 Weiyang Qu, Xi'an Shi	461 202	1 448	877	94. 75	0. 07	0. 61	31. 28	Y
732	西安市雁塔区 Yanta Qu, Xi'an Shi	882 760	1 939	1 509	84. 37	2. 37	0. 78	3. 39	
733	西安市高陵区 Gaoling Qu, Xi'an Shi	340 327	806	479	63. 28	0. 00	0. 59	-9. 45	Y
734	西安市鄠邑区 Huyi Qu, Xi'an Shi	578 584	1 120	774	56. 34	21. 07	0. 69	—	
735	铜川市王益区 Wangyi Qu, Tongchuan Shi	203 357	371	318	75. 74	0. 54	0. 86	-12. 19	
736	铜川市耀州区 Yaozhou Qu, Tongchuan Shi	331 941	663	93	74. 96	0. 00	0. 14	61. 10	
737	宝鸡市金台区 Jintai Qu, Baoji Shi	384 448	710	446	89. 01	1. 27	0. 63	-25. 24	

续表

序号 No.	肿瘤登记处 Cancer registries	人口数 Population	发病数 New cases	死亡数 Deaths	MV%	DCO%	M/I	发病率变化 Change for CR %	接受 Accepted
738	宝鸡市陈仓区 Chencang Qu,Baoji Shi	438 717	789	532	76. 17	0. 00	0. 67	188. 40	
739	凤翔县 Fengxiang Xian	483 471	915	724	71. 91	1. 31	0. 79	9. 84	Y
740	岐山县 Qishan Xian	462 499	836	604	75. 24	0. 60	0. 72	29. 01	
741	眉县 Mei Xian	304 700	564	307	56. 74	0. 53	0. 54	11. 68	
742	陇县 Long Xian	273 297	506	346	97. 63	1. 19	0. 68	10. 04	
743	千阳县 Qianyang Xian	128 326	258	154	88. 76	0. 39	0. 60	-6. 31	Y
744	麟游县 Linyou Xian	87 821	182	91	63. 19	0. 00	0. 50	3. 51	
745	泾阳县 Jingyang Xian	528 117	1 100	696	63. 55	0. 09	0. 63	20. 51	Y
746	渭南市临渭区 Linwei Qu, Weinan Shi	744 429	1 586	1 061	63. 49	1. 39	0. 67	5. 52	Y
747	渭南市华州区 Huazhou Qu,Weinan Shi	327 904	685	490	54. 01	0. 29	0. 72	3. 01	Y
748	潼关县 Tongguan Xian	158 399	280	169	61. 43	1. 07	0. 60	3. 75	Y
749	大荔县 Dali Xian	701 100	1 559	940	65. 75	0. 00	0. 60	43. 72	Y
750	合阳县 Heyang Xian	441 200	732	452	59. 15	0. 27	0. 62	0. 58	
751	澄城县 Chengcheng Xian	391 535	660	433	79. 24	0. 00	0. 66	32. 53	
752	蒲城县 Pucheng Xian	752 792	1 423	1 077	76. 11	0. 56	0. 76	29. 32	
753	富平县 Fuping Xian	754 700	1 443	1 021	78. 86	0. 14	0. 71	10. 41	Y
754	华阴市 Huayin Shi	263 107	454	301	73. 35	0. 66	0. 66	0. 69	
755	延安市宝塔区 Baota Qu, Yan' an Shi	481 420	809	473	95. 80	0. 74	0. 58	49. 39	
756	富县 Fu Xian	159 298	320	135	77. 50	0. 31	0. 42	154. 93	
757	黄陵县 Huangling Xian	126 583	132	102	95. 45	0. 00	0. 77	-10. 14	
758	汉中市汉台区 Hantai Qu, Hanzhong Shi	541 426	1 325	687	66. 49	1. 74	0. 52	275. 71	Y
759	城固县 Chenggu Xian	557 070	1 038	680	79. 87	0. 48	0. 66	8. 49	Y
760	宁强县 Ningqiang Xian	326 273	969	392	50. 98	0. 00	0. 40	327. 72	
761	绥德县 Suide Xian	359 281	506	417	29. 84	1. 38	0. 82	12. 76	
762	安康市汉滨区 Hanbin Qu, Ankang Shi	978 469	1 845	1 118	80. 49	4. 01	0. 61	-2. 39	Y
763	汉阴县 Hanyin Xian	247 932	341	219	90. 62	0. 00	0. 64	-13. 45	
764	石泉县 Shiquan Xian	172 919	281	166	61. 92	0. 00	0. 59	—	
765	宁陕县 Ningshan Xian	71 138	173	130	89. 02	0. 58	0. 75	-11. 03	Y
766	紫阳县 Ziyang Xian	286 675	736	503	85. 19	0. 82	0. 68	1. 57	Y

续表

序号 No.	肿瘤登记处 Cancer registries	人口数 Population	发病数 New cases	死亡数 Deaths	MV%	DCO%	M/I	发病率变化 Change for CR %	接受 Accepted
767	镇坪县 Zhenping Xian	51 386	153	56	54. 90	0. 00	0. 37	—	
768	旬阳县 Xunyang Xian	460 219	835	544	76. 29	0. 00	0. 65	-23. 27	
769	商洛市商州区 Shangzhou Qu, Shangluo Shi	564 767	1 643	1 227	70. 36	0. 00	0. 75	37. 38	Y
770	镇安县 Zhen'an Xian	277 800	564	386	99. 29	0. 00	0. 68	17. 34	
771	兰州市城关区 Chengguan Qu, Lanzhou Shi	957 085	3 186	719	74. 20	1. 51	0. 23	30. 40	
772	兰州市七里河区 Qilihe Qu, Lanzhou Shi	575 122	1 488	288	69. 29	0. 00	0. 19	-9. 40	
773	兰州市西固区 Xigu Qu, Lanzhou Shi	323 935	1 116	587	54. 21	2. 78	0. 53	-5. 32	Y
774	兰州市安宁区 Anning Qu, Lanzhou Shi	190 305	485	75	78. 56	0. 21	0. 15	-10. 86	
775	兰州市红古区 Honggu Qu, Lanzhou Shi	144 298	303	56	79. 54	0. 00	0. 18	-14. 04	
776	白银市白银区 Baiyin Qu, Baiyin Shi	307 626	865	431	49. 83	1. 62	0. 50	—	Y
777	白银市平川区 Pingchuan Qu, Baiyin Shi	209 800	301	143	58. 47	9. 63	0. 48	—	
778	靖远县 Jingyuan Xian	457 375	927	411	35. 17	0. 00	0. 44	-3. 24	
779	景泰县 Jingtai Xian	239 576	622	417	69. 45	2. 41	0. 67	10. 61	Y
780	天水市秦州区 Qinzhou Qu, Tianshui Shi	660 600	1 073	50	95. 25	0. 19	0. 05	—	
781	天水市麦积区 Maiji Qu, Tianshui Shi	559 987	1 108	74	80. 96	0. 18	0. 07	70. 02	
782	武威市凉州区 Liangzhou Qu, Wuwei Shi	1 069 627	3 322	1 814	78. 09	0. 27	0. 55	0. 57	Y
783	民勤县 Minqin Xian	242 161	707	375	70. 01	0. 28	0. 53	—	Y
784	古浪县 Gulang Xian	388 803	1 024	115	65. 72	0. 00	0. 11	—	
785	天祝藏族自治县 Tianzhu Zangzu Zizhixian	179 100	538	183	66. 73	0. 56	0. 34	—	
786	张掖市甘州区 Ganzhou Qu, Zhangye Shi	517 685	1 494	824	71. 82	0. 27	0. 55	-5. 60	Y
787	高台县 Gaotai Xian	145 314	550	173	47. 27	15. 82	0. 31	—	
788	静宁县 Jingning Xian	484 219	1 493	863	71. 67	1. 00	0. 58	16. 69	Y
789	敦煌市 Dunhuang Shi	145 314	339	199	71. 09	0. 59	0. 59	-7. 94	Y
790	庆城县 Qingcheng Xian	268 841	543	244	34. 62	1. 10	0. 45	161. 62	

序号 No.	肿瘤登记处 Cancer registries	人口数 Population	发病数 New cases	死亡数 Deaths	MV%	DCO%	M/I	发病率变化 Change for CR %	接受 Accepted
791	临洮县 Lintao Xian	501 606	446	428	25. 11	26. 46	0. 96	-46. 22	
792	临潭县 Lintan Xian	139 854	216	152	80. 56	0. 00	0. 70	-39. 05	
793	西宁市 Xining Shi	976 802	2 778	1 321	71. 17	1. 08	0. 48	4. 58	Y
794	大通回族土族自治县 Datong Huizu Tuzu Zizhixian	466 698	691	369	68. 31	0. 58	0. 53	7. 81	
795	西宁市湟中县 Huangzhong Xian, Xining Shi	481 813	922	616	67. 68	0. 00	0. 67	5. 85	Y
796	海东市乐都区 Ledu Qu, Haidong Shi	288 436	585	370	48. 89	0. 00	0. 63	13. 27	Y
797	民和回族土族自治县 Minhe Huizu Tuzu Zizhixian	436 136	701	496	55. 06	0. 14	0. 71	22. 82	
798	互助土族自治县 Huzhu Tuzu Zizhixian	401 540	721	579	55. 89	0. 00	0. 80	5. 80	Y
799	循化撒拉族自治县 Xunhua Salarzu Zizhixian	161 611	302	242	92. 72	0. 00	0. 80	38. 47	Y
800	海南藏族自治州 Hainan Zangzu Zizhizhou	472 849	1 076	647	47. 68	0. 56	0. 60	19. 78	Y
801	银川市兴庆区 Xingqing Qu, Yinchuan Shi	745 635	1 960	675	82. 04	5. 10	0. 34	—	
802	银川市西夏区 Xixia Qu, Yinchuan Shi	361 936	853	364	52. 64	2. 81	0. 43	—	
803	银川市金凤区 Jinfeng Qu, Yinchuan Shi	310 619	790	331	76. 33	1. 01	0. 42	—	Y
804	贺兰县 Helan Xian	236 112	642	320	59. 97	3. 43	0. 50	17. 37	Y
805	石嘴山市大武口区 Dawukou Qu, Shizuishan Shi	259 775	807	484	79. 43	0. 50	0. 60	9. 63	Y
806	石嘴山市惠农区 Huinong Qu, Shizuishan Shi	172 226	584	344	69. 86	0. 68	0. 59	14. 88	Y
807	平罗县 Pingluo Xian	312 087	583	435	60. 72	0. 34	0. 75	5. 42	Y
808	青铜峡市 Qingtongxia Shi	288 512	607	346	76. 94	0. 49	0. 57	-12. 88	Y
809	固原市原州区 Yuanzhou Qu, Guyuan Shi	418 684	929	524	85. 47	8. 61	0. 56	—	Y
810	中卫市沙坡头区 Shapotou Qu, Zhongwei Shi	403 151	1 092	654	58. 52	0. 00	0. 60	—	
811	中宁县 Zhongning Xian	331 963	484	340	80. 58	1. 45	0. 70	-22. 01	
812	乌鲁木齐市天山区 Tianshan Qu, Urumqi Shi	471 876	1 524	758	74. 61	1. 51	0. 50	-4. 47	Y

续表

序号 No.	肿瘤登记处 Cancer registries	人口数 Population	发病数 New cases	死亡数 Deaths	MV%	DCO%	M/I	发病率变化 Change for CR %	接受 Accepted
813	乌鲁木齐市米东区 Midong Qu, Urumqi Shi	250 456	501	36	74. 85	2. 59	0. 07	-7. 05	
814	克拉玛依市 Karamay Shi	305 521	1 073	473	72. 32	1. 40	0. 44	21. 69	Y
815	第二师 Di'ershi	210 011	281	224	23. 84	1. 42	0. 80	27. 25	
816	库尔勒市 Korla Shi	458 067	228	0	84. 65	0. 88	0. 00	-67. 75	
817	和田市 Hotan Shi	421 582	211	49	89. 10	0. 00	0. 23	-26. 82	
818	和田县 Hotan Xian	351 898	104	57	85. 58	0. 00	0. 55	-44. 09	
819	第七师 Diqishi	134 488	380	224	76. 05	0. 00	0. 59	5. 54	Y
820	新源县 Xinyuan Xian	295 942	386	289	70. 21	0. 00	0. 75	-24. 90	
821	第八师 Dibashi	594 836	1 819	929	66. 36	3. 13	0. 51	1. 30	Y

4 本年报收录登记地区的选取与数据质量评价

4.1 年报收录登记地区的选取

国家癌症中心审核了 821 个登记地区提交的 2017 年登记资料，经质量控制，554 个肿瘤登记地区的数据被本年报收录，覆盖了全国 31 个省（自治区、直辖市）及新疆生产建设兵团（未包括香港、澳门特别行政区、台湾省）。该数据作为全国肿瘤登记地区样本数据，用于分析中国癌症的发病与死亡。

4.2 全国登记地区数据质量评价指标

554 个肿瘤登记地区合计病理诊断比例为 67. 77%，只有死亡医学证明书比例为 1. 53%，死亡/发病比为 0. 59；全国城市登记地区合计病理诊断比例为 69. 97%，只有死亡医学证明书比例为 1. 62%，死亡/发病比为 0. 56；全国农村登记地区合计病理诊断比例为 65. 47 %，只有死亡医学证明书比例为 1. 44%，死亡/发病比为 0. 62（表 3-3）。

4 Coverage and data quality of cancer registries in this annual report

4.1 Coverage of cancer registries in this annual report

Among 821 cancer registries which provided cancer data to NCC, 554 cancer registries'data were included in this annual report, covering all 31 provinces (autonomous regions and municipalities) and Xinjiang Production and Construction Corps in China (data of Hong Kong SAR, Macao SAR and Taiwan Province is not included). The qualified data were included in the final database for further analysis.

4.2 Evaluation of data quality

Among the 554 cancer registries, the MV%, DCO%, M/I was 67. 77%, 1. 53% and 0. 59, respectively. In urban cancer registries, the MV%, DCO% and M/I was 69. 97%, 1. 62% and 0. 56, respectively. In rural cancer registries, the MV%, DCO% and M/I was 65. 47%, 1. 44% and 0. 62, respectively (Table 3-3).

表 3-3 中国肿瘤登记地区合计数据质量评价

Table 3-3 Quality indicators of the qualified national cancer registries

部位 Site	ICD-10 编码范围	全国合计 All			城市 Urban			农村 Rural		
		MV%	DCO%	M/I	MV%	DCO%	M/I	MV%	DCO%	M/I
口腔和咽喉(除外鼻咽癌)Oral cavity & pharynx but nasopharynx	C00-C10, C12-C14	74. 74	1. 11	0. 54	77. 36	1. 20	0. 53	71. 75	1. 01	0. 55
鼻咽癌 Nasopharynx	C11	72. 45	1. 29	0. 50	72. 95	1. 48	0. 50	72. 00	1. 11	0. 49
食管 Esophagus	C15	72. 54	1. 47	0. 75	71. 92	1. 78	0. 76	72. 92	1. 28	0. 75
胃 Stomach	C16	73. 25	1. 92	0. 72	73. 48	1. 95	0. 68	73. 07	1. 89	0. 75
结直肠肛门 Colon, rectum & anus	C18-C21	77. 10	1. 06	0. 47	78. 35	1. 17	0. 47	75. 47	0. 92	0. 48
肝脏 Liver	C22	42. 09	2. 75	0. 86	41. 71	3. 10	0. 86	42. 40	2. 47	0. 86
胆囊及其他 Gallbladder etc.	C23-C24	49. 71	1. 69	0. 73	50. 31	1. 91	0. 73	48. 99	1. 42	0. 72
胰腺 Pancreas	C25	42. 53	2. 20	0. 87	43. 03	2. 44	0. 89	41. 92	1. 92	0. 85
喉 Larynx	C32	72. 66	1. 46	0. 58	75. 76	1. 44	0. 55	68. 84	1. 48	0. 63
气管,支气管,肺 Trachea, bronchus & lung	C33-C34	58. 67	1. 89	0. 76	61. 18	2. 04	0. 75	56. 17	1. 75	0. 78
其他胸腔器官 Other thoracic organs	C37-C38	57. 64	1. 05	0. 68	60. 85	1. 29	0. 68	53. 67	0. 75	0. 68
骨 Bone	C40-C41	45. 54	2. 36	0. 70	46. 90	2. 88	0. 70	44. 50	1. 97	0. 70
皮肤黑色素瘤 Melanoma of skin	C43	93. 69	0. 55	0. 72	92. 66	0. 59	0. 67	94. 87	0. 50	0. 78
乳房 Breast	C50	84. 56	0. 49	0. 22	86. 25	0. 52	0. 21	82. 25	0. 44	0. 24
子宫颈 Cervix uteri	C53	82. 90	0. 76	0. 31	83. 77	0. 75	0. 29	82. 15	0. 78	0. 33
子宫体及子宫部位不明 Uterus & unspecified	C54-C55	81. 07	0. 63	0. 24	83. 80	0. 63	0. 22	78. 22	0. 62	0. 26
卵巢 Ovary	C56	75. 58	0. 94	0. 44	76. 60	1. 32	0. 47	74. 39	0. 49	0. 41
前列腺 Prostate	C61	70. 33	0. 94	0. 41	73. 24	0. 97	0. 39	65. 33	0. 89	0. 44
睾丸 Testis	C62	73. 21	0. 86	0. 27	76. 18	1. 00	0. 24	69. 62	0. 69	0. 31
肾及泌尿系统不明 Kidney & unspecified urinary organs	C64-C66, C68	71. 89	0. 93	0. 36	74. 03	1. 03	0. 35	68. 18	0. 77	0. 37
膀胱 Bladder	C67	74. 23	1. 15	0. 41	76. 23	1. 30	0. 40	71. 56	0. 95	0. 43
脑,神经系统 Brain & central nervous system	C70-C72	48. 78	1. 94	0. 50	52. 85	2. 08	0. 46	44. 85	1. 81	0. 53
甲状腺 Thyroid gland	C73	89. 88	0. 25	0. 04	92. 04	0. 32	0. 04	85. 62	0. 12	0. 06
淋巴瘤 Lymphoma	C81-85, C88, C90,C96	93. 79	0. 77	0. 55	93. 28	0. 86	0. 53	94. 42	0. 66	0. 56
白血病 Leukemia	C91-C95	93. 27	0. 98	0. 57	92. 56	1. 15	0. 55	94. 03	0. 80	0. 60
不明及其他癌症 Other and unspectified	O&U	61. 53	2. 19	0. 52	63. 53	2. 50	0. 52	59. 18	1. 83	0. 53
所有部位合计 All sites	C00-96, D32-33, D42-43, D45-47	67. 77	1. 53	0. 59	69. 97	1. 62	0. 56	65. 47	1. 44	0. 62

第四章 2017年中国肿瘤登记地区癌症发病与死亡

本年报收录的肿瘤登记处覆盖人口436 336 955人,占2017年中国总人口(1 400 110 000)的31.16%。本年报收录的数据反映了目前我国癌症的发病和死亡情况,为我国的癌症防治与研究提供了基础数据。

1 中国肿瘤登记地区覆盖人口

2017年纳入年报的中国肿瘤登记地区覆盖人口436 336 955人(男性221 134 960人,女性215 201 995人),占全国2017年末人口数的31.16%。其中城市人口213 246 283人(男性107 014 376人,女性106 231 907人),占全国登记地区人口的48.87%;农村人口223 090 672人(男性114 120 584,女性108 970 088人),占全国登记地区人口的51.13 %(表4-1a,图4-1)。

东部登记地区覆盖人口197 913 056人(男性99 508 519人,女性98 404 537人),占全国登记地区人口的45.36 %;中部登记地区覆盖人口115 080 139人(男性58 819 171人,女性56 260 968人),占全国登记地区人口的26.37%;西部登记地区覆盖人口123 343 760人(男性62 807 270人,女性60 536 490人),占全国登记地区人口的28.27%(表4-1b,图4-1)。

Chapter 4 Cancer incidence and mortality in the registration areas of China, 2017

In this annual report, a total of 436 336 955 people were covered in the registration system in China, accounting for 31.16% of the total population (1 400 110 000) in China in 2017. This annual report represented the current status of cancer incidence and mortality rates in China and provided the basic data for cancer prevention and control.

1 Population coverage in cancer registration areas of China

The population covered by cancer registration areas included in the annual report in 2017 was 436 336 955 (221 134 960 males and 215 201 995 females), which accounted for 31.16% of the total population at the end of 2017. There were 213 246 283 people in urban areas (107 014 376 males and 106 231 907 females) and 223 090 672 people in the rural areas (114 120 584 males and 108 970 088 females), accounting for 48.87% and 51.13% of the covered population in all cancer registration areas, respectively (Table 4-1a, Figure 4-1).

The population covered by cancer registration in eastern areas was 197 913 056 (99 508 519 males and 98 404 537 females), which accounted for 45.36% of the covered population in all cancer registration areas. The population covered by the cancer registration in the central areas was 115 080 139 (58 819 171 males and 56 260 968 females), which accounted for 26.37% of the population in all cancer registration areas. The population covered by the cancer registration in western areas was 123 343 760 (62 807 270 males and 60 536 490 females), which accounted for 28.27% of the population in all cancer registration areas (Table 4-1b, Figure 4-1).

表 4-1a 2017 年中国肿瘤登记地区覆盖人口

Table 4-1a Population in all cancer registration areas of China, 2017

年龄组/岁 Age group/ years	全国 All areas			城市地区 Urban areas			农村地区 Rural areas		
	合计 All	男性 Male	女性 Female	合计 All	男性 Male	女性 Female	合计 All	男性 Male	女性 Female
Total	436 336 955	221 134 960	215 201 995	213 246 283	107 014 376	106 231 907	223 090 672	114 120 584	108 970 088
0~	4 653 648	2 465 356	2 188 292	2 253 504	1 185 888	1 067 616	2 400 144	1 279 468	1 120 676
1~	19 735 402	10 544 615	9 190 787	9 354 770	4 947 284	4 407 486	10 380 632	5 597 331	4 783 301
5~	24 034 832	12 744 732	11 290 100	10 924 785	5 773 347	5 151 438	13 110 047	6 971 385	6 138 662
10~	21 588 488	11 546 149	10 042 339	9 467 325	5 021 749	4 445 576	12 121 163	6 524 400	5 596 763
15~	23 266 394	12 216 721	11 049 673	10 298 582	5 355 681	4 942 901	12 967 812	6 861 040	6 106 772
20~	29 014 896	14 815 642	14 199 254	13 439 991	6 848 472	6 591 519	15 574 905	7 967 170	7 607 735
25~	33 333 111	16 839 085	16 494 026	16 221 263	8 064 002	8 157 261	17 111 848	8 775 083	8 336 765
30~	31 957 806	16 005 637	15 952 169	16 663 399	8 213 210	8 450 189	15 294 407	7 792 427	7 501 980
35~	33 496 246	16 837 620	16 658 626	17 135 841	8 493 079	8 642 762	16 360 405	8 344 541	8 015 864
40~	35 065 408	17 691 143	17 374 265	17 062 350	8 514 801	8 547 549	18 003 058	9 176 342	8 826 716
45~	39 300 205	19 764 144	19 536 061	19 186 102	9 605 967	9 580 135	20 114 103	10 158 177	9 955 926
50~	32 891 678	16 694 834	16 196 844	16 323 797	8 273 165	8 050 632	16 567 881	8 421 669	8 146 212
55~	27 318 505	13 778 674	13 539 831	13 891 567	6 983 197	6 908 370	13 426 938	6 795 477	6 631 461
60~	26 394 347	13 250 102	13 144 245	13 531 239	6 725 573	6 805 666	12 863 108	6 524 529	6 338 579
65~	19 479 486	9 698 625	9 780 861	9 734 324	4 802 175	4 932 149	9 745 162	4 896 450	4 848 712
70~	13 536 013	6 654 237	6 881 776	6 650 361	3 225 767	3 424 594	6 885 652	3 428 470	3 457 182
75~	9 963 871	4 725 730	5 238 141	5 032 828	2 352 833	2 679 995	4 931 043	2 372 897	2 558 146
80~	6 726 575	3 027 487	3 699 088	3 554 380	1 597 447	1 956 933	3 172 195	1 430 040	1 742 155
85+	4 580 044	1 834 427	2 745 617	2 519 875	1 030 739	1 489 136	2 060 169	803 688	1 256 481

表 4-1b 2017 年中国肿瘤登记地区东、中、西部地区覆盖人口

Table 4-1b Population in eastern, central and western areas in cancer registration areas of China, 2017

年龄组/岁 Age group/years	东部地区 Eastern areas			中部地区 Central areas			西部地区 Western areas		
	合计 All	男性 Male	女性 Female	合计 All	男性 Male	女性 Female	合计 All	男性 Male	女性 Female
合计	197 913 056	99 508 519	98 404 537	115 080 139	58 819 171	56 260 968	123 343 760	62 807 270	60 536 490
0~	2 174 751	1 147 428	1 027 323	1 248 851	667 439	581 412	1 230 046	650 489	579 557
1~	9 044 722	4 809 743	4 234 979	5 564 809	3 018 665	2 546 144	5 125 871	2 716 207	2 409 664
5~	10 365 793	5 513 220	4 852 573	7 070 860	3 771 422	3 299 438	6 598 179	3 460 090	3 138 089
10~	8 583 881	4 578 657	4 005 224	6 352 370	3 443 477	2 908 893	6 652 237	3 524 015	3 128 222
15~	8 595 522	4 522 483	4 073 039	6 592 264	3 502 489	3 089 775	8 078 608	4 191 749	3 886 859
20~	11 375 320	5 871 999	5 503 321	8 224 511	4 204 980	4 019 531	9 415 065	4 738 663	4 676 402
25~	15 685 416	7 913 847	7 771 569	9 136 146	4 619 400	4 516 746	8 511 549	4 305 838	4 205 711
30~	15 601 862	7 728 572	7 873 290	8 669 426	4 375 721	4 293 705	7 686 518	3 901 344	3 785 174
35~	14 744 845	7 321 648	7 423 197	8 965 461	4 549 704	4 415 757	9 785 940	4 966 268	4 819 672
40~	14 279 717	7 103 875	7 175 842	9 665 339	4 919 355	4 745 984	11 120 352	5 667 913	5 452 439
45~	17 151 584	8 561 926	8 589 658	10 149 497	5 131 145	5 018 352	11 999 124	6 071 073	5 928 051
50~	16 484 416	8 301 148	8 183 268	8 030 544	4 083 469	3 947 075	8 376 718	4 310 217	4 066 501
55~	12 976 908	6 537 978	6 438 930	6 793 975	3 446 714	3 347 261	7 547 622	3 793 982	3 753 640
60~	13 666 922	6 805 879	6 861 043	6 008 665	3 030 540	2 978 125	6 718 760	3 413 683	3 305 077
65~	9 742 852	4 807 475	4 935 377	4 486 601	2 244 783	2 241 818	5 250 033	2 646 367	2 603 666
70~	6 487 159	3 148 577	3 338 582	3 210 934	1 589 198	1 621 736	3 837 920	1 916 462	1 921 458
75~	4 800 884	2 249 771	2 551 113	2 447 438	1 158 269	1 289 169	2 715 549	1 317 690	1 397 859
80~	3 545 615	1 564 758	1 980 857	1 504 677	679 017	825 660	1 676 283	783 712	892 571
85+	2 604 887	1 019 535	1 585 352	957 771	383 384	574 387	1 017 386	431 508	585 878

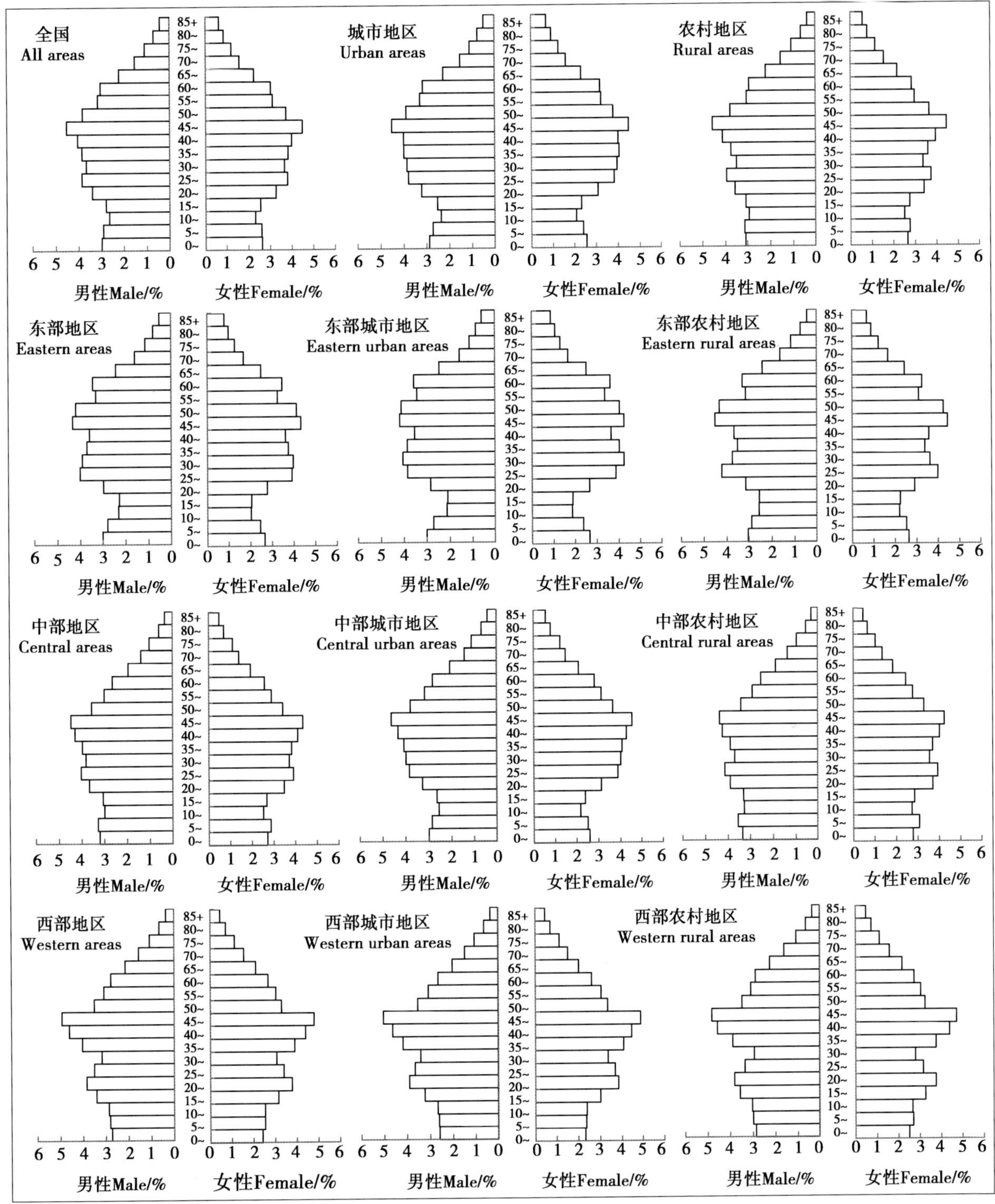

图 4-1　中国肿瘤登记地区人口金字塔

Figure 4-1　Population pyramid in cancer registration areas of China

2 中国肿瘤登记地区全部癌症发病与死亡

2.1 中国肿瘤登记地区全部癌症发病情况

2017年中国肿瘤登记地区新发病例数1 281 357例(男性711 618例,女性569 739例),其中城市地区的新发病例数674 037例,占52.60%,农村地区607 320例,占47.40%。东部地区660 824例,占新发病例数的51.57%;中部地区301 319例,占新发病例数的23.52%;西部地区319 214例,占新发病例数的24.91%(表4-2)。

中国肿瘤登记地区发病率为293.66/10万(男性321.80/10万,女性264.75/10万),中标率188.10/10万,世标率183.68/10万,累积率(0~74岁)为21.07%。城市地区发病率为316.08/10万(男性341.22/10万,女性290.77/10万),中标率196.53/10万,世标率191.54/10万,累积率(0~74岁)为21.82%。农村地区发病率为272.23/10万(男性303.60/10万,女性239.38/10万),中标率179.48/10万,世标率175.66/10万,累积率(0~74岁)为20.32%。城市与农村相比,城市男女的发病率、中标率、世标率、累积率均高于农村地区男女相应的指标(表4-2)。

东部地区发病率为333.90/10万(男性358.05/10万,女性309.47/10万),中标率200.01/10万,世标率194.36/10万,累积率(0~74岁)为22.16%。中部地区发病率为261.83/10万(男性284.08/10万,女性238.58/10万),中标率183.32/10万,世标率179.69/10万,累积率(0~74岁)为20.82%。西部地区发病率为258.80/10万(男性299.70/10万,女性216.37/10万),中标率173.15/10万,世标率170.02/10万,累积率(0~74岁)为19.54%。东中西部地区相比,东部地区的男性和女性发病率、中标率、世标率和累积率均高于中部和西部地区。西部地区的女性发病率、中标率、世标率和累积率均低于东部和中部地区(表4-2)。

2 Incidence and mortality for all cancer sites in the registration areas of China

2.1 Incidence for all cancer sites in the registration areas of China

In 2017, there were 1 281 357 new cases (711 618 males and 569 739 females) in cancer registration areas of China. Among all the new cases, 674 037 (52.60%) came from urban areas, and 607 320 (47.40%) were from rural areas. There were 660 824 (51.57%) cases in eastern areas, 301 319 (23.52%) cases in the central areas, and 319 214 (24.91%) cases in western areas (Table 4-2).

The incidence rate for all cancer sites was 293.66 per 100 000 in 2017 (321.80 per 100 000 in males, and 264.75 per 100 000 in females). The ASR China was 188.10 per 100 000, and the ASR World was 183.68 per 100 000. The cumulative rate (0-74 years old) was 21.07%. The incidence rate in the urban areas was 316.08 per 100 000 in 2017 (341.22 per 100 000 in males and 290.77 per 100 000 in females). The ASR China was 196.53 per 100 000, and the ASR world was 191.54 per 100 000. The cumulative rate (0-74 years old) was 21.82%. The incidence rate in the rural areas was 272.23 per 100 000 (303.60 per 100 000 in males and 239.38 per 100 000 in females). The ASR China was 179.48 per 100 000, and the ASR world was 175.66 per 100 000. The cumulative rate (0-74 years old) was 20.32%. The incidence rate, ASR China, ASR World, and the cumulative rate of all cancer sites were higher in the urban areas than those in the rural areas for both sexes (Table 4-2).

The incidence rate in eastern areas was 333.90 per 100 000 (358.05 per 100 000 in males and 309.47 per 100 000 in females). The ASR China was 200.01 per 100 000, and the ASR world was 194.36 per 100 000. The cumulative rate (0-74 years old) was 22.16%. The incidence rate in the central areas was 261.83 per 100 000 in 2017 (284.08 per 100 000 in males and 238.58 per 100 000 in females). The ASR China was 183.32 per 100 000, and the ASR World was 179.69 per 100 000. The cumulative rate (0-74 years old) was 20.82%. The incidence rate in western areas was 258.80 per 100 000 (299.70 per 100 000 in males and 216.37 per 100 000 in females). The ASR China was 173.15 per 100 000, and the ASR World was 170.02 per 100 000. The cumulative rate (0-74 years old) was 19.54%. The incidence rate, ASR China, ASR World, and the cumulative rate of both males and females in eastern areas were higher than those in central and western areas. The incidence rate, ASR China, ASR World, and cumulative rate for females in western areas were lower than those in eastern and central areas (Table 4-2).

表 4-2 2017 年中国肿瘤登记地区全部癌症发病情况

Table 4-2 Incidence rate for all cancer sites in the registration areas of China,2017

地区 Area	性别 Sex	病例数 No. cases	发病率 Incidence rate/ 100 000^{-1}	中标率 ASR China/ 100 000^{-1}	世标率 ASR World/ 100 000^{-1}	累积率 Cum. rate 0~74/%
全国 All areas	合计 Both	1 281 357	293. 66	188. 10	183. 68	21. 07
	男性 Male	711 618	321. 80	206. 07	204. 34	24. 06
	女性 Female	569 739	264. 75	172. 02	164. 93	18. 15
城市地区 Urban areas	合计 Both	674 037	316. 08	196. 53	191. 54	21. 82
	男性 Male	365 150	341. 22	210. 69	208. 81	24. 47
	女性 Female	308 887	290. 77	184. 56	176. 50	19. 30
农村地区 Rural areas	合计 Both	607 320	272. 23	179. 48	175. 66	20. 32
	男性 Male	346 468	303. 60	201. 30	199. 70	23. 66
	女性 Female	260 852	239. 38	159. 11	153. 05	16. 97
东部地区 Eastern areas	合计 Both	660 824	333. 90	200. 01	194. 36	22. 16
	男性 Male	356 294	358. 05	212. 27	209. 88	24. 64
	女性 Female	304 530	309. 47	190. 07	181. 20	19. 80
中部地区 Central areas	合计 Both	301 319	261. 83	183. 32	179. 69	20. 82
	男性 Male	167 092	284. 08	201. 51	200. 37	23. 85
	女性 Female	134 227	238. 58	166. 94	160. 78	17. 82
西部地区 Western areas	合计 Both	319 214	258. 80	173. 15	170. 02	19. 54
	男性 Male	188 232	299. 70	200. 42	199. 25	23. 37
	女性 Female	130 982	216. 37	146. 66	141. 56	15. 66

2. 2 中国肿瘤登记地区全部癌症年龄别发病率

2017 年中国肿瘤登记地区全部癌症的年龄别发病率在 0~29 岁时处于较低水平,30~34 岁年龄组发病率快速上升,为 62. 72/10 万,80~84 岁年龄组发病率处于最高水平,为 1 465. 77/10 万,85 岁及以上年龄组的发病率有所下降,为 1 313. 11/10 万。城市和农村地区的癌症年龄别发病率变化模式基本相同。除 5~9 岁年龄组农村发病率略高于城市以外,城市发病率均高于农村。城市男性癌症发病率在 5~14、45~54 和 65~69 岁年龄组的发病率低于农村,其他年龄组高于农村;城市女性各年龄组癌症发病率均高于农村(表 4-3a,图 4-2)。

东部、中部和西部地区的年龄别发病率均在 80~84 岁年龄组达到最高,85 岁及以上年龄组时有所下降。除少数几个年龄组外,东部地区男女性年龄组发病率均高于中部和西部地区。三个区域的城市癌症发病率均高于农村,分城乡、分性别的年龄别发病率曲线基本类似(表 4-3b,图 4-2)。

2. 2 Age-specific incidence rates for all cancer sites in the registration areas of China

In 2017, incidence rate for all cancer sites was relatively low in the age group of 0-29 years, and dramatically increased from age group 30-34 years old (62. 72 per 100 100), and reached the peak at the age of 80-84 years old (1 465. 77 per 100 000) and then decreased slightly after 85 years old (1 313. 11 per 100 000). The overall trends of the age-specific incidence in urban areas were similar as that in rural areas. The incidence rate in urban areas was higher than that in rural areas except the age group of 5-9. The incidence rates for males in urban areas were lower than those in rural areas in the age group of 5-14, 45-54 and 65-69, and higher in other age groups, and the incidence rates for females were higher in urban areas than those in rural areas across all age groups (Table 4-3a, Figure 4-2).

The age-specific incidence rates in eastern, central and western areas reached peak at the age group of 80-84 years old, and declined after 85-year-old. Overall, the incidence rates in eastern areas were higher than those in central and western areas for both sexes. The incidence rates in urban areas were higher than those in rural areas in the all three geographic areas and the age-specific incidence curves by urban and rural areas and by sex are basically similar (Table 4-3b, Figure 4-2).

表 4-3a　2017 年中国肿瘤登记地区癌症年龄别发病率

Table 4-3a　Age-specific incidence rates for all cancer sites in the registration areas of China, 2017

单位：100 000⁻¹

年龄组/岁 Age group/years	全国 All areas			城市地区 Urban areas			农村地区 Rural areas		
	合计 All	男性 Male	女性 Female	合计 All	男性 Male	女性 Female	合计 All	男性 Male	女性 Female
合计	293.66	321.80	264.75	316.08	341.22	290.77	272.23	303.60	239.38
0~	14.76	14.97	14.53	17.08	17.54	16.58	12.58	12.58	12.58
1~	11.44	12.68	10.01	12.19	13.46	10.75	10.76	11.99	9.32
5~	7.94	8.59	7.21	7.89	8.21	7.53	7.99	8.91	6.94
10~	9.16	10.17	8.00	9.33	10.14	8.41	9.03	10.19	7.67
15~	11.35	11.70	10.96	11.86	12.29	11.39	10.94	11.24	10.61
20~	17.72	14.24	21.35	19.58	15.67	23.64	16.12	13.02	19.36
25~	38.21	28.30	48.34	43.02	31.42	54.48	33.66	25.42	42.33
30~	62.72	45.55	79.95	70.78	49.63	91.34	53.95	41.26	67.13
35~	88.19	62.00	114.66	98.10	66.43	129.23	77.80	57.50	98.94
40~	147.78	109.53	186.72	159.21	112.96	205.29	136.94	106.35	168.75
45~	235.99	191.75	280.75	243.16	187.24	299.22	229.16	196.01	262.98
50~	403.66	383.11	424.84	415.05	381.73	449.29	392.43	384.47	400.66
55~	433.43	477.67	388.41	472.35	510.08	434.21	393.16	444.35	340.69
60~	713.41	858.26	567.40	733.41	867.20	601.20	692.37	849.04	531.10
65~	920.62	1 162.71	680.57	930.97	1 162.45	705.60	910.29	1 162.97	655.12
70~	1 112.03	1 435.54	799.21	1 135.76	1 463.71	826.84	1 089.11	1 409.03	771.84
75~	1 322.67	1 730.51	954.73	1 364.38	1 770.08	1 008.21	1 280.09	1 691.27	898.70
80~	1 465.77	1 913.60	1 099.24	1 543.03	1 998.19	1 171.48	1 379.20	1 819.11	1 018.11
85+	1 313.11	1 789.88	994.57	1 398.40	1 899.12	1 051.82	1 208.78	1 649.77	926.72

表 4-3b　2017 年中国不同肿瘤登记地区癌症年龄别发病率

Table 4-3b　Age-specific incidence rates for all cancer sites in different registration areas of China, 2017

单位:100 000^{-1}

年龄组/岁 Age group/ years	东部地区 Eastern areas			中部地区 Central areas			西部地区 Western areas		
	合计 All	男性 Male	女性 Female	合计 All	男性 Male	女性 Female	合计 All	男性 Male	女性 Female
合计	333.90	358.05	309.47	261.83	284.08	238.58	258.80	299.70	216.37
0~	18.62	20.48	16.55	11.05	8.69	13.76	11.71	11.68	11.73
1~	12.55	13.91	11.00	10.64	11.93	9.11	10.34	11.34	9.21
5~	8.31	8.78	7.77	7.92	8.94	6.76	7.40	7.92	6.82
10~	9.58	10.31	8.74	9.54	10.77	8.08	8.25	9.39	6.97
15~	13.09	13.16	13.01	10.57	10.56	10.58	10.13	11.07	9.11
20~	21.93	17.08	27.11	15.88	12.51	19.41	14.23	12.26	16.23
25~	43.71	31.17	56.48	35.58	25.63	45.76	30.91	25.87	36.07
30~	72.23	49.54	94.51	52.99	38.26	68.01	54.39	45.83	63.22
35~	108.09	71.83	143.86	78.40	54.27	103.27	67.17	54.61	80.11
40~	168.08	113.99	221.62	132.55	98.08	168.27	134.95	113.87	156.87
45~	253.70	192.05	315.16	232.12	184.89	280.41	213.95	197.12	231.19
50~	391.07	354.70	427.97	408.58	382.66	435.39	423.71	438.26	408.29
55~	503.18	534.74	471.13	392.69	429.74	354.53	350.18	422.85	276.72
60~	719.91	846.08	594.75	710.92	854.30	565.02	702.42	886.05	512.76
65~	939.23	1 168.62	715.79	962.89	1 221.05	704.38	849.98	1 102.49	593.32
70~	1 165.98	1 501.19	849.85	1 101.86	1 426.88	783.36	1 029.33	1 334.86	724.61
75~	1 412.14	1 838.63	1 036.02	1 270.55	1 671.11	910.66	1 211.47	1 598.10	847.01
80~	1 539.99	2 006.64	1 171.36	1 464.04	1 917.48	1 091.13	1 310.34	1 724.49	946.70
85+	1 332.34	1 818.57	1 019.65	1 280.37	1 732.21	978.78	1 294.69	1 773.32	942.18

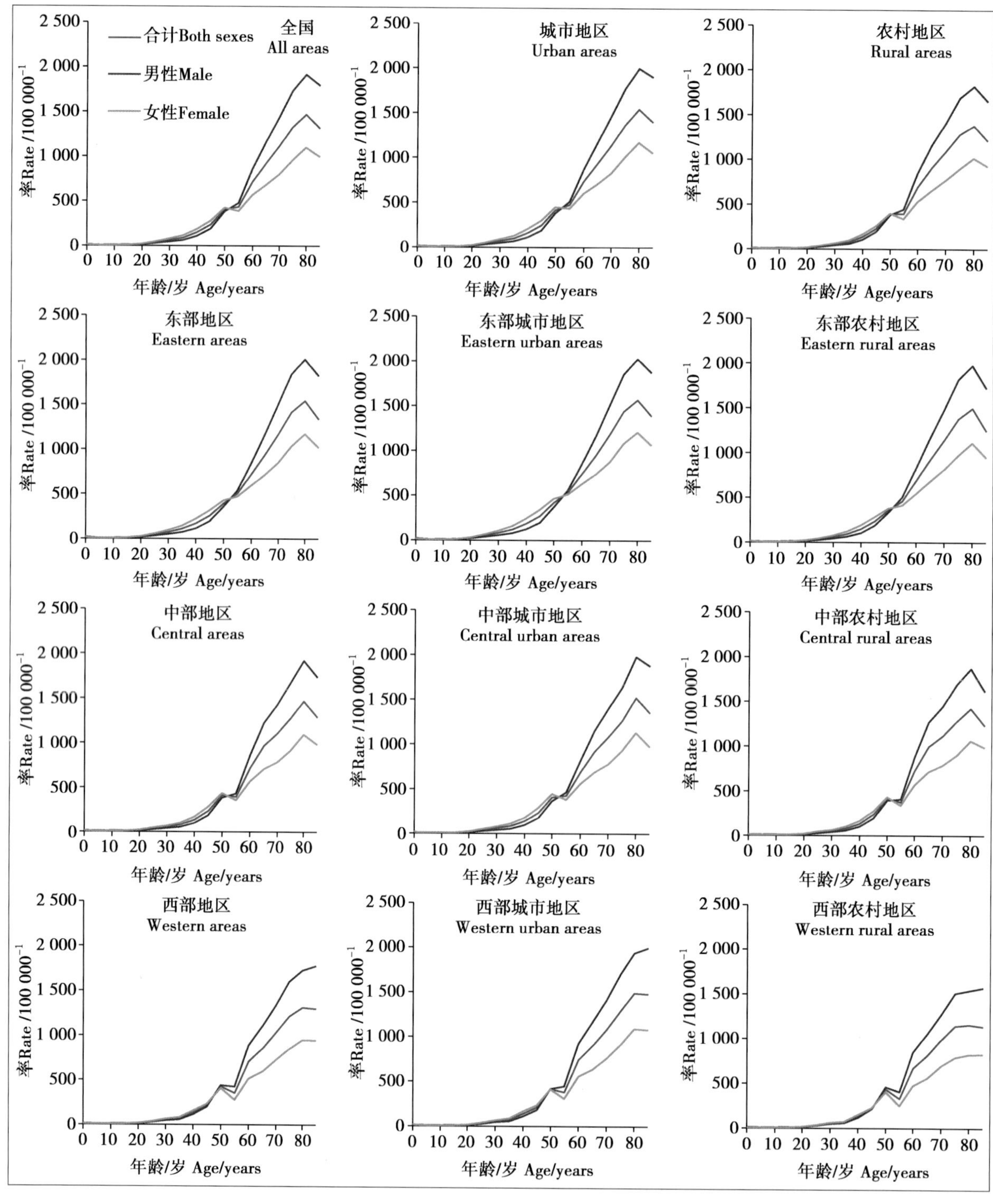

图 4-2 2017 年中国肿瘤登记地区癌症年龄别发病率

Figure 4-2 Age-specific incidence rates for all cancer sites in the registration areas of China,2017

2.3 中国肿瘤登记地区全部癌症死亡情况

2017年中国肿瘤登记地区报告癌症死亡772 968例(男性494 330例,女性278 638例),其中城市地区386 265例,占全国癌症死亡的49.97%,农村地区386 703例,占全国癌症死亡的50.03%。东部地区382 166例,占全国癌症死亡的49.44%;中部地区187 718例,占全国癌症死亡的24.29%;西部地区203 084例,占全国癌症死亡的26.27%(表4-4)。

中国肿瘤登记地区2017年癌症死亡率为177.15/10万(男性223.54/10万,女性129.48/10万),中标率104.20/10万,世标率103.47/10万,累积率(0~74岁)为11.65%。城市地区死亡率为181.14/10万(男性229.00/10万,女性132.92/10万),中标率101.43/10万,世标率100.74/10万,累积率(0~74岁)为11.19%。农村地区死亡率为173.34/10万(男性218.42/10万,女性126.12/10万),中标率106.86/10万,世标率106.05/10万,累积率(0~74岁)为12.11%。城市与农村相比,城市地区男性和女性死亡率均高于农村,而城市男性和女性的中标率、世标率和累积率均低于农村(表4-4)。

东部、中部和西部地区死亡率分别为193.10/10万(男性242.00/10万,女性143.65/10万)、163.12万(男性203.63/10万,女性120.77/10万)和164.65/10万(男性212.95/10万,女性114.53/10万)。东部地区的中标率为102.34/10万、中部地区107.47/10万、西部地区104.65/10万。东部地区的世标率为101.36/10万、中部地区106.76/10万、西部地区104.39/10万。东部、中部和西部地区累积率(0~74岁)分别为11.33%、12.20%和11.82%。东部地区男女的死亡率均高于中部和西部,男女合计的中标率、世标率和累积率均低于中部和西部地区(表4-4)。

2.3 Mortality for all cancer sites in the registration areas of China

In 2017, there were 772 968 cancer deaths (494 330 males and 278 638 females) in the registration areas of China. Among those, 386 265 (49.97%) came from urban areas, and 386 703 (50.03%) came from rural areas. There were 382166 (49.44%) death cases in eastern areas, 187 718 (24.29%) in central areas and 203 084 (26.27%) in western areas (Table 4-4).

The mortality rate of all cancer sites was 177.15 per 100 000 in 2017 (223.54 per 100 000 in males and 129.48 per 100 000 in females). The ASR China was 104.20 per 100 000, and the ASR World was 103.47 per 100 000. The cumulative rate (0-74 years old) was 11.65%. The mortality for all cancer sites in urban areas was 181.14 per 100 000 (229.00 per 100 000 in males and 132.92 per 100 000 in females). The ASR China was 101.43 per 100 000, and the ASR World was 100.74 per 100 000. The cumulative rate (0-74 years old) was 11.19%. The mortality for all cancer sites in rural areas was 173.34 per 100 000 in 2017 (218.42 per 100 000 in males and 126.12 per 100 000 in females). The ASR China was 106.86 per 100 000, and the ASR World was 106.05 per 100 000. The cumulative rate (0-74 years old) was 12.11%. The mortality rates for all cancer sites in urban areas were higher than those in rural areas for both sexes. The ASR China, ASR World and cumulative rates of all cancer sites were lower in urban areas than those in rural areas for both sexes (Table 4-4).

The mortality rates for all cancer sites in eastern, central and western areas were 193.10 per 100 000 (242.00 per 100 000 in males and 143.65 per 100 000 in females), 163.12 per 100 000 (203.63 per 100 000 in males and 120.77 per 100 000 in females), and 164.65 per 100 000 (212.95 per 100 000 in males and 114.53 per 100 000 in females), respectively. The ASR China were 102.34 per 100 000 in eastern areas, 107.47 per 100 000 in central areas, and 104.65 per 100 000 in western areas, respectively. The ASR World were 101.36 per 100 000 in eastern areas, 106.76 per 100 000 in central areas, and 104.39 per 100 000 in western areas. The cumulative rates (0-74 years old) in the eastern, central and western areas were 11.33%, 12.20% and 11.82%, respectively. The mortality rate for all cancer sites in eastern areas was higher than that in central and western areas for both sexes. The ASR China, ASR World and cumulative rates were the lowest in eastern areas for both sexes combined (Table 4-4).

表 4-4 2017 年中国肿瘤登记地区全部癌症死亡情况

Table 4-4 Mortality for all cancer sites in the registration areas of China,2017

地区 Area	性别 Sex	死亡数 No. deaths	粗率 Crude rate/ 100 000^{-1}	中标率 ASR China/ 100 000^{-1}	世标率 ASR World/ 100 000^{-1}	累积率 Cum. rate 0~74/%
全国 All areas	合计 Both	772 968	177. 15	104. 20	103. 47	11. 65
	男性 Male	494 330	223. 54	137. 23	136. 84	15. 54
	女性 Female	278 638	129. 48	72. 77	71. 77	7. 80
城市地区 Urban areas	合计 Both	386 265	181. 14	101. 43	100. 74	11. 19
	男性 Male	245 064	229. 00	133. 80	133. 59	15. 04
	女性 Female	141 201	132. 92	71. 14	70. 06	7. 46
	合计 Both	386 703	173. 34	106. 86	106. 05	12. 11
农村地区 Rural areas	男性 Male	249 266	218. 42	140. 43	139. 81	16. 03
	女性 Female	137 437	126. 12	74. 34	73. 44	8. 15
东部地区 Eastern areas	合计 Both	382 166	193. 10	102. 34	101. 36	11. 33
	男性 Male	240 808	242. 00	134. 66	134. 04	15. 12
	女性 Female	141 358	143. 65	72. 34	71. 08	7. 64
中部地区 Central areas	合计 Both	187 718	163. 12	107. 47	106. 76	12. 20
	男性 Male	119 773	203. 63	140. 41	140. 00	16. 10
	女性 Female	67 945	120. 77	75. 95	75. 01	8. 30
西部地区 Western areas	合计 Both	203 084	164. 65	104. 65	104. 39	11. 82
	男性 Male	133 749	212. 95	138. 97	139. 08	15. 87
	女性 Female	69 335	114. 53	70. 67	70. 14	7. 69

2. 4 中国肿瘤登记地区全部癌症年龄别死亡率

中国肿瘤登记地区癌症年龄别死亡率在 25~29 岁组为 8. 43/10 万(男性 9. 29/10 万,女性 7. 55/10 万),在 40~44 岁年龄组时达到 46. 07/10 万,在这以后死亡率随年龄增长而明显升高,在 85 岁以上年龄组达最高,死亡率为 1 462. 63/10 万。城乡年龄别死亡率的变化模式基本相似,城市地区和农村地区的癌症死亡率均在 85 岁及以上年龄组达到最高,死亡率分别为 1 549. 52/10 万和 1 356. 35/10 万。城市多数年龄组的死亡率低于农村(表 4-5a,图 4-3)。

东部、中部和西部地区的年龄别癌症死亡率曲线与全国的基本一致。东部、中部和西部地区男女年龄别死亡率均在 85 岁以后达到高峰,死亡率分别为 1 497. 45/10 万、1 437. 19/10 万和 1 397. 40/10 万。在 0~64 岁的各个组别中,西部多数年龄组的死亡率高于东部和中部,65~74 岁年龄组以中部最高,而 75 岁以上的年龄组以东部地区最高。三个区域的城市癌症死亡率均高于农村,城市与农村的年龄别死亡率曲线基本相似(表 4-5b,图 4-3)。

2. 4 Age-specific mortality rates for all cancer sites in the registration areas of China

The age-specific mortality rate for all cancer sites was 8. 43 per 100 000(9. 29 per 100 000 in males and 7. 55 per 100 000 in females) in the 25-29 age group and 46. 07 per 100 000 in the 40-44 age group. The mortality rate increased significantly after the age group of 40-44 years old and reached the peak in the 85+ age group, with a mortality rate of 1 462. 63/100 000. The trends of age-specific mortality in urban and rural areas were similar, the mortality rate in urban areas and rural areas reaches the highest in the age group of 85 years and above, with a mortality rate of 1 549. 52 per 100 000 and 1 356. 35 per 100 000, respectively. Most age groups had lower mortality rates in urban areas than in rural areas(Table 4-5a, Figure 4-3).

The trends of age-specific mortality rates in different areas(eastern areas, central areas, and western areas) were similar to those of the overall country. The age-specific mortality rates for both sexes in eastern, central and western areas reached peak after 85 years old, with mortality rates of 1 497. 45 per 100 000, 1 437. 19 per 100 000 and 1 397. 40 per 100 000, respectively. Most age groups in the age range of 0-64 had the highest mortality rate in western areas. The mortality rate was the highest in the central areas in the 65-74 age group, and it was the highest in eastern areas in above 75 years old age groups. The trends of the age-specific mortality rates were similar in urban and rural areas, although the rates in urban areas were generally higher than those in rural areas in all three geographic areas(Table 4-5b, Figure 4-3).

表 4-5a　2017 年中国肿瘤登记地区癌症年龄别死亡率

Table 4-5a　Age-specific mortality rates for all cancer sites in the registration areas of China,2017

单位：100 000^{-1}

年龄组/岁 Age group/years	全国 All areas			城市地区 Urban areas			农村地区 Rural areas		
	合计 All	男性 Male	女性 Female	合计 All	男性 Male	女性 Female	合计 All	男性 Male	女性 Female
合计	177.15	223.54	129.48	181.14	229.00	132.92	173.34	218.42	126.12
0~	11.52	12.45	10.46	5.99	5.99	5.99	16.71	18.45	14.72
1~	4.02	4.58	3.37	3.93	4.16	3.68	4.09	4.95	3.09
5~	3.22	3.73	2.65	3.08	3.78	2.31	3.34	3.70	2.93
10~	3.58	4.10	2.98	3.57	4.06	3.01	3.58	4.12	2.95
15~	4.23	5.19	3.18	4.03	4.80	3.20	4.40	5.49	3.16
20~	4.44	5.16	3.70	4.15	4.98	3.29	4.69	5.31	4.05
25~	8.43	9.29	7.55	7.54	8.31	6.78	9.27	10.19	8.31
30~	14.75	16.53	12.96	13.55	14.82	12.32	16.05	18.33	13.69
35~	22.75	25.27	20.21	20.99	22.57	19.43	24.60	28.02	21.05
40~	46.07	53.70	38.30	44.17	50.29	38.07	47.88	56.86	38.53
45~	86.40	103.66	68.94	80.29	94.85	65.69	92.23	112.00	72.07
50~	171.14	215.51	125.41	163.31	204.30	121.18	178.86	226.52	129.59
55~	211.55	283.56	138.27	213.75	289.24	137.44	209.27	277.73	139.12
60~	390.46	533.33	246.44	371.24	513.12	231.03	410.69	554.17	262.99
65~	573.15	783.00	365.06	546.09	752.49	345.12	600.17	812.92	385.34
70~	785.25	1 060.17	519.43	758.76	1 035.20	498.37	810.85	1 083.66	540.30
75~	1 078.32	1 443.84	748.55	1 072.58	1 427.64	760.86	1 084.17	1 459.90	735.65
80~	1 383.32	1 830.20	1 017.58	1 431.14	1 875.56	1 068.36	1 329.74	1 779.53	960.53
85+	1 462.63	2 011.36	1 096.00	1 549.52	2 122.75	1 152.75	1 356.35	1 868.51	1 028.75

表 4-5b 2017 年中国不同肿瘤登记地区癌症年龄别死亡率

Table 4-5b Age-specific mortality rates for all cancer sites in different registration areas of China,2017

单位:100 000⁻¹

年龄组/岁 Age group/ years	东部地区 Eastern areas			中部地区 Central areas			西部地区 Western areas		
	合计 All	男性 Male	女性 Female	合计 All	男性 Male	女性 Female	合计 All	男性 Male	女性 Female
合计	193.10	242.00	143.65	163.12	203.63	120.77	164.65	212.95	114.53
0~	6.16	6.97	5.26	4.40	3.90	4.99	28.21	30.90	25.19
1~	3.60	4.05	3.09	4.10	4.77	3.30	4.66	5.30	3.94
5~	3.24	3.90	2.49	3.31	3.71	2.85	3.11	3.50	2.68
10~	3.29	3.87	2.62	3.67	4.07	3.20	3.86	4.43	3.23
15~	4.05	4.89	3.12	4.02	4.80	3.14	4.60	5.84	3.27
20~	4.16	4.94	3.33	4.28	4.71	3.83	4.93	5.82	4.02
25~	7.10	7.20	7.00	9.61	10.80	8.39	9.61	11.50	7.68
30~	12.80	13.68	11.94	14.55	16.18	12.88	18.93	22.56	15.19
35~	21.52	22.10	20.95	23.37	25.47	21.20	24.04	29.76	18.15
40~	42.74	48.07	37.46	43.45	50.51	36.14	52.62	63.52	41.30
45~	78.86	92.32	65.44	90.00	104.95	74.73	94.14	118.58	69.11
50~	148.43	185.61	110.71	179.44	219.05	138.46	207.89	269.73	142.33
55~	227.17	302.07	151.11	204.09	269.33	136.92	191.41	264.60	117.43
60~	365.03	499.05	232.09	412.52	553.04	269.53	422.46	584.18	255.43
65~	548.09	751.97	349.50	635.29	858.08	412.21	566.53	775.67	353.96
70~	794.48	1 079.22	525.94	808.99	1 090.61	533.01	749.81	1 003.62	496.65
75~	1 134.81	1 519.84	795.26	1 074.59	1 452.17	735.36	981.79	1 306.76	675.46
80~	1 469.20	1 951.36	1 088.32	1 407.28	1 869.32	1 027.30	1 180.17	1 554.40	851.58
85+	1 497.45	2 068.20	1 130.41	1 437.19	1 989.13	1 068.79	1 397.40	1 896.84	1 029.57

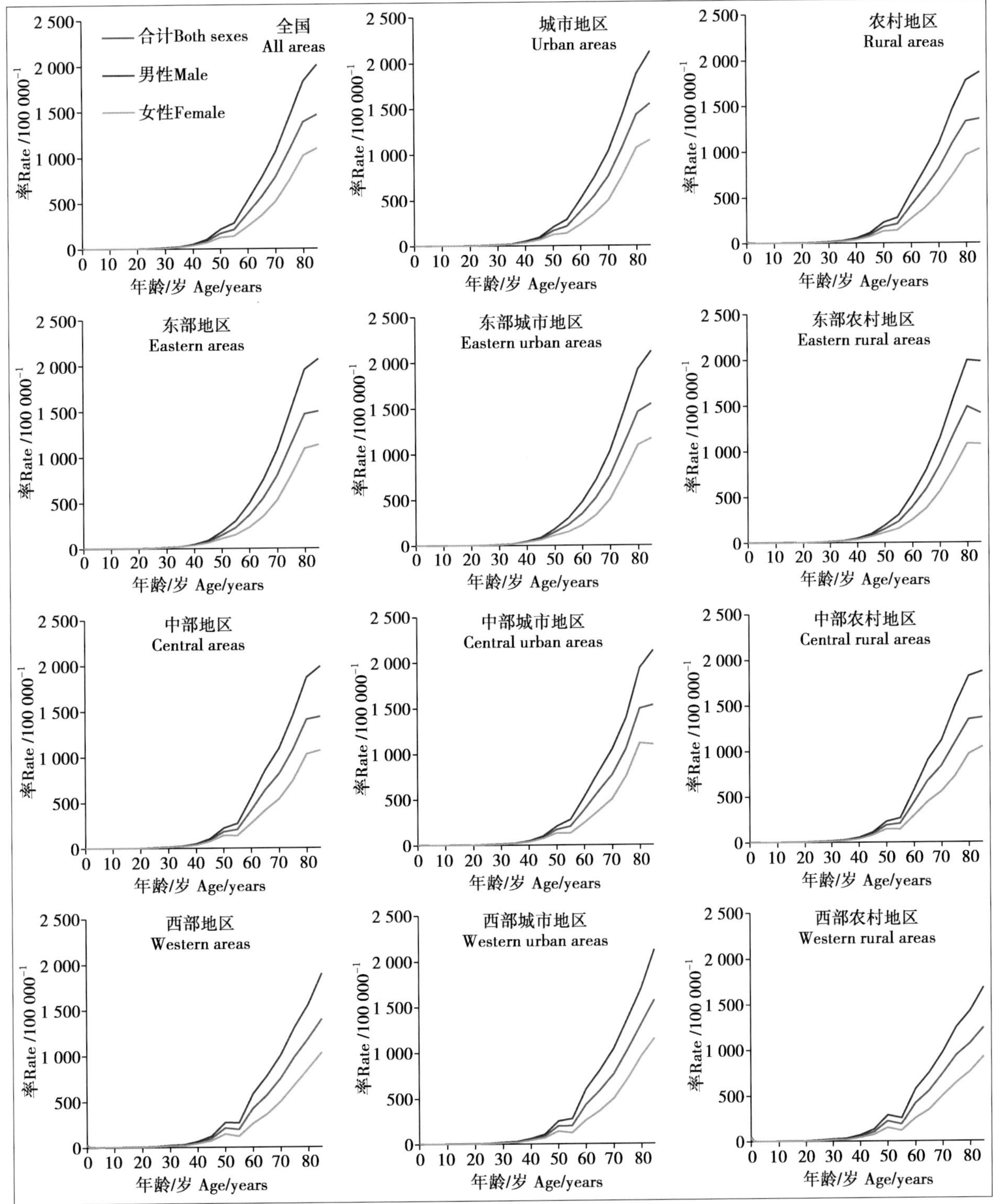

图 4-3　2017 年中国肿瘤登记地区癌症年龄别死亡率

Figure 4-3　Age-specific mortality rates for all cancer sites in the registration areas of China, 2017

2.5 中国不同肿瘤登记地区全部癌症发病和死亡情况

总体而言，七大区发病率与死亡率相差不大。华南地区男性发病率和死亡率均最高，华北地区男性发病率和死亡率最低；华南地区女性发病率最高，西南地区女性发病率最低；东北地区女性死亡率最高，西南地区女性死亡率最低。城市地区男女合计的发病率与死亡率相差不大。华南城市地区男性癌症发病率最高，华北城市男性发病率最低；华南城市地区女性发病率最高，西南城市地区女性发病率最低。东北城市地区男性死亡率最高，华东城市地区男性死亡率最低；东北城市地区女性死亡率最高。华南农村地区男性发病率和死亡率最高，西北农村地区男性发病率和死亡率最低；华南地区农村女性发病率最高，西南地区农村女性发病率最低；东北地区农村女性死亡率最高，西南地区农村女性死亡率最低（图 4-4）。

2.5 Incidence and mortality for all cancer sites in different registration areas of China

In general, there was little difference among the seven administrative districts for the incidence and mortality rates. The incidence and mortality rates were highest in South China and lowest in North China for males. For females, the incidence rate was highest in South China and lowest in Southwest China, and the mortality was highest in Northeast China and lowest in Southwest China. There was little difference of the incidence and mortality rates in the urban areas for both sexes. The incidence rate in the urban areas was highest in South China and lowest in North China for males, and highest in South China and lowest in Southwest for females. The mortality rate in the urban areas was highest in Northeast China and lowest in East China for males, and highest in Northeast China for females. In the rural areas, the incidence rate and mortality rate of males were highest in South China, the incidence and mortality rate were lowest in Northwest China. For females, the incidence rate was highest in South China and lowest in Northwest China, and the mortality rate was highest in Northeast China and lowest in Southwest China (Figure 4-4).

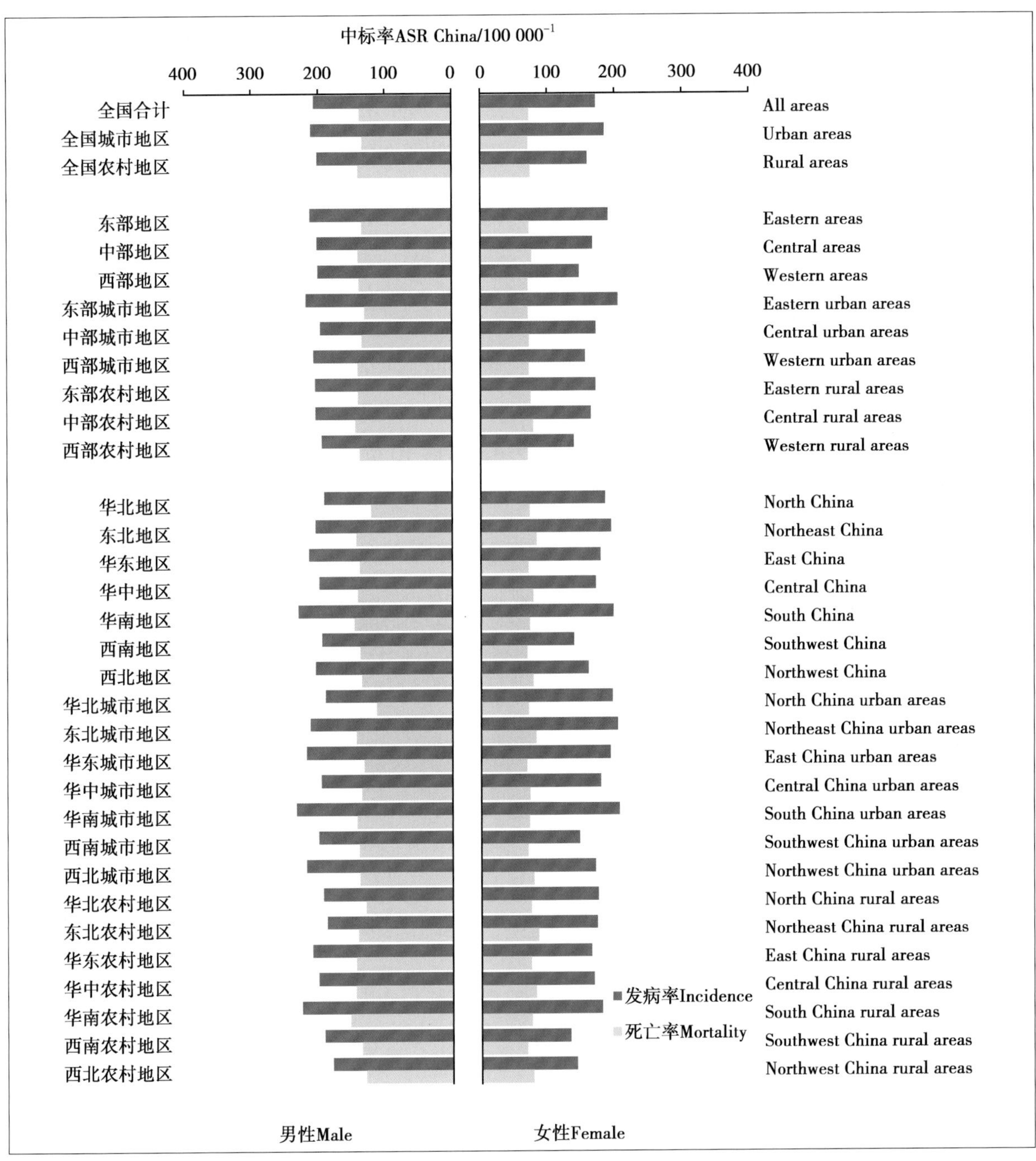

图 4-4　2017 年中国不同肿瘤登记地区癌症发病率和死亡率

Figure 4-4　Incidence and mortality for all cancer sites in different registration areas of China, 2017

3 中国肿瘤登记地区前 10 位癌症发病与死亡

3.1 中国肿瘤登记地区前 10 位癌症发病情况

中国肿瘤登记地区癌症发病第 1 位的是肺癌，其次为女性乳腺癌、结直肠癌、胃癌和肝癌。男性发病第 1 位癌症为肺癌，其次为肝癌、胃癌、结直肠癌和食管癌；女性发病第 1 位癌症为肺癌，其次为乳腺癌、结直肠癌、甲状腺癌和胃癌（表 4-6，图 4-5a，图 4-5b）。

3 Top ten leading causes of new cancer cases and deaths in the registration areas of China

3.1 Top ten leading causes of new cancer cases in the registration areas of China

Lung cancer was the most common cancer in cancer registration areas of China, followed by female breast cancer, colorectal cancer, stomach cancer and liver cancer. The top five cancers in males were lung cancer, liver cancer, stomach cancer, colorectal cancer, and esophageal cancer. The most common cancer in females was lung cancer, followed by breast cancer, colorectal cancer, thyroid cancer and stomach cancer (Table 4-6, Figure 4-5a, Figure 4-5b).

表 4-6 2017 年中国肿瘤登记地区前 10 位癌症发病率

Table 4-6 Incidence rates of top ten leading cancer sites in the registration areas of China, 2017

单位：100 000^{-1}

顺位 Rank	合计 All				男性 Male				女性 Female			
	部位 Site	粗率 Crude rate	世标率 ASR World	中标率 ASR China	部位 Site	粗率 Crude rate	世标率 ASR World	中标率 ASR China	部位 Site	粗率 Crude rate	世标率 ASR World	中标率 ASR China
1	肺 Lung	62.95	37.28	37.29	肺 Lung	82.28	50.56	50.36	肺 Lung	43.09	24.54	24.77
2	乳腺 Breast	42.51	28.11	30.08	肝 Liver	41.05	26.53	27.08	乳腺 Breast	42.51	28.11	30.08
3	结直肠 Colon-rectum	28.96	17.32	17.54	胃 Stomach	38.99	24.05	24.04	结直肠 Colon-rectum	24.34	13.96	14.21
4	胃 Stomach	28.24	16.78	16.88	结直肠 Colon-rectum	33.45	20.81	20.98	甲状腺 Thyroid	21.43	15.71	18.10
5	肝 Liver	28.17	17.50	17.82	食管 Esophagus	27.85	17.14	16.91	胃 Stomach	17.18	9.75	9.99
6	食管 Esophagus	19.23	11.25	11.14	前列腺 Prostate	11.57	6.54	6.64	子宫颈 Cervix	17.07	11.35	12.28
7	子宫颈 Cervix	17.07	11.35	12.28	膀胱 Bladder	9.26	5.56	5.59	肝 Liver	14.93	8.53	8.61
8	甲状腺 Thyroid	13.91	10.30	11.94	胰腺 Pancreas	8.02	4.91	4.92	食管 Esophagus	10.37	5.52	5.54
9	前列腺 Prostate	11.57	6.54	6.64	淋巴瘤 Lymphoma	7.36	4.99	5.07	子宫体 Uterus	10.06	6.56	6.79
10	子宫体 Uterus	10.06	6.56	6.79	脑 Brain	7.14	5.26	5.37	脑 Brain	8.45	5.75	5.87

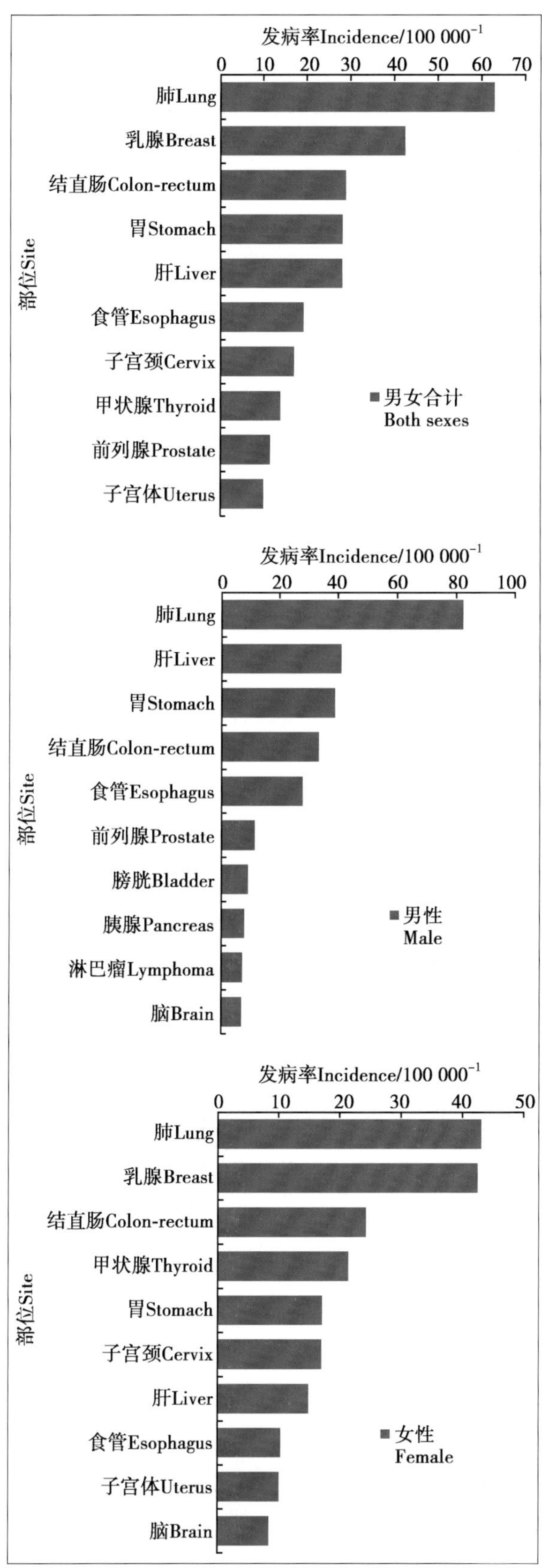

图 4-5a 2017 年中国肿瘤登记地区前 10 位癌症发病率

Figure 4-5a Incidence rates of top ten leading cancer sites in the registration areas of China, 2017

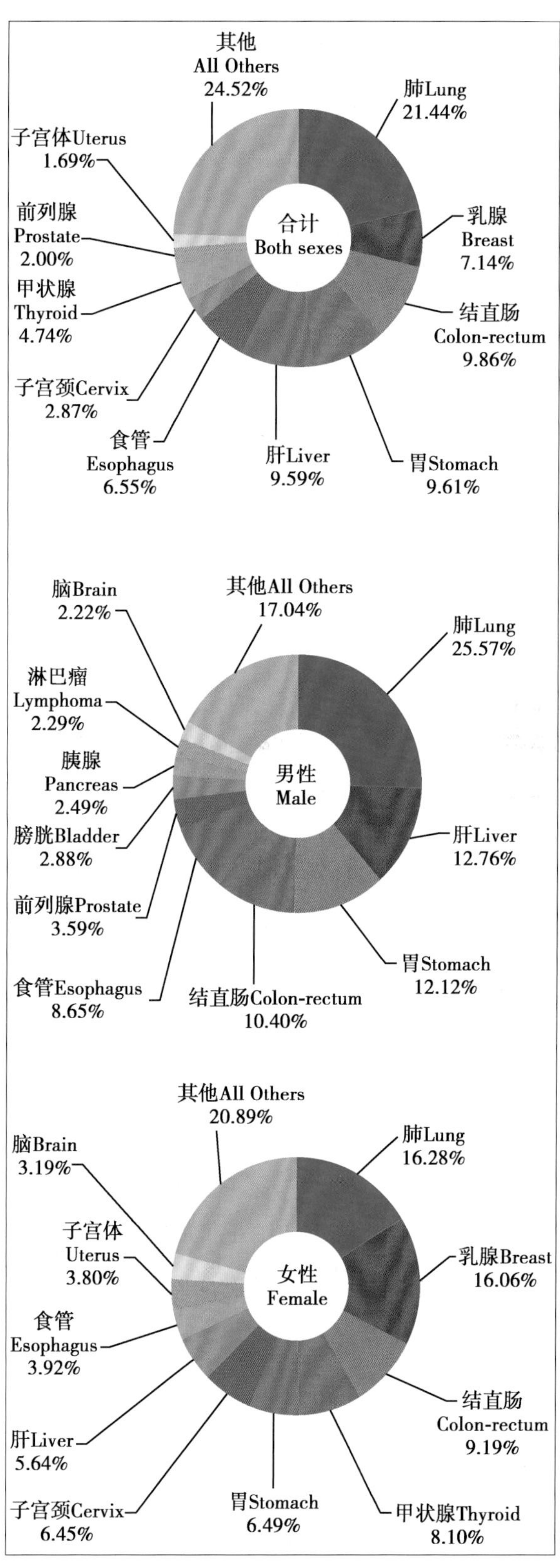

图 4-5b 2017 年中国肿瘤登记地区前 10 位癌症发病构成

Figure 4-5b Distribution of top ten leading causes of new cancer cases in the registration areas of China, 2017

3.2 中国肿瘤登记地区前 10 位癌症死亡情况

中国肿瘤登记地区男女合计和男性癌症死亡第 1 位的均为肺癌,其次为肝癌、胃癌、食管癌和结直肠癌;女性死亡第 1 位癌症为肺癌,其次为肝癌、胃癌、结直肠癌和乳腺癌(表 4-7,图 4-6a,图 4-6b)。

3.2 Top ten leading causes of cancer deaths in the registration areas of China

For both sexes combined and males, lung cancer was the leading cause of cancer deaths, followed by liver cancer, stomach cancer, esophageal cancer and colorectal cancer. For females, the top five leading causes of cancer deaths were lung cancer, liver cancer, stomach cancer, colorectal cancer and breast cancer (Table 4-7, Figure 4-6a, Figure 4-6b).

表 4-7 2017 年中国肿瘤登记地区前 10 位癌症死亡率

Table 4-7 Mortality rates of top ten leading cancer sites in the registration areas of China, 2017

单位:100 000^{-1}

顺位 Rank	合计 All				男性 Male				女性 Female			
	部位 Site	粗率 Crude rate	世标率 ASR World	中标率 ASR China	部位 Site	粗率 Crude rate	世标率 ASR World	中标率 ASR China	部位 Site	粗率 Crude rate	世标率 ASR World	中标率 ASR China
1	肺 Lung	49.28	28.08	28.14	肺 Lung	67.83	40.76	40.71	肺 Lung	30.22	16.01	16.16
2	肝 Liver	24.91	15.20	15.41	肝 Liver	36.12	23.07	23.43	肝 Liver	13.39	7.41	7.47
3	胃 Stomach	20.89	11.81	11.95	胃 Stomach	28.72	17.12	17.25	胃 Stomach	12.85	6.78	6.93
4	食管 Esophagus	15.21	8.55	8.53	食管 Esophagus	22.03	13.22	13.13	结直肠 Colon-rectum	11.73	6.10	6.20
5	结直肠 Colon-rectum	14.08	7.84	7.92	结直肠 Colon-rectum	16.37	9.71	9.75	乳腺 Breast	9.76	5.98	6.17
6	乳腺 Breast	9.76	5.98	6.17	胰腺 Pancreas	7.23	4.37	4.37	食管 Esophagus	8.20	4.06	4.10
7	胰腺 Pancreas	6.40	3.64	3.66	前列腺 Prostate	4.83	2.61	2.56	子宫颈 Cervix	5.55	3.42	3.56
8	子宫颈 Cervix	5.55	3.42	3.56	淋巴瘤 Lymphoma	4.38	2.78	2.81	胰腺 Pancreas	5.54	2.94	2.96
9	前列腺 Prostate	4.83	2.61	2.56	脑 Brain	4.37	3.09	3.11	卵巢 Ovary	3.60	2.21	2.25
10	脑 Brain	3.95	2.70	2.72	白血病 Leukemia	4.19	3.13	3.11	脑 Brain	3.53	2.31	2.32

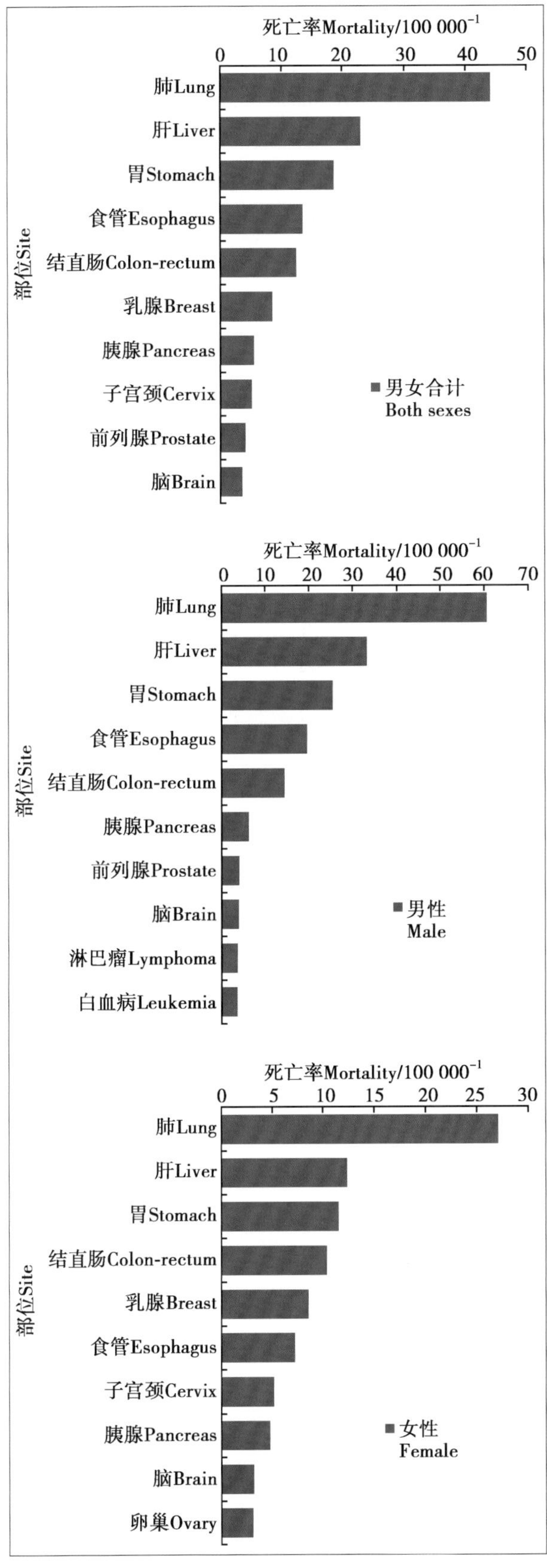

图 4-6a 2017 年中国肿瘤登记地区前 10 位癌症死亡率

Figure 4-6a Mortality rates of top ten leading cancer sites in the registration areas of China, 2017

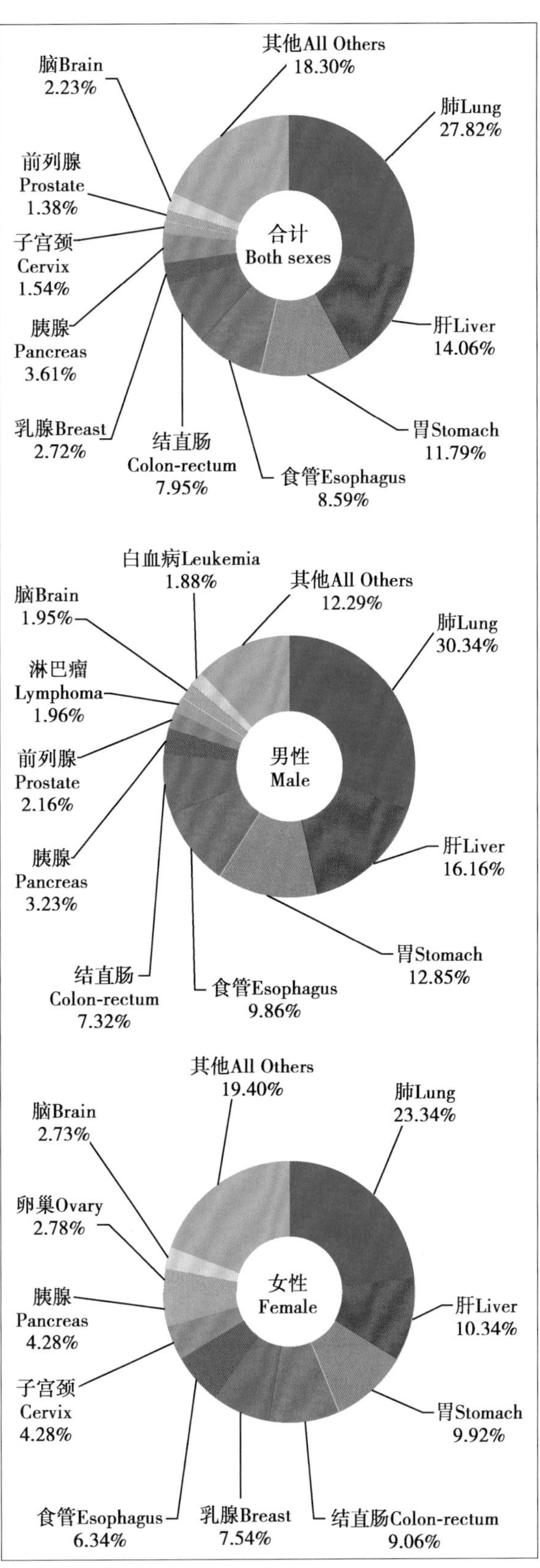

图 4-6b 2017 年中国肿瘤登记地区前 10 位癌症死亡构成

Figure 4-6b Distribution of top ten leading causes of cancer deaths in the registration areas of China, 2017

3.3 中国城市肿瘤登记地区前 10 位癌症发病情况

中国城市肿瘤登记地区癌症发病第 1 位的是肺癌，其次为女性乳腺癌、结直肠癌、肝癌和胃癌。男性癌症发病第 1 位的是肺癌，其次为结直肠癌、肝癌、胃癌和食管癌；女性癌症发病第 1 位的是乳腺癌，其次为肺癌、甲状腺癌、结直肠癌和子宫颈癌（表 4-8，图 4-7a，图 4-7b）。

3.3 Top ten leading causes of new cancer cases in urban registration areas of China

Lung cancer was the most common cancer in urban areas of China, followed by female breast cancer, colorectal cancer, liver cancer and stomach cancer. In males, lung cancer was the most common cancer, followed by colorectal cancer, liver cancer, stomach cancer and esophageal cancer. In females, breast cancer was the most common cancer, followed by lung cancer, thyroid cancer, colorectal cancer and cervix cancer (Table 4-8, Figure 4-7a, Figure 4-7b).

表 4-8 2017 年中国城市肿瘤登记地区前 10 位癌症发病率

Table 4-8 Incidence rates of top ten leading cancer sites in urban registration areas of China, 2017

单位：$100\ 000^{-1}$

顺位 Rank	合计 All				男性 Male				女性 Female			
	部位 Site	粗率 Crude rate	世标率 ASR World	中标率 ASR China	部位 Site	粗率 Crude rate	世标率 ASR World	中标率 ASR China	部位 Site	粗率 Crude rate	世标率 ASR World	中标率 ASR China
1	肺 Lung	66.08	37.67	37.65	肺 Lung	85.90	50.75	50.43	乳腺 Breast	50.57	32.44	34.49
2	乳腺 Breast	50.57	32.44	34.49	结直肠 Colon-rectum	40.53	24.17	24.30	肺 Lung	46.11	25.34	25.61
3	结直肠 Colon-rectum	34.65	19.86	20.07	肝 Liver	39.26	24.51	24.92	甲状腺 Thyroid	28.81	20.78	24.02
4	肝 Liver	26.68	15.99	16.23	胃 Stomach	36.36	21.56	21.55	结直肠 Colon-rectum	28.73	15.78	16.06
5	胃 Stomach	26.31	15.06	15.17	食管 Esophagus	22.50	13.38	13.18	子宫颈 Cervix	16.53	10.80	11.70
6	甲状腺 Thyroid	19.07	13.88	16.18	前列腺 Prostate	15.46	8.35	8.49	胃 Stomach	16.19	8.90	9.14
7	子宫颈 Cervix	16.53	10.80	11.70	膀胱 Bladder	11.15	6.40	6.42	肝 Liver	14.01	7.64	7.71
8	前列腺 Prostate	15.46	8.35	8.49	甲状腺 Thyroid	9.39	6.96	8.30	子宫体 Uterus	10.89	6.93	7.14
9	食管 Esophagus	14.86	8.40	8.31	胰腺 Pancreas	9.15	5.36	5.35	脑 Brain	9.04	5.99	6.11
10	子宫体 Uterus	10.89	6.93	7.14	淋巴瘤 Lymphoma	8.60	5.64	5.74	卵巢 Ovary	8.65	5.69	5.97

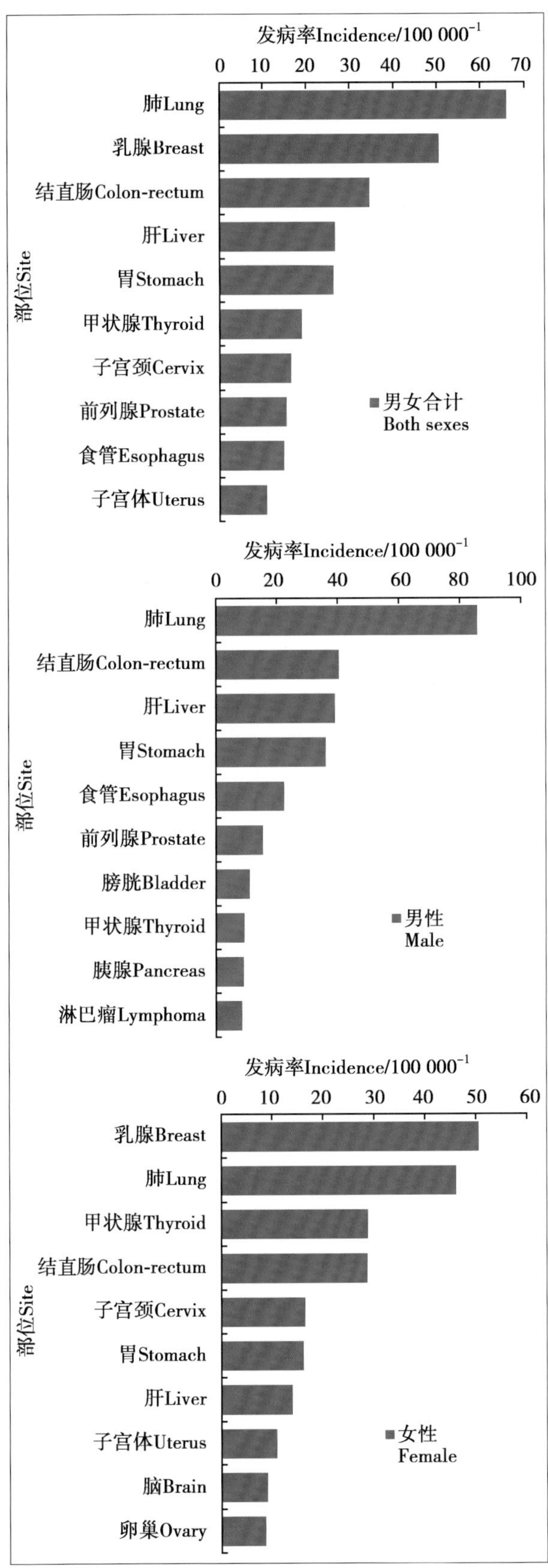

图 4-7a 2017 年中国城市肿瘤登记地区前 10 位癌症发病率

Figure 4-7a Incidence rates of top ten leading cancer sites in urban registration areas of China, 2017

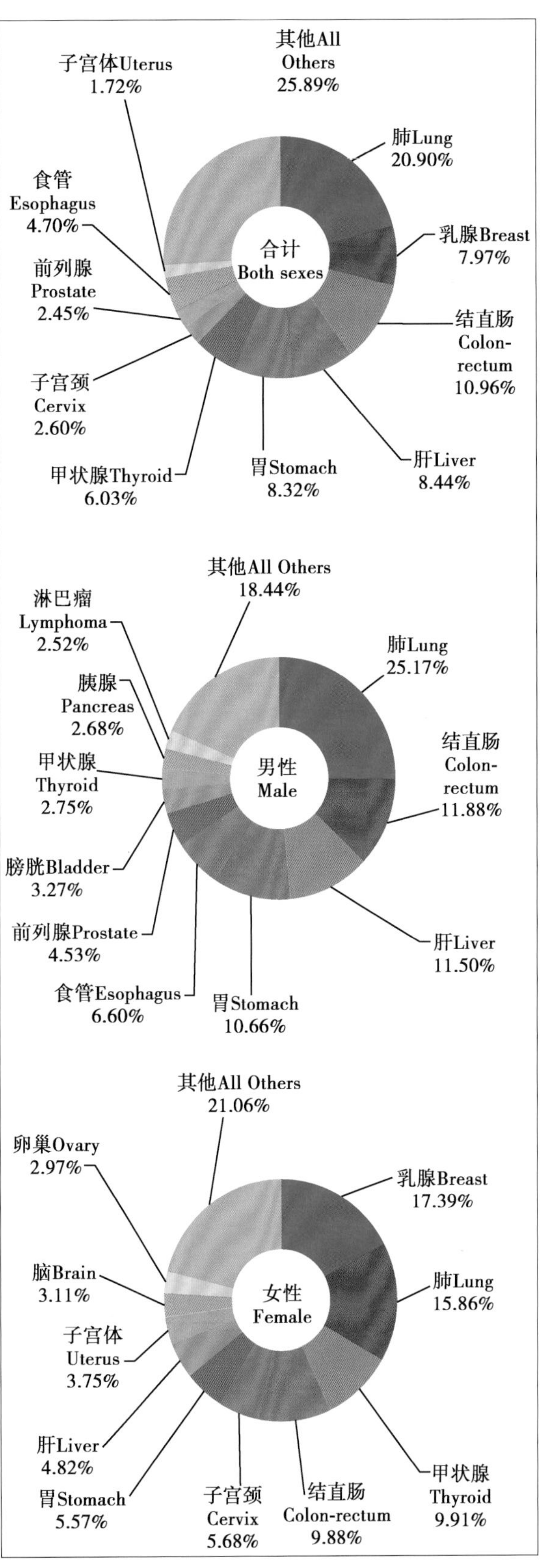

图 4-7b 2017 年中国城市肿瘤登记地区前 10 位癌症发病构成

Figure 4-7b Distribution of top ten leading causes of new cancer cases in urban registration areas of China, 2017

3.4 中国城市肿瘤登记地区前 10 位癌症死亡情况

中国城市肿瘤登记地区合计癌症死亡第 1 位的为肺癌，其次为肝癌、胃癌、结直肠癌和食管癌。男性癌症死亡第 1 位的为肺癌，其次为肝癌、胃癌、结直肠癌和食管癌；女性癌症死亡率第 1 位的为肺癌，其次为结直肠癌、肝癌、胃癌和乳腺癌（表 4-9，图 4-8a，图 4-8b）。

3.4 Top ten leading causes of cancer deaths in urban registration areas of China

Lung cancer was the leading cause of cancer death in urban areas of China, followed by cancers of liver, stomach, colorectum and esophagus. In males, lung cancer was the leading cause of cancer deaths, followed by liver cancer, stomach cancer, colorectal cancer and esophageal cancer. In females, lung cancer ranked as the leading cancer cause of cancer death, followed by colorectal cancer, liver cancer, stomach cancer and breast cancer (Table 4-9, Figure 4-8a, Figure 4-8b).

表 4-9 2017 年中国城市肿瘤登记地区前 10 位癌症死亡率

Table 4-9 Mortality rates of top ten leading cancer sites in urban registration areas of China, 2017

单位：100 000^{-1}

顺位 Rank	合计 All				男性 Male				女性 Female			
	部位 Site	粗率 Crude rate	世标率 ASR World	中标率 ASR China	部位 Site	粗率 Crude rate	世标率 ASR World	中标率 ASR China	部位 Site	粗率 Crude rate	世标率 ASR World	中标率 ASR China
1	肺 Lung	50.89	27.58	27.64	肺 Lung	70.62	40.49	40.41	肺 Lung	31.01	15.48	15.68
2	肝 Liver	23.70	13.85	14.04	肝 Liver	34.69	21.26	21.57	结直肠 Colon-rectum	13.73	6.70	6.80
3	胃 Stomach	18.62	10.03	10.17	胃 Stomach	25.76	14.62	14.74	肝 Liver	12.64	6.63	6.70
4	结直肠 Colon-rectum	16.81	8.84	8.91	结直肠 Colon-rectum	19.86	11.15	11.18	胃 Stomach	11.43	5.77	5.93
5	食管 Esophagus	12.01	6.51	6.48	食管 Esophagus	18.23	10.55	10.46	乳腺 Breast	11.25	6.55	6.74
6	乳腺 Breast	11.25	6.55	6.74	胰腺 Pancreas	8.46	4.89	4.88	胰腺 Pancreas	6.51	3.27	3.31
7	胰腺 Pancreas	7.49	4.06	4.08	前列腺 Prostate	6.21	3.10	3.04	食管 Esophagus	5.74	2.67	2.70
8	前列腺 Prostate	6.21	3.10	3.04	淋巴瘤 Lymphoma	4.99	3.00	3.04	子宫颈 Cervix	5.13	3.09	3.23
9	子宫颈 Cervix	5.13	3.09	3.23	膀胱 Bladder	4.63	2.40	2.36	卵巢 Ovary	4.27	2.52	2.57
10	卵巢 Ovary	4.27	2.52	2.57	白血病 Leukemia	4.41	3.13	3.10	胆囊 Gallbladder	3.68	1.80	1.82

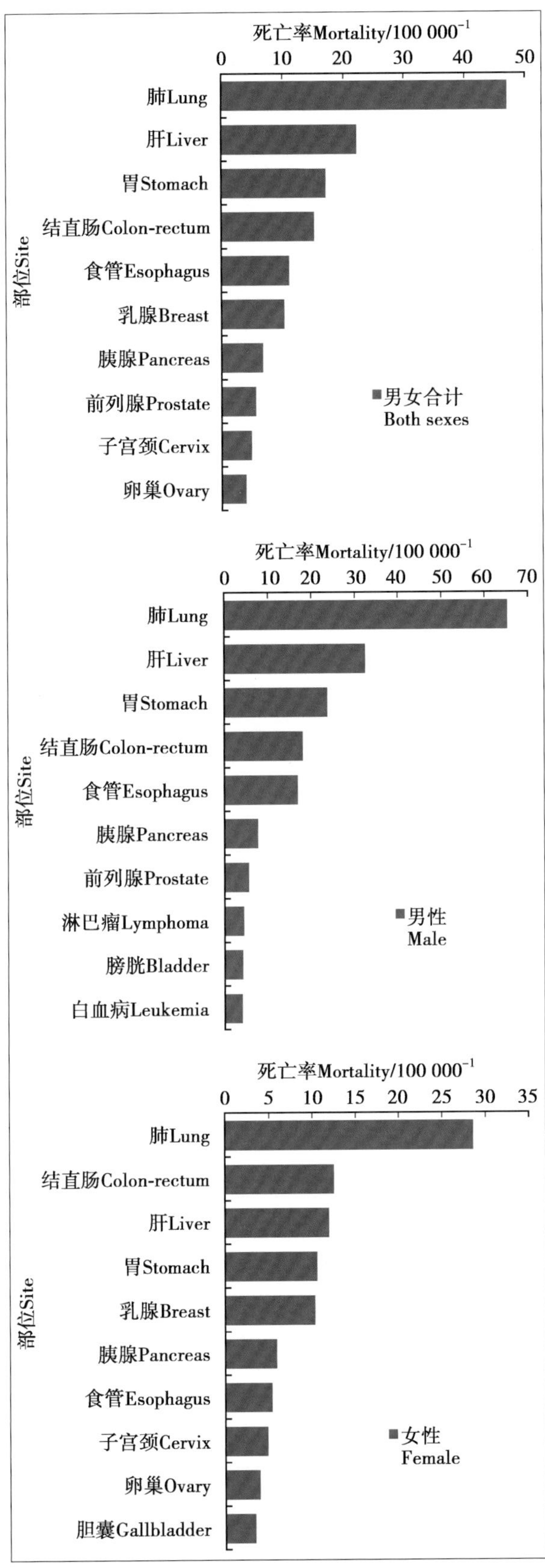

图 4-8a 2017 年中国城市肿瘤登记地区前 10 位癌症死亡率

Figure 4-8a Mortality rates of top ten leading cancer sites in urban registration areas of China,2017

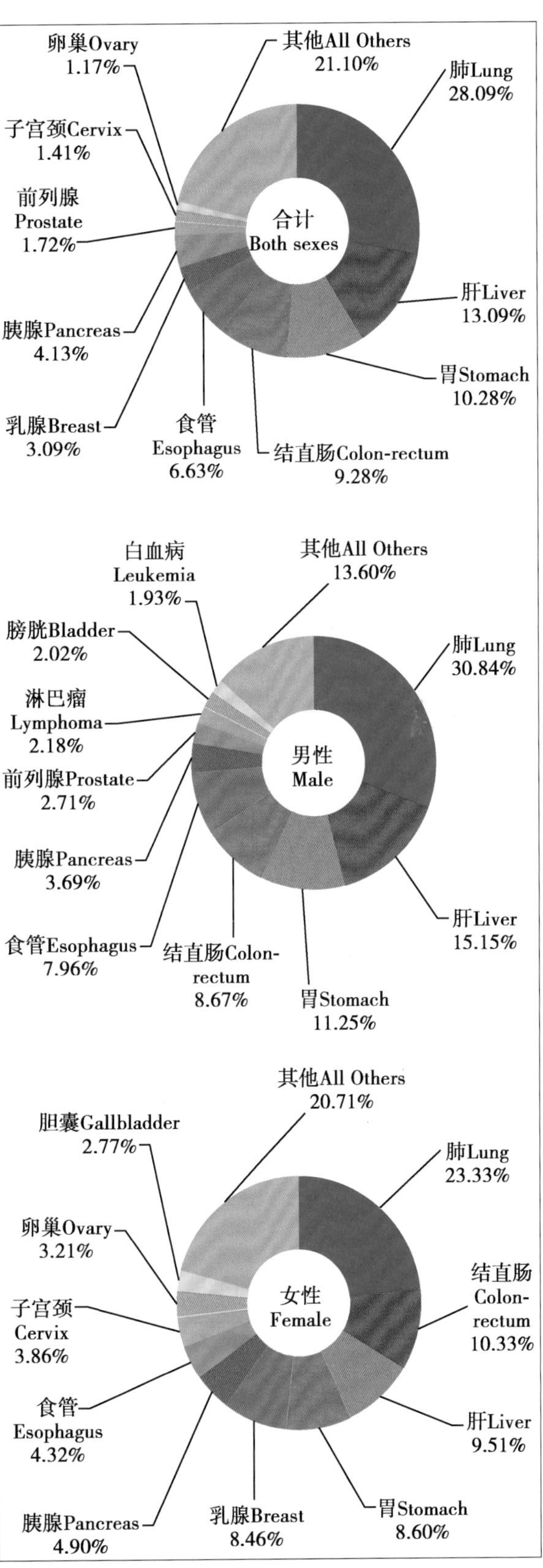

图 4-8b 2017 年中国城市肿瘤登记地区前 10 位癌症死亡构成

Figure 4-8b Distribution of top ten leading causes of cancer deaths in urban registration areas of China,2017

3.5 中国农村肿瘤登记地区前10位癌症发病情况

中国农村肿瘤登记地区合计发病第1位癌症为肺癌，其次为女性乳腺癌、胃癌、肝癌和结直肠癌。男性发病第1位癌症为肺癌，其次为肝癌、胃癌、食管癌和结直肠癌；女性发病第1位癌症为肺癌，其次为乳腺癌、结直肠癌、胃癌和子宫颈癌（表4-10，图4-9a，图4-9b）。

3.5 Top ten leading causes of new cancer cases in rural registration areas of China

Lung cancer was the most common cancer in rural areas of China, followed by cancers of female breast, stomach, liver and colon-rectum. In males, lung cancer was the most common cancer, followed by liver cancer, stomach cancer, esophageal cancer and colorectal cancer. In females, lung cancer was the most common cancer, followed by breast cancer, colorectal cancer, stomach cancer and cervical cancer (Table 4-10, Figure 4-9a, Figure 4-9b).

表4-10 2017年中国农村肿瘤登记地区前10位癌症发病率

Table 4-10 Incidence rates of top ten leading cancer sites in rural registration areas of China, 2017

单位：100 000^{-1}

顺位 Rank	合计 All				男性 Male				女性 Female			
	部位 Site	粗率 Crude rate	世标率 ASR World	中标率 ASR China	部位 Site	粗率 Crude rate	世标率 ASR World	中标率 ASR China	部位 Site	粗率 Crude rate	世标率 ASR World	中标率 ASR China
1	肺 Lung	59.97	36.84	36.91	肺 Lung	78.89	50.33	50.26	肺 Lung	40.15	23.69	23.89
2	乳腺 Breast	34.64	23.66	25.55	肝 Liver	42.72	28.53	29.21	乳腺 Breast	34.64	23.66	25.55
3	胃 Stomach	30.08	18.52	18.62	胃 Stomach	41.46	26.54	26.51	结直肠 Colon-rectum	20.06	12.06	12.29
4	肝 Liver	29.59	19.02	19.41	食管 Esophagus	32.86	20.93	20.65	胃 Stomach	18.15	10.62	10.86
5	结直肠 Colon-rectum	23.52	14.70	14.93	结直肠 Colon-rectum	26.81	17.40	17.62	子宫颈 Cervix	17.60	11.91	12.87
6	食管 Esophagus	23.40	14.16	14.02	前列腺 Prostate	7.92	4.69	4.77	肝 Liver	15.83	9.44	9.54
7	子宫颈 Cervix	17.60	11.91	12.87	膀胱 Bladder	7.50	4.71	4.75	甲状腺 Thyroid	14.24	10.56	12.04
8	子宫体 Uterus	9.24	6.17	6.43	脑 Brain	6.98	5.27	5.41	食管 Esophagus	13.50	7.48	7.49
9	甲状腺 Thyroid	8.98	6.73	7.70	胰腺 Pancreas	6.96	4.44	4.48	子宫体 Uterus	9.24	6.17	6.43
10	前列腺 Prostate	7.92	4.69	4.77	白血病 Leukemia	6.40	5.40	5.25	脑 Brain	7.87	5.51	5.63

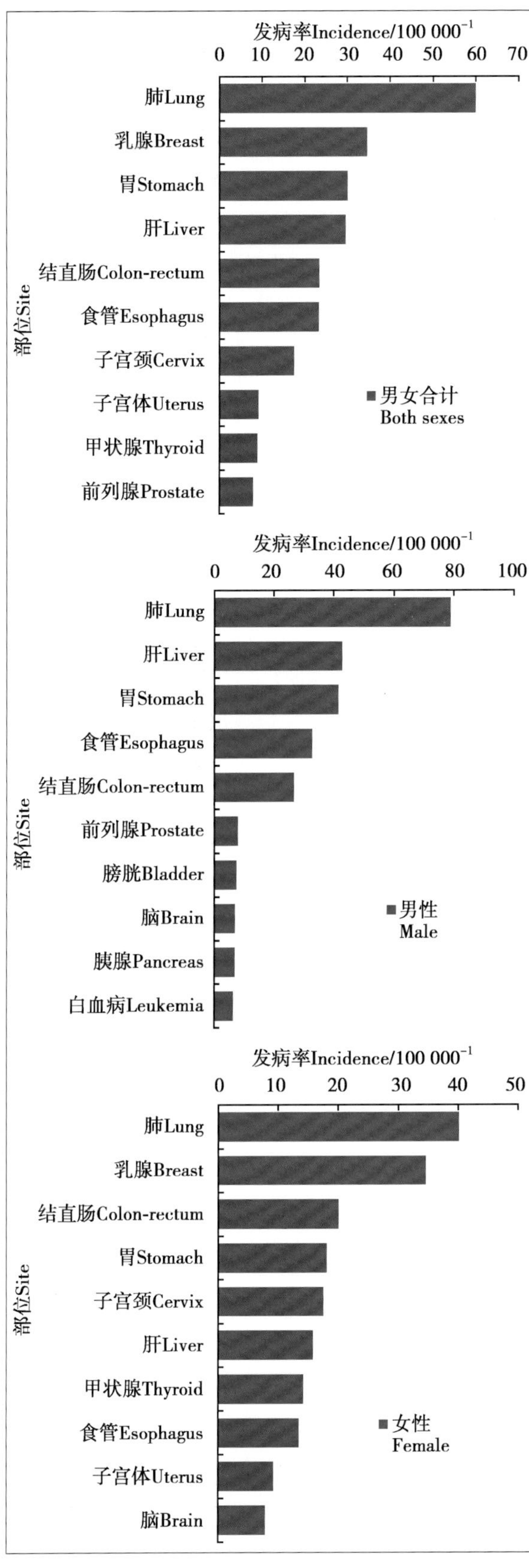

图 4-9a 2017 年中国农村肿瘤登记地区前 10 位癌症发病率

Figure 4-9a Incidence rates of top ten leading cancer sites in rural registration areas of China, 2017

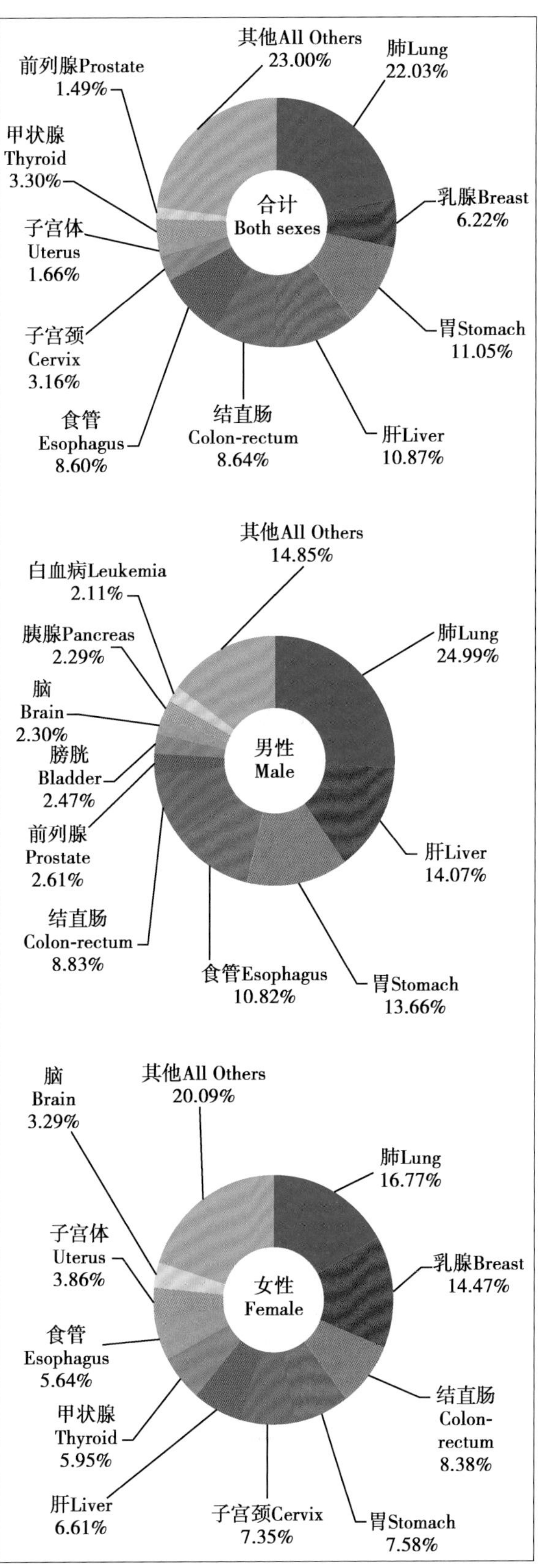

图 4-9b 2017 年中国农村肿瘤登记地区前 10 位癌症发病构成

Figure 4-9b Distribution of top ten leading causes of new cancer cases in rural registration areas of China, 2017

3.6 中国农村肿瘤登记地区前 10 位癌症死亡情况

中国农村肿瘤登记地区合计癌症死亡第 1 位的是肺癌，其次为肝癌、胃癌、食管癌和结直肠癌。男性癌症死亡第 1 位的是肺癌，其次为肝癌、胃癌、食管癌和结直肠癌；女性癌症死亡第 1 位的是肺癌，其次为胃癌、肝癌、食管癌和结直肠癌（表 4-11，图 4-10a，图 4-10b）。

3.6 Top ten leading causes of cancer deaths in rural registration areas of China

Lung cancer was the leading cause of cancer death in rural areas of China, followed by cancers of liver, stomach, esophagus and colorectum. In males, lung cancer was the leading cause of cancer death, followed by liver cancer, stomach cancer, esophageal cancer and colorectal cancer. In females, lung cancer ranked as the leading cause of cancer death, followed by stomach cancer, liver cancer, esophageal cancer and colorectal cancer (Table 4-11, Figure 4-10a, Figure 4-10b).

表 4-11 2017 年中国农村肿瘤登记地区前 10 位癌症死亡率

Table 4-11 Mortality rates of top ten leading cancer sites in rural registration areas of China, 2017

单位：100 000^{-1}

顺位 Rank	合计 All				男性 Male				女性 Female			
	部位 Site	粗率 Crude rate	世标率 ASR World	中标率 ASR China	部位 Site	粗率 Crude rate	世标率 ASR World	中标率 ASR China	部位 Site	粗率 Crude rate	世标率 ASR World	中标率 ASR China
1	肺 Lung	47.74	28.54	28.59	肺 Lung	65.21	40.97	40.96	肺 Lung	29.44	16.53	16.62
2	肝 Liver	26.06	16.55	16.79	肝 Liver	37.47	24.86	25.28	胃 Stomach	14.23	7.83	7.96
3	胃 Stomach	23.07	13.63	13.75	胃 Stomach	31.50	19.63	19.75	肝 Liver	14.11	8.21	8.27
4	食管 Esophagus	18.28	10.66	10.63	食管 Esophagus	25.60	15.95	15.84	食管 Esophagus	10.60	5.53	5.57
5	结直肠 Colon-rectum	11.48	6.77	6.88	结直肠 Colon-rectum	13.10	8.18	8.27	结直肠 Colon-rectum	9.78	5.44	5.55
6	乳腺 Breast	8.30	5.37	5.56	胰腺 Pancreas	6.07	3.84	3.86	乳腺 Breast	8.30	5.37	5.56
7	子宫颈 Cervix	5.95	3.76	3.90	脑 Brain	4.44	3.24	3.27	子宫颈 Cervix	5.95	3.76	3.90
8	胰腺 Pancreas	5.35	3.20	3.22	白血病 Leukemia	3.99	3.11	3.12	胰腺 Pancreas	4.60	2.58	2.60
9	脑 Brain	4.02	2.83	2.85	淋巴瘤 Lymphoma	3.82	2.55	2.57	脑 Brain	3.57	2.40	2.42
10	前列腺 Prostate	3.55	2.06	2.04	前列腺 Prostate	3.55	2.06	2.04	白血病 Leukemia	3.00	2.25	2.23

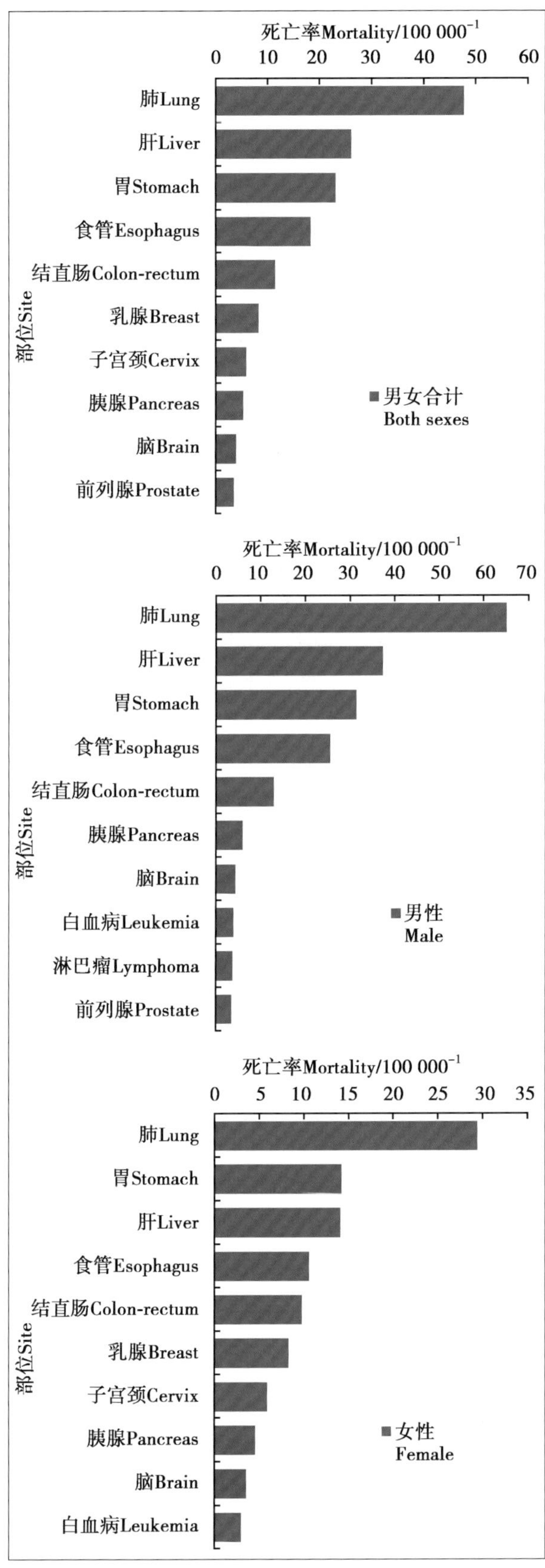

图 4-10a 2017 年中国农村肿瘤登记地区前 10 位癌症死亡率

Figure 4-10a Mortality rates of top ten leading cancer sites in rural registration areas of China,2017

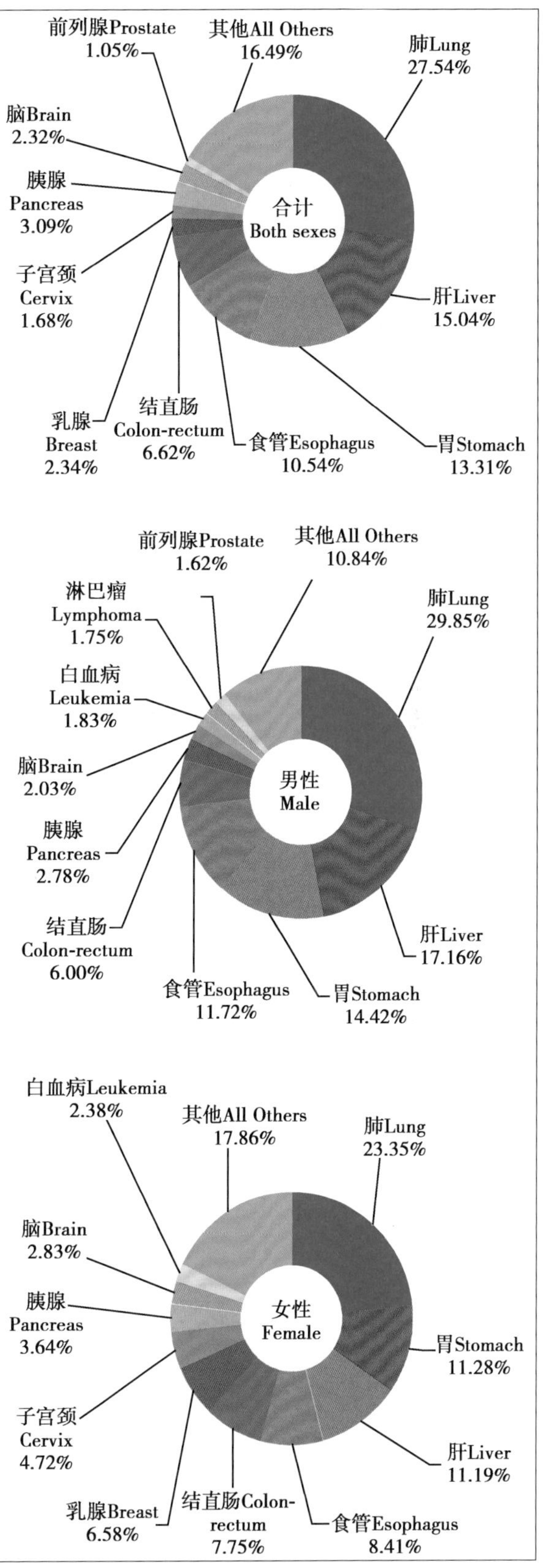

图 4-10b 2017 年中国农村肿瘤登记地区前 10 位癌症死亡构成

Figure 4-10b Distribution of top ten leading causes of cancer deaths in rural registration areas of China,2017

3.7 中国东部肿瘤登记地区前 10 位癌症发病情况

中国东部肿瘤登记地区合计发病第 1 位癌症为肺癌，其次为女性乳腺癌、结直肠癌、胃癌和肝癌。男性发病第 1 位癌症为肺癌，其次为胃癌、结直肠癌、肝癌和食管癌；女性发病第 1 位癌症为乳腺癌，其次为肺癌、甲状腺癌、结直肠癌和胃癌（表 4-12，图 4-11a，图 4-11b）。

3.7 Top ten leading causes of new cancer cases in eastern registration areas of China

Lung cancer was the most common cancer in eastern areas of China, followed by female breast cancer, colorectal cancer, stomach cancer and liver cancer. In males, lung cancer was the most common cancer, followed by stomach cancer, colorectal cancer, liver cancer and esophageal cancer. In females, breast cancer was the most common cancer, followed by lung cancer, colorectal cancer, thyroid cancer and stomach cancer(Table 4-12, Figure 4-11a, Figure 4-11b).

表 4-12　2017 年中国东部肿瘤登记地区前 10 位癌症发病率

Table 4-12　Incidence rates of top ten leading cancer sites in eastern registration areas of China, 2017

单位：100 000^{-1}

顺位 Rank	合计 All				男性 Male				女性 Female			
	部位 Site	粗率 Crude rate	世标率 ASR World	中标率 ASR China	部位 Site	粗率 Crude rate	世标率 ASR World	中标率 ASR China	部位 Site	粗率 Crude rate	世标率 ASR World	中标率 ASR China
1	肺 Lung	69.61	37.64	37.79	肺 Lung	87.81	49.25	49.17	乳腺 Breast	52.74	33.30	35.61
2	乳腺 Breast	52.74	33.30	35.61	胃 Stomach	43.57	24.52	24.59	肺 Lung	51.20	26.80	27.17
3	结直肠 Colon-rectum	34.54	18.87	19.10	结直肠 Colon-rectum	40.08	22.89	23.06	甲状腺 Thyroid	31.53	22.76	26.32
4	胃 Stomach	31.36	16.98	17.15	肝 Liver	38.82	23.32	23.68	结直肠 Colon-rectum	28.93	15.06	15.34
5	肝 Liver	26.52	15.20	15.41	食管 Esophagus	27.77	15.52	15.34	胃 Stomach	19.01	9.85	10.13
6	甲状腺 Thyroid	20.71	15.14	17.64	前列腺 Prostate	15.71	8.09	8.23	子宫颈 Cervix	15.44	9.92	10.81
7	食管 Esophagus	19.25	10.14	10.07	膀胱 Bladder	11.54	6.32	6.36	肝 Liver	14.08	7.25	7.33
8	前列腺 Prostate	15.71	8.09	8.23	胰腺 Pancreas	10.03	5.59	5.61	子宫体 Uterus	11.66	7.16	7.39
9	子宫颈 Cervix	15.44	9.92	10.81	甲状腺 Thyroid	10.02	7.52	8.95	食管 Esophagus	10.64	5.01	5.05
10	子宫体 Uterus	11.66	7.16	7.39	淋巴瘤 Lymphoma	9.18	5.77	5.88	脑 Brain	10.02	6.46	6.59

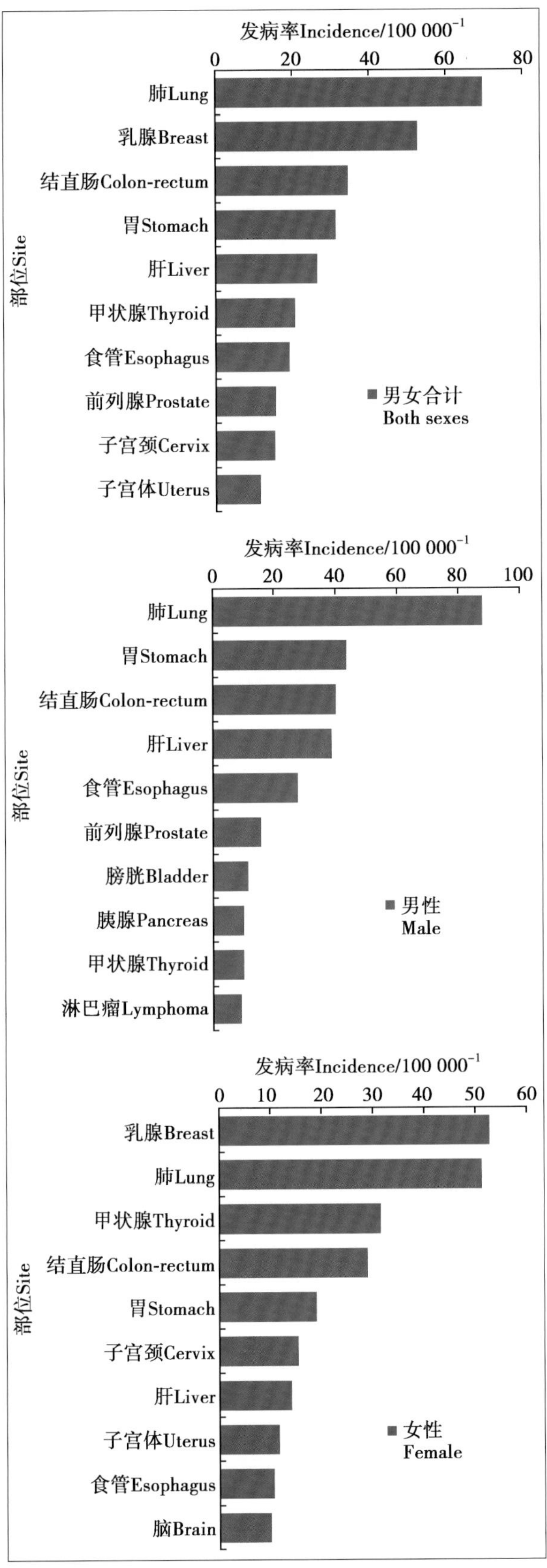

图 4-11a 2017 年中国东部肿瘤登记地区前 10 位癌症发病率

Figure 4-11a Incidence rates of top ten leading cancer sites in eastern registration areas of China, 2017

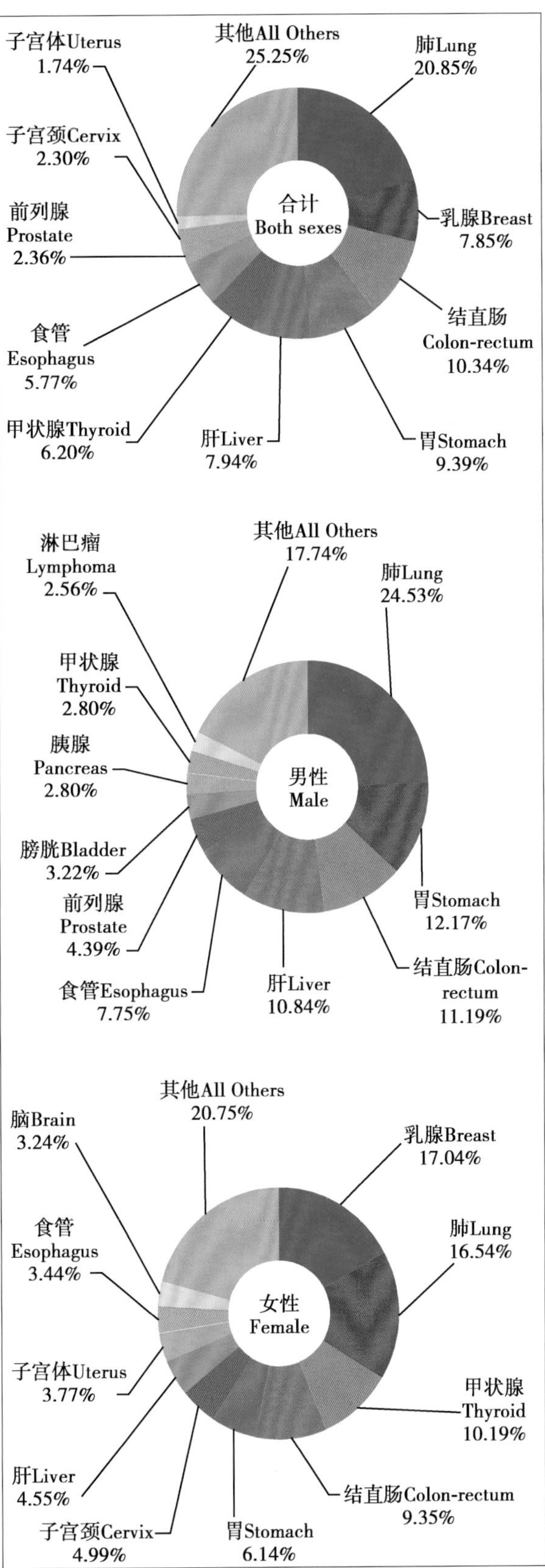

图 4-11b 2017 年中国东部肿瘤登记地区前 10 位癌症发病构成

Figure 4-11b Distribution of top ten leading causes of new cancer cases in eastern registration areas of China, 2017

3.8 中国东部肿瘤登记地区前10位癌症死亡情况

中国东部肿瘤登记地区男女合计癌症死亡第1位的为肺癌，其次为肝癌、胃癌、结直肠癌和食管癌；男性癌症死亡第1位的是肺癌，其次是肝癌、胃癌、食管癌和结直肠癌；女性癌症死亡第1位的是肺癌，其次为胃癌、结直肠癌、肝癌和乳腺癌（表4-13，图4-12a，图4-12b）。

3.8 Top ten leading causes of cancer deaths in eastern registration areas of China

Lung cancer was the leading cause of cancer death in eastern areas of China, followed by liver cancer, stomach cancer, colorectal cancer and esophageal cancer. In males, lung cancer was the leading cause of cancer death, followed by liver cancer, stomach cancer, esophageal cancer and colorectal cancer. In females, lung cancer was still the leading cause of cancer death, followed by stomach cancer, colorectal cancer, liver cancer and breast cancer (Table 4-13, Figure 4-12a, Figure 4-12b).

表4-13 2017年中国东部肿瘤登记地区前10位癌症死亡率

Table 4-13 Mortality rates of top ten leading cancer sites in eastern registration areas of China, 2017

单位：$100\ 000^{-1}$

顺位 Rank	合计 All				男性 Male				女性 Female			
	部位 Site	粗率 Crude rate	世标率 ASR World	中标率 ASR China	部位 Site	粗率 Crude rate	世标率 ASR World	中标率 ASR China	部位 Site	粗率 Crude rate	世标率 ASR World	中标率 ASR China
1	肺 Lung	53.27	27.19	27.38	肺 Lung	72.31	39.22	39.32	肺 Lung	34.03	16.03	16.28
2	肝 Liver	23.88	13.33	13.50	肝 Liver	34.78	20.50	20.77	胃 Stomach	13.80	6.52	6.72
3	胃 Stomach	22.76	11.53	11.75	胃 Stomach	31.62	16.98	17.21	结直肠 Colon-rectum	13.76	6.29	6.40
4	结直肠 Colon-rectum	16.34	8.09	8.17	食管 Esophagus	22.93	12.42	12.39	肝 Liver	12.86	6.36	6.44
5	食管 Esophagus	15.94	8.00	8.02	结直肠 Colon-rectum	18.90	10.07	10.12	乳腺 Breast	11.47	6.41	6.59
6	乳腺 Breast	11.47	6.41	6.59	胰腺 Pancreas	9.25	5.07	5.09	食管 Esophagus	8.86	3.83	3.91
7	胰腺 Pancreas	8.28	4.24	4.26	前列腺 Prostate	6.19	2.94	2.89	胰腺 Pancreas	7.30	3.44	3.48
8	前列腺 Prostate	6.19	2.94	2.89	淋巴瘤 Lymphoma	5.36	3.08	3.11	子宫颈 Cervix	4.71	2.71	2.83
9	子宫颈 Cervix	4.71	2.71	2.83	膀胱 Bladder	4.86	2.37	2.33	卵巢 Ovary	4.28	2.42	2.46
10	淋巴瘤 Lymphoma	4.52	2.46	2.50	白血病 Leukemia	4.73	3.23	3.22	胆囊 Gallbladder	3.92	1.79	1.81

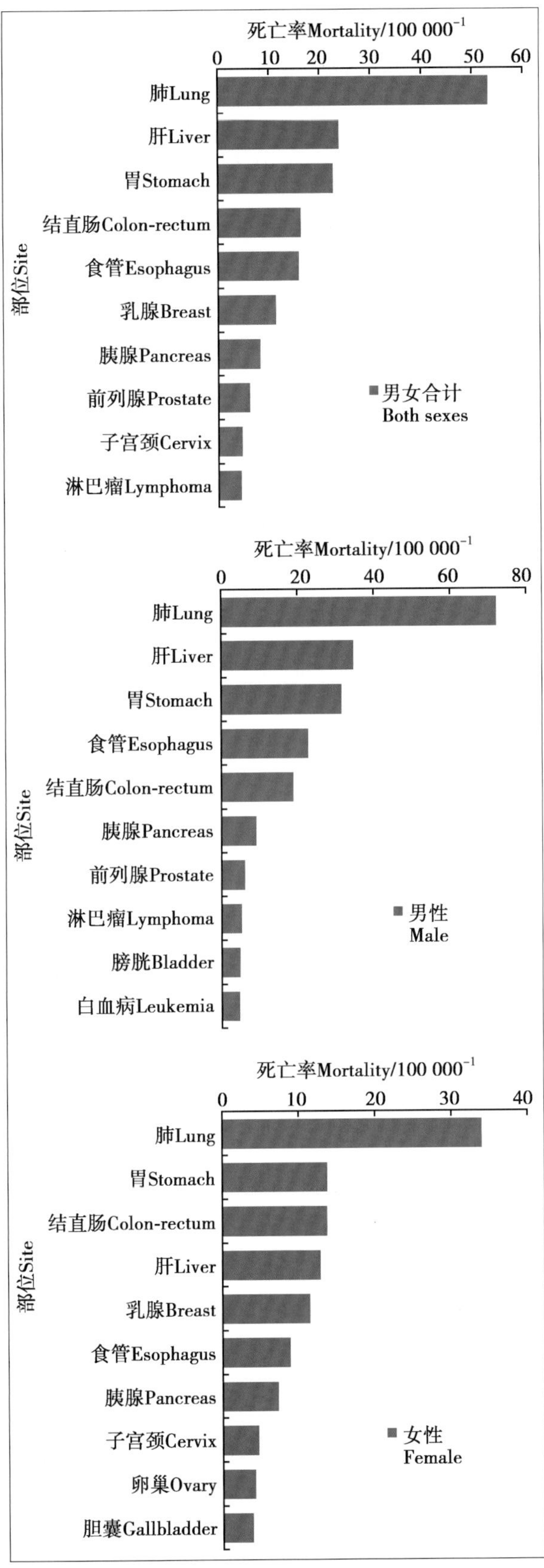

图 4-12a　2017 年中国东部肿瘤登记地区前 10 位癌症死亡率

Figure 4-12a　Mortality rates of top ten leading cancer sites in eastern registration areas of China,2017

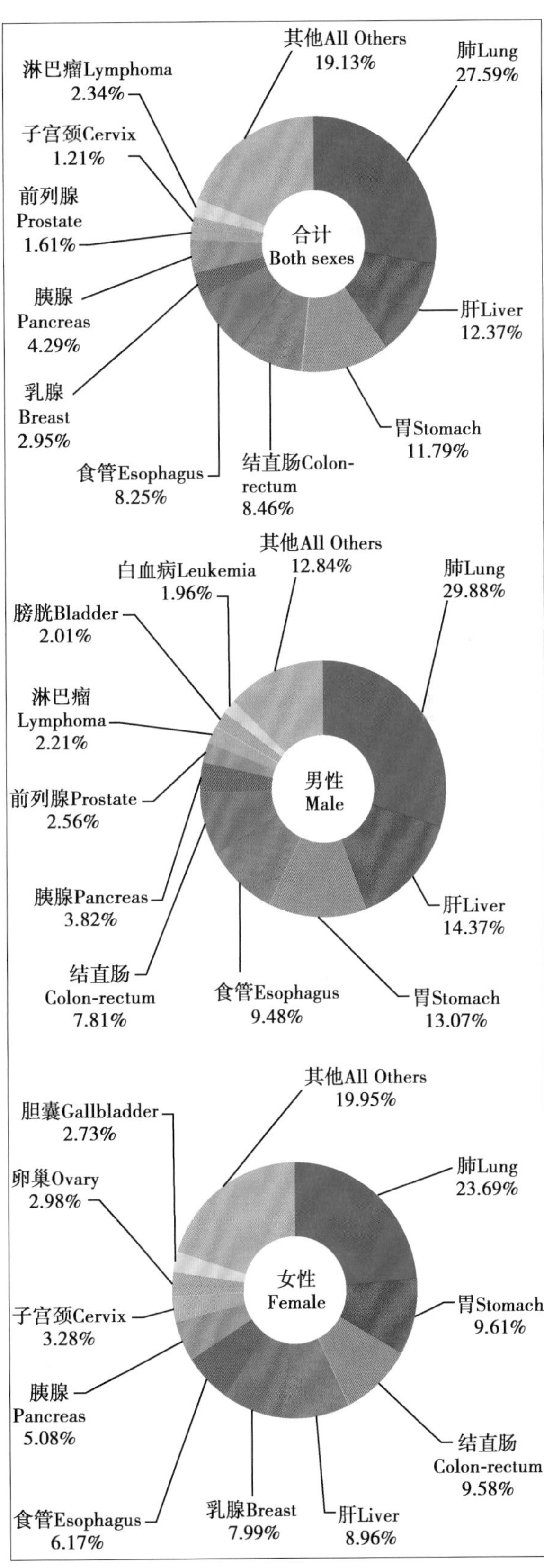

图 4-12b　2017 年中国东部肿瘤登记地区前 10 位癌症死亡构成

Figure 4-12b　Distribution of top ten leading causes of cancer deaths in eastern registration areas of China,2017

3.9 中国中部肿瘤登记地区前10位癌症发病情况

中国中部肿瘤登记地区男女合计发病第1位癌症为肺癌，其次为女性乳腺癌、胃癌、肝癌和结直肠癌。男性发病第1位癌症为肺癌，其次为胃癌、肝癌、结直肠癌和食管癌；女性发病第1位癌症为乳腺癌，其次为肺癌、子宫颈癌、结直肠癌和胃癌（表4-14，图4-13a，图4-13b）。

3.9 Top ten leading causes of new cancer cases in central registration areas of China

Lung cancer was the most common cancer in the central areas of China, followed by female breast cancer, stomach cancer, liver cancer and colorectal cancer. In males, lung cancer was the most common cancer, followed by stomach cancer, liver cancer, colorectal cancer and esophageal cancer. In females, breast cancer was the most common cancer, followed by lung cancer, cervical cancer, colorectal cancer and stomach cancer (Table 4-14, Figure 4-13a, Figure 4-13b).

表4-14 2017年中国中部肿瘤登记地区前10位癌症发病率

Table 4-14 Incidence rates of top ten leading cancer sites in central registration areas of China, 2017

单位：100 000^{-1}

顺位 Rank	合计 All				男性 Male				女性 Female			
	部位 Site	粗率 Crude rate	世标率 ASR World	中标率 ASR China	部位 Site	粗率 Crude rate	世标率 ASR World	中标率 ASR China	部位 Site	粗率 Crude rate	世标率 ASR World	中标率 ASR China
1	肺 Lung	55.99	36.94	36.84	肺 Lung	76.18	52.50	52.23	乳腺 Breast	38.42	26.97	28.91
2	乳腺 Breast	38.42	26.97	28.91	胃 Stomach	39.28	27.28	27.18	肺 Lung	34.88	21.88	21.98
3	胃 Stomach	28.81	19.15	19.22	肝 Liver	39.00	27.56	28.08	子宫颈 Cervix	19.87	13.86	14.91
4	肝 Liver	27.80	18.88	19.18	结直肠 Colon-rectum	25.84	18.03	18.20	结直肠 Colon-rectum	19.86	12.76	12.96
5	结直肠 Colon-rectum	22.92	15.35	15.54	食管 Esophagus	24.78	17.16	16.96	胃 Stomach	17.86	11.23	11.47
6	子宫颈 Cervix	19.87	13.86	14.91	前列腺 Prostate	7.50	4.84	4.91	肝 Liver	16.08	10.19	10.28
7	食管 Esophagus	18.24	11.97	11.87	膀胱 Bladder	7.33	4.99	5.01	甲状腺 Thyroid	16.02	11.98	13.60
8	甲状腺 Thyroid	10.19	7.70	8.78	脑 Brain	6.48	5.08	5.15	食管 Esophagus	11.40	6.89	6.89
9	子宫体 Uterus	9.22	6.45	6.73	淋巴瘤 Lymphoma	6.05	4.53	4.59	子宫体 Uterus	9.22	6.45	6.73
10	前列腺 Prostate	7.50	4.84	4.91	胰腺 Pancreas	5.93	4.08	4.09	卵巢 Ovary	7.10	5.12	5.35

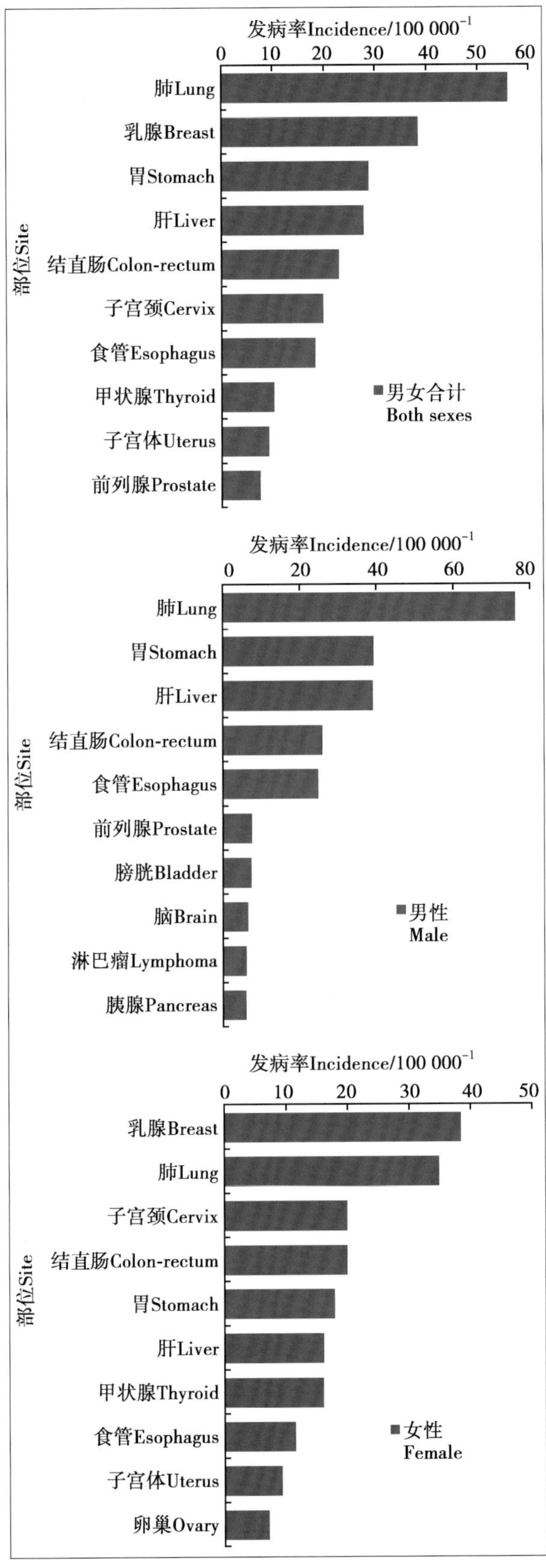

图 4-13a 2017 年中国中部肿瘤登记地区前 10 位癌症发病率

Figure 4-13a Incidence rates of top ten leading cancer sites in central registration areas of China,2017

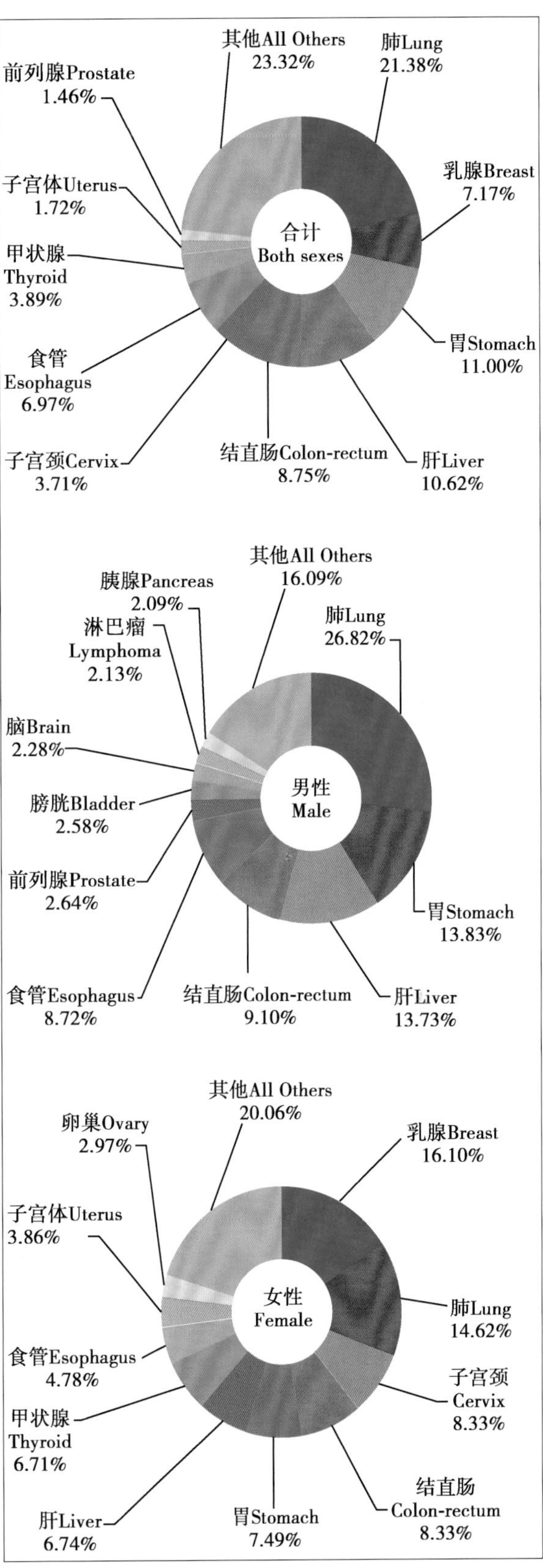

图 4-13b 2017 年中国中部肿瘤登记地区前 10 位癌症发病构成

Figure 4-13b Distribution of top ten leading causes of new cancer cases in central registration areas of China,2017

3.10 中国中部肿瘤登记地区前 10 位癌症死亡情况

中国中部肿瘤登记地区癌症死亡第 1 位的是肺癌，其次为肝癌、胃癌、食管癌和结直肠癌。男性癌症死亡第 1 位的是肺癌，其次是肝癌、胃癌、食管癌和结直肠癌；女性癌症死亡第 1 位的是肺癌，其次为肝癌、胃癌、结直肠癌和乳腺癌（表 4-15，图 4-14a，图 4-14b）。

3.10 Top ten leading causes of cancer deaths in central registration areas of China

Lung cancer was the leading cause of cancer death in the central areas of China, followed by liver cancer, stomach cancer, esophageal cancer and colorectal cancer. In males, lung cancer was the leading cause of cancer death, followed by liver cancer, stomach cancer, esophageal cancer and colorectal cancer. In females, lung cancer was still the leading cause of cancer death, followed by liver cancer, stomach cancer, colorectal cancer and breast cancer (Table 4-15, Figure 4-14a, Figure 4-14b).

表 4-15 2017 年中国中部肿瘤登记地区前 10 位癌症死亡率

Table 4-15 Mortality rates of top ten leading cancer sites in central registration areas of China, 2017

单位：100 000⁻¹

顺位 Rank	合计 All				男性 Male				女性 Female			
	部位 Site	粗率 Crude rate	世标率 ASR World	中标率 ASR China	部位 Site	粗率 Crude rate	世标率 ASR World	中标率 ASR China	部位 Site	粗率 Crude rate	世标率 ASR World	中标率 ASR China
1	肺 Lung	45.01	28.88	28.89	肺 Lung	63.30	42.92	42.85	肺 Lung	25.89	15.43	15.51
2	肝 Liver	24.59	16.48	16.67	肝 Liver	34.56	24.25	24.57	肝 Liver	14.17	8.75	8.81
3	胃 Stomach	21.70	13.86	13.97	胃 Stomach	29.34	19.82	19.90	胃 Stomach	13.71	8.16	8.29
4	食管 Esophagus	13.80	8.73	8.70	食管 Esophagus	18.98	12.86	12.77	结直肠 Colon-rectum	9.99	5.96	6.09
5	结直肠 Colon-rectum	11.75	7.45	7.57	结直肠 Colon-rectum	13.43	9.04	9.14	乳腺 Breast	9.09	6.14	6.36
6	乳腺 Breast	9.09	6.14	6.36	胰腺 Pancreas	5.31	3.65	3.65	食管 Esophagus	8.39	4.76	4.78
7	子宫颈 Cervix	6.49	4.30	4.45	脑 Brain	4.10	3.13	3.14	子宫颈 Cervix	6.49	4.30	4.45
8	胰腺 Pancreas	4.69	3.04	3.05	淋巴瘤 Lymphoma	3.79	2.70	2.73	胰腺 Pancreas	4.03	2.44	2.46
9	脑 Brain	3.73	2.76	2.77	白血病 Leukemia	3.76	3.05	3.05	脑 Brain	3.34	2.39	2.40
10	前列腺 Prostate	3.45	2.16	2.13	前列腺 Prostate	3.45	2.16	2.13	卵巢 Ovary	3.23	2.17	2.20

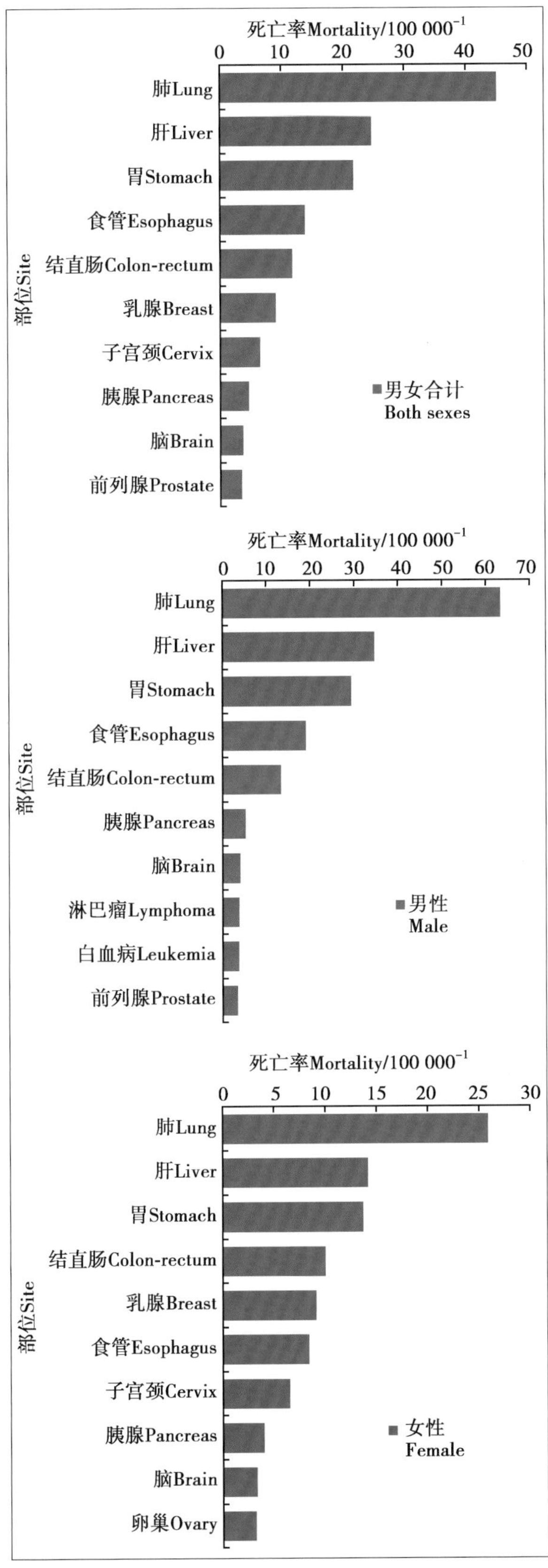

图 4-14a 2017 年中国中部肿瘤登记地区前 10 位癌症死亡率

Figure 4-14a Mortality rates of top ten leading cancer sites in central registration areas of China, 2017

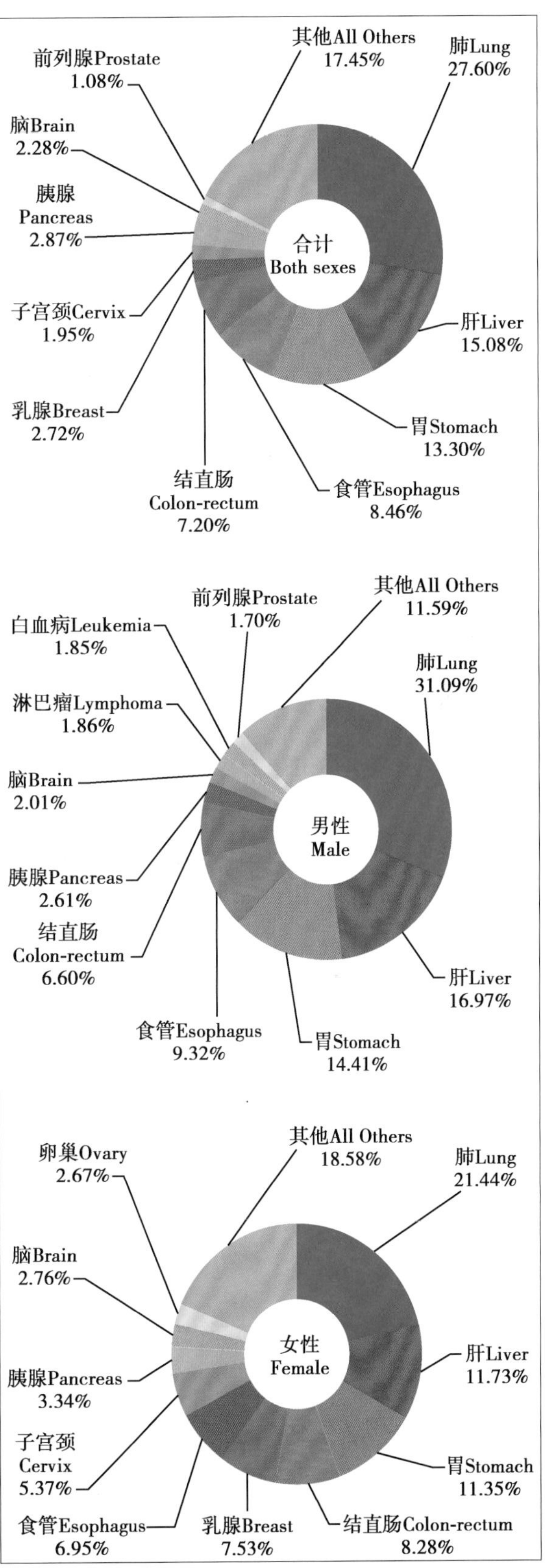

图 4-14b 2017 年中国中部肿瘤登记地区前 10 位癌症死亡构成

Figure 4-14b Distribution of top ten leading causes of cancer deaths in central registration areas of China, 2017

3.11 中国西部肿瘤登记地区前10位癌症发病情况

中国西部肿瘤登记地区合计发病第1位癌症为肺癌，其次为肝癌、女性乳腺癌、结直肠癌、胃癌。男性发病第1位癌症为肺癌，其次为肝癌、胃癌、食管癌和结直肠癌；女性发病第1位癌症为肺癌，其次为乳腺癌、结直肠癌、子宫颈癌和肝癌（表4-16，图4-15a，图4-15b）。

3.11 Top ten leading causes of new cancer cases in western registration areas of China

Lung cancer was the most common cancer in the western areas of China, followed by cancers of liver cancer, female breast cancer, colorectal cancer and stomach cancer. In males, lung cancer was the most common cancer, followed by liver cancer, stomach cancer, esophageal cancer and colorectal cancer. In females, lung cancer was the most common cancer, followed by breast cancer, colorectal cancer, cervical cancer and liver cancer (Table 4-16, Figure 4-15a, Figure 4-15b).

表4-16 2017年中国西部肿瘤登记地区前10位癌症发病率

Table 4-16 Incidence rates of top ten leading cancer sites in western registration areas of China, 2017

单位：100 000⁻¹

顺位 Rank	合计 All				男性 Male				女性 Female			
	部位 Site	粗率 Crude rate	世标率 ASR World	中标率 ASR China	部位 Site	粗率 Crude rate	世标率 ASR World	中标率 ASR China	部位 Site	粗率 Crude rate	世标率 ASR World	中标率 ASR China
1	肺 Lung	58.78	37.18	37.05	肺 Lung	79.24	51.49	51.10	肺 Lung	37.54	22.94	23.07
2	肝 Liver	31.15	20.47	20.95	肝 Liver	46.48	31.32	32.16	乳腺 Breast	29.67	20.27	21.77
3	乳腺 Breast	29.67	20.27	21.77	胃 Stomach	31.46	20.47	20.38	结直肠 Colon-rectum	21.04	13.02	13.29
4	结直肠 Colon-rectum	25.64	16.26	16.49	食管 Esophagus	30.86	20.12	19.73	子宫颈 Cervix	17.13	11.72	12.62
5	胃 Stomach	22.68	14.38	14.41	结直肠 Colon-rectum	30.08	19.54	19.74	肝 Liver	15.25	9.45	9.53
6	食管 Esophagus	20.12	12.70	12.49	前列腺 Prostate	8.82	5.23	5.30	胃 Stomach	13.58	8.30	8.46
7	子宫颈 Cervix	17.13	11.72	12.62	膀胱 Bladder	7.47	4.71	4.73	甲状腺 Thyroid	10.05	7.51	8.67
8	前列腺 Prostate	8.82	5.23	5.30	胰腺 Pancreas	6.79	4.39	4.40	食管 Esophagus	8.97	5.28	5.24
9	子宫体 Uterus	8.24	5.60	5.82	脑 Brain	6.60	5.01	5.15	子宫体 Uterus	8.24	5.60	5.82
10	卵巢 Ovary	6.90	4.84	5.11	鼻咽 Nasopharynx	6.07	4.24	4.54	脑 Brain	7.21	5.13	5.25

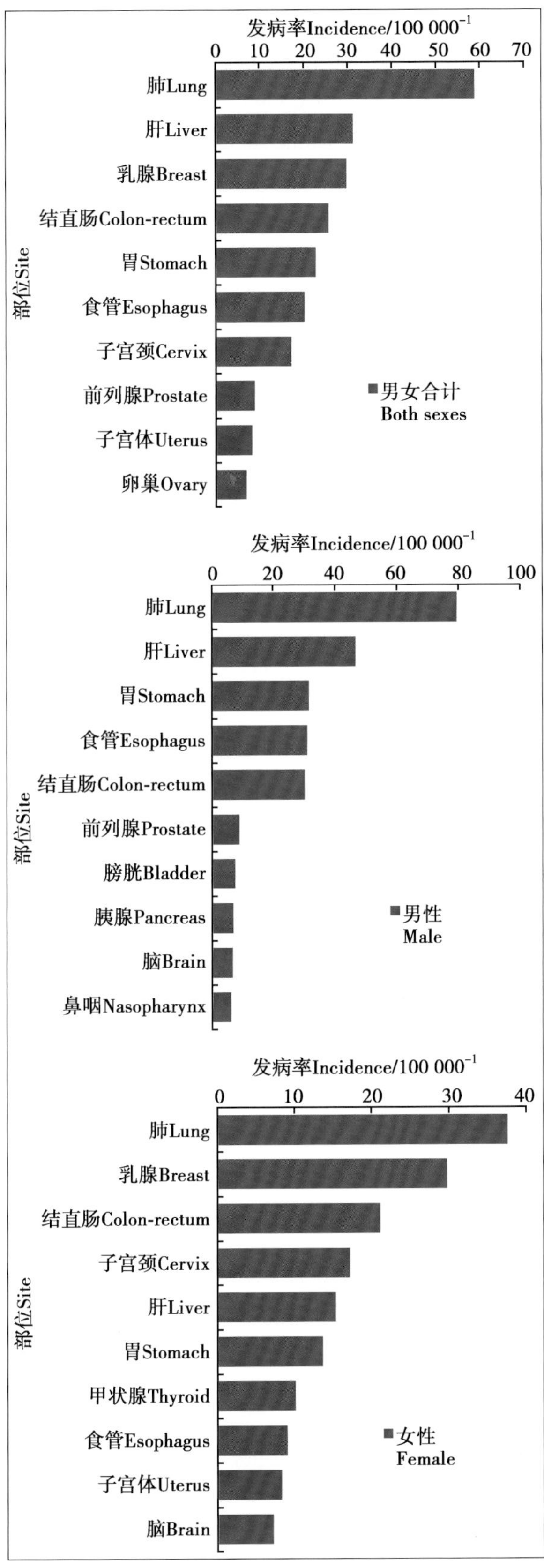

图 4-15a 2017 年中国西部肿瘤登记地区前 10 位癌症发病率

Figure 4-15a Incidence rates of top ten leading cancer sites in western registration areas of China,2017

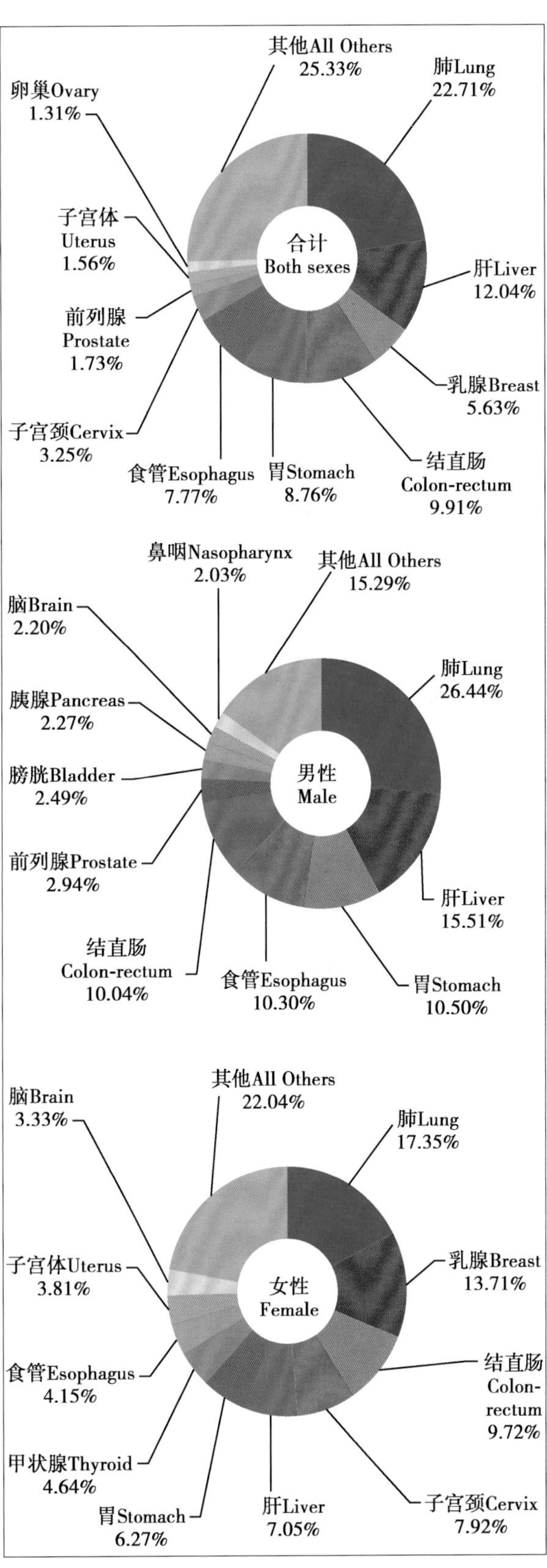

图 4-15b 2017 年中国西部肿瘤登记地区前 10 位癌症发病构成

Figure 4-15b Distribution of top ten leading causes of new cancer cases in western registration areas of China,2017

3.12 中国西部肿瘤登记地区前 10 位癌症死亡情况

中国西部肿瘤登记地区癌症死亡第 1 位的为肺癌，其次为肝癌、胃癌、食管癌和结直肠癌。男性癌症死亡第 1 位的是肺癌，其次是肝癌、胃癌、食管癌和结直肠癌；女性癌症死亡第 1 位的是肺癌，其次为肝癌、胃癌、结直肠癌和乳腺癌（表 4-17，图 4-16a，图 4-16b）。

3.12 Top ten leading causes of cancer deaths in western registration areas of China

Lung cancer was the leading cause of cancer death in the western areas of China, followed by liver cancer, stomach cancer, esophageal cancer and colorectal cancer. In males, lung cancer ranked as the leading cause of cancer death, followed by liver cancer, stomach cancer, esophageal cancer and colorectal cancer. In females, lung cancer was also the leading cause of cancer death, followed by liver cancer, stomach cancer, colorectal cancer and breast cancer (Table 4-17, Figure 4-16a, Figure 4-16b).

表 4-17 2017 年中国西部肿瘤登记地区前 10 位癌症死亡率

Table 4-17 Mortality rates of top ten leading cancer sites in western registration areas of China, 2017

单位：$100\ 000^{-1}$

顺位 Rank	合计 All				男性 Male				女性 Female			
	部位 Site	粗率 Crude rate	世标率 ASR World	中标率 ASR China	部位 Site	粗率 Crude rate	世标率 ASR World	中标率 ASR China	部位 Site	粗率 Crude rate	世标率 ASR World	中标率 ASR China
1	肺 Lung	46.85	29.09	28.92	肺 Lung	64.97	41.78	41.43	肺 Lung	28.05	16.54	16.53
2	肝 Liver	26.85	17.50	17.76	肝 Liver	39.72	26.64	27.14	肝 Liver	13.50	8.23	8.24
3	胃 Stomach	17.15	10.56	10.57	胃 Stomach	23.55	15.05	15.01	胃 Stomach	10.51	6.10	6.16
4	食管 Esophagus	15.36	9.44	9.33	食管 Esophagus	23.46	15.04	14.81	结直肠 Colon-rectum	10.03	5.83	5.90
5	结直肠 Colon-rectum	12.62	7.66	7.72	结直肠 Colon-rectum	15.12	9.57	9.59	乳腺 Breast	7.59	5.00	5.18
6	乳腺 Breast	7.59	5.00	5.18	胰腺 Pancreas	5.81	3.73	3.72	食管 Esophagus	6.96	3.90	3.88
7	子宫颈 Cervix	6.03	3.96	4.09	脑 Brain	4.53	3.35	3.38	子宫颈 Cervix	6.03	3.96	4.09
8	胰腺 Pancreas	4.97	3.07	3.07	前列腺 Prostate	3.98	2.36	2.31	胰腺 Pancreas	4.09	2.42	2.43
9	前列腺 Prostate	3.98	2.36	2.31	白血病 Leukemia	3.74	3.00	2.97	脑 Brain	3.37	2.37	2.37
10	脑 Brain	3.96	2.86	2.88	淋巴瘤 Lymphoma	3.38	2.31	2.34	卵巢 Ovary	2.85	1.87	1.92

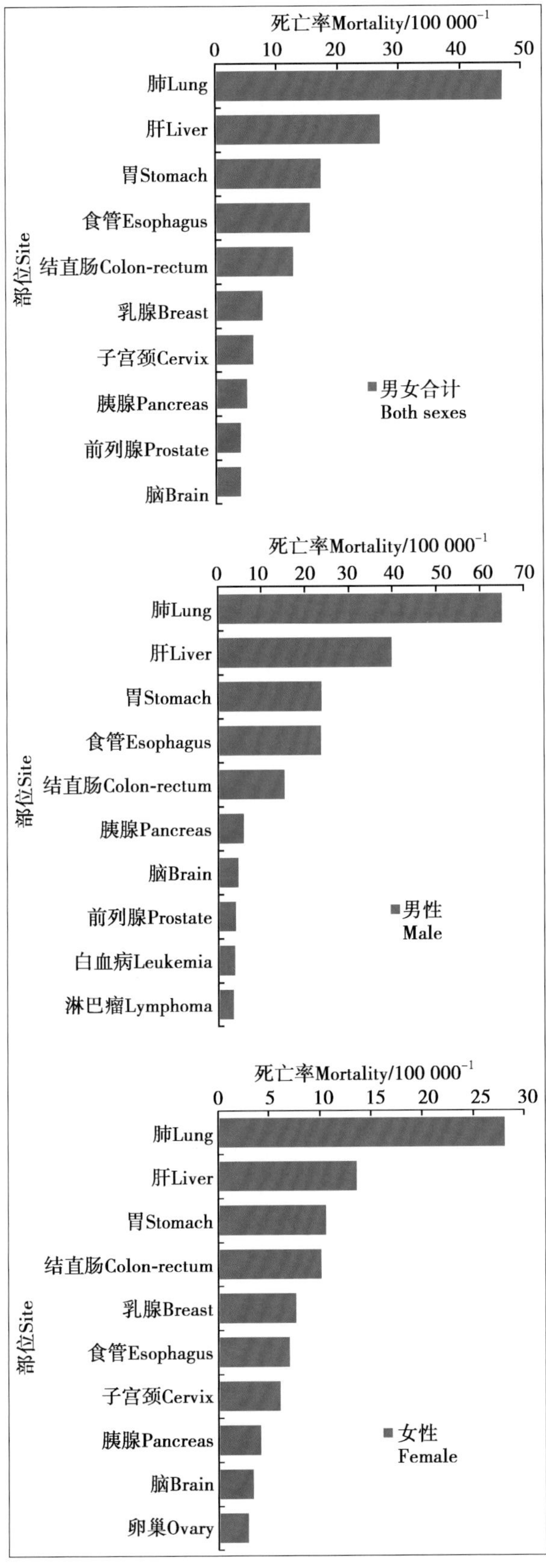

图 4-16a 2017 年中国西部肿瘤登记地区前 10 位癌症死亡率

Figure 4-16a Mortality rates of top ten leading cancer sites in western registration areas of China,2017

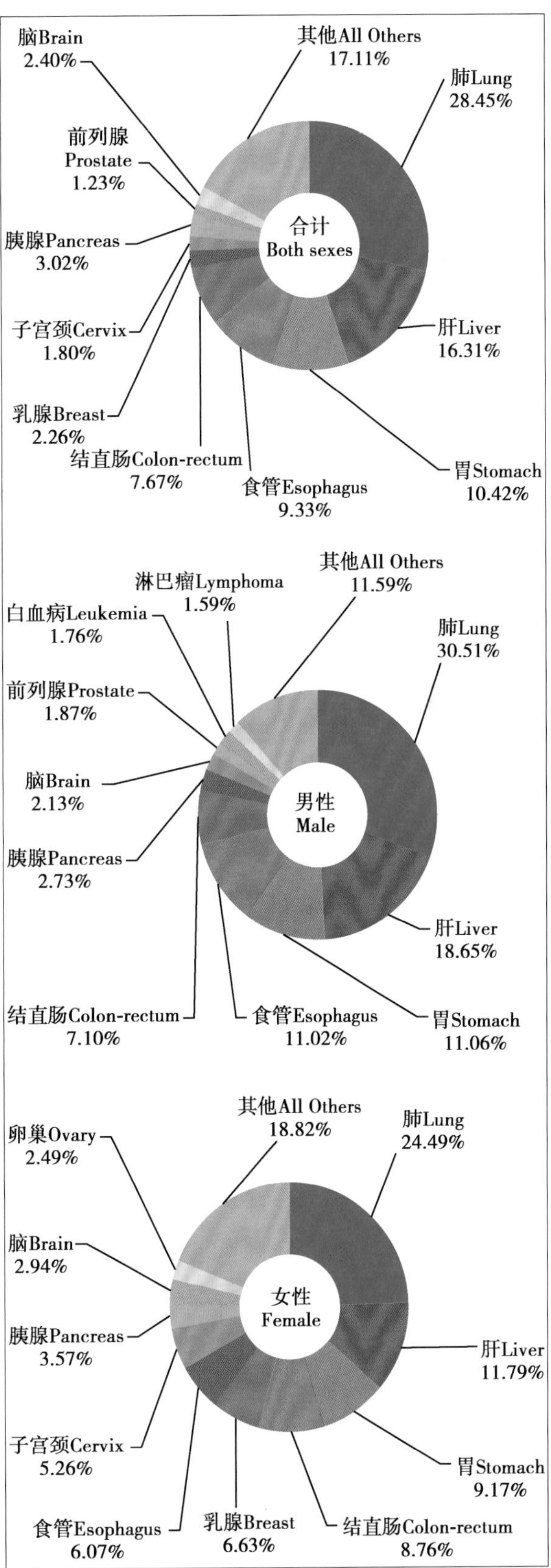

图 4-16b 2017 年中国西部肿瘤登记地区前 10 位癌症死亡构成

Figure 4-16b Distribution of top ten leading causes of cancer deaths in western registration areas of China,2017

第五章 各部位癌症的发病与死亡

Chapter 5 Cancer incidence and mortality by site

1 口腔和咽(除外鼻咽)

2017 年口腔癌和咽癌位居中国肿瘤登记地区癌症发病谱第 19 位。新发病例数为 16 597 例,占全部癌症发病的 1.30%;其中男性 11 524 例,女性 5 073 例,城市地区 9 146 例,农村地区 7 451 例。发病率为 3.80/10 万,中标发病率为 2.46/10 万,世标发病率为 2.42/10 万;男性中标发病率为女性的 2.27 倍,城市中标发病率为农村的 1.19 倍。0~74 岁累积发病率为 0.28%(表 5-1a)。

口腔癌和咽癌位居中国肿瘤登记地区癌症死亡谱第 17 位。口腔癌和咽癌死亡病例 8 752 例,占全部癌症死亡数的 1.13%;其中男性 6 401 例,女性 2 351 例,城市地区 4 659 例,农村地区 4 093 例。死亡率为 2.01/10 万,中标和世标死亡率均为 1.19/10 万;男性中标死亡率为女性的 2.98 倍,城市中标死亡率为农村的 1.09 倍。0~74 岁累积死亡率为 0.14%(表 5-1b)。

口腔癌和咽癌年龄别发病率和死亡率在 40 岁以前均处于较低水平,40 岁之后开始快速上升,男性上升速度快于女性。男性发病率在 80~84 岁组达到高峰,女性在 85 岁及以上年龄组达到高峰,死亡率均在 85 岁及以上年龄组达到高峰(图 5-1a)。

1 Oral cavity & pharynx(except nasopharynx)

Oral cavity and pharyngeal cancer were the 19th most common cancer in the registration areas of China in 2017. There were 16 597 new cases diagnosed as oral cavity and pharyngeal cancer(11 524 males and 5 073 females,9 146 in urban areas and 7 451 in rural areas), accounting for 1.30% of all new cancer cases. The crude incidence rate was 3.80 per 100 000, with ASR China 2.46 per 100 000 and ASR World 2.42 per 100 000,respectively. The incidence of ASR China was 2.27 times in males as that in females,and was 1.19 times in urban areas as that in rural areas. The cumulative incidence rate for subjects aged 0 to 74 years was 0.28%(Table 5-1a).

Oral cavity and pharyngeal cancer were the 17th most common cause of cancer deaths in the registration areas of China. A total of 8 752 cases died of oral cavity and pharyngeal cancer(6 401 males and 2 351 females,4 659 in urban areas and 4 093 in rural areas),accounting for 1.13% of all cancer deaths. The crude mortality rate was 2.01 per 100 000,with ASR China 1.19 per 100 000 and the same as ASR World. The mortality of ASR China was 2.98 times in males as that in females,and was 1.09 times in urban areas as that in rural areas. The cumulative mortality rate for subjects aged 0 to 74 years was 0.14%(Table 5-1b).

The age-specific incidence and mortality rates for oral cavity and pharyngeal cancer were low before 40 years old, but increased sharply thereafter. The age-specific rates increased faster in males than that in females. The age-specific incidence rates were the highest in the age group of 80-84 years in males and 85+ years in females, and the mortality rates peaked at the age group of 85+ years for both sexes (Figure 5-1a).

城市地区口腔癌和咽癌发病和死亡率均略高于农村。东中西部地区间差异不大，男性中标发病率中部地区最高，中标死亡率西部和中部地区最高，女性东部地区中标发病率最高，西部地区死亡率最高。在七大行政区中，男性和女性口腔癌和咽癌的中标发病率均在华南地区最高，中标死亡率男性在东北地区最高，女性在西北地区最高（表 5-1a，表 5-1b，图 5-1b）。

全部口腔癌和咽癌新发病例中，有明确亚部位病例数占 93.63%，其中口腔是最常见的发病部位，占 28.05%；其次是舌、唾液腺和下咽，分别占全部口腔癌和咽癌的 21.07%、15.66% 和 12.89%（图 5-1c）。

The incidence and mortality rates of oral cavity and pharyngeal cancer were slightly higher in urban areas than that in rural areas. The incidence rate (ASR China) was the highest in the central areas in males, and the mortality rate (ASR China) were the highest in the western and central areas in males. The incidence and mortality (ASR China) were the highest in the eastern areas and western areas in females, respectively. Among the seven administrative districts, the incidence rates (ASR China) were the highest in South China for both sexes, and the mortality rates (ASR China) were the highest in Northeast China in males and in Northwest China in females, respectively (Table 5-1a, Table 5-1b, Figure 5-1b).

There were 93.63% of oral cavity and pharyngeal cancer cases having specific subsite information. The proportions for cancers of mouth, tongue, salivary glands, and hypopharynx were 28.05%, 21.07%, 15.66%, and 12.89%, respectively (Figure 5-1c).

表 5-1a　2017 年中国肿瘤登记地区口腔癌和咽癌发病情况

Table 5-1a　Incidence of oral cavity and pharyngeal cancer in the registration areas of China,2017

地区 Area	性别 Sex	病例数 No. cases	粗率 Crude rate/ 100 000⁻¹	构成比 Freq./%	中标率 ASR China/ 100 000⁻¹	世标率 ASR World/ 100 000⁻¹	累积率 Cum. rate 0~74/%	顺位 Rank
合计	合计 Both	16 597	3.80	1.30	2.46	2.42	0.28	19
All	男性 Male	11 524	5.21	1.62	3.43	3.39	0.40	14
	女性 Female	5 073	2.36	0.89	1.51	1.46	0.16	18
城市地区	合计 Both	9 146	4.29	1.36	2.67	2.63	0.30	19
Urban areas	男性 Male	6 361	5.94	1.74	3.75	3.72	0.43	14
	女性 Female	2 785	2.62	0.90	1.62	1.56	0.17	18
农村地区	合计 Both	7 451	3.34	1.23	2.25	2.21	0.26	20
Rural areas	男性 Male	5 163	4.52	1.49	3.09	3.06	0.36	13
	女性 Female	2 288	2.10	0.88	1.40	1.35	0.15	18
东部地区	合计 Both	8 195	4.14	1.24	2.48	2.44	0.28	19
Eastern areas	男性 Male	5 572	5.60	1.56	3.40	3.38	0.40	14
	女性 Female	2 623	2.67	0.86	1.59	1.52	0.17	18
中部地区	合计 Both	4 023	3.50	1.34	2.52	2.46	0.28	18
Central areas	男性 Male	2 853	4.85	1.71	3.58	3.50	0.40	12
	女性 Female	1 170	2.08	0.87	1.46	1.41	0.16	17
西部地区	合计 Both	4 379	3.55	1.37	2.38	2.35	0.27	18
Western areas	男性 Male	3 099	4.93	1.65	3.32	3.30	0.39	13
	女性 Female	1 280	2.11	0.98	1.44	1.40	0.15	18

表 5-1b　2017 年中国肿瘤登记地区口腔癌和咽癌死亡情况

Table 5-1b　Mortality of oral cavity and pharyngeal cancer in the registration areas of China,2017

地区 Area	性别 Sex	死亡数 No. deaths	粗率 Crude rate/ 100 000⁻¹	构成比 Freq./%	中标率 ASR China/ 100 000⁻¹	世标率 ASR World/ 100 000⁻¹	累积率 Cum. rate 0~74/%	顺位 Rank
合计	合计 Both	8 752	2.01	1.13	1.19	1.19	0.14	17
All	男性 Male	6 401	2.89	1.29	1.79	1.80	0.21	12
	女性 Female	2 351	1.09	0.84	0.60	0.59	0.06	18
城市	合计 Both	4 659	2.18	1.21	1.24	1.24	0.14	18
Urban areas	男性 Male	3 413	3.19	1.39	1.89	1.90	0.22	13
	女性 Female	1 246	1.17	0.88	0.61	0.60	0.06	17
农村	合计 Both	4 093	1.83	1.06	1.14	1.13	0.13	17
Rural areas	男性 Male	2 988	2.62	1.20	1.70	1.69	0.20	12
	女性 Female	1 105	1.01	0.80	0.59	0.58	0.06	18
东部地区	合计 Both	4 263	2.15	1.12	1.15	1.15	0.13	18
Eastern areas	男性 Male	3 073	3.09	1.28	1.74	1.75	0.20	14
	女性 Female	1 190	1.21	0.84	0.58	0.57	0.06	17
中部地区	合计 Both	2 059	1.79	1.10	1.21	1.19	0.14	17
Central areas	男性 Male	1 537	2.61	1.28	1.84	1.82	0.22	12
	女性 Female	522	0.93	0.77	0.58	0.56	0.06	19
西部地区	合计 Both	2 430	1.97	1.20	1.25	1.25	0.14	18
Western areas	男性 Male	1 791	2.85	1.34	1.84	1.87	0.22	13
	女性 Female	639	1.06	0.92	0.65	0.64	0.07	17

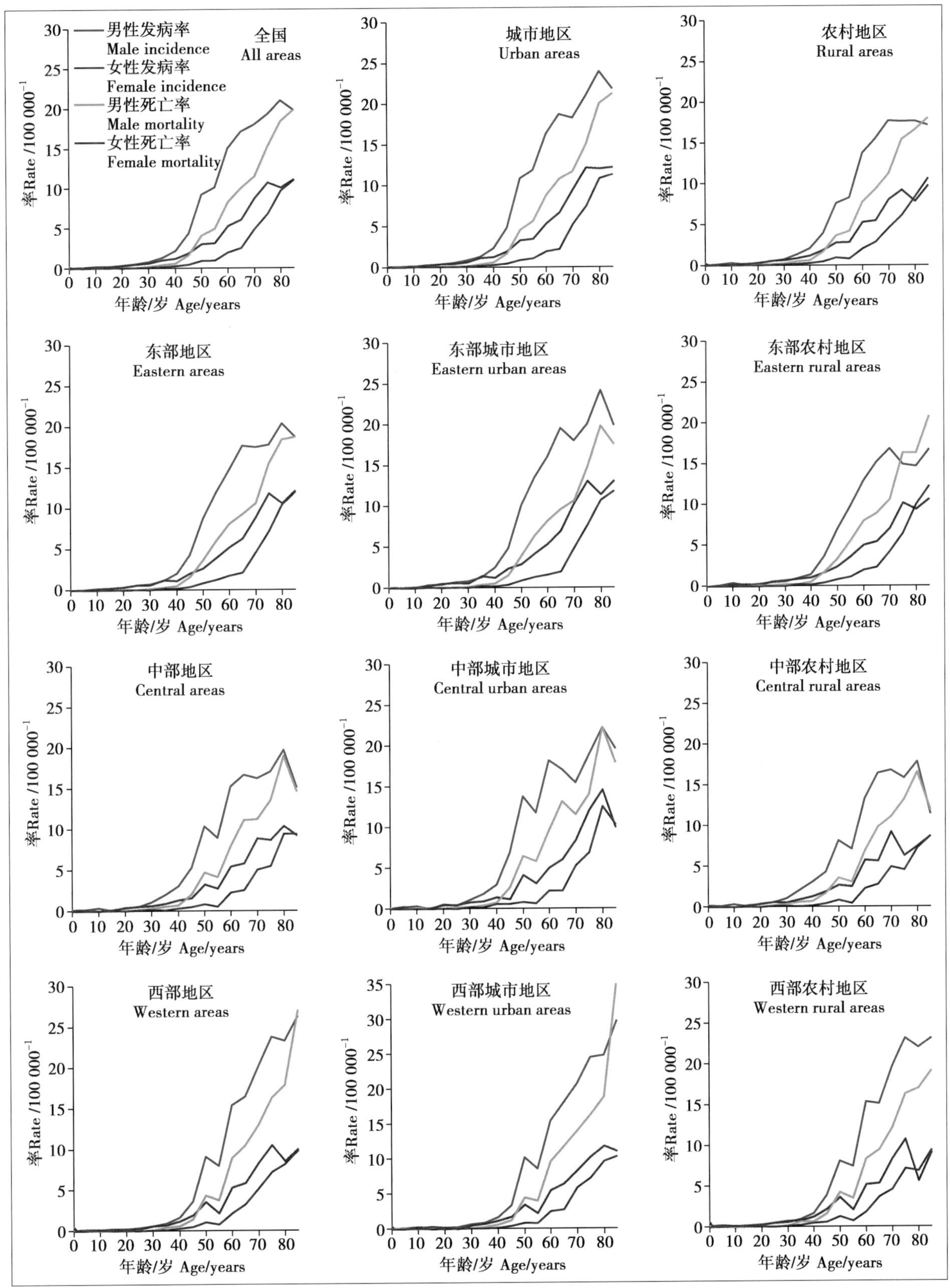

图 5-1a 2017 年中国肿瘤登记地区口腔癌和咽癌年龄别发病率和死亡率

Figure 5-1a Age-specific incidence and mortality rates of oral cavity and pharyngeal cancer in the registration areas of China, 2017

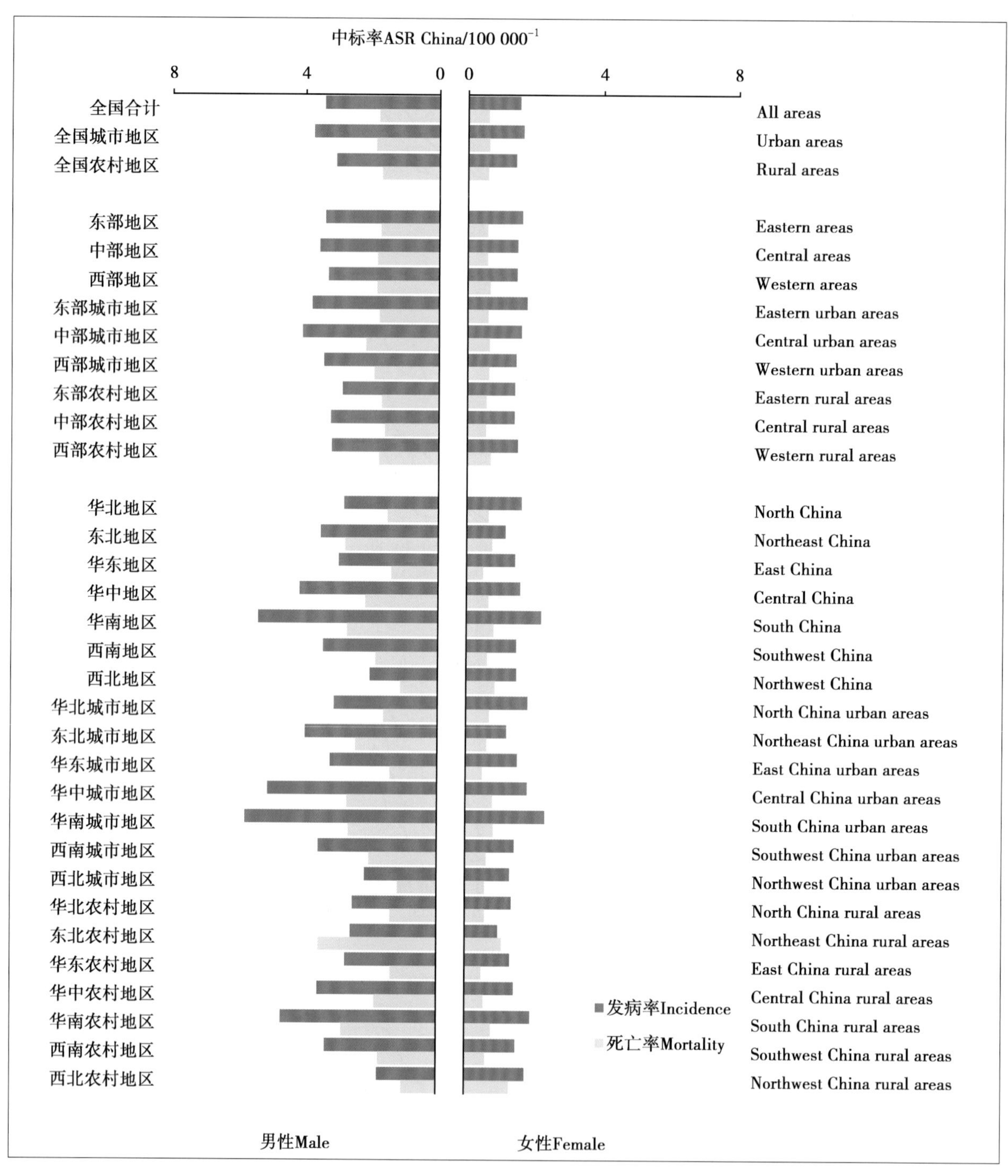

图 5-1b　2017 年中国肿瘤登记不同地区口腔癌和咽癌发病率和死亡率

Figure 5-1b　Incidence and mortality rates of oral cavity and pharyngeal cancer in different registration areas of China, 2017

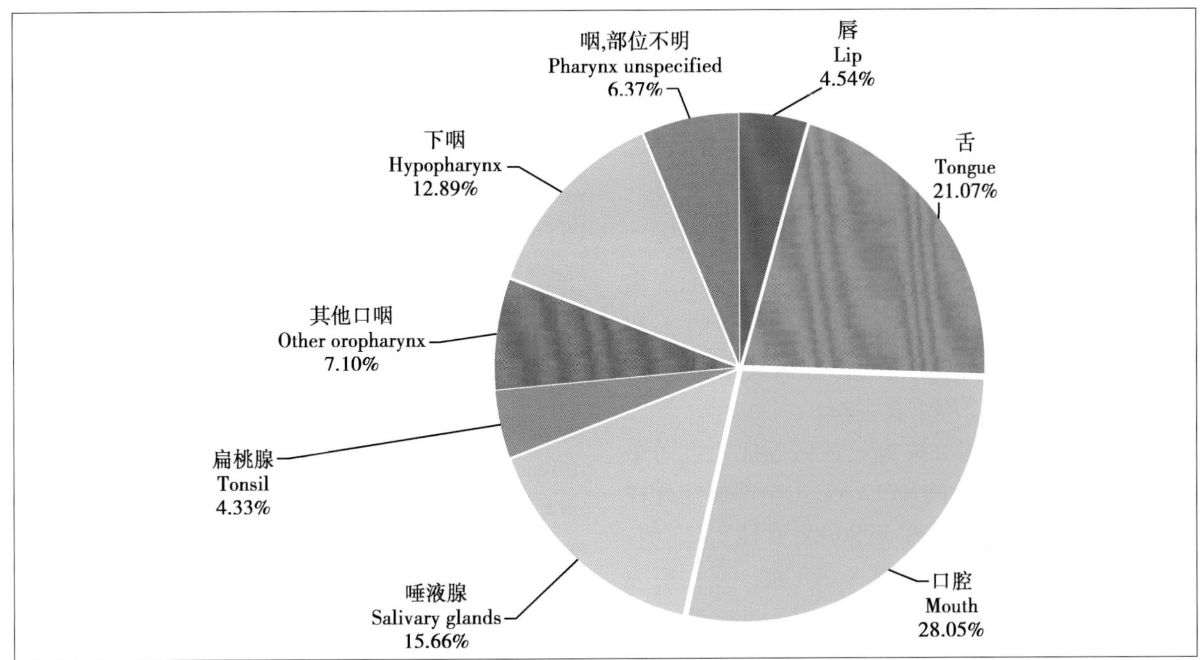

图 5-1c　2017 年中国肿瘤登记地区口腔癌和咽癌亚部位分布

Figure 5-1c　Subsite distribution of oral cavity and pharyngeal cancer in the registration areas of China,2017

2 鼻咽

2017 年鼻咽癌位居中国肿瘤登记地区癌症发病谱第 20 位。新发病例 15 838 例，占全部癌症发病的 1. 24%。其中男性 11 185 例，女性 4 653 例；城市地区 7 940 例，农村地区 7 898 例。发病率为 3. 63/10 万，中标发病率为 2. 64/10 万，世标发病率为 2. 47/10 万；男性中标发病率为女性的 2. 38 倍，城市地区中标发病率与农村地区接近。0～74 岁累积发病率为 0. 27%（表 5-2a）。

鼻咽癌位居中国肿瘤登记地区癌症死亡谱第 19 位。鼻咽癌死亡病例 8 212 例，占全部癌症死亡人数的 1. 06%。其中男性 5 990 例，女性 2 222 例；城市地区 4 134 例，农村地区 4 078 例。死亡率为 1. 88/10 万，中标死亡率 1. 24/10 万，世标死亡率 1. 20/10 万；男性中标死亡率为女性的 2. 79 倍，城市地区中标死亡率与农村地区接近。0～74 岁累积死亡率为 0. 14%（表 5-2b）。

鼻咽癌年龄别发病率和死亡率男性明显高于女性。发病率在 20 岁之前处于较低水平，20 岁以后开始快速上升，在 55～59 岁组有所下降，随后上升，男性和女性均在 65～69 岁组出现最高峰，随后下降。鼻咽癌年龄别死亡率男性和女性 30 岁之前均处于较低水平，随后快速上升，男性 75～79 岁组达到高峰，女性 85+岁组达到高峰（图 5-2a）。

城市鼻咽癌发病率和死亡率与农村接近。中标发病率和死亡率均是西部地区最高，东部和中部地区相似。在七大行政区中，华南地区发病率和死亡率均最高，华北地区最低（表 5-2a，表 5-2b，图 5-2b）。

2 Nasopharynx

Nasopharyngeal cancer was the 20th most common cancer in the registration areas of China in 2017. There were 15 838 new cases of nasopharyngeal cancer (11 185 males and 4 653 females, 7 940 in urban areas and 7 898 in rural areas), accounting for 1. 24% of all new cancer cases. The crude incidence rate was 3. 63 per 100 000, with ASR China 2. 64 per 100 000 and ASR World 2. 47 per 100 000, respectively. The incidence of ASR China in males was 2. 38 times as that in females, while in urban areas it was close to that in rural areas. The cumulative incidence rate for subjects aged 0 to 74 years was 0. 27% (Table 5-2a).

Nasopharyngeal cancer was the 19th most common cause of cancer deaths. A total of 8 212 cases died of nasopharyngeal cancer (5 990 males and 2 222 females, 4 134 in urban areas and 4 078 in rural areas), accounting for 1. 06% of all cancer deaths. The crude mortality rate was 1. 88 per 100 000, with ASR China 1. 24 per 100 000 and ASR World 1. 20 per 100 000, respectively. The ASR China in males was 2. 79 times as that in females, while in urban areas it was close to that in rural areas. The cumulative mortality rate for subjects aged 0 to 74 years was 0. 14% (Table 5-2b).

The age-specific incidence and mortality rates of nasopharyngeal cancer were higher in males than that in females. For both sexes, the age-specific incidence rates were low before 20 years old but increased sharply since then, until the age group of 50-54 years. The incidence rates slightly decreased at the age group of 55-59 years, then increased to the peak age group of 65-69 years for both sexes, and declined afterwards. For both sexes, the age-specific mortality rates were low before 30 years old and increased fast thereafter, with a peak age group of 75-79 years in males and 85+ years in females (Figure 5-2a).

The incidence and mortality rates of nasopharyngeal cancer in urban areas were closed to that in rural areas. The incidence and mortality rates (ASR China) were the highest in the western areas, and similar in the eastern and central areas. Among the seven administrative districts, the incidence and mortality rates (ASR China) were the highest in South China and the lowest in North China (Table 5-2a, Table 5-2b, Figure 5-2b).

表 5-2a　2017 年中国肿瘤登记地区鼻咽癌发病情况

Table 5-2a　Incidence of nasopharyngeal cancer in the registration areas of China, 2017

地区 Area	性别 Sex	病例数 No. cases	粗率 Crude rate/ $100\ 000^{-1}$	构成比 Freq./%	中标率 ASR China/ $100\ 000^{-1}$	世标率 ASR World/ $100\ 000^{-1}$	累积率 Cum. rate 0~74/%	顺位 Rank
合计	合计 Both	15 838	3. 63	1. 24	2. 64	2. 47	0. 27	20
All	男性 Male	11 185	5. 06	1. 57	3. 72	3. 47	0. 38	15
	女性 Female	4 653	2. 16	0. 82	1. 57	1. 45	0. 16	19
城市地区	合计 Both	7 940	3. 72	1. 18	2. 66	2. 48	0. 27	20
Urban areas	男性 Male	5 651	5. 28	1. 55	3. 80	3. 54	0. 39	15
	女性 Female	2 289	2. 15	0. 74	1. 53	1. 42	0. 15	19
农村地区	合计 Both	7 898	3. 54	1. 30	2. 63	2. 46	0. 26	18
Rural areas	男性 Male	5 534	4. 85	1. 60	3. 64	3. 41	0. 37	12
	女性 Female	2 364	2. 17	0. 91	1. 60	1. 49	0. 16	17
东部地区	合计 Both	6 876	3. 47	1. 04	2. 48	2. 29	0. 24	20
Eastern areas	男性 Male	4 908	4. 93	1. 38	3. 53	3. 27	0. 35	15
	女性 Female	1 968	2. 00	0. 65	1. 44	1. 31	0. 14	19
中部地区	合计 Both	3 499	3. 04	1. 16	2. 31	2. 18	0. 24	20
Central areas	男性 Male	2 462	4. 19	1. 47	3. 22	3. 06	0. 34	15
	女性 Female	1 037	1. 84	0. 77	1. 38	1. 30	0. 14	19
西部地区	合计 Both	5 463	4. 43	1. 71	3. 28	3. 07	0. 33	17
Western areas	男性 Male	3 815	6. 07	2. 03	4. 54	4. 24	0. 46	10
	女性 Female	1 648	2. 72	1. 26	1. 99	1. 88	0. 20	16

表 5-2b　2017 年中国肿瘤登记地区鼻咽癌死亡情况

Table 5-2b　Mortality of nasopharyngeal cancer in the registration areas of China, 2017

地区 Area	性别 Sex	死亡数 No. deaths	粗率 Crude rate/ $100\ 000^{-1}$	构成比 Freq./%	中标率 ASR China/ $100\ 000^{-1}$	世标率 ASR World/ $100\ 000^{-1}$	累积率 Cum. rate 0~74/%	顺位 Rank
合计	合计 Both	8 212	1. 88	1. 06	1. 24	1. 20	0. 14	19
All	男性 Male	5 990	2. 71	1. 21	1. 83	1. 77	0. 21	14
	女性 Female	2 222	1. 03	0. 80	0. 65	0. 63	0. 07	19
城市地区	合计 Both	4 134	1. 94	1. 07	1. 23	1. 20	0. 14	19
Urban areas	男性 Male	3 054	2. 85	1. 25	1. 87	1. 81	0. 21	15
	女性 Female	1 080	1. 02	0. 76	0. 61	0. 59	0. 07	18
农村地区	合计 Both	4 078	1. 83	1. 05	1. 24	1. 20	0. 14	18
Rural areas	男性 Male	2 936	2. 57	1. 18	1. 79	1. 74	0. 20	13
	女性 Female	1 142	1. 05	0. 83	0. 69	0. 67	0. 08	16
东部地区	合计 Both	3 808	1. 92	1. 00	1. 19	1. 15	0. 14	19
Eastern areas	男性 Male	2 852	2. 87	1. 18	1. 81	1. 76	0. 21	15
	女性 Female	956	0. 97	0. 68	0. 58	0. 55	0. 06	19
中部地区	合计 Both	1 808	1. 57	0. 96	1. 11	1. 08	0. 13	18
Central areas	男性 Male	1 281	2. 18	1. 07	1. 60	1. 55	0. 18	14
	女性 Female	527	0. 94	0. 78	0. 63	0. 61	0. 07	18
西部地区	合计 Both	2 596	2. 10	1. 28	1. 45	1. 41	0. 16	16
Western areas	男性 Male	1 857	2. 96	1. 39	2. 05	2. 00	0. 23	12
	女性 Female	739	1. 22	1. 07	0. 83	0. 81	0. 09	15

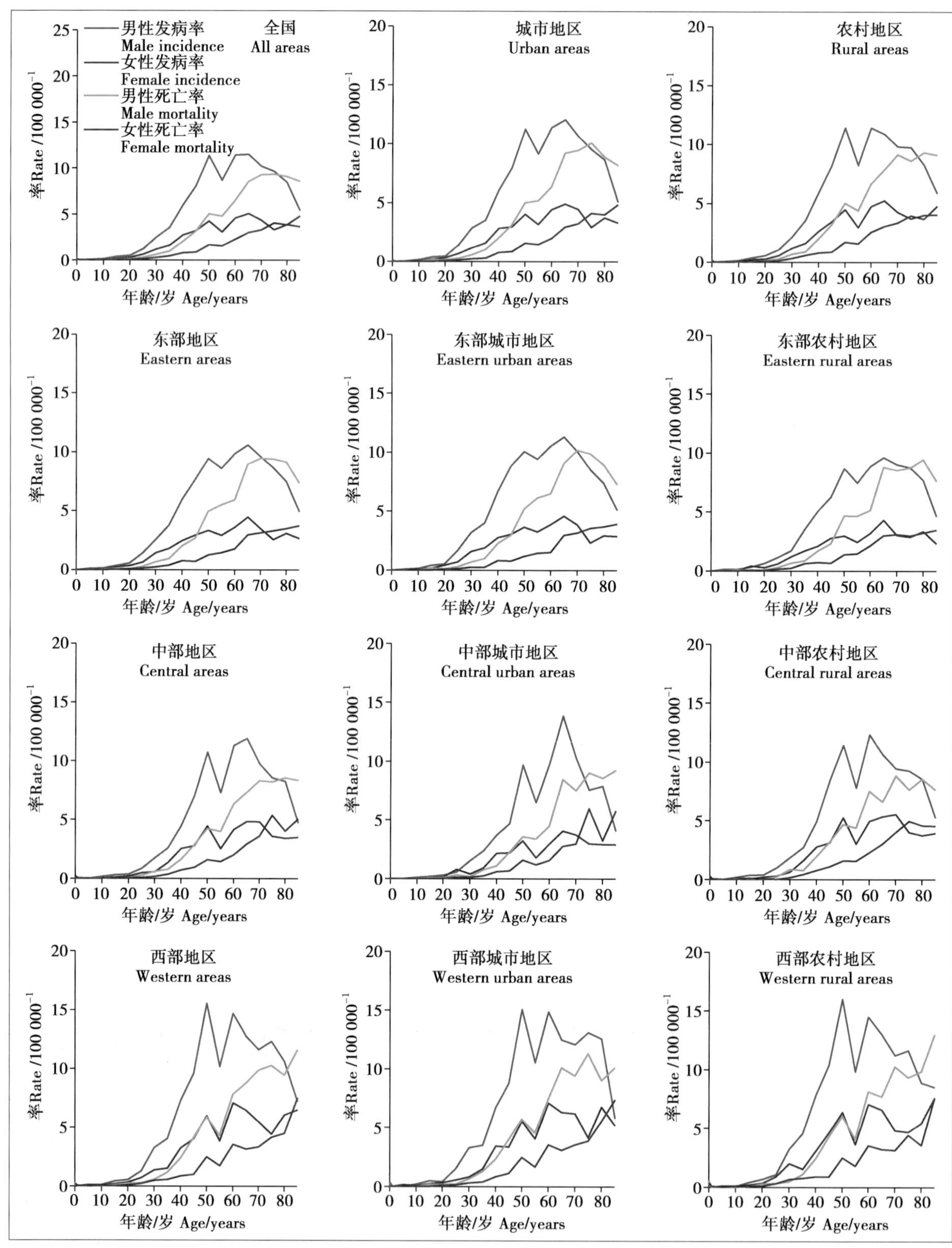

图 5-2a 2017 年中国肿瘤登记地区鼻咽癌年龄别发病率和死亡率

Figure 5-2a Age-specific incidence and mortality rates of nasopharyngeal cancer in the registration areas of China, 2017

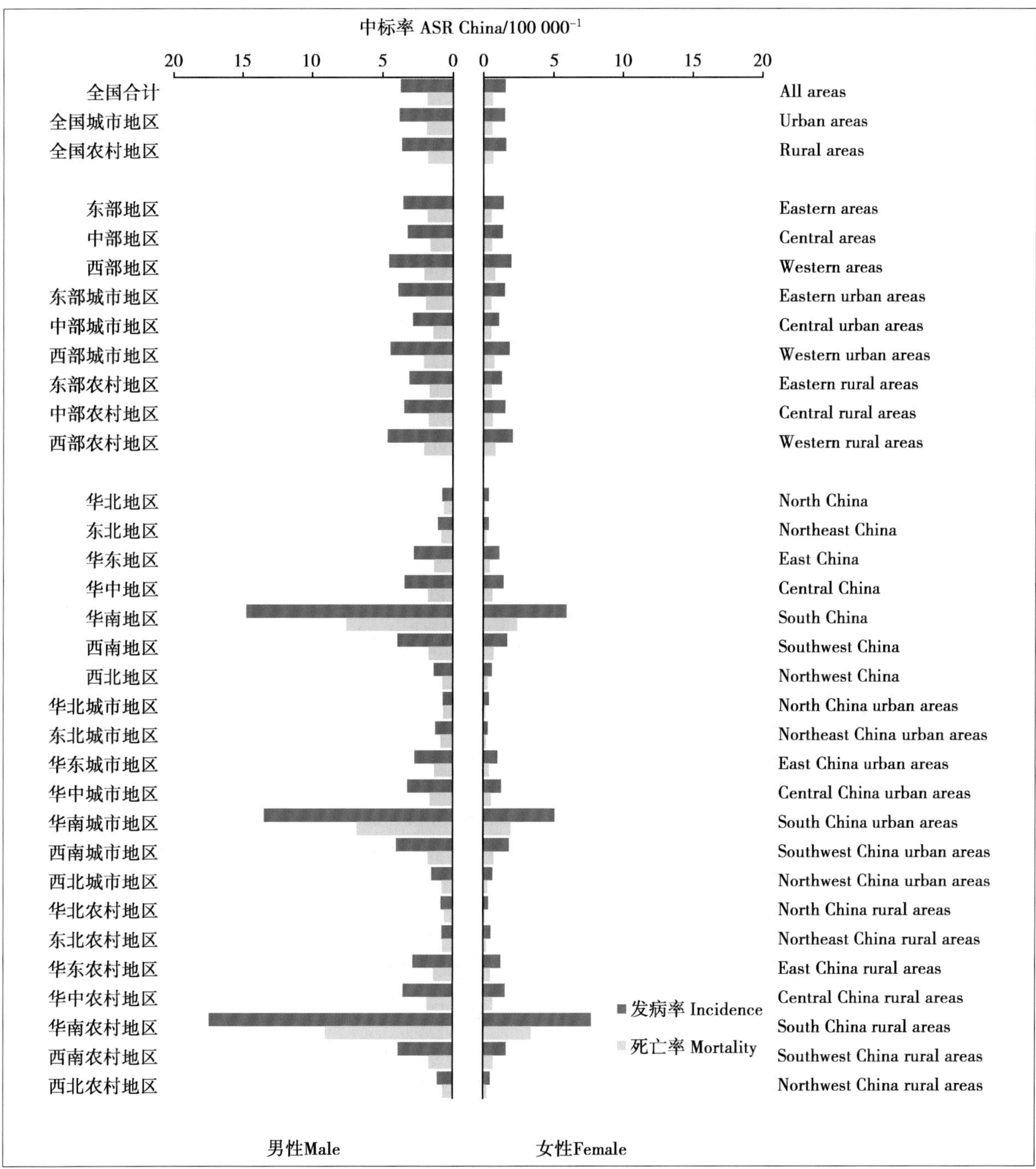

图 5-2b 2017 年中国肿瘤登记不同地区鼻咽癌发病率和死亡率
Figure 5-2b Incidence and mortality rates of nasopharyngeal cancer in different registration areas of China,2017

3 食管

2017 年中国肿瘤登记地区食管癌位居癌症发病谱第 6 位。新发病例数为 83 901 例,占全部癌症发病的 6.55%;其中男性 61 585 例,女性 22 316 例,城市地区 31 690 例,农村地区 52 211 例。食管癌发病率为 19.23/10 万,中标发病率为 11.14/10 万,世标发病率为 11.25/10 万;男性中标发病率为女性的 3.05 倍,农村中标发病率为城市的 1.69 倍。0~74 岁累积发病率为 1.43%(表 5-3a)。

2017 年中国肿瘤登记地区食管癌位居癌症死亡谱第 4 位。食管癌死亡病例 66 371 例,占全部癌症死亡的 8.59%;其中男性 48 719 例,女性 17 652 例,城市地区 25 601 例,农村地区 40 770 例。食管癌死亡率为 15.21/10 万,中标死亡率 8.53/10 万,世标死亡率 8.55/10 万;男性中标死亡率为女性的 3.20 倍,农村中标死亡率为城市的 1.64 倍。0~74 岁累积死亡率为 1.02%(表 5-3b)。

食管癌年龄别发病率和死亡率在 40 岁之前处于较低水平,自 40 岁之后快速上升。男女发病率均于 80~84 岁达到高峰,死亡率均在 85 岁之后达到高峰。男性各年龄别发病率和死亡率均明显高于女性(图 5-3a)。

3 Esophagus

Esophageal cancer was the 6th most common cancer in the registration areas of China in 2017. There were 83 901 new cases of esophageal cancer(61 585 males and 22 316 females, 31 690 in urban areas and 52 211 in rural areas), accounting for 6.55% of new cases of all cancers. The crude incidence rate was 19.23 per 100 000, with ASR China 11.14 per 100 000 and ASR World 11.25 per 100 000, respectively. Subgroup analyses showed that the incidence of ASR China was 3.05 times in males as that in females, and was 1.69 times in rural areas as that in urban areas. The cumulative incidence rate for subjects aged 0 to 74 years was 1.43%(Table 5-3a).

Esophageal cancer was the 4th most common cause of cancer deaths in the registration areas of China in 2017. A total of 66 371 cases died of esophageal cancer(48 719 males and 17 652 females, 25 601 in urban areas and 40 770 in rural areas), accounting for 8.59% of all cancer deaths. The crude mortality rate was 15.21 per 100 000, with ASR China 8.53 per 100 000 and ASR World 8.55 per 100 000, respectively. Subgroup analyses showed that the mortality of ASR China was 3.20 times in males as that in females, and was 1.64 times in rural areas as that in urban areas. The cumulative mortality rate for subjects aged 0 to 74 years was 1.02%(Table 5-3b).

The age-specific incidence and mortality rates of esophageal cancer were relatively low before 40 years old and increased dramatically since then. The age-specific incidence rates were the highest in the age group of 80-84 years for both sexes. The mortality rates peaked in age group of 85+ years for both sexes. The age-specific incidence and mortality rates were generally higher in males than those in females (Figure 5-3a).

农村食管癌的发病率和死亡率均高于城市。男性中标发病率和死亡率西部地区最高，东部地区最低，女性中标发病率和死亡率在中部地区最高，发病率东部地区最低，死亡率西部地区最低。七大行政区中，男性中标发病率在西南地区最高，东北地区最低，死亡率在华东地区最高，华南地区最低；女性中标发病率和死亡率在华中地区最高，东北地区最低(表 5-3a，表 5-3b，图 5-3b)。

食管癌病例中有明确亚部位信息的占 31.61%，其中 46.78%的病例发生在食管中段，其次是食管上段占 24.15%，食管癌下段占 21.61%，交搭跨越占 7.46%(图 5-3c)。

全部食管癌病例中有明确组织学类型的病例占 66.12%，其中鳞状细胞癌是最主要的病理类型，占 84.20%；其次是腺癌，占 10.96%；腺鳞癌占 1.14%(图 5-3d)。

The incidence and mortality rates of esophageal cancer were higher in rural areas than those in urban areas. The incidence and mortality rates (ASR China) in males were the highest in the western areas and the lowest in eastern areas. The incidence and mortality rates (ASR China) in females were the highest in the central areas, and the lowest in the eastern and western areas, respectively. Among the seven administrative districts, the incidence rates (ASR China) in males were the highest in Southwest China and the lowest in Northeast China, and the mortality rates (ASR China) were the highest in East China and the lowest in South China. The incidence and mortality rates (ASR China) in females were the highest in Central China and the lowest in Northeast China (Table 5-3a, Table 5-3b, Figure 5-3b).

There were 31.61% of esophageal cancer cases having specific subsite information. Esophageal cancer occurred most frequently in the middle third of the esophagus (46.78%), followed by upper third (24.15%), lower third (21.61%) and overlapping esophagus (7.46%) (Figure 5-3c).

About 66.12% of the esophageal cancer cases had morphological verification. Among those, esophageal squamous cell carcinoma was the most common type, accounting for 84.20% of all cases, followed by adenocarcinoma (10.96%) and adenosquamous carcinoma (1.14%) (Figure 5-3d).

表 5-3a 2017 年中国肿瘤登记地区食管癌发病情况

Table 5-3a Incidence of esophageal cancer in the registration areas of China, 2017

地区 Area	性别 Sex	病例数 No. cases	粗率 Crude rate/ $100\ 000^{-1}$	构成比 Freq./%	中标率 ASR China/ $100\ 000^{-1}$	世标率 ASR World/ $100\ 000^{-1}$	累积率 Cum. rate 0~74/%	顺位 Rank
合计	合计 Both	83 901	19.23	6.55	11.14	11.25	1.43	6
All	男性 Male	61 585	27.85	8.65	16.91	17.14	2.20	5
	女性 Female	22 316	10.37	3.92	5.54	5.52	0.67	8
城市地区	合计 Both	31 690	14.86	4.70	8.31	8.40	1.06	9
Urban areas	男性 Male	24 082	22.50	6.60	13.18	13.38	1.71	5
	女性 Female	7 608	7.16	2.46	3.65	3.63	0.43	11
农村地区	合计 Both	52 211	23.40	8.60	14.02	14.16	1.80	6
Rural areas	男性 Male	37 503	32.86	10.82	20.65	20.93	2.68	4
	女性 Female	14 708	13.50	5.64	7.49	7.48	0.91	8
东部地区	合计 Both	38 097	19.25	5.77	10.07	10.14	1.28	7
Eastern areas	男性 Male	27 629	27.77	7.75	15.34	15.52	1.96	5
	女性 Female	10 468	10.64	3.44	5.05	5.01	0.60	9
中部地区	合计 Both	20 990	18.24	6.97	11.87	11.97	1.52	7
Central areas	男性 Male	14 574	24.78	8.72	16.96	17.16	2.20	5
	女性 Female	6 416	11.40	4.78	6.89	6.89	0.84	8
西部地区	合计 Both	24 814	20.12	7.77	12.49	12.70	1.64	6
Western areas	男性 Male	19 382	30.86	10.30	19.73	20.12	2.61	4
	女性 Female	5 432	8.97	4.15	5.24	5.28	0.65	8

表 5-3b 2017 年中国肿瘤登记地区食管癌死亡情况

Table 5-3b Mortality of esophageal cancer in the registration areas of China, 2017

地区 Area	性别 Sex	死亡数 No. deaths	粗率 Crude rate/ $100\ 000^{-1}$	构成比 Freq./%	中标率 ASR China/ $100\ 000^{-1}$	世标率 ASR World/ $100\ 000^{-1}$	累积率 Cum. rate 0~74/%	顺位 Rank
合计	合计 Both	66 371	15.21	8.59	8.53	8.55	1.02	4
All	男性 Male	48 719	22.03	9.86	13.13	13.22	1.60	4
	女性 Female	17 652	8.20	6.34	4.10	4.06	0.44	6
城市地区	合计 Both	25 601	12.01	6.63	6.48	6.51	0.77	5
Urban areas	男性 Male	19 504	18.23	7.96	10.46	10.55	1.28	5
	女性 Female	6 097	5.74	4.32	2.70	2.67	0.28	7
农村地区	合计 Both	40 770	18.28	10.54	10.63	10.66	1.27	4
Rural areas	男性 Male	29 215	25.60	11.72	15.84	15.95	1.91	4
	女性 Female	11 555	10.60	8.41	5.57	5.53	0.61	4
东部地区	合计 Both	31 539	15.94	8.25	8.02	8.00	0.94	5
Eastern areas	男性 Male	22 819	22.93	9.48	12.39	12.42	1.48	4
	女性 Female	8 720	8.86	6.17	3.91	3.83	0.41	6
中部地区	合计 Both	15 885	13.80	8.46	8.70	8.73	1.04	4
Central areas	男性 Male	11 165	18.98	9.32	12.77	12.86	1.55	4
	女性 Female	4 720	8.39	6.95	4.78	4.76	0.53	6
西部地区	合计 Both	18 947	15.36	9.33	9.33	9.44	1.16	4
Western areas	男性 Male	14 735	23.46	11.02	14.81	15.04	1.86	4
	女性 Female	4 212	6.96	6.07	3.88	3.90	0.44	6

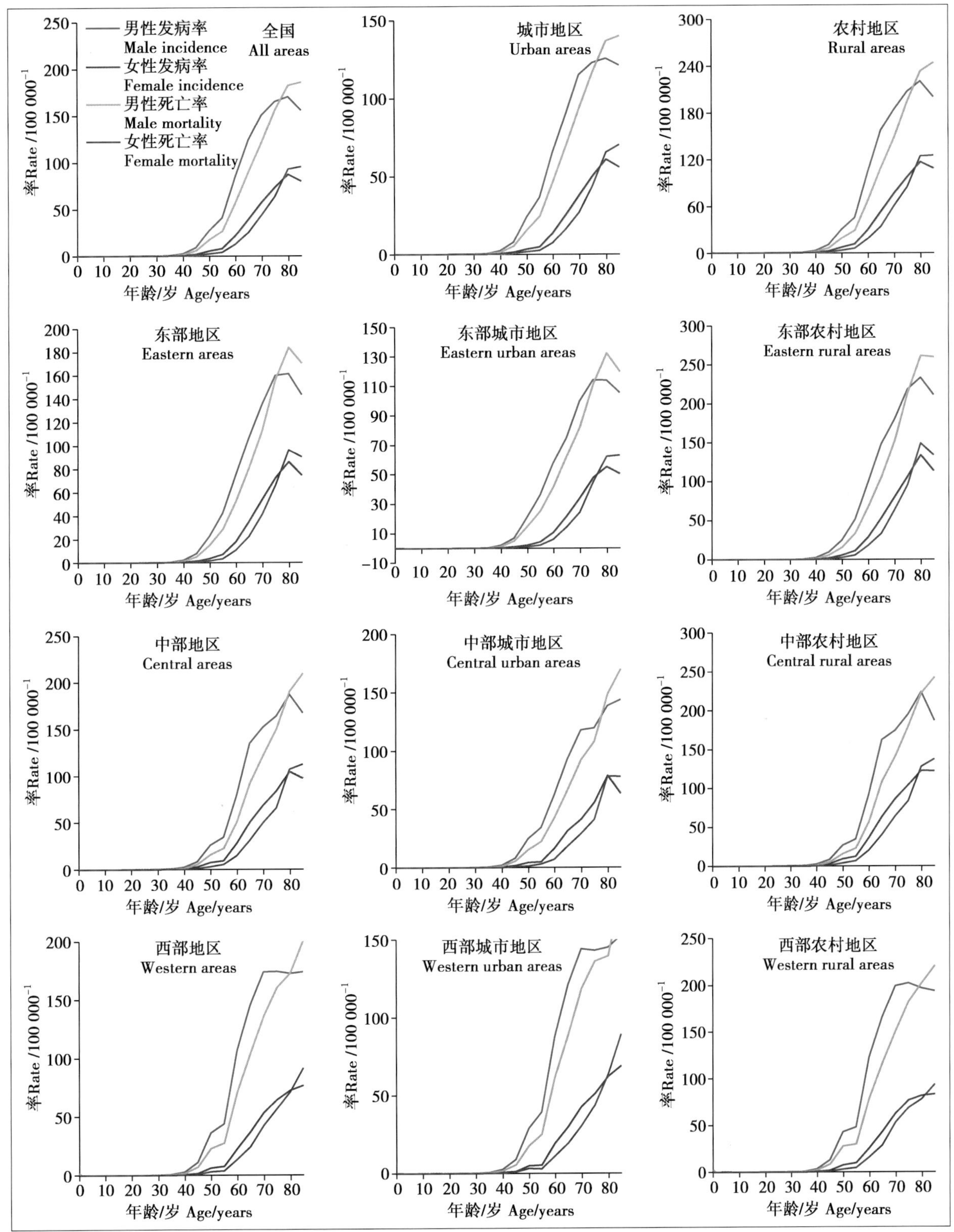

图 5-3a　2017 年中国肿瘤登记地区食管癌年龄别发病率和死亡率

Figure 5-3a　Age-specific incidence and mortality rates of esophageal cancer in the registration areas of China, 2017

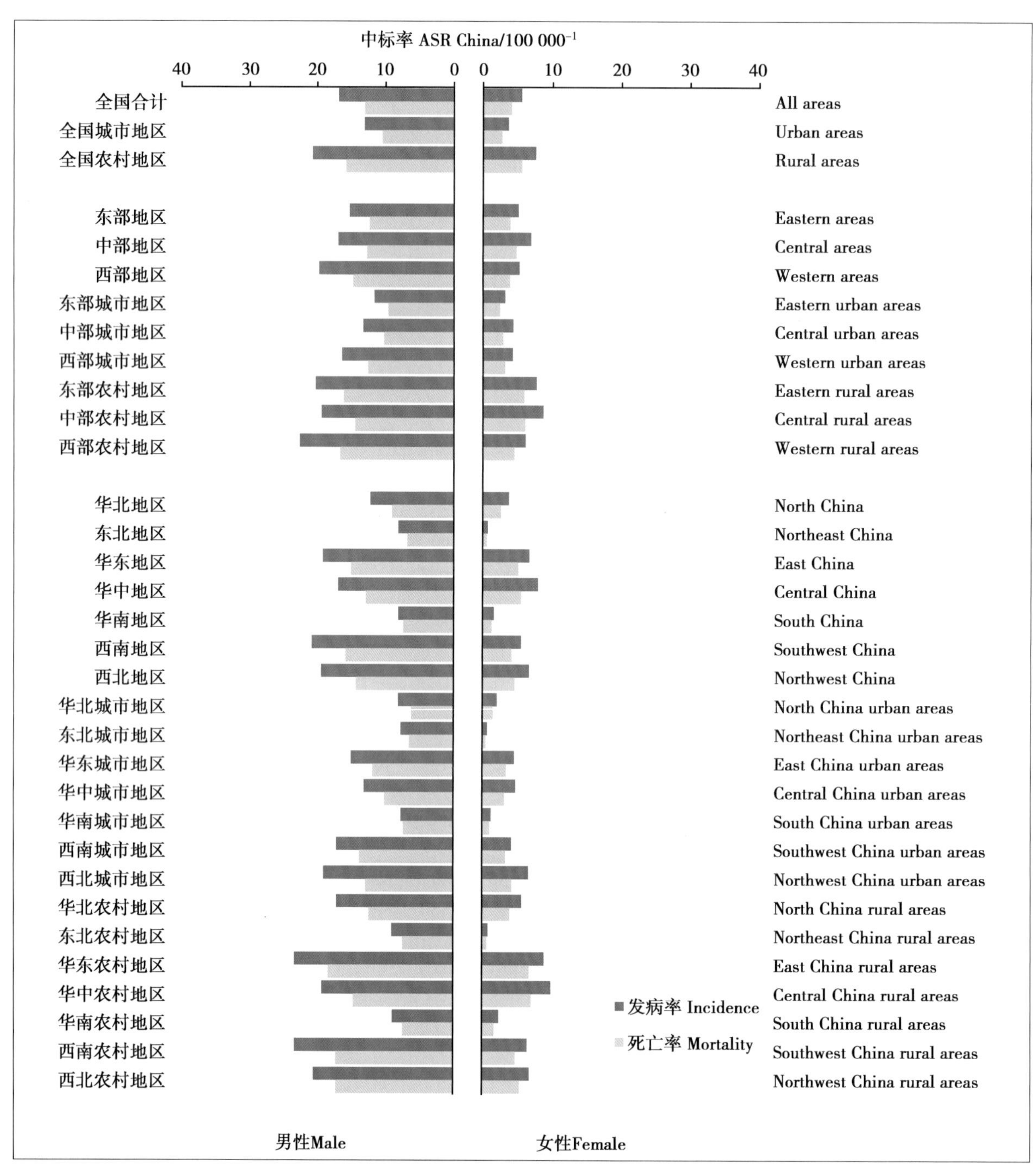

图 5-3b 2017 年中国肿瘤登记地区分城乡食管癌发病率和死亡率

Figure 5-3b Incidence and mortality rates of esophageal cancer in different registration areas of China, 2017

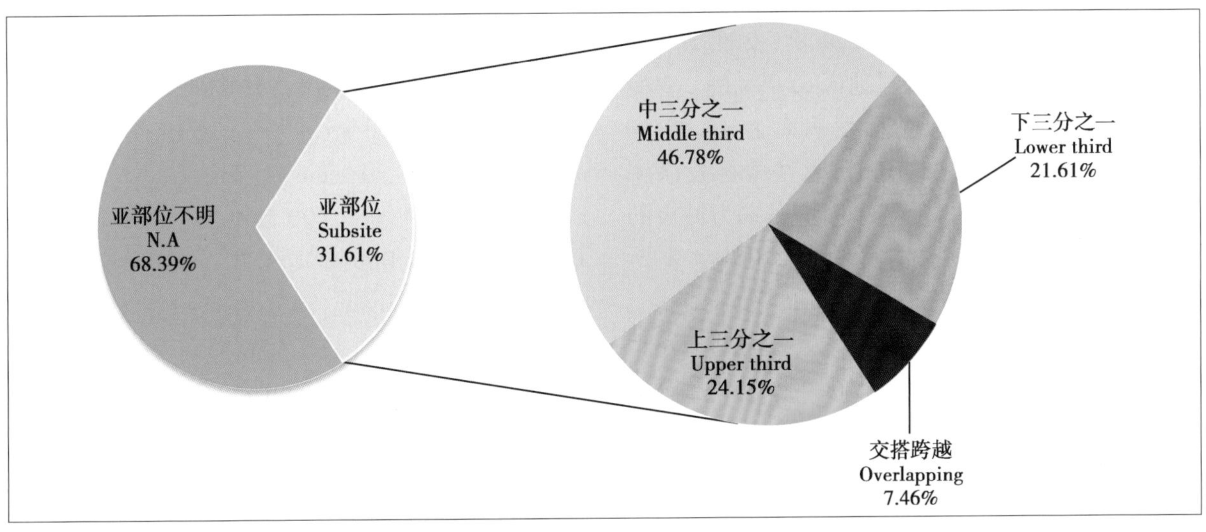

图 5-3c 2017 年中国肿瘤登记地区食管癌亚部位分布情况
Figure 5-3c Subsite distribution of esophageal cancer in the registration areas of China,2017

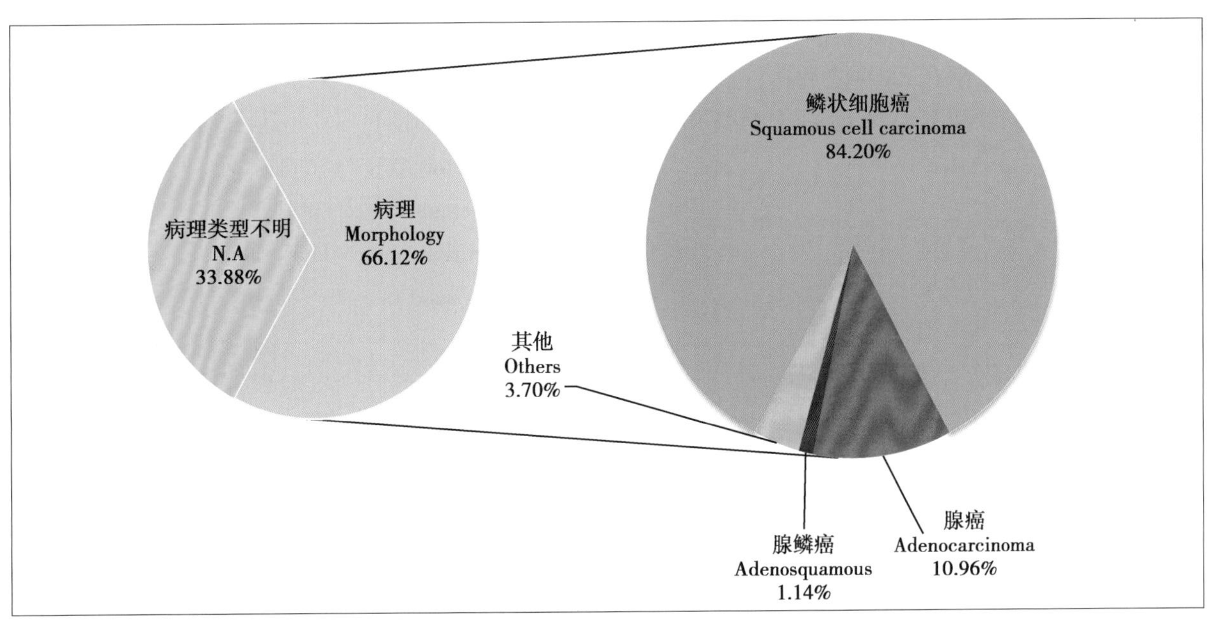

图 5-3d 2017 年中国肿瘤登记地区食管癌病理分型情况
Figure 5-3d Morphological distribution of esophageal cancer in the registration areas of China,2017

4 胃

2017 年中国肿瘤登记地区胃癌位居癌症发病谱第 4 位。新发病例数为 123 200 例，占全部癌症发病的 9.61%；其中男性 86 224 例，女性 36 976 例，城市地区 56 101 例，农村地区 67 099 例。胃癌发病率为 28.24/10 万，中标发病率为 16.88/10 万，世标发病率为 16.78/10 万；男性中标发病率为女性的 2.41 倍，农村地区中标发病率为城市的 1.23 倍。0～74 岁累积发病率为 2.06%（表 5-4a）。

2017 年中国肿瘤登记地区胃癌位居癌症死亡谱第 3 位。胃癌死亡病例 91 166 例，占全部癌症死亡的 11.79%；其中男性 63 514 例，女性 27 652 例，城市地区 39 707 例，农村地区 51 459 例。胃癌死亡率为 20.89/10 万，中标死亡率 11.95/10 万，世标死亡率 11.81/10 万；男性中标死亡率为女性的 2.49 倍，农村地区中标死亡率为城市的 1.35 倍。0～74 岁累积死亡率为 1.35%（表 5-4b）。

胃癌年龄别发病率和死亡率在 40 岁之前处于较低水平，40 岁后快速上升，男女发病率均于 80～84 岁组达到高峰，男性死亡率在 80～84 岁组达到高峰，女性死亡率在 85 岁之后达到高峰。男性各年龄别发病率和死亡率均高于女性（图 5-4a）。

4 Stomach

Stomach cancer was the 4th most common cancer in the registration areas of China in 2017. There were 123 200 new cases of stomach cancer (86 224 males and 36 976 females, 56 101 in urban areas and 67 099 in rural areas), accounting for 9.61% of new cases of all cancers. The crude incidence rate was 28.24 per 100 000, with ASR China 16.88 per 100 000 and ASR World 16.78 per 100 000, respectively. Subgroup analyses showed that the incidence of ASR China was 2.41 times in males as that in females, and was 1.23 times in rural areas as that in urban areas. The cumulative incidence rate for subjects aged 0 to 74 years was 2.06% (Table 5-4a).

Stomach cancer was the 3rd most common cause of cancer deaths in 2017. A total of 91 166 cases died of stomach cancer in 2017 (63 514 males and 27 652 females, 39 707 in urban areas and 51 459 in rural areas), accounting for 11.79% of all cancer deaths. The crude mortality rate was 20.89 per 100 000, with ASR China 11.95 per 100 000 and ASR World 11.81 per 100 000, respectively. Subgroup analyses showed that the mortality of ASR China was 2.49 times in males as that in females, and was 1.35 times in rural areas as that in urban areas. The cumulative mortality rate for subjects aged 0 to 74 years was 1.35% (Table 5-4b).

The age-specific incidence and mortality rates of stomach cancer were relatively low before 40 years old and increased rapidly since then. The incidence rates in age group of 80-84 years were the highest in both sexes. The mortality rates peaked at age group of 80-84 years in males and 85+ years in females. Age-specific incidence and mortality rates in males were generally higher than those in females across all age groups (Figure 5-4a).

农村胃癌的发病率和死亡率均高于城市。中标发病率和死亡率均以中部地区最高，其次是东部地区，西部地区最低。七大行政区中，西北地区男性和女性中标发病率和死亡率最高，华南地区最低（表 5-4a，表 5-4b，图 5-4b）。

全部胃癌病例中有明确亚部位信息的病例占 40.48%。其中贲门病例最多，占 41.10%，其次是幽门窦（19.19%）、胃体（16.62%）、胃底（8.53%）、胃小弯（6.92%）、交搭跨越（4.79%）、幽门（1.45%）和胃大弯（1.41%）（图 5-4c）。

全部胃癌病例中有明确组织学类型的病例占 66.49%，其中腺癌是最主要的病理类型，占 89.47%；其次是鳞状细胞癌（4.35%），其他类型（3.82%），类癌（0.55%）和腺鳞癌（0.20%）（图 5-4d）。

The incidence and mortality rates of stomach cancer were higher in rural areas than those in urban areas. The incidence and mortality rates (ASR China) were the highest in the central areas, followed by the eastern areas and western areas. Among the seven administrative districts, the incidence and mortality rates (ASR China) were the highest in Northwest China and the lowest in South China for both sexes (Table 5-4a, Table 5-4b, Figure 5-4b).

About 40.48% of the stomach cancer cases had complete information on subsite. Among those, cardia was the most common subsite and accounted for 41.10% of the total cases, followed by pyloric antrum (19.19%), body (16.62%), fundus (8.53%), lesser curvature (6.92%), overlapping (4.79%), pylorus (1.45%) and greater curvature (1.41%) (Figure 5-4c).

About 66.49% of the stomach cancer cases had morphological verification. Among those, adenocarcinoma was the most common histological type, accounting for 89.47% of all cases, followed by squamous cell carcinoma (4.35%), other type (3.82%), carcinoid (0.55%) and adenosquamous carcinoma (0.20%) (Figure 5-4d).

表 5-4a 2017 年中国肿瘤登记地区胃癌发病情况

Table 5-4a Incidence of stomach cancer in the registration areas of China,2017

地区 Area	性别 Sex	病例数 No. cases	粗率 Crude rate/ 100 000^{-1}	构成比 Freq./%	中标率 ASR China/ 100 000^{-1}	世标率 ASR World/ 100 000^{-1}	累积率 Cum. rate 0~74/%	顺位 Rank
合计	合计 Both	123 200	28. 24	9. 61	16. 88	16. 78	2. 06	4
All	男性 Male	86 224	38. 99	12. 12	24. 04	24. 05	3. 00	3
	女性 Female	36 976	17. 18	6. 49	9. 99	9. 75	1. 13	5
城市地区	合计 Both	56 101	26. 31	8. 32	15. 17	15. 06	1. 83	5
Urban areas	男性 Male	38 907	36. 36	10. 66	21. 55	21. 56	2. 67	4
	女性 Female	17 194	16. 19	5. 57	9. 14	8. 90	1. 02	6
农村地区	合计 Both	67 099	30. 08	11. 05	18. 62	18. 52	2. 28	3
Rural areas	男性 Male	47 317	41. 46	13. 66	26. 51	26. 54	3. 31	3
	女性 Female	19 782	18. 15	7. 58	10. 86	10. 62	1. 23	4
东部地区	合计 Both	62 063	31. 36	9. 39	17. 15	16. 98	2. 08	4
Eastern areas	男性 Male	43 357	43. 57	12. 17	24. 59	24. 52	3. 04	2
	女性 Female	18 706	19. 01	6. 14	10. 13	9. 85	1. 14	5
中部地区	合计 Both	33 158	28. 81	11. 00	19. 22	19. 15	2. 37	3
Central areas	男性 Male	23 107	39. 28	13. 83	27. 18	27. 28	3. 44	2
	女性 Female	10 051	17. 86	7. 49	11. 47	11. 23	1. 30	5
西部地区	合计 Both	27 979	22. 68	8. 76	14. 41	14. 38	1. 75	5
Western areas	男性 Male	19 760	31. 46	10. 50	20. 38	20. 47	2. 54	3
	女性 Female	8 219	13. 58	6. 27	8. 46	8. 30	0. 95	6

表 5-4b 2017 年中国肿瘤登记地区胃癌死亡情况

Table 5-4b Mortality of stomach cancer in the registration areas of China,2017

地区 Area	性别 Sex	死亡数 No. deaths	粗率 Crude rate/ 100 000^{-1}	构成比 Freq./%	中标率 ASR China/ 100 000^{-1}	世标率 ASR World/ 100 000^{-1}	累积率 Cum. rate 0~74/%	顺位 Rank
合计	合计 Both	91 166	20. 89	11. 79	11. 95	11. 81	1. 35	3
All	男性 Male	63 514	28. 72	12. 85	17. 25	17. 12	1. 98	3
	女性 Female	27 652	12. 85	9. 92	6. 93	6. 78	0. 72	3
城市地区	合计 Both	39 707	18. 62	10. 28	10. 17	10. 03	1. 13	3
Urban areas	男性 Male	27 563	25. 76	11. 25	14. 74	14. 62	1. 67	3
	女性 Female	12 144	11. 43	8. 60	5. 93	5. 77	0. 60	4
农村地区	合计 Both	51 459	23. 07	13. 31	13. 75	13. 63	1. 57	3
Rural areas	男性 Male	35 951	31. 50	14. 42	19. 75	19. 63	2. 29	3
	女性 Female	15 508	14. 23	11. 28	7. 96	7. 83	0. 85	2
东部地区	合计 Both	45 044	22. 76	11. 79	11. 75	11. 53	1. 30	3
Eastern areas	男性 Male	31 465	31. 62	13. 07	17. 21	16. 98	1. 94	3
	女性 Female	13 579	13. 80	9. 61	6. 72	6. 52	0. 69	2
中部地区	合计 Both	24 969	21. 70	13. 30	13. 97	13. 86	1. 62	3
Central areas	男性 Male	17 257	29. 34	14. 41	19. 90	19. 82	2. 34	3
	女性 Female	7 712	13. 71	11. 35	8. 29	8. 16	0. 90	3
西部地区	合计 Both	21 153	17. 15	10. 42	10. 57	10. 56	1. 21	3
Western areas	男性 Male	14 792	23. 55	11. 06	15. 01	15. 05	1. 77	3
	女性 Female	6 361	10. 51	9. 17	6. 16	6. 10	0. 64	3

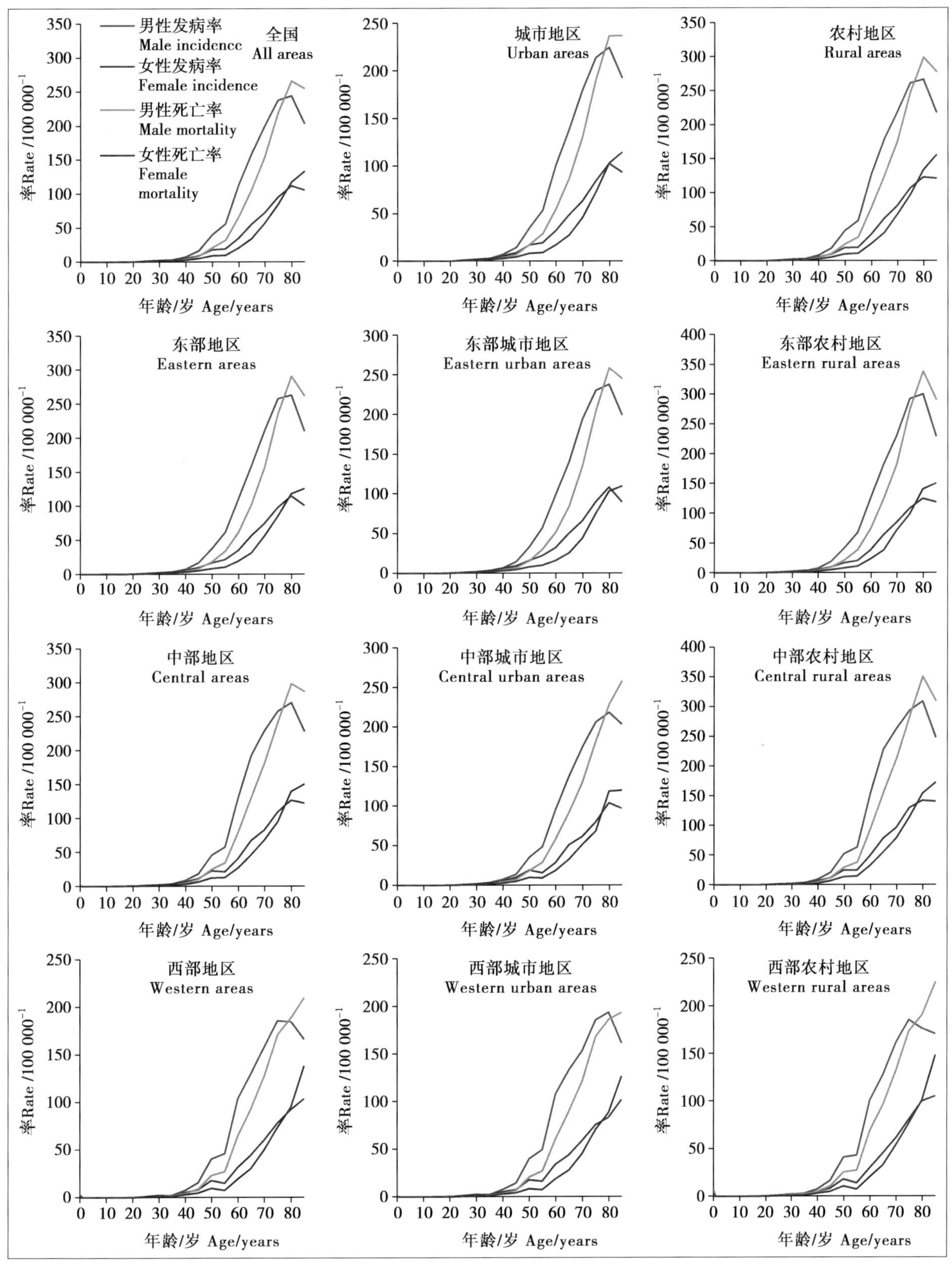

图 5-4a　2017 年中国肿瘤登记地区胃癌年龄别发病率和死亡率

Figure 5-4a　Age-specific incidence and mortality rates of stomach cancer in the registration areas of China, 2017

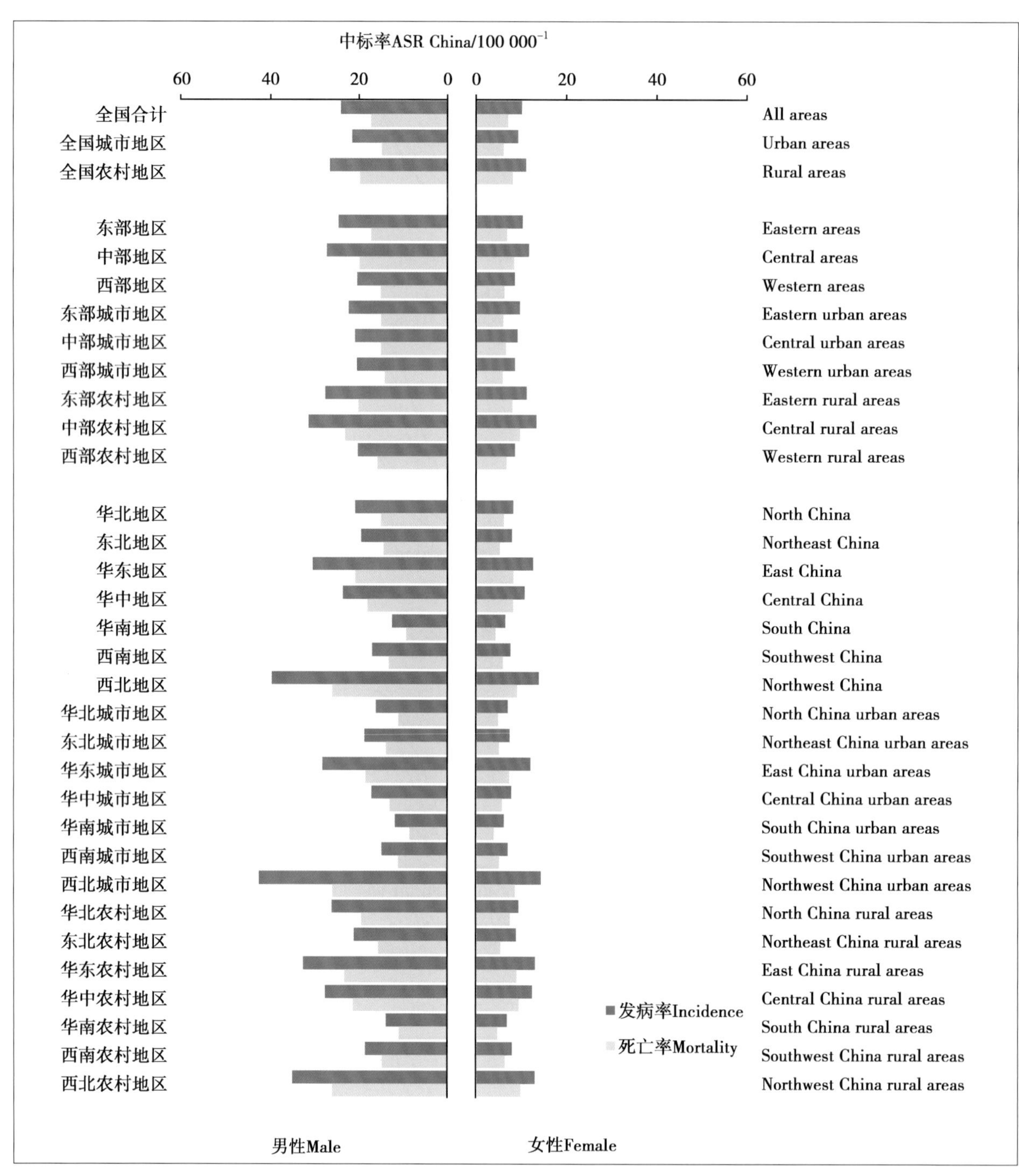

图 5-4b 2017 年中国肿瘤登记地区分城乡胃癌发病率和死亡率

Figure 5-4b Incidence and mortality rates of stomach cancer in different registration areas of China, 2017

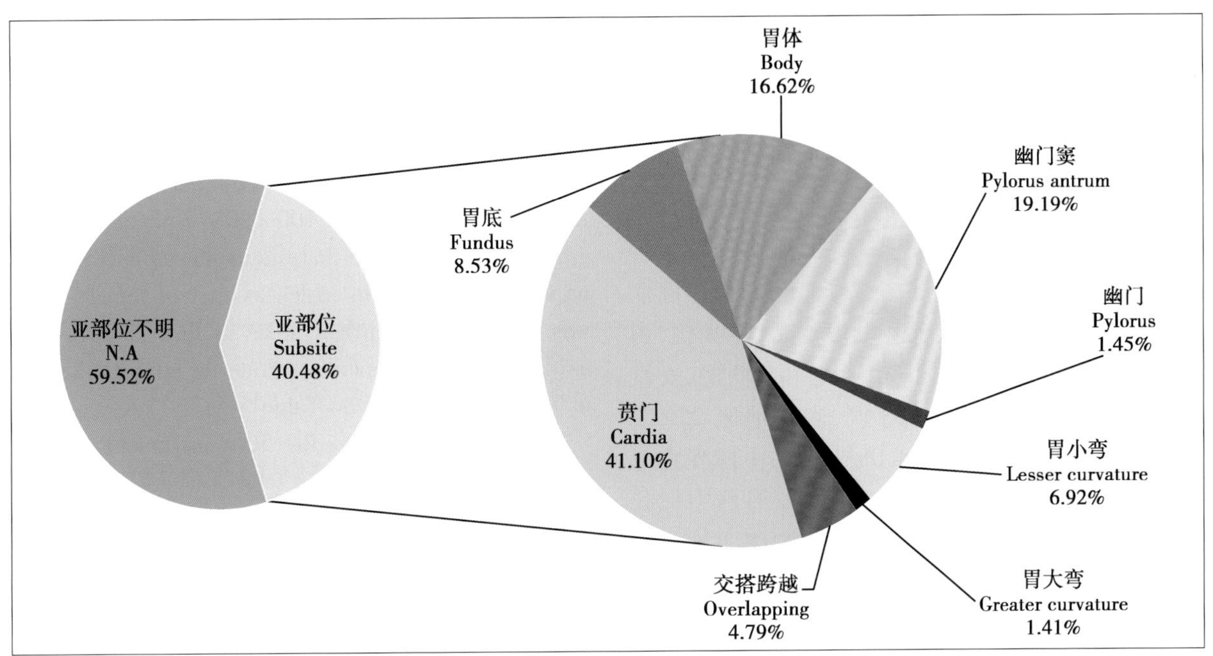

图 5-4c　2017 年中国肿瘤登记地区胃癌亚部位分布情况

Figure 5-4c　Subsite distribution of stomach cancer in the registration areas of China,2017

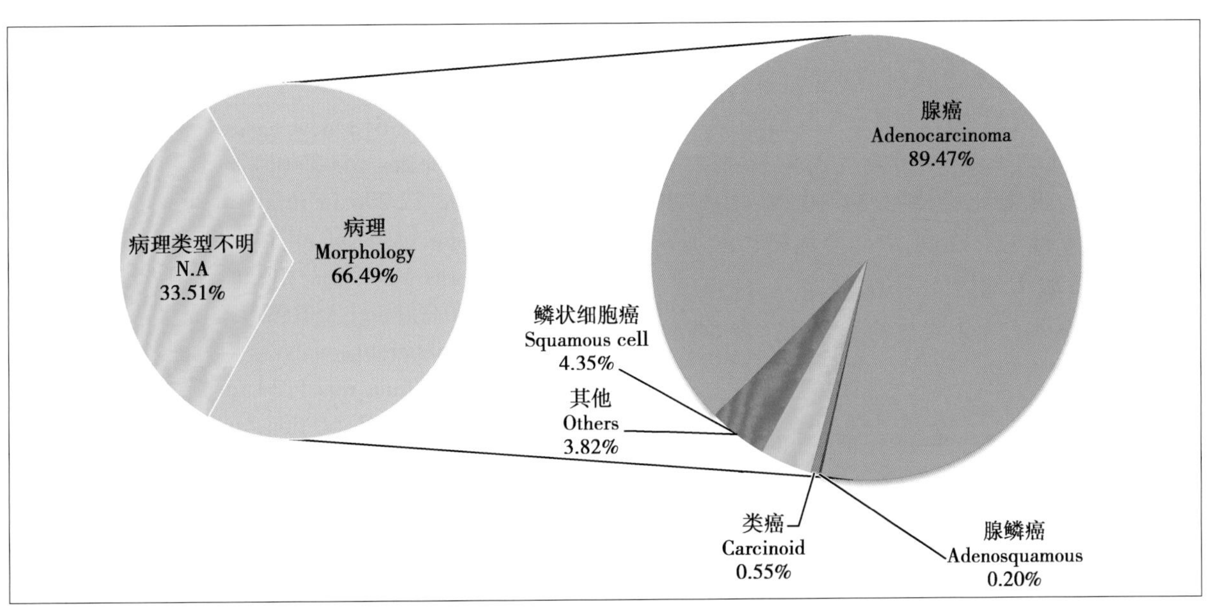

图 5-4d　2017 年中国肿瘤登记地区胃癌病理分型情况

Figure 5-4d　Morphological distribution of stomach cancer in the registration areas of China,2017

5 结直肠

2017 年中国肿瘤登记地区结直肠癌位居癌症发病谱第 3 位。新发病例数为 126 356 例，占全部癌症发病的 9.86%；其中男性 73 974 例，女性 52 382 例，城市地区 73 896 例，农村地区 52 460 例。发病率为 28.96/10 万，中标发病率为 17.54/10 万，世标发病率 17.32/10 万；男性中标发病率为女性的 1.48 倍，城市中标发病率为农村的 1.34 倍。0~74 岁累积发病率为 2.06%（表 5-5a）。

2017 年中国肿瘤登记地区结直肠癌位居癌症死亡谱第 5 位。结直肠癌死亡病例 61 440 例，占全部癌症死亡的 7.95%；其中男性 36 203 例，女性 25 237 例，城市地区 35 838 例，农村地区 25 602 例。结直肠癌死亡率为 14.08/10 万，中标死亡率 7.92/10 万，世标死亡率 7.84/10 万；男性中标死亡率为女性的 1.57 倍，城市中标死亡率为农村的 1.30 倍。0~74 岁累积死亡率为 0.83%（表 5-5b）。

结肠癌新发病例数为 61 613 例，占全部癌症发病的 4.81%，发病率为 14.12/10 万，中标发病率为 8.54/10 万，世标发病率 8.40/10 万；其中男性 34 556 例，女性 27 057 例，男性中标发病率为女性的 1.34 倍；城市地区 39 317 例，农村地区 22 296 例，城市中标发病率为农村的 1.66 倍（表 5-5c）。结肠癌死亡病例数为 27 904 例，占全部癌症死亡的 3.61%，死亡率为 6.40/10 万，中标死亡率为 3.57/10 万，世标死亡率 3.54/10 万；其中男性 15 662 例，女性 12 242 例，男性中标死亡率为女性的 1.41 倍；城市地区 18 105 例，农村地区 9 799 例，城市中标死亡率为农村的 1.69 倍（表 5-5d）。

5 Colon-rectum

Colorectal cancer was the 3rd most common cancer in the registration areas of China in 2017. There were 126 356 new cases of colorectal cancer (73 974 males and 52 382 females, 73 896 in urban areas and 52 460 rural areas), accounting for 9.86% of new cases of all cancers. The crude incidence rate was 28.96 per 100 000, with ASR China 17.54 per 100 000 and ASR World 17.32 per 100 000, respectively. Subgroup analyses showed that the incidence of ASR China was 1.48 times in males as that in females, and was 1.34 times in urban areas as that in rural areas. The cumulative incidence rate for subjects aged 0 to 74 years was 2.06% (Table 5-5a).

Colorectal cancer was the 5th most common cause of cancer deaths in 2017. A total of 61 440 cases died of colorectal cancer (36 203 males and 25 237 females, 35 838 in urban areas and 25 602 in rural areas), accounting for 7.95% of all cancer deaths. The crude mortality rate was 14.08 per 100 000, with ASR China 7.92 per 100 000 and ASR World 7.84 per 100 000, respectively. Subgroup analyses showed that the mortality of ASR China was 1.57 times in males as that in females, and was 1.30 times in urban areas as that in rural areas. The cumulative mortality rate for subjects aged 0 to 74 years was 0.83% (Table 5-5b).

There were 61 613 new cases of colon cancer in 2017 (34 556 males and 27 057 females, 39 317 in urban areas and 22 296 in rural areas), accounting for 4.81% of new cases of all cancers. The crude incidence rate was 14.12 per 100 000, with ASR China 8.54 per 100 000 and ASR World 8.40 per 100 000, respectively. Subgroup analyses showed that the incidence of ASR China was 1.34 times in males as that in females, and was 1.66 times in urban areas as that in rural areas (Table 5-5c). A total of 27 904 cases died of colon cancer (15 662 males and 12 242 in females, 18 105 in urban areas and 9 799 in rural areas), accounting for 3.61% of all cancer deaths. The crude mortality rate was 6.40 per 100 000, with ASR China 3.57 per 100 000 and ASR World 3.54 per 100 000, respectively. Subgroup analyses showed that the mortality of ASR China was 1.41 times in males as that in females, and was 1.69 times in urban areas as that in rural areas (Table 5-5d).

直肠癌新发病例数为 63 185 例，占全部癌症发病的 4. 93%，发病率为 14. 48/10 万，中标发病率为 8. 78/10 万，世标发病率 8. 71/10 万；其中男性 38 503 例，女性 24 682 例，男性中标发病率为女性的 1. 62 倍；城市地区 33 852 例，农村地区 29 333 例，城市中标发病率为农村的 1. 11 倍（表 5-5e）。直肠癌死亡病例数为 32 402 例，占全部癌症死亡的 4. 19%，死亡率为 7. 43/10 万，中标死亡率为 4. 20/10 万，世标死亡率 4. 15/10 万；其中男性 19 831 例，女性 12 571 例，男性中标死亡率为女性的 1. 72 倍；城市地区 17 158 例，农村地区 15 244 例，城市中标死亡率为农村的 1. 05 倍（表 5-5f）。

结直肠癌年龄别发病率和死亡率在男性和女性中均随年龄呈上升趋势，40～44 岁组之后上升明显，发病率在 80～84 岁组达高峰；死亡率在 85 岁以上组达到高峰，男性各年龄别发病率和死亡率均明显高于女性（图 5-5a）。

城市地区结直肠癌的发病率和死亡率均高于农村地区；中标发病率和死亡率东部地区最高，西部地区略高于中部地区（表 5-5a，表 5-5b，图 5-5a）。七大行政区中，发病率男性和女性均华南地区最高，西北地区最低。死亡率男性和女性均东北地区最高，西北地区最低（图 5-5b）。

在全部结肠癌病例中，有明确亚部位的病例占 57. 42%，其中乙状结肠发生癌症的比例最高，占 42. 09%，其次是升结肠、横结肠和降结肠，分别占 23. 85%、8. 91%和 8. 09%（图 5-5c）。

There were 63 185 new cases of rectal cancer in 2017 (38 503 males and 24 682 females, 33 852 in urban areas and 29 333 in rural areas), accounting for 4. 93% of new cases of all cancers. The crude incidence rate was 14. 48 per 100 000, with ASR China 8. 78 per 100 000 and ASR World 8. 71 per 100 000, respectively. Subgroup analyses showed that the incidence of ASR China was 1. 62 times in males as that in females, and was 1. 11 times in urban areas as that in rural areas (Table 5-5e). A total of 32 402 cases died of rectal cancer (19 831 males and 12 571 females, 17 158 in urban areas and 15 244 in rural areas), accounting for 4. 19% of all cancer deaths. The crude mortality rate was 7. 43 per 100 000, with ASR China 4. 20 per 100 000 and ASR World 4. 15 per 100 000, respectively. Subgroup analyses showed that the mortality of ASR China was 1. 72 times in males as that in females, and was 1. 05 times in urban areas as that in rural areas (Table 5-5f).

The age-specific incidence and mortality rates of colorectal cancer increased with age in both sexes, especially after age of 40 years, and reached thepeak at the age group of 80-84 years for the incidence rates and at the age group of 85 + years for the mortality rates peaked at the age group of 85+ years in both sexes. Age-specific incidence and mortality rates in males were generally higher than those in females across all age groups (Figure 5-5a).

The incidence and mortality rates of colorectal cancer were higher in urban areas than those in rural areas. The incidence and mortality rates (ASR China) were the highest in the eastern areas, and the rates in the western areas were slightly higher than those in the central areas (Table 5-5a, Table 5-5b, Figure 5-5a). Among the seven administrative districts, the incidence rates (ASR China) were the highest in South China and the lowest in Northwest China for both sexes. The mortality rates (ASR China) were the highest in Northeast China and the lowest in Northwest China for both sexes (Figure 5-5b).

Approximately 57. 42% of the colon cancer cases had complete information onsubsite. Among those, sigmoid colon was the most common subsite (42. 09%), followed by ascending colon (23. 85%), transverse colon (8. 91%) and descending colon (8. 09%) (Figure 5-5c).

表 5-5a　2017 年中国肿瘤登记地区结直肠癌发病情况
Table 5-5a　Incidence of colorectal cancer in the registration areas of China, 2017

地区 Area	性别 Sex	病例数 No. cases	粗率 Crude rate/ 100 000⁻¹	构成比 Freq./%	中标率 ASR China/ 100 000⁻¹	世标率 ASR World/ 100 000⁻¹	累积率 Cum. rate 0~74/%	顺位 Rank
合计	合计 Both	126 356	28. 96	9. 86	17. 54	17. 32	2. 06	3
All	男性 Male	73 974	33. 45	10. 40	20. 98	20. 81	2. 50	4
	女性 Female	52 382	24. 34	9. 19	14. 21	13. 96	1. 63	3
城市地区	合计 Both	73 896	34. 65	10. 96	20. 07	19. 86	2. 36	3
Urban areas	男性 Male	43 376	40. 53	11. 88	24. 30	24. 17	2. 90	2
	女性 Female	30 520	28. 73	9. 88	16. 06	15. 78	1. 83	4
农村地区	合计 Both	52 460	23. 52	8. 64	14. 93	14. 70	1. 76	5
Rural areas	男性 Male	30 598	26. 81	8. 83	17. 62	17. 40	2. 09	5
	女性 Female	21 862	20. 06	8. 38	12. 29	12. 06	1. 42	3
东部地区	合计 Both	68 353	34. 54	10. 34	19. 10	18. 87	2. 24	3
Eastern areas	男性 Male	39 884	40. 08	11. 19	23. 06	22. 89	2. 76	3
	女性 Female	28 469	28. 93	9. 35	15. 34	15. 06	1. 74	4
中部地区	合计 Both	26 376	22. 92	8. 75	15. 54	15. 35	1. 84	5
Central areas	男性 Male	15 200	25. 84	9. 10	18. 20	18. 03	2. 17	4
	女性 Female	11 176	19. 86	8. 33	12. 96	12. 76	1. 51	4
西部地区	合计 Both	31 627	25. 64	9. 91	16. 49	16. 26	1. 93	4
Western areas	男性 Male	18 890	30. 08	10. 04	19. 74	19. 54	2. 32	5
	女性 Female	12 737	21. 04	9. 72	13. 29	13. 02	1. 52	3

表 5-5b　2017 年中国肿瘤登记地区结直肠癌死亡情况
Table 5-5b　Mortality of colorectal cancer in the registration areas of China, 2017

地区 Area	性别 Sex	死亡数 No. deaths	粗率 Crude rate/ 100 000⁻¹	构成比 Freq./%	中标率 ASR China/ 100 000⁻¹	世标率 ASR World/ 100 000⁻¹	累积率 Cum. rate 0~74/%	顺位 Rank
合计	合计 Both	61 440	14. 08	7. 95	7. 92	7. 84	0. 83	5
All	男性 Male	36 203	16. 37	7. 32	9. 75	9. 71	1. 03	5
	女性 Female	25 237	11. 73	9. 06	6. 20	6. 10	0. 62	4
城市地区	合计 Both	35 838	16. 81	9. 28	8. 91	8. 84	0. 92	4
Urban areas	男性 Male	21 254	19. 86	8. 67	11. 18	11. 15	1. 19	4
	女性 Female	14 584	13. 73	10. 33	6. 80	6. 70	0. 66	2
农村地区	合计 Both	25 602	11. 48	6. 62	6. 88	6. 77	0. 74	5
Rural areas	男性 Male	14 949	13. 10	6. 00	8. 27	8. 18	0. 89	5
	女性 Female	10 653	9. 78	7. 75	5. 55	5. 44	0. 58	5
东部地区	合计 Both	32 348	16. 34	8. 46	8. 17	8. 09	0. 83	4
Eastern areas	男性 Male	18 808	18. 90	7. 81	10. 12	10. 07	1. 05	5
	女性 Female	13 540	13. 76	9. 58	6. 40	6. 29	0. 62	3
中部地区	合计 Both	13 523	11. 75	7. 20	7. 57	7. 45	0. 82	5
Central areas	男性 Male	7 900	13. 43	6. 60	9. 14	9. 04	0. 99	5
	女性 Female	5 623	9. 99	8. 28	6. 09	5. 96	0. 65	4
西部地区	合计 Both	15 569	12. 62	7. 67	7. 72	7. 66	0. 83	5
Western areas	男性 Male	9 495	15. 12	7. 10	9. 59	9. 57	1. 04	5
	女性 Female	6 074	10. 03	8. 76	5. 90	5. 83	0. 62	4

表 5-5c 2017 年中国肿瘤登记地区结肠癌发病情况

Table5-5c Incidence of colon cancer in the registration areas of China, 2017

地区 Area	性别 Sex	病例数 No. cases	粗率 Crude rate/ 100 000^{-1}	构成比 Freq. /%	中标率 ASR China/ 100 000^{-1}	世标率 ASR World/ 100 000^{-1}	累积率 Cum. rate 0~74/%
合计	合计 Both	61 613	14. 12	4. 81	8. 54	8. 40	0. 99
All	男性 Male	34 556	15. 63	4. 86	9. 81	9. 69	1. 14
	女性 Female	27 057	12. 57	4. 75	7. 31	7. 17	0. 83
城市地区	合计 Both	39 317	18. 44	5. 83	10. 63	10. 47	1. 23
Urban areas	男性 Male	22 051	20. 61	6. 04	12. 33	12. 21	1. 44
	女性 Female	17 266	16. 25	5. 59	9. 02	8. 84	1. 02
农村地区	合计 Both	22 296	9. 99	3. 67	6. 40	6. 27	0. 74
Rural areas	男性 Male	12 505	10. 96	3. 61	7. 27	7. 14	0. 85
	女性 Female	9 791	8. 99	3. 75	5. 54	5. 42	0. 64
东部地区	合计 Both	36 563	18. 47	5. 53	10. 18	10. 02	1. 18
Eastern areas	男性 Male	20 400	20. 50	5. 73	11. 80	11. 66	1. 39
	女性 Female	16 163	16. 43	5. 31	8. 65	8. 48	0. 98
中部地区	合计 Both	12 424	10. 80	4. 12	7. 32	7. 20	0. 85
Central areas	男性 Male	6 921	11. 77	4. 14	8. 28	8. 17	0. 96
	女性 Female	5 503	9. 78	4. 10	6. 39	6. 27	0. 75
西部地区	合计 Both	12 626	10. 24	3. 96	6. 65	6. 50	0. 76
Western areas	男性 Male	7 235	11. 52	3. 84	7. 63	7. 50	0. 87
	女性 Female	5 391	8. 91	4. 12	5. 68	5. 52	0. 64

表 5-5d 2017 年中国肿瘤登记地区结肠癌死亡情况

Table 5-5d Mortality of colon cancer in the registration areas of China, 2017

地区 Area	性别 Sex	死亡数 No. deaths	粗率 Crude rate/ 100 000^{-1}	构成比 Freq. /%	中标率 ASR China/ 100 000^{-1}	世标率 ASR World/ 100 000^{-1}	累积率 Cum. rate 0~74/%
合计	合计 Both	27 904	6. 40	3. 61	3. 57	3. 54	0. 36
All	男性 Male	15 662	7. 08	3. 17	4. 21	4. 19	0. 44
	女性 Female	12 242	5. 69	4. 39	2. 98	2. 93	0. 29
城市地区	合计 Both	18 105	8. 49	4. 69	4. 46	4. 42	0. 45
Urban areas	男性 Male	10 167	9. 50	4. 15	5. 32	5. 31	0. 55
	女性 Female	7 938	7. 47	5. 62	3. 66	3. 61	0. 35
农村地区	合计 Both	9 799	4. 39	2. 53	2. 64	2. 60	0. 28
Rural areas	男性 Male	5 495	4. 82	2. 20	3. 06	3. 02	0. 33
	女性 Female	4 304	3. 95	3. 13	2. 25	2. 21	0. 24
东部地区	合计 Both	16 461	8. 32	4. 31	4. 14	4. 09	0. 41
Eastern areas	男性 Male	9 147	9. 19	3. 80	4. 92	4. 89	0. 51
	女性 Female	7 314	7. 43	5. 17	3. 43	3. 37	0. 33
中部地区	合计 Both	5 965	5. 18	3. 18	3. 33	3. 28	0. 35
Central areas	男性 Male	3 321	5. 65	2. 77	3. 84	3. 80	0. 41
	女性 Female	2 644	4. 70	3. 89	2. 86	2. 80	0. 30
西部地区	合计 Both	5 478	4. 44	2. 70	2. 71	2. 69	0. 29
Western areas	男性 Male	3 194	5. 09	2. 39	3. 22	3. 22	0. 34
	女性 Female	2 284	3. 77	3. 29	2. 21	2. 18	0. 23

表 5-5e 2017 年中国肿瘤登记地区直肠癌发病情况
Table 5-5e Incidence of rectal cancer in the registration areas of China, 2017

地区 Area	性别 Sex	病例数 No. cases	粗率 Crude rate/ 100 000^{-1}	构成比 Freq./%	中标率 ASR China/ 100 000^{-1}	世标率 ASR World/ 100 000^{-1}	累积率 Cum. rate 0~74/%
合计 All	合计 Both	63 185	14.48	4.93	8.78	8.71	1.05
	男性 Male	38 503	17.41	5.41	10.91	10.86	1.32
	女性 Female	24 682	11.47	4.33	6.73	6.63	0.78
城市地区 Urban areas	合计 Both	33 852	15.87	5.02	9.25	9.20	1.11
	男性 Male	20 902	19.53	5.72	11.73	11.72	1.43
	女性 Female	12 950	12.19	4.19	6.88	6.78	0.80
农村地区 Rural areas	合计 Both	29 333	13.15	4.83	8.30	8.20	0.99
	男性 Male	17 601	15.42	5.08	10.07	9.99	1.21
	女性 Female	11 732	10.77	4.50	6.56	6.46	0.76
东部地区 Eastern areas	合计 Both	31 184	15.76	4.72	8.75	8.68	1.05
	男性 Male	19 143	19.24	5.37	11.06	11.03	1.35
	女性 Female	12 041	12.24	3.95	6.55	6.44	0.75
中部地区 Central areas	合计 Both	13 569	11.79	4.50	8.00	7.94	0.97
	男性 Male	8 054	13.69	4.82	9.64	9.59	1.18
	女性 Female	5 515	9.80	4.11	6.39	6.32	0.75
西部地区 Western areas	合计 Both	18 432	14.94	5.77	9.55	9.47	1.13
	男性 Male	11 306	18.00	6.01	11.75	11.68	1.40
	女性 Female	7 126	11.77	5.44	7.38	7.28	0.86

表 5-5f 2017 年中国肿瘤登记地区直肠癌死亡情况
Table 5-5f Mortality of rectal cancer in the registration areas of China, 2017

地区 Area	性别 Sex	死亡数 No. deaths	粗率 Crude rate/ 100 000^{-1}	构成比 Freq./%	中标率 ASR China/ 100 000^{-1}	世标率 ASR World/ 100 000^{-1}	累积率 Cum. rate 0~74/%
合计 All	合计 Both	32 402	7.43	4.19	4.20	4.15	0.45
	男性 Male	19 831	8.97	4.01	5.35	5.32	0.58
	女性 Female	12 571	5.84	4.51	3.12	3.07	0.32
城市地区 Urban areas	合计 Both	17 158	8.05	4.44	4.31	4.27	0.46
	男性 Male	10 708	10.01	4.37	5.66	5.65	0.61
	女性 Female	6 450	6.07	4.57	3.05	3.01	0.31
农村地区 Rural areas	合计 Both	15 244	6.83	3.94	4.08	4.02	0.44
	男性 Male	9 123	7.99	3.66	5.03	4.98	0.54
	女性 Female	6 121	5.62	4.45	3.19	3.12	0.33
东部地区 Eastern areas	合计 Both	15 544	7.85	4.07	3.95	3.91	0.41
	男性 Male	9 479	9.53	3.94	5.10	5.08	0.54
	女性 Female	6 065	6.16	4.29	2.89	2.84	0.28
中部地区 Central areas	合计 Both	7 292	6.34	3.88	4.09	4.02	0.45
	男性 Male	4 411	7.50	3.68	5.10	5.04	0.56
	女性 Female	2 881	5.12	4.24	3.13	3.06	0.34
西部地区 Western areas	合计 Both	9 566	7.76	4.71	4.76	4.71	0.52
	男性 Male	5 941	9.46	4.44	6.01	5.98	0.66
	女性 Female	3 625	5.99	5.23	3.54	3.49	0.37

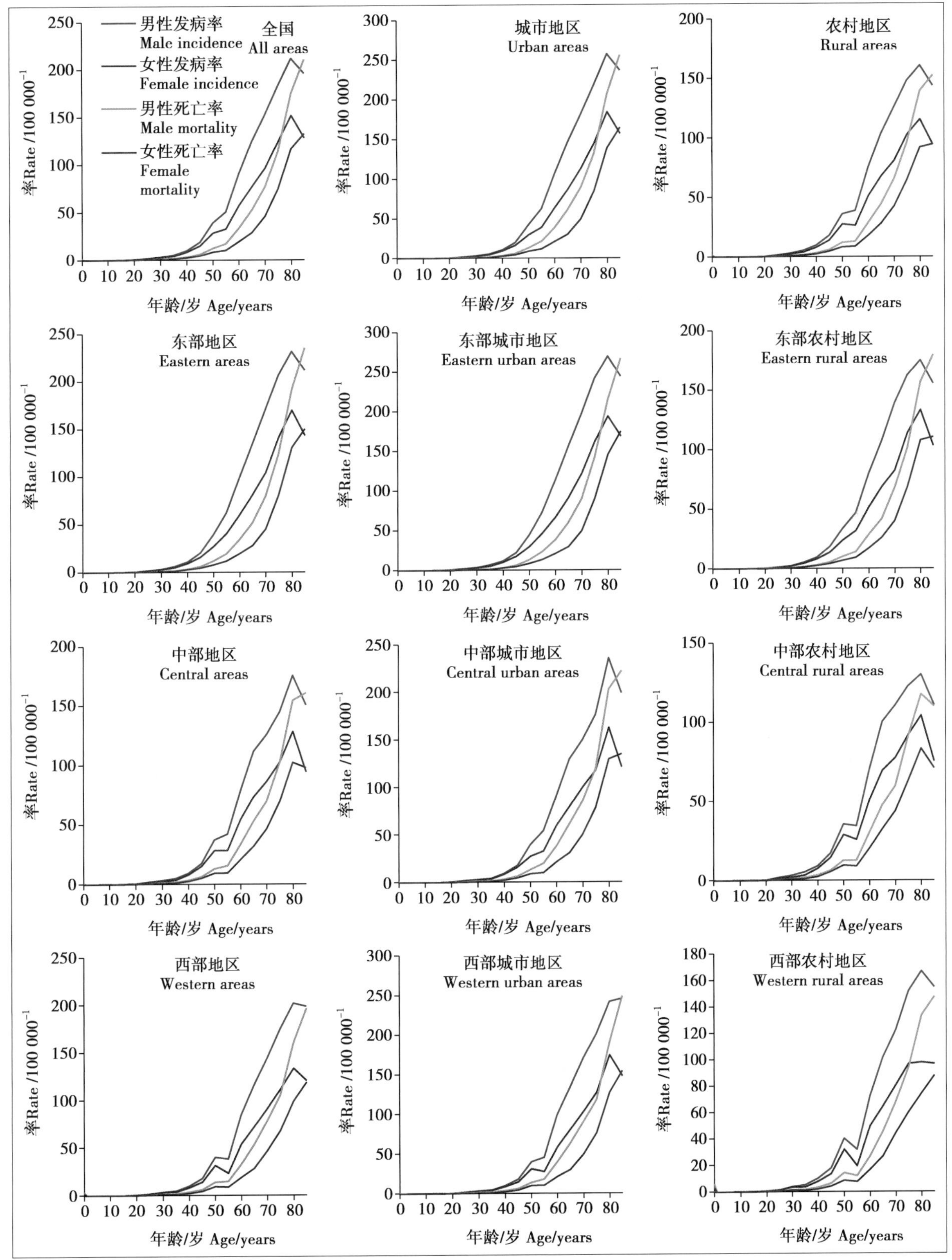

图 5-5a　2017 年中国肿瘤登记地区结直肠癌年龄别发病率和死亡率
Figure 5-5a　Age-specific incidence and mortality rates of colorectal cancer in the registration areas of China, 2017

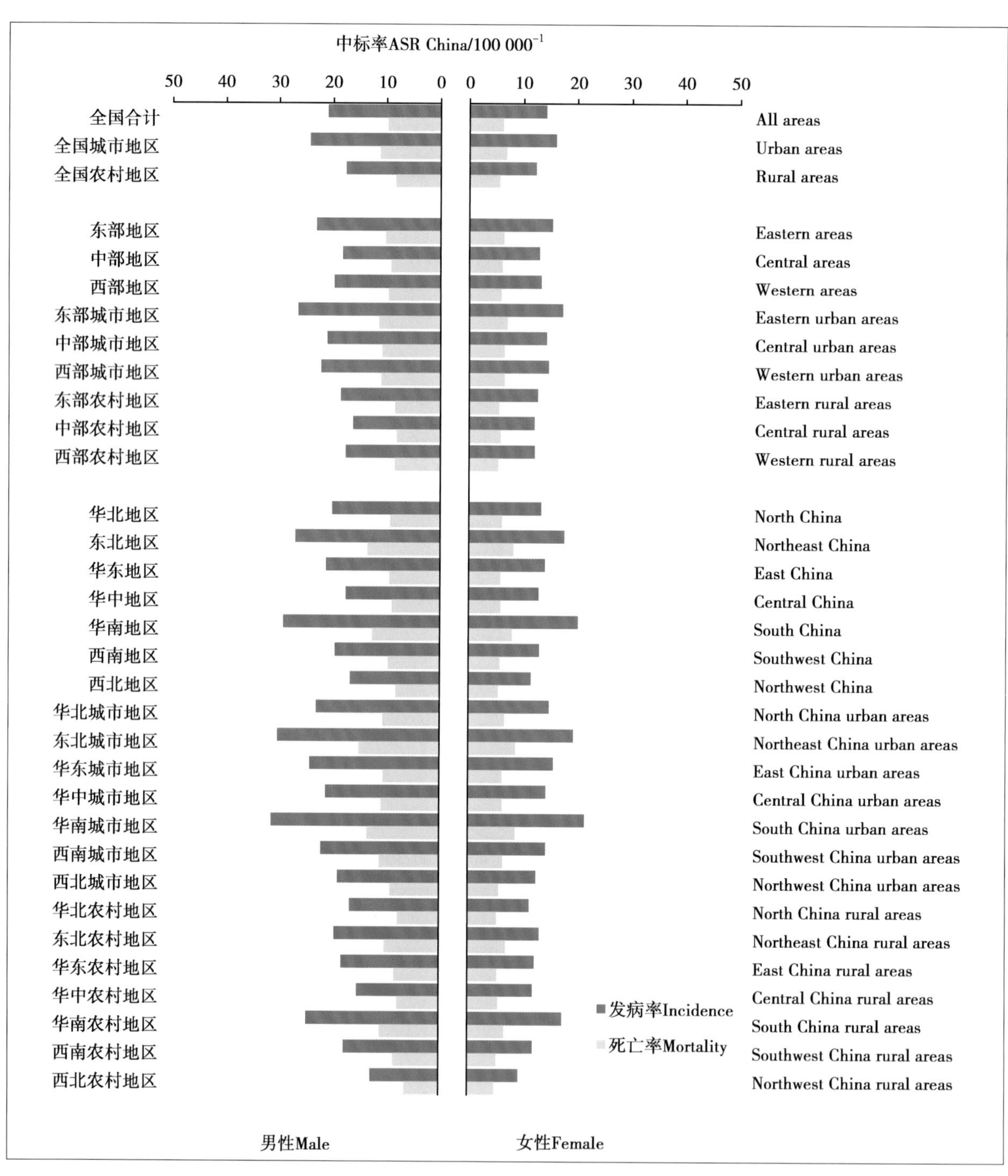

图 5-5b　2017 年中国肿瘤登记地区分城乡结直肠癌发病率和死亡率
Figure 5-5b　Incidence and mortality rates of colorectal cancer in different registration areas of China, 2017

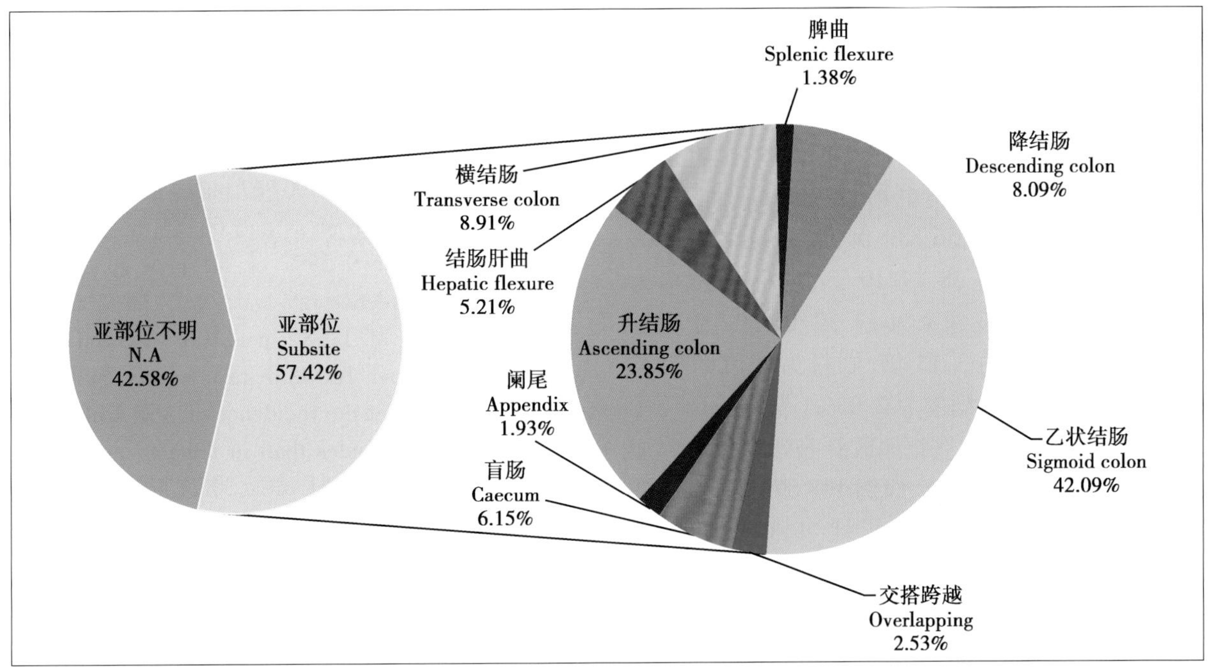

图 5-5c　2017 年中国肿瘤登记地区结肠癌亚部位分布情况
Figure 5-5c　Subsite distribution of colon cancer in the registration areas of China,2017

6 肝

2017 年中国肿瘤登记地区肝癌发病位居癌症发病谱第 5 位。新发病例数为 122 898 例，占全部癌症发病的 9.59%；其中男性 90 767 例，女性 32 131 例，城市地区 56 889 例，农村地区 66 009 例。肝癌发病率为 28.17/10 万，中标发病率为 17.82/10 万，世标发病率为 17.50/10 万。中标发病率男性为女性的 3.15 倍，农村为城市的 1.20 倍。0~74 岁累积发病率为 2.03%（表 5-6a）。

2017 年中国肿瘤登记地区肝癌死亡位居癌症死亡谱第 2 位。肝癌死亡病例 108 691 例，占全部癌症死亡的 14.06%；其中男性 79 885 例，女性 28 806 例，城市地区 50 549 例，农村地区 58 142 例。死亡率为 24.91/10 万，中标死亡率 15.41/10 万，世标死亡率 15.20/10 万。中标死亡率男性为女性的 3.14 倍，农村为城市的 1.20 倍。0~74 岁累积死亡率为 1.74%（表 5-6b）。

肝癌的年龄别发病率和死亡率呈明显的性别差异。男性、女性发病率分别自 30~34 岁和 40~44 岁组开始上升，至 85 岁以上年龄组达到高峰。男性、女性死亡率曲线趋势分别与男女性发病率趋势相似（图 5-6a）。

肝癌的发病率和死亡率呈现地域差异。农村地区发病率和死亡率高于城市地区，西部地区高于中部和东部地区。七大行政区中，发病率和死亡率男性在华南地区为最高，女性在西北地区和华中地区为最高。华北地区的男性和女性的发病率和死亡率均为最低（表 5-6a，表 5-6b，图 5-6a，图 5-6b）。

6 Liver

Liver cancer was the fifth most common cancer in the registration areas of China in 2017. There were 122 898 new cases of liver cancer (90 767 males and 32 131 females, 56 889 in urban areas and 66 009 in rural areas), accounting for 9.59% of all new cancer cases. The crude incidence rate was 28.17 per 100 000, with ASR China of 17.82 per 100 000 and ASR World of 17.50 per 100 000, respectively. Subgroup analyses showed that the incidence of ASR China was 3.15 times high in males than in females, and it was 1.20 times high in rural areas than in urban areas. The cumulative incidence rate of 0 to 74 years old was 2.03% (Table 5-6a).

Liver cancer was the second most common cause of cancer deaths in the registration areas of China in 2017. A total of 108 691 cases died of liver cancer (79 885 males and 28 806 females, 50 549 in urban areas and 58 142 in rural areas), accounting for 14.06% of all cancer deaths. The crude mortality rate was 24.91 per 100 000, with ASR China of 15.41 per 100 000 and ASR World of 15.20 per 100 000, respectively. Subgroup analyses showed that the mortality of ASR China was 3.14 times high in males than in females, and it was 1.20 times high in rural areas than in urban areas. The cumulative mortality rate of 0 to 74 years old was 1.74% (Table 5-6b).

Trends of age-specific incidence and mortality rates showed differences between males and females. The age-specific incidence rates increased rapidly since 30-34 in males and 40-44 years in females, reaching peak both at the age group of 85+ years. The curve trends of age-specific mortality rate in males and females were similar as that of age-specific incidence (Figure 5-6a).

The incidence and mortality rates of liver cancer varied by geographical areas. Both incidence and mortality rates were higher in rural areas than in urban areas. Western areas had the higher rates of incidence and mortality (ASR China). Among the seven administrative districts, South China had the highest incidence and mortality rate (ASR China) for males, and Northwest and Central China had highest rates for females. North China had the lowest incidence and mortality rates both for males and females (Table 5-6a, Table 5-6b, Figure 5-6a, Figure 5-6b).

表 5-6a 2017 年中国肿瘤登记地区肝癌发病情况

Table 5-6a Incidence of liver cancer in registration areas of China, 2017

地区 Area	性别 Sex	病例数 No. cases	粗率 Crude rate/ 100 000^{-1}	构成比 Freq./%	中标率 ASR China/ 100 000^{-1}	世标率 ASR World/ 100 000^{-1}	累积率 Cum. rate 0~74/%	顺位 Rank
合计	合计 Both	122 898	28. 17	9. 59	17. 82	17. 50	2. 03	5
All	男性 Male	90 767	41. 05	12. 76	27. 08	26. 53	3. 07	2
	女性 Female	32 131	14. 93	5. 64	8. 61	8. 53	0. 98	7
城市地区	合计 Both	56 889	26. 68	8. 44	16. 23	15. 99	1. 85	4
Urban areas	男性 Male	42 010	39. 26	11. 50	24. 92	24. 51	2. 84	3
	女性 Female	14 879	14. 01	4. 82	7. 71	7. 64	0. 87	7
农村地区	合计 Both	66 009	29. 59	10. 87	19. 41	19. 02	2. 20	4
Rural areas	男性 Male	48 757	42. 72	14. 07	29. 21	28. 53	3. 29	2
	女性 Female	17 252	15. 83	6. 61	9. 54	9. 44	1. 10	6
东部地区	合计 Both	52 491	26. 52	7. 94	15. 41	15. 20	1. 76	5
Eastern areas	男性 Male	38 634	38. 82	10. 84	23. 68	23. 32	2. 71	4
	女性 Female	13 857	14. 08	4. 55	7. 33	7. 25	0. 83	7
中部地区	合计 Both	31 987	27. 80	10. 62	19. 18	18. 88	2. 20	4
Central areas	男性 Male	22 942	39. 00	13. 73	28. 08	27. 56	3. 20	3
	女性 Female	9 045	16. 08	6. 74	10. 28	10. 19	1. 18	6
西部地区	合计 Both	38 420	31. 15	12. 04	20. 95	20. 47	2. 35	2
Western areas	男性 Male	29 191	46. 48	15. 51	32. 16	31. 32	3. 58	2
	女性 Female	9 229	15. 25	7. 05	9. 53	9. 45	1. 09	5

表 5-6b 2017 年中国肿瘤登记地区肝癌死亡情况

Table 5-6b Mortality of liver cancer in registration areas of China, 2017

地区 Area	性别 Sex	死亡数 No. deaths	粗率 Crude rate/ 100 000^{-1}	构成比 Freq./%	中标率 ASR China/ 100 000^{-1}	世标率 ASR World/ 100 000^{-1}	累积率 Cum. rate 0~74/%	顺位 Rank
合计	合计 Both	108 691	24. 91	14. 06	15. 41	15. 20	1. 74	2
All	男性 Male	79 885	36. 12	16. 16	23. 43	23. 07	2. 65	2
	女性 Female	28 806	13. 39	10. 34	7. 47	7. 41	0. 84	2
城市地区	合计 Both	50 549	23. 70	13. 09	14. 04	13. 85	1. 59	2
Urban areas	男性 Male	37 123	34. 69	15. 15	21. 57	21. 26	2. 45	2
	女性 Female	13 426	12. 64	9. 51	6. 70	6. 63	0. 74	3
农村地区	合计 Both	58 142	26. 06	15. 04	16. 79	16. 55	1. 90	2
Rural areas	男性 Male	42 762	37. 47	17. 16	25. 28	24. 86	2. 84	2
	女性 Female	15 380	14. 11	11. 19	8. 27	8. 21	0. 94	3
东部地区	合计 Both	47 270	23. 88	12. 37	13. 50	13. 33	1. 54	2
Eastern areas	男性 Male	34 611	34. 78	14. 37	20. 77	20. 50	2. 37	2
	女性 Female	12 659	12. 86	8. 96	6. 44	6. 36	0. 72	4
中部地区	合计 Both	28 299	24. 59	15. 08	16. 67	16. 48	1. 89	2
Central areas	男性 Male	20 327	34. 56	16. 97	24. 57	24. 25	2. 78	2
	女性 Female	7 972	14. 17	11. 73	8. 81	8. 75	0. 99	2
西部地区	合计 Both	33 122	26. 85	16. 31	17. 76	17. 50	1. 98	2
Western areas	男性 Male	24 947	39. 72	18. 65	27. 14	26. 64	3. 01	2
	女性 Female	8 175	13. 50	11. 79	8. 24	8. 23	0. 93	2

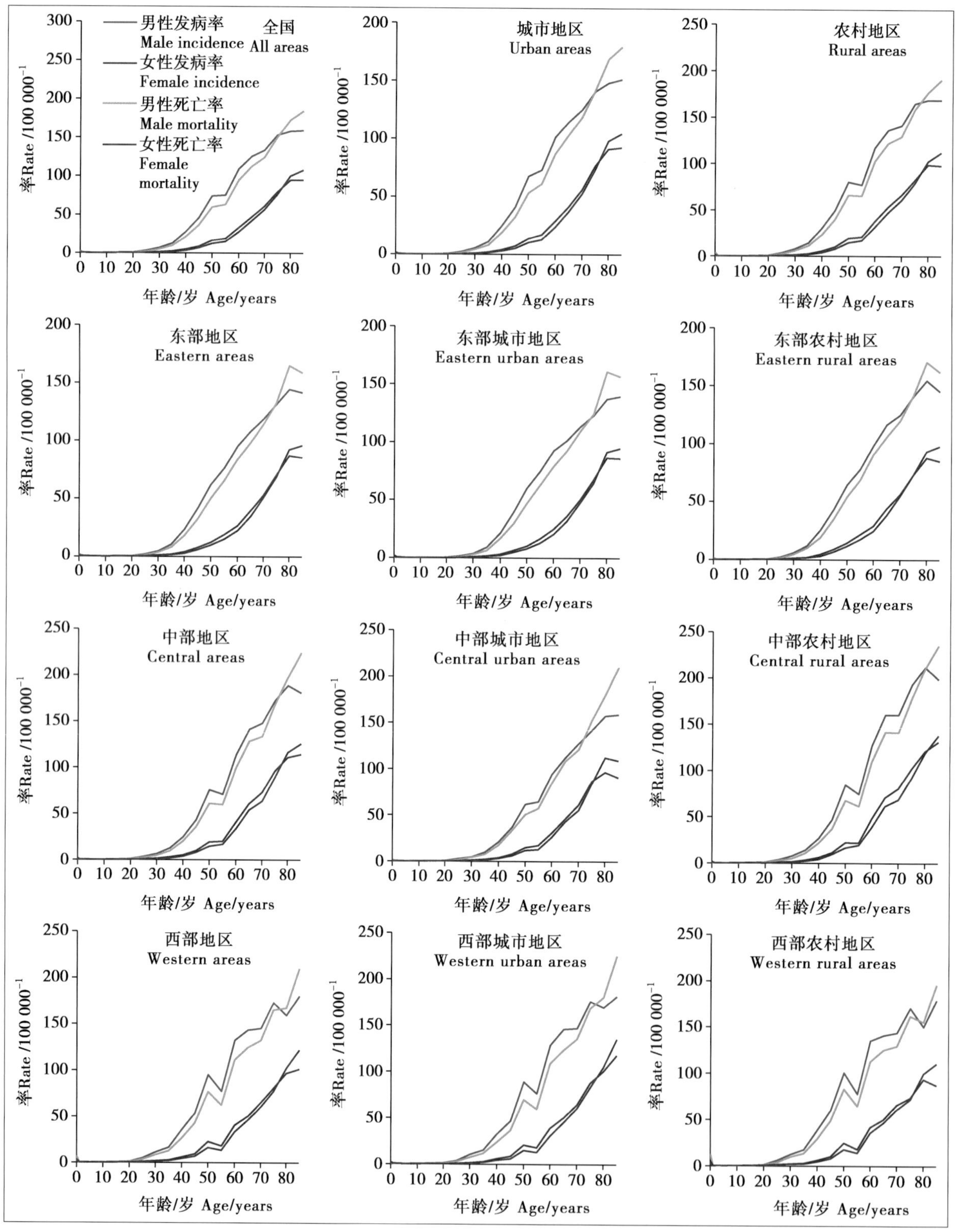

图 5-6a 2017 年中国肿瘤登记地区肝癌年龄别发病率和死亡率

Figure 5-6a Age-specific incidence and mortality rates of liver cancer in registration areas of China, 2017

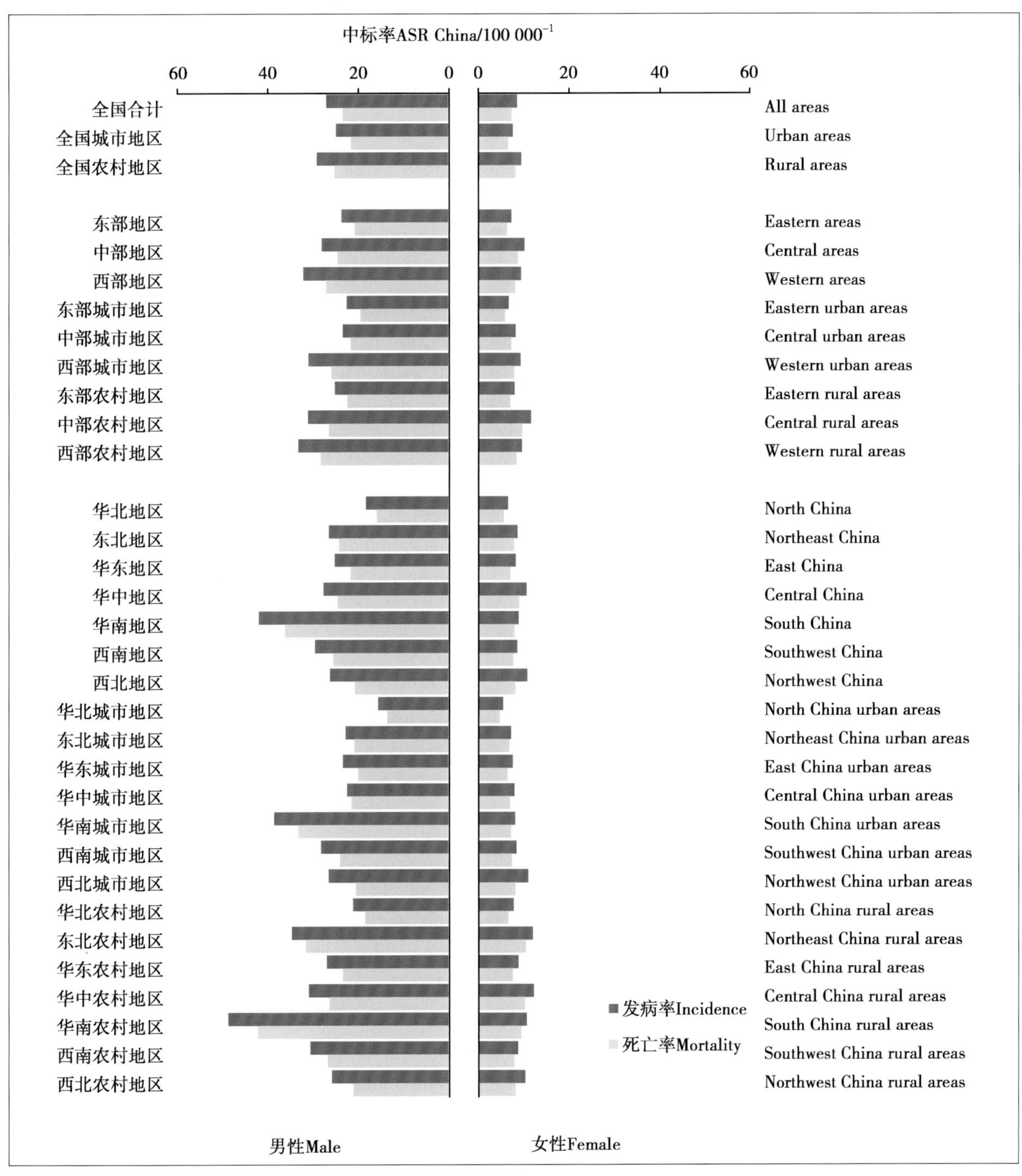

图 5-6b 2017 年中国肿瘤登记地区分城乡肝癌发病率和死亡率

Figure 5-6b Incidence and mortality rates of liver cancer in different registration areas of China, 2017

7 胆囊

2017年中国肿瘤登记地区胆囊癌位居癌症发病谱第18位。新发病例数为17 442例，占全部癌症发病的1.36%；其中男性8 206例，女性9 236例，城市地区9 760例，农村地区7 682例。发病率为4.00/10万，中标发病率为2.30/10万，世标发病率为2.30/10万。中标发病率男性与女性基本相同，城市为农村的1.21倍。0~74岁累积发病率为0.27%（表5-7a）。

2017年中国肿瘤登记地区胆囊癌位居癌症死亡谱第14位。胆囊癌死亡病例为13 178例，占全部癌症死亡的1.70%；其中男性6 149例，女性7 029例，城市地区7 386例，农村地区5 792例。胆囊癌死亡率为3.02/10万，中标死亡率为1.68/10万，世标死亡率为1.68/10万；女性中标死亡率与男性接近，城市地区中标死亡率为农村地区的1.20倍，0~74岁累积死亡率为0.18%（表5-7b）。

中国肿瘤登记地区胆囊癌年龄别发病率和死亡率在40岁之前处于较低水平，40~44岁年龄组开始呈显著上升趋势。男性发病率于85岁及以上年龄组达到高峰，女性发病率于80~84岁组达到高峰，男女死亡率均于85岁及以上年龄组达到高峰。男性与女性年龄别发病（死亡）率较为接近（图5-7a）。

城市地区胆囊癌发病和死亡率高于农村地区，东部地区高于中部和西部地区。在七大行政区中，男性和女性发病率和死亡率均在西北地区最高，男性在西南地区最低，女性在华南地区最低（表5-7a，表5-7b，图5-7b）。

7 Gallbladder

The incidence of gallbladder cancer ranked 18th among all cancer types in the registration areas of China in 2017. There were 17 442 new cases of gallbladder cancer(8 206 males and 9 236 females, 9 760 in urban areas and 7 682 in rural areas), accounting for 1.36% of all new cancer cases. The crude incidence rate was 4.00 per 100 000, with ASR China 2.30 per 100 000 and ASR World 2.30 per 100 000, respectively. Subgroup analyses showed that the incidence of ASR China in males was similar to that in females, and it was 1.21 times in urban areas as that in rural areas. The cumulative incidence rate of 0 to 74 years old was 0.27%(Table 5-7a).

The mortality rate of gallbladder cancer ranked 14th among different causes of cancer death in the registration areas of China in 2017. There were 13 178 cases dying of gallbladder cancer in 2017(6 149 males and 7 029 females, 7 386 in urban areas and 5 792 in rural areas), accounting for 1.70% of all cancer deaths. The crude mortality rate was 3.02 per 100 000, with ASR China 1.68 per 100 000 and ASR World 1.68 per 100 000, respectively. Subgroup analyses showed that the mortality of ASR China in males and females were similar, and it was 1.20 times in urban areas as that in rural areas. The cumulative mortality rate of 0 to 74 years old was 0.18%(Table 5-7b).

The age-specific incidence and mortality rates were relatively low before 40 years old, and increased rapidly since then. The age-specific incidence rates peaked at the age group of 85+ years in males and 80-84 years for females, respectively. Both for males and females, the age-specific incidence and mortality rate were similar(Figure 5-7a).

The incidence and mortality rates of gallbladder cancer were higher in urban areas than those in rural areas. Eastern areas had thehighest incidence and mortality rates(ASR China), followed by central and the western areas. Among seven administrative districts, the rates were highest in Northwest both for males and females, and lowest in Southwest for males and South China for females(Table 5-7a, Table 5-7b, Figure 5-7b).

表 5-7a　2017 年中国肿瘤登记地区胆囊癌发病情况

Table 5-7a　Incidence of gallbladder cancer in registration areas of China,2017

地区 Area	性别 Sex	病例数 No. cases	粗率 Crude rate/ 100 000^{-1}	构成比 Freq./%	中标率 ASR China/ 100 000^{-1}	世标率 ASR World/ 100 000^{-1}	累积率 Cum. rate 0~74/%	顺位 Rank
合计	合计 Both	17 442	4.00	1.36	2.30	2.30	0.27	18
All	男性 Male	8 206	3.71	1.15	2.25	2.26	0.27	16
	女性 Female	9 236	4.29	1.62	2.35	2.34	0.27	15
城市地区	合计 Both	9 760	4.58	1.45	2.52	2.51	0.29	18
Urban areas	男性 Male	4 632	4.33	1.27	2.51	2.52	0.29	16
	女性 Female	5 128	4.83	1.66	2.53	2.51	0.29	16
农村地区	合计 Both	7 682	3.44	1.26	2.08	2.08	0.25	19
Rural areas	男性 Male	3 574	3.13	1.03	1.98	1.99	0.24	16
	女性 Female	4 108	3.77	1.57	2.17	2.15	0.26	15
东部地区	合计 Both	9 644	4.87	1.46	2.54	2.52	0.29	18
Eastern areas	男性 Male	4 764	4.79	1.34	2.65	2.65	0.31	16
	女性 Female	4 880	4.96	1.60	2.42	2.40	0.27	16
中部地区	合计 Both	3 815	3.32	1.27	2.15	2.16	0.26	19
Central areas	男性 Male	1 653	2.81	0.99	1.92	1.94	0.24	17
	女性 Female	2 162	3.84	1.61	2.37	2.37	0.28	15
西部地区	合计 Both	3 983	3.23	1.25	2.01	2.01	0.24	19
Western areas	男性 Male	1 789	2.85	0.95	1.83	1.83	0.21	17
	女性 Female	2 194	3.62	1.68	2.19	2.18	0.26	15

表 5-7b　2017 年中国肿瘤登记地区胆囊癌死亡情况

Table 5-7b　Mortality of gallbladder cancer inregistration areas of China,2017

地区 Area	性别 Sex	死亡数 No. deaths	粗率 Crude rate/ 100 000^{-1}	构成比 Freq./%	中标率 ASR China/ 100 000^{-1}	世标率 ASR World/ 100 000^{-1}	累积率 Cum. rate 0~74/%	顺位 Rank
合计	合计 Both	13 178	3.02	1.70	1.68	1.68	0.18	14
All	男性 Male	6 149	2.78	1.24	1.65	1.65	0.18	13
	女性 Female	7 029	3.27	2.52	1.71	1.70	0.18	11
城市地区	合计 Both	7 386	3.46	1.91	1.83	1.82	0.20	14
Urban areas	男性 Male	3 478	3.25	1.42	1.83	1.84	0.20	12
	女性 Female	3 908	3.68	2.77	1.82	1.80	0.19	10
农村地区	合计 Both	5 792	2.60	1.50	1.53	1.52	0.17	14
Rural areas	男性 Male	2 671	2.34	1.07	1.46	1.46	0.17	14
	女性 Female	3 121	2.86	2.27	1.59	1.58	0.18	12
东部地区	合计 Both	7 472	3.78	1.96	1.89	1.87	0.20	14
Eastern areas	男性 Male	3 617	3.63	1.50	1.95	1.95	0.22	12
	女性 Female	3 855	3.92	2.73	1.81	1.79	0.19	10
中部地区	合计 Both	2 944	2.56	1.57	1.62	1.61	0.18	14
Central areas	男性 Male	1 320	2.24	1.10	1.52	1.52	0.18	13
	女性 Female	1 624	2.89	2.39	1.71	1.69	0.19	11
西部地区	合计 Both	2 762	2.24	1.36	1.36	1.36	0.15	15
Western areas	男性 Male	1 212	1.93	0.91	1.22	1.22	0.13	14
	女性 Female	1 550	2.56	2.24	1.50	1.50	0.17	12

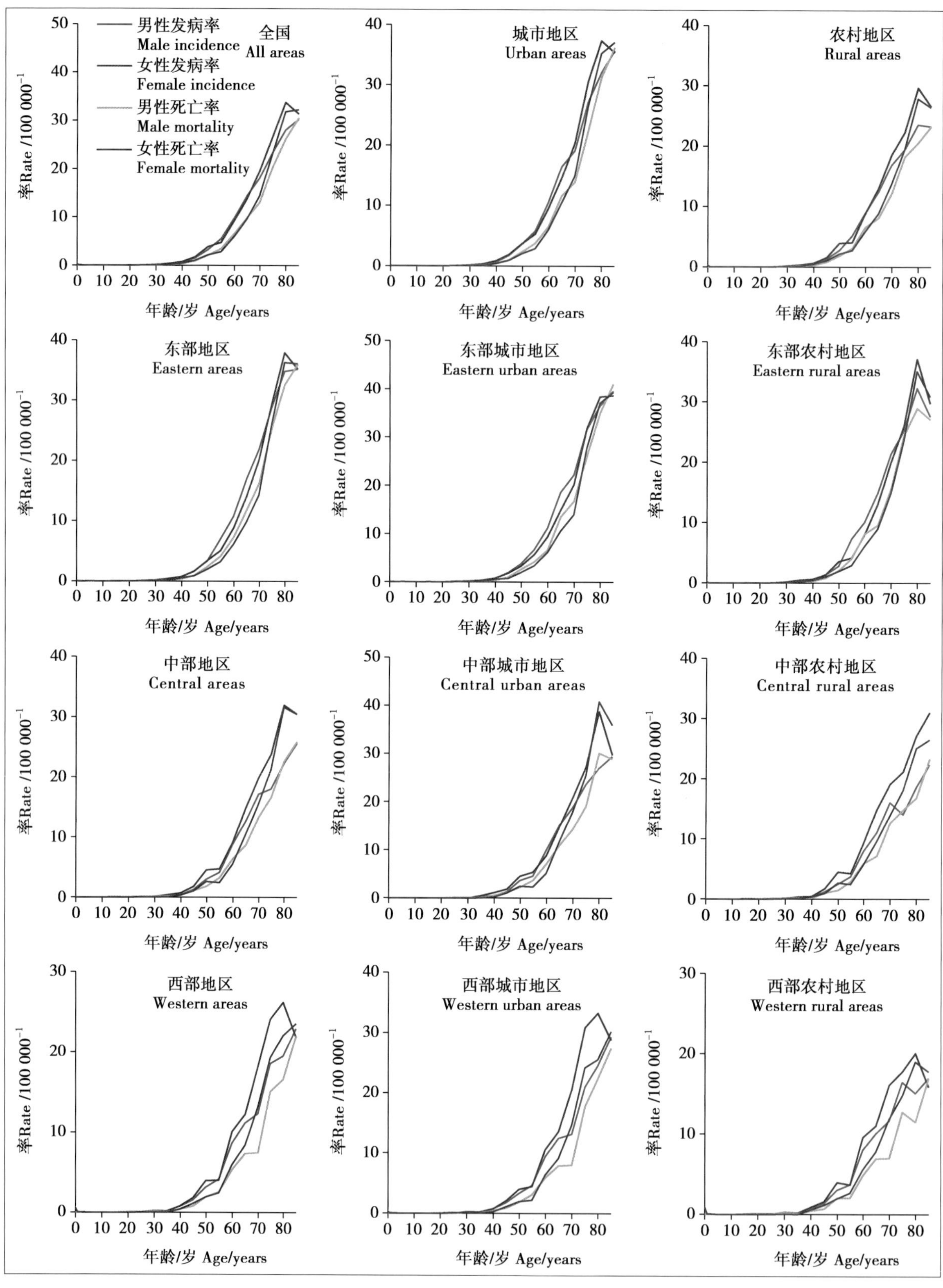

图 5-7a　2017 年中国肿瘤登记地区胆囊癌年龄别发病率和死亡率

Figure 5-7a　Age-specific incidence and mortality rates of gallbladder cancer in registration areas of China, 2017

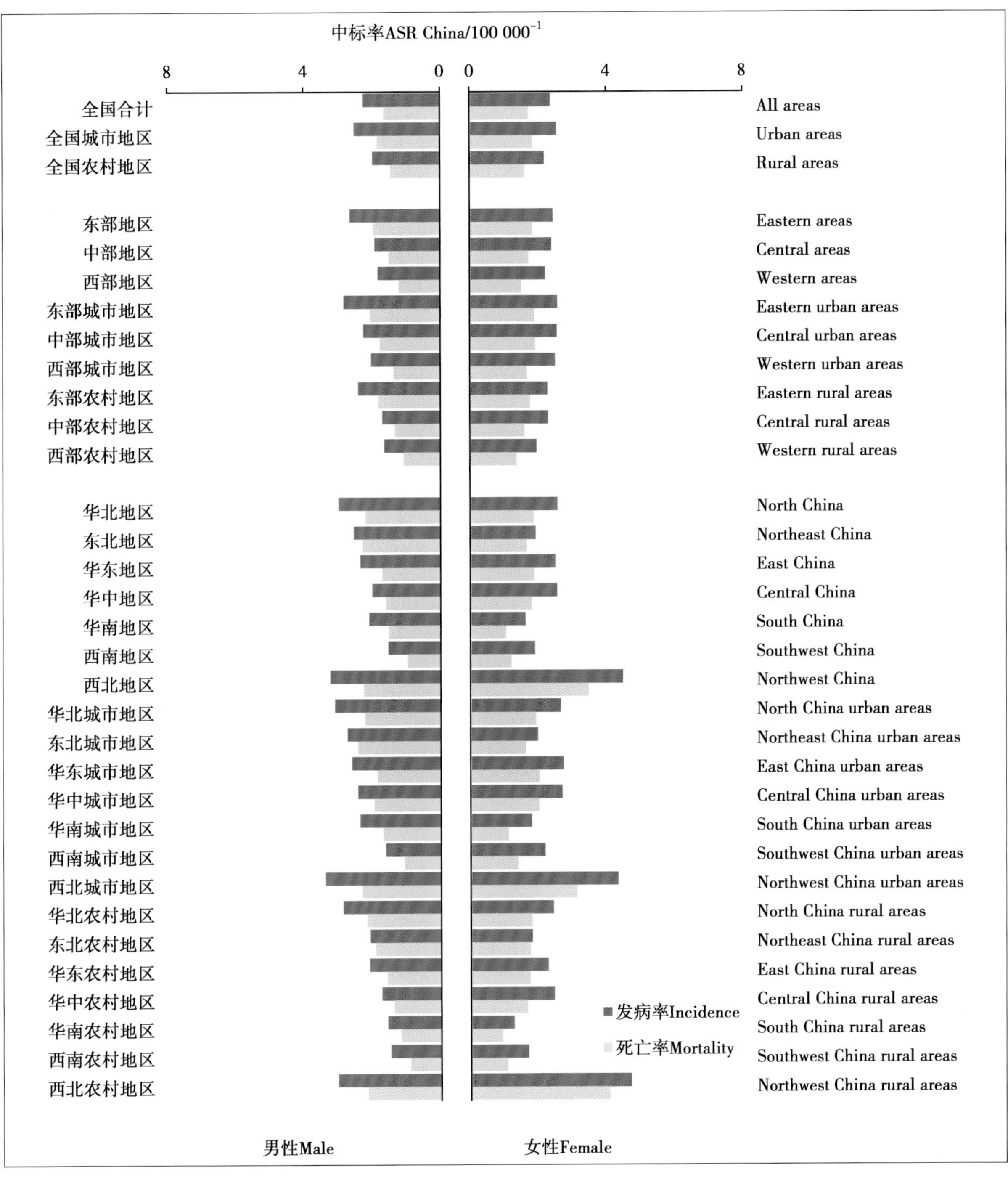

图 5-7b 2017 年中国肿瘤登记地区分城乡胆囊癌发病率和死亡率

Figure 5-7b Incidence and mortality rates of gallbladder cancer in different registration areas of China,2017

8 胰腺

2017 年中国肿瘤登记地区胰腺癌位居癌症发病谱第 13 位。新发病例数为 30 869 例,占全部癌症发病的 2. 41%;其中男性 17 732 例,女性 13 137 例,城市地区 17 284 例,农村地区 13 585 例。发病率为 7. 07/10 万,中标发病率为 4. 13/10 万,世标发病率为 4. 11/10 万。男性中标发病率为女性的 1. 46 倍,城市中标发病率为农村的 1. 21 倍。0 ~ 74 岁累积发病率为 0. 48%(表 5-8a)。

2017 年中国肿瘤登记地区胰腺癌位居癌症死亡谱第 7 位。因胰腺癌死亡病例 27 907 例,占全部癌症死亡的 3. 61%;其中男性 15 979 例,女性 11 928 例,城市地区 15 968 例,农村地区 11 939 例。胰腺癌死亡率为 6. 40/10 万,中标死亡率 3. 66/10 万,世标死亡率 3. 64/10 万。男性中标死亡率为女性的 1. 48 倍,城市中标死亡率为农村的 1. 27 倍。0 ~ 74 岁累积死亡率为 0. 42%(表 5-8b)。

胰腺癌年龄别发病率和死亡率在 44 岁之前均处于较低水平,自 45 ~ 49 岁组快速上升,分别在 85 岁及以上和 80 ~ 84 岁年龄组达到顶峰,男性高于女性(图 5-8a)。

城市地区胰腺癌的发病率和死亡率均高于农村地区。东部地区中标发病率和死亡率高于中部和西部地区。七大行政区中,东北地区最高,华南地区最低(表 5-8a,表 5-8b,图 5-8b)。

31. 79%的胰腺癌病例报告了明确亚部位信息。各亚部位的胰腺癌比例构成如下:胰头占 52. 50%、胰岛[朗格汉斯岛]占 20. 35%、胰体占 10. 66%、胰尾占 8. 11%、交搭跨越占 3. 96%,胰管占 2. 60%(图 5-8c)。

8 Pancreas

The incidence of pancreatic cancer ranked 13th among all cancer types in the registration areas of China in 2017. There were 30 869 new cases of pancreatic cancer (17 732 males and 13 137 females, 17 284 in urban areas and 13 585 in rural areas), accounting for 2. 41% of new cases. The crude incidence rate was 7. 07 per 100 000, with ASR China 4. 13 per 100 000 and ASR World 4. 11 per 100 000, respectively. Subgroup analyses showed that the incidence of ASR China was 1. 46 times in males as high as that in females, and it was 1. 21 times in urban areas as high as that in rural areas. The cumulative incidence rate for subjects aged from 0 to 74 years old was 0. 48% (Table 5-8a).

Pancreatic cancer was the 7th leading cause of cancer death in the registration areas of China in 2017. A total of 27 907 cases died of pancreatic cancer (15 979 males and 11 928 females, 15 968 in urban areas and 11 939 in rural areas), accounting for 3. 61% of all cancer deaths. The crude mortality rate was 6. 40 per 100 000, with ASR China 3. 66 per 100 000 and ASR World 3. 64 per 100 000, respectively. Subgroup analyses showed that the mortality of ASR China was 1. 48 times in males as high as that in females, and it was 1. 27 times in urban areas as high as that in rural areas. The cumulative mortality rate for subjects aged from 0 to 74 years old was 0. 42% (Table 5-8b).

The age-specific incidence and mortality rates were relatively low before 44 years old and increased rapidly from the age group of 45-49 years old, peaked at the age group of 80-84 and 85+ years old, respectively. The incidence and mortality rates in males were generally higher than those in females (Figure 5-8a).

The incidenceand mortality rates of pancreatic cancer were higher in urban areas than that in rural areas. Eastern areas had the higher incidence and mortality rates (ASR China) than central and western areas. Among the seven administraitve districts, the highest pancreatic cancer incidence and mortality (ASR China) were shown in Northeast China, and the lowest in South China (Table 5-8a, Table 5-8b, Figure 5-8b).

There were 31. 79% of pancreatic cancer cases with specific subsite information. Among those, 52. 50% of cases occurred in head, followed by islets of Langerhans (20. 35%), body (10. 66%), tail (8. 11%), overlapping (3. 96%) and pancreatic duct (2. 60%) (Figure 5-8c).

表 5-8a 2017 年中国肿瘤登记地区胰腺癌发病情况
Table 5-8a Incidence of pancreatic cancer in the registration areas of China, 2017

地区 Area	性别 Sex	病例数 No. cases	粗率 Crude rate/ 100 000⁻¹	构成比 Freq. /%	中标率 ASR China/ 100 000⁻¹	世标率 ASR World/ 100 000⁻¹	累积率 Cum. rate 0~74/%	顺位 Rank
合计	合计 Both	30 869	7.07	2.41	4.13	4.11	0.48	13
All	男性 Male	17 732	8.02	2.49	4.92	4.91	0.58	8
	女性 Female	13 137	6.10	2.31	3.37	3.34	0.39	12
城市地区	合计 Both	17 284	8.11	2.56	4.51	4.50	0.52	13
Urban areas	男性 Male	9 789	9.15	2.68	5.35	5.36	0.63	9
	女性 Female	7 495	7.06	2.43	3.71	3.67	0.42	12
农村地区	合计 Both	13 585	6.09	2.24	3.74	3.71	0.44	13
Rural areas	男性 Male	7 943	6.96	2.29	4.48	4.44	0.53	9
	女性 Female	5 642	5.18	2.16	3.01	2.98	0.35	12
东部地区	合计 Both	17 633	8.91	2.67	4.71	4.67	0.55	12
Eastern areas	男性 Male	9 980	10.03	2.80	5.61	5.59	0.66	8
	女性 Female	7 653	7.78	2.51	3.85	3.80	0.44	12
中部地区	合计 Both	6 053	5.26	2.01	3.47	3.45	0.41	15
Central areas	男性 Male	3 486	5.93	2.09	4.09	4.08	0.49	10
	女性 Female	2 567	4.56	1.91	2.87	2.85	0.33	14
西部地区	合计 Both	7 183	5.82	2.25	3.65	3.64	0.43	13
Western areas	男性 Male	4 266	6.79	2.27	4.40	4.39	0.51	8
	女性 Female	2 917	4.82	2.23	2.91	2.89	0.34	12

表 5-8b 2017 年中国肿瘤登记地区胰腺癌死亡情况
Table 5-8b Mortality of pancreatic cancer in the registration areas of China, 2017

地区 Area	性别 Sex	死亡数 No. deaths	粗率 Crude rate/ 100 000⁻¹	构成比 Freq. /%	中标率 ASR China/ 100 000⁻¹	世标率 ASR World/ 100 000⁻¹	累积率 Cum. rate 0~74/%	顺位 Rank
合计	合计 Both	27 907	6.40	3.61	3.66	3.64	0.42	7
All	男性 Male	15 979	7.23	3.23	4.37	4.37	0.51	6
	女性 Female	11 928	5.54	4.28	2.96	2.94	0.33	8
城市地区	合计 Both	15 968	7.49	4.13	4.08	4.06	0.47	7
Urban areas	男性 Male	9 049	8.46	3.69	4.88	4.89	0.57	6
	女性 Female	6 919	6.51	4.90	3.31	3.27	0.37	6
农村地区	合计 Both	11 939	5.35	3.09	3.22	3.20	0.38	8
Rural areas	男性 Male	6 930	6.07	2.78	3.86	3.84	0.45	6
	女性 Female	5 009	4.60	3.64	2.60	2.58	0.30	8
东部地区	合计 Both	16 385	8.28	4.29	4.26	4.24	0.49	7
Eastern areas	男性 Male	9 205	9.25	3.82	5.09	5.07	0.59	6
	女性 Female	7 180	7.30	5.08	3.48	3.44	0.39	7
中部地区	合计 Both	5 393	4.69	2.87	3.05	3.04	0.36	8
Central areas	男性 Male	3 123	5.31	2.61	3.65	3.65	0.44	6
	女性 Female	2 270	4.03	3.34	2.46	2.44	0.28	8
西部地区	合计 Both	6 129	4.97	3.02	3.07	3.07	0.35	8
Western areas	男性 Male	3 651	5.81	2.73	3.72	3.73	0.43	6
	女性 Female	2 478	4.09	3.57	2.43	2.42	0.28	8

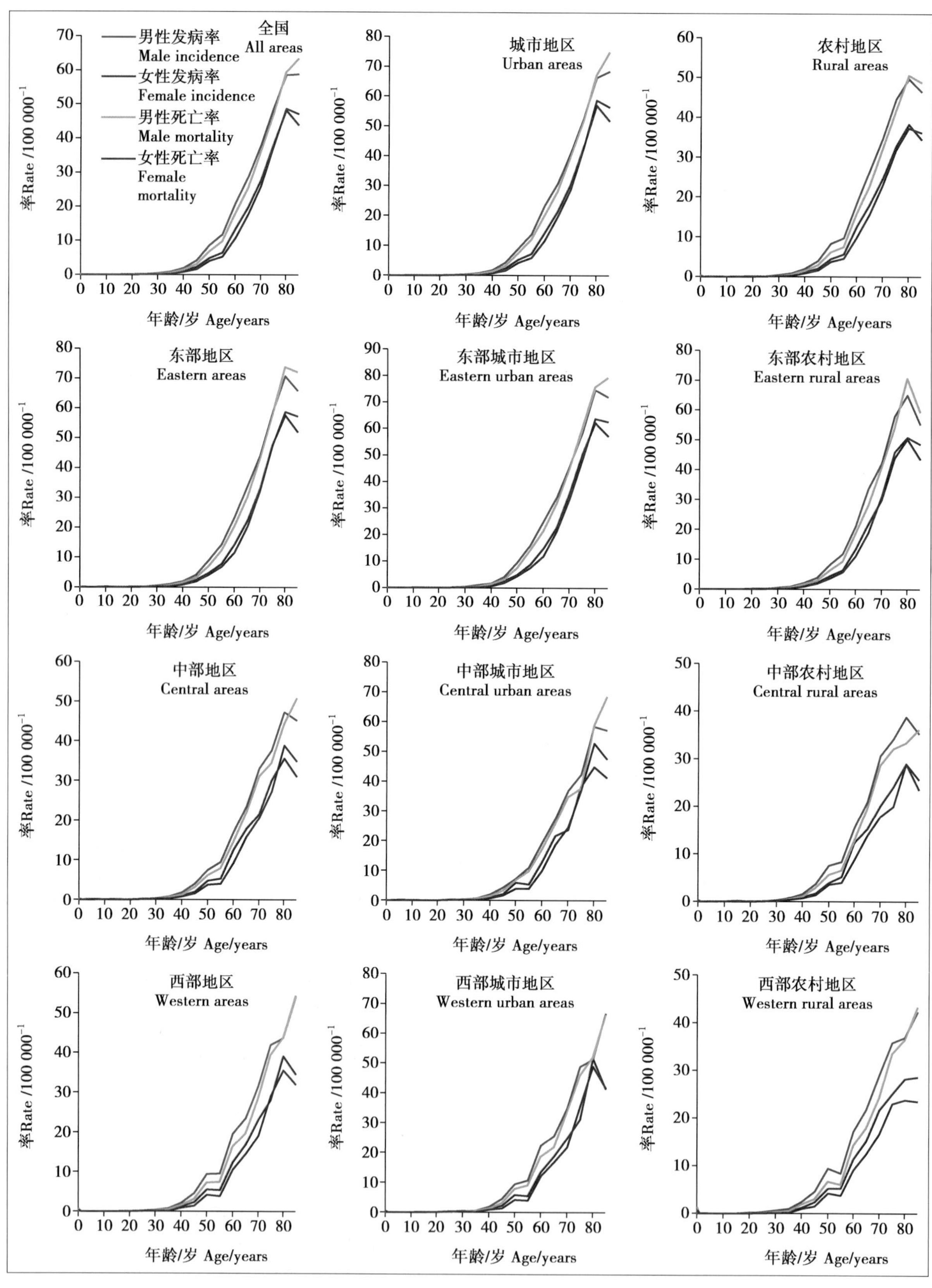

图 5-8a　2017 年中国肿瘤登记地区胰腺癌年龄别发病率和死亡率

Figure 5-8a　Age-specific incidence and mortality rates of pancreatic cancer in the registration areas of China, 2017

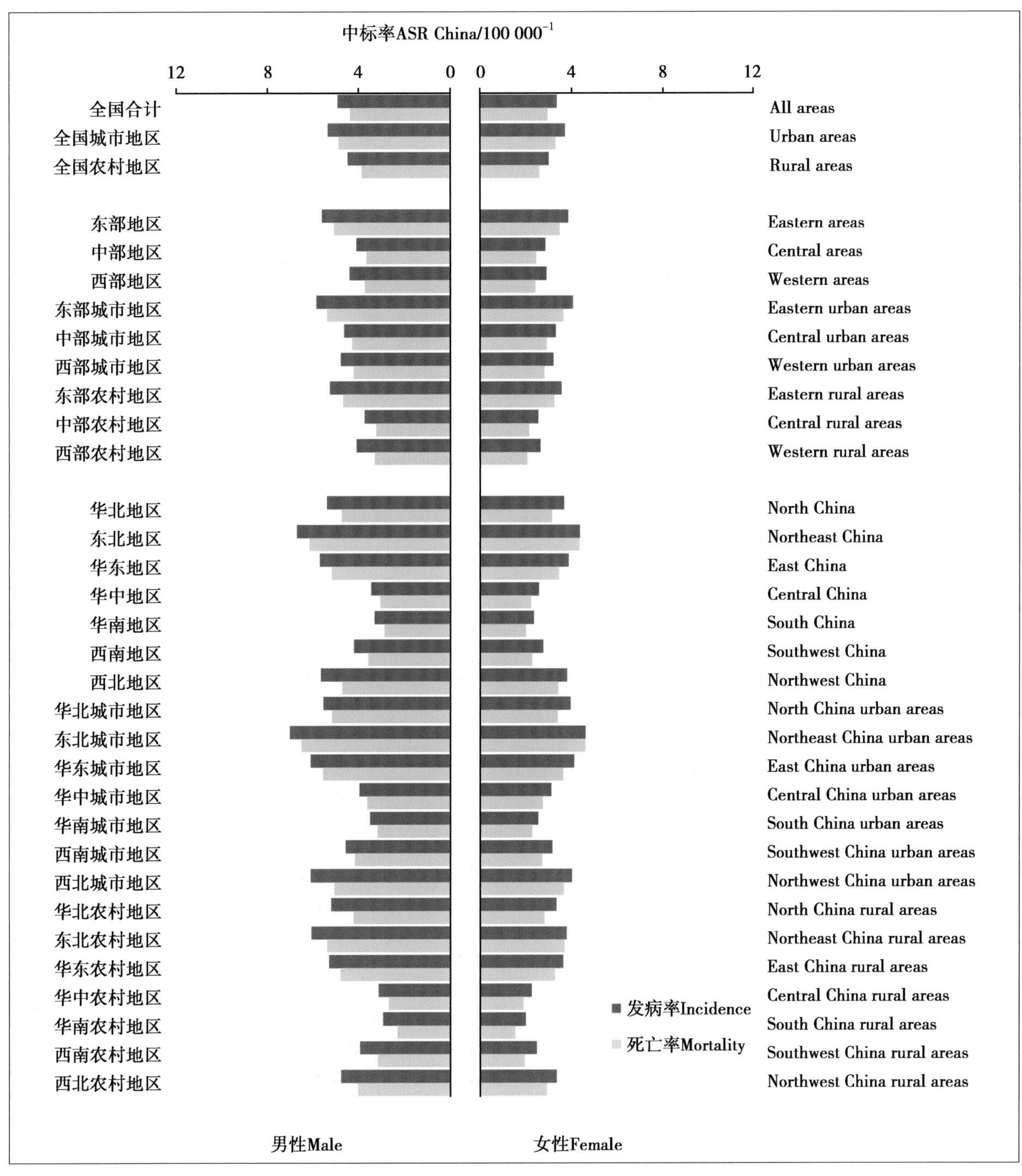

图 5-8b 2017 年中国肿瘤登记地区分城乡胰腺癌发病率和死亡率
Figure 5-8b Incidence and mortality rates of pancreatic cancer in different registration areas of China,2017

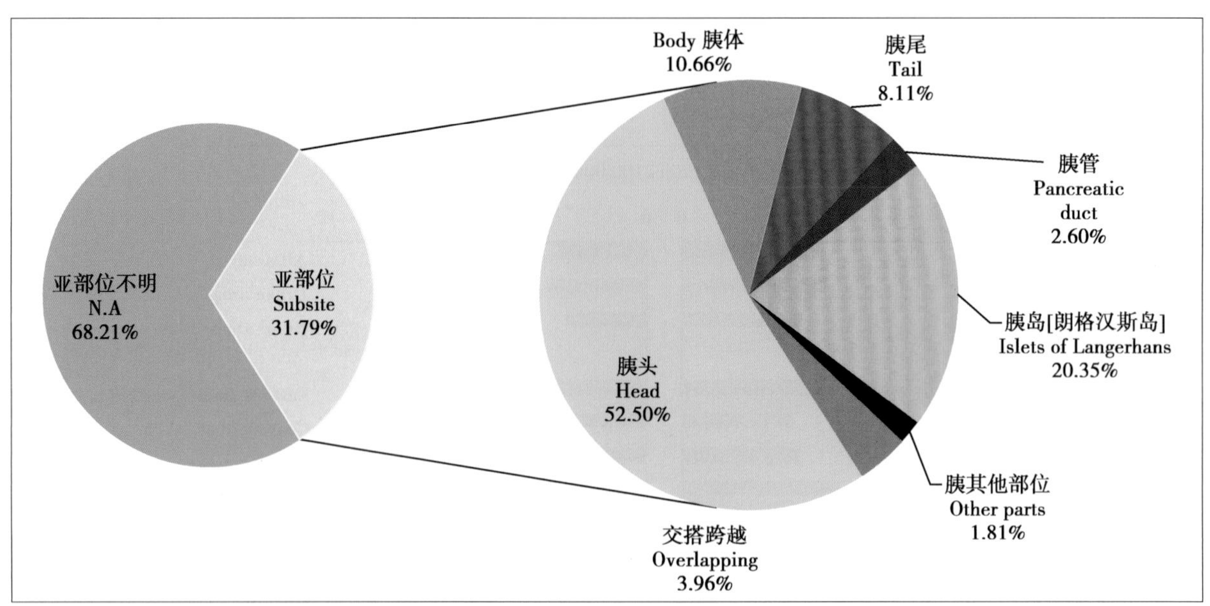

图 5-8c 2017 年中国肿瘤登记地区胰腺癌亚部位分布情况
Figure 5-8c Subsite distribution of pancreatic cancer in the registration areas of China,2017

9 喉

2017 年,中国肿瘤登记地区喉癌位居癌症发病谱第 21 位。新发病例数为 8 016 例,占全部癌症发病的 0.63%;其中男性 7 290 例,女性 726 例,城市地区 4 541 例,农村地区 3 475 例。喉癌发病率为 1.84/10 万,中标发病率为 1.11/10 万,世标发病率为 1.13/10 万;男性中标发病率为女性的 10.33 倍,城市中标发病率为农村的 1.27 倍。0~74 岁累积发病率为 0.14%(表 5-9a)。

2017 年,中国肿瘤登记地区喉癌位居癌症死亡谱第 21 位。喉癌死亡病例 4 712 例,占全部癌症死亡的 0.61%;其中男性 3 947 例,女性 765 例,城市地区 2 531 例,农村地区 2 181 例。喉癌死亡率为 1.08/10 万,中标死亡率和世标死亡率均为 0.62/10 万;男性中标死亡率为女性的 5.70 倍,城市中标死亡率稍高于农村。0~74 岁累积死亡率为 0.07%(表 5-9b)。

喉癌年龄别发病率、年龄别死亡率呈现性别差异。男性年龄别发病率和死亡率在 0~39 岁处于较低水平,40~44 岁组后显著上升;女性在 0~49 岁处于较低水平,50~54 岁组后上升。各年龄组男性发病率和死亡率一般高于女性(图 5-9a)。

城市地区喉癌发病率和死亡率均高于农村地区。中部地区中标发病率最高。七大行政区中,男性喉癌的发病率和死亡率华南地区最高,西北地区最低;女性发病率和死亡率最高的是西北地区和华中地区;发病率和死亡率华东地区最低(表 5-9a,表 5-9b,图 5-9b)。

9 Larynx

In 2017, the incidence of laryngeal cancer ranked 21st among all cancer types in cancer registration areas of China. There were 8 016 new cases diagnosed with laryngeal cancer(7 290 males and 726 females, 4 541 in urban areas and 3 475 in rural areas), accounting for 0.63% of new cancer cases. The crude incidence rate was 1.84 per 100 000, with ASR China and ASR World 1.11 per 100 000 and 1.13 per 100 000, respectively. The incidence rate of ASR China in males was 10.33 times as high as that in females. The incidence rate of ASR China in urban areas was 1.27 folds as high as that in rural areas. The cumulative incidence rate for subjects aged 0 to 74 years was 0.14%(Table 5-9a).

Laryngeal cancer ranked 21st among all causes of cancer death in 2017. A total of 4 712 cases died of laryngeal cancer(3 947 males and 765 females, 2 531 in urban areas and 2 181 in rural areas), accounting for 0.61% of all cancer deaths. The crude mortality rate was 1.08 per 100 000, The ASR China and ASR World were both 0.62 per 100 000. The mortality rate of ASR China in males was 5.70 times as high as that in females. The mortality rate of ASR China in urban areas was slightly higher than that in rural areas. The cumulative mortality rate for subjects aged 0 to 74 years was 0.07%(Table 5-9b).

The age-specific incidence and mortality rates showed differences between males and females. The incidence and mortality rates for males were relatively low in 0-39 years old, but increased sharply since then. For females, the age-specific rates were relatively low in 0-49 years old and increased since then. Age-specific incidence and mortality rates in males were generally higher than those in females(Figure 5-9a).

The incidence and mortality rates of laryngeal cancer in urban areas were higher than those in rural areas. Central areas had the highest incidence rate of ASR China. Among the seven administrative districts, for males, South China had the highest incidence and mortality rates, while Northwest China had the lowest rates. For females, the highest incidence and mortality rate was in Northwest China and in Central China; the lowest incidence and mortality rate was in East China (Table 5-9a, Table 5-9b, Figure 5-9b).

表 5-9a 2017 年中国肿瘤登记地区喉癌发病情况
Table 5-9a Incidence of laryngeal cancer in registration areas of China, 2017

地区 Area	性别 Sex	病例数 No. cases	粗率 Crude rate/ 100 000^{-1}	构成比 Freq./%	中标率 ASR China/ 100 000^{-1}	世标率 ASR World/ 100 000^{-1}	累积率 Cum. rate 0~74/%	顺位 Rank
合计	合计 Both	8 016	1. 84	0. 63	1. 11	1. 13	0. 14	21
All	男性 Male	7 290	3. 30	1. 02	2. 04	2. 07	0. 26	17
	女性 Female	726	0. 34	0. 13	0. 20	0. 20	0. 02	23
城市地区	合计 Both	4 541	2. 13	0. 67	1. 24	1. 26	0. 16	21
Urban areas	男性 Male	4 178	3. 90	1. 14	2. 33	2. 37	0. 30	17
	女性 Female	363	0. 34	0. 12	0. 19	0. 19	0. 02	23
农村地区	合计 Both	3 475	1. 56	0. 57	0. 98	0. 99	0. 13	22
Rural areas	男性 Male	3 112	2. 73	0. 90	1. 75	1. 77	0. 23	17
	女性 Female	363	0. 33	0. 14	0. 21	0. 20	0. 02	23
东部地区	合计 Both	3 886	1. 96	0. 59	1. 08	1. 10	0. 14	21
Eastern areas	男性 Male	3 609	3. 63	1. 01	2. 06	2. 10	0. 27	17
	女性 Female	277	0. 28	0. 09	0. 15	0. 15	0. 02	23
中部地区	合计 Both	2 025	1. 76	0. 67	1. 18	1. 19	0. 15	22
Central areas	男性 Male	1 819	3. 09	1. 09	2. 14	2. 17	0. 27	16
	女性 Female	206	0. 37	0. 15	0. 25	0. 24	0. 03	23
西部地区	合计 Both	2 105	1. 71	0. 66	1. 09	1. 11	0. 14	22
Western areas	男性 Male	1 862	2. 96	0. 99	1. 93	1. 96	0. 24	16
	女性 Female	243	0. 40	0. 19	0. 25	0. 25	0. 03	23

表 5-9b 2017 年中国肿瘤登记地区喉癌死亡情况
Table 5-9b Mortality of laryngeal cancer in registration areas of China, 2017

地区 Area	性别 Sex	死亡数 No. deaths	粗率 Crude rate/ 100 000^{-1}	构成比 Freq./%	中标率 ASR China/ 100 000^{-1}	世标率 ASR World/ 100 000^{-1}	累积率 Cum. rate 0~74/%	顺位 Rank
合计	合计 Both	4 712	1. 08	0. 61	0. 62	0. 62	0. 07	21
All	男性 Male	3 947	1. 78	0. 80	1. 07	1. 08	0. 13	16
	女性 Female	765	0. 36	0. 27	0. 19	0. 19	0. 02	22
城市地区	合计 Both	2 531	1. 19	0. 66	0. 65	0. 65	0. 08	21
Urban areas	男性 Male	2 156	2. 01	0. 88	1. 15	1. 17	0. 14	16
	女性 Female	375	0. 35	0. 27	0. 17	0. 17	0. 02	22
农村地区	合计 Both	2 181	0. 98	0. 56	0. 59	0. 59	0. 07	21
Rural areas	男性 Male	1 791	1. 57	0. 72	0. 99	1. 00	0. 12	17
	女性 Female	390	0. 36	0. 28	0. 20	0. 20	0. 02	21
东部地区	合计 Both	2 251	1. 14	0. 59	0. 59	0. 59	0. 07	21
Eastern areas	男性 Male	1 874	1. 88	0. 78	1. 02	1. 03	0. 12	16
	女性 Female	377	0. 38	0. 27	0. 18	0. 18	0. 02	23
中部地区	合计 Both	1 205	1. 05	0. 64	0. 68	0. 69	0. 08	21
Central areas	男性 Male	1 003	1. 71	0. 84	1. 16	1. 18	0. 14	16
	女性 Female	202	0. 36	0. 30	0. 22	0. 22	0. 02	22
西部地区	合计 Both	1 256	1. 02	0. 62	0. 63	0. 63	0. 07	21
Western areas	男性 Male	1 070	1. 70	0. 80	1. 09	1. 10	0. 13	16
	女性 Female	186	0. 31	0. 27	0. 17	0. 17	0. 02	22

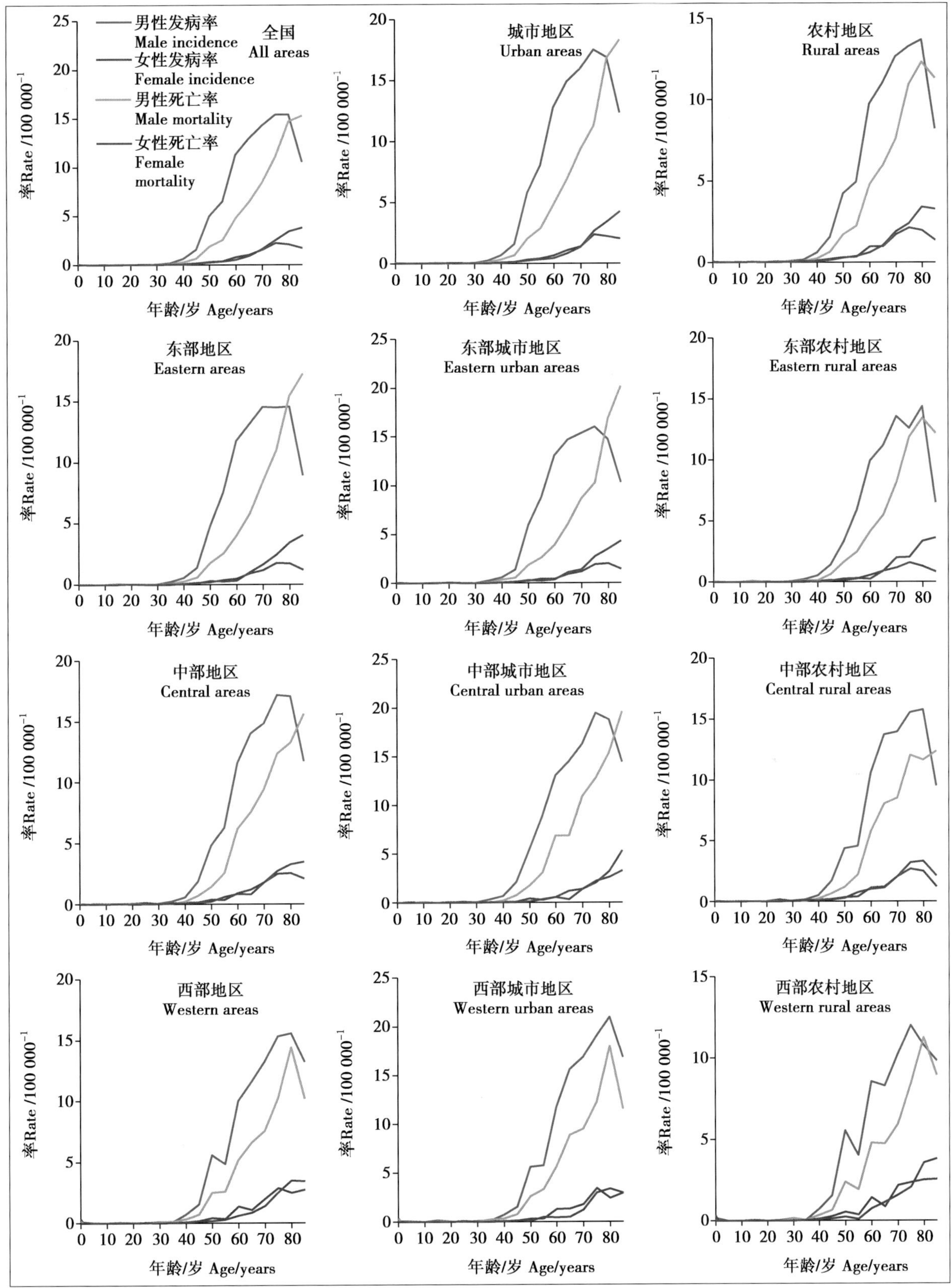

图 5-9a　2017 年中国肿瘤登记地区喉癌年龄别发病率和死亡率

Figure 5-9a　Age-specific incidence and mortality rates of laryngeal cancer in registration areas of China, 2017

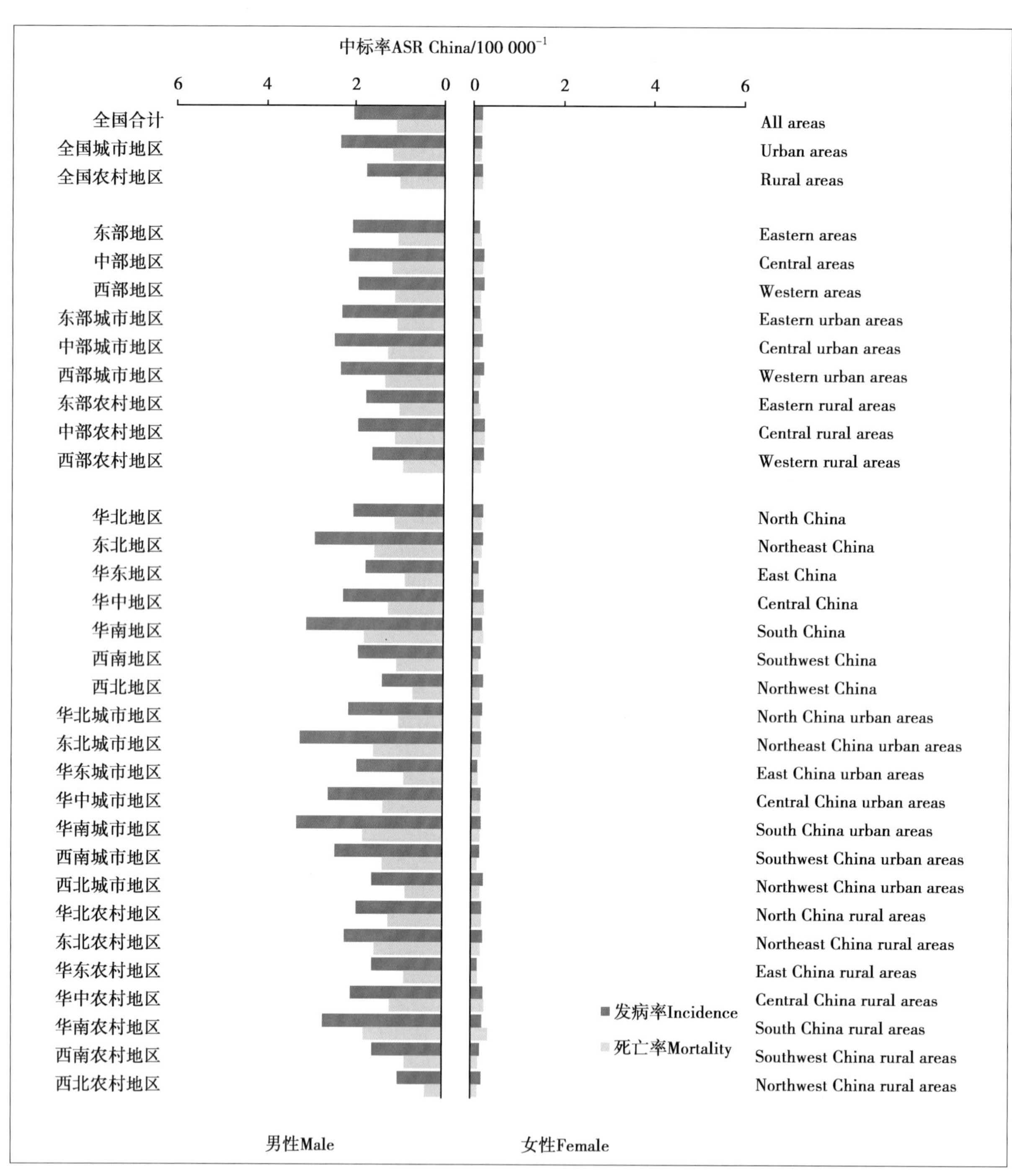

图 5-9b　2017 年中国肿瘤登记不同地区喉癌发病率和死亡率

Figure 5-9b　Incidence and mortality rates of laryngeal cancer in different registration areas of China,2017

10 肺

2017 年,中国肿瘤登记地区肺癌位居癌症发病谱第 1 位。新发病例数为 274 690 例,占全部癌症发病的 21.44%;其中男性 181 959 例,女性 92 731 例,城市地区 140 904 例,农村地区 133 786 例。肺癌发病率为 62.95/10 万,中标发病率为 37.29/10 万,世标发病率为 37.28/10 万;男性中标发病率为女性的 2.03 倍,城市中标发病率为农村的 1.02 倍。0~74 岁累积发病率为 4.57%(表 5-10a)。

2017 年,中国肿瘤登记地区肺癌位居癌症死亡谱第 1 位。肺癌死亡病例 215 025 例,占全部癌症死亡的 27.82%;其中男性 149 992 例,女性 65 033 例,城市地区 108 521 例,农村地区 106 504 例。肺癌死亡率为 49.28/10 万,中标死亡率为 28.14/10 万,世标死亡率为 28.08/10 万;男性中标死亡率为女性的 2.52 倍,城市中标死亡率与农村接近。0~74 岁累积死亡率为 3.29%(表 5-10b)。

肺癌年龄别发病率和死亡率在 40 岁之前均处于较低水平,自 40~44 岁组开始快速上升,男性和女性发病率均在 80~84 岁组达到高峰,男性死亡率在 85 岁及以上组达到高峰,女性在 80~84 岁组达到高峰,男性上升速度快于女性。40~44 岁组后,男性各年龄别发病率和死亡率均明显高于女性(图 5-10a)。

10 Lung

In 2017, lung cancer was the most frequently diagnosed cancer in registration areas of China. There were 274 690 new cases diagnosed as lung cancer (181 959 males and 92 731 females, 140 904 in urban areas and 133 786 in rural areas), accounting for 21.44% of new cases of all cancers. The crude incidence rate was 62.95 per 100 000, with the ASR China and ASR World were 37.29 and 37.28 per 100 000, respectively. The incidence rate of ASR China was 2.03 and 1.02 folds in males and in urban areas as those in females and in rural areas, respectively. The cumulative incidence rate for subjects aged 0 to 74 years was 4.57% (Table 5-10a).

Lung cancer was the leading cause of cancer death in 2017. A total of 215 025 cases died of lung cancer (149 992 males and 65 033 females, 108 521 in urban areas and 106 504 in rural areas), accounting for 27.82% of all cancer deaths. The crude mortality rate was 49.28 per 100 000, with the ASR China and ASR World were 28.14 and 28.08 per 100 000, respectively. The mortality rate of ASR China was 2.52 folds in males as that in females, while the ASR China in urban areas was similar to that in rural areas. The cumulative mortality rate for subjects aged 0 to 74 years was 3.29% (Table 5-10b).

The age-specific incidence and mortality rates of lung cancer were relatively low before 40 years old and increased dramatically since then. The age-specific incidence rate for both males and females peaked at age group of 80-84 years, while the age-specific mortality rate peaked at age group of 85+ years and 80-84 years for males and females, respectively. Incidence and mortality rates in males increased faster than those in females. Age-specific incidence and mortality rates in males were generally higher than those in females since the age group of 40-44 years (Figure 5-10a).

城市地区肺癌的发病率和死亡率略高于农村地区。东部地区中标发病率和西部地区接近，略高于中部地区；中标死亡率以西部地区最高，其次是中部地区，东部地区最低。在七大行政区中，女性发病率和死亡率均是东北地区最高，西北地区最低，男性发病、死亡率华中地区最高，西北地区男性发病率和死亡率均最低（表 5-10a，表 5-10b，图 5-10b）。

全部肺癌病例中有明确亚部位的病例占 28.76%，其中主要在肺上叶，占 48.97%，其次是肺下叶（29.45%）和肺中叶（12.05%），主支气管仅占 6.42%（图 5-10c）。

全部肺癌病例中有明确组织学类型的病例占 52.95%，其中腺癌是主要的病理类型，占 56.76%，其次是鳞状细胞癌（26.58%）和小细胞癌（10.61%）（图 5-10d）。

The incidence and mortality rates of lung cancer in urban areas were slightly higherthan those in rural areas. The incidence rate of ASR China in eastern areas was close to western areas and slightly higher than the central areas. Western areas had the highest mortality rate of ASR China, followed by central areas and eastern areas. Among the seven administrative districts, the incidence and mortality rates of lung cancer for females were highest in Northeast China and lowest in Northwest China. While Central China had the highest incidence and mortality rate of ASR China for males, but the lowest incidence and mortality rate of ASR China for lung cancer of males was in Northwest China (Table 5-10a, Table 5-10b, Figure 5-10b).

About 28.76% cases of lung cancer had specified subsite. Among those, lung cancer occurred more frequently in upper lobe (48.97%), followed by lower lobe (29.45%), middle lobe (12.05%) and main bronchus (6.42%) (Figure 5-10c).

About 52.95% cases of lung cancer had morphological verification. Among those, adenocarcinoma was the most common histological type, accounting for 56.76% of all cases, followed by squamous cell carcinoma (26.58%) and small cell carcinoma (10.61%) (Figure 5-10d).

表 5-10a 2016 年中国肿瘤登记地区肺癌发病情况
Table 5-10a Incidence of lung cancer in the registration areas of China, 2016

地区 Area	性别 Sex	病例数 No. cases	粗率 Crude rate/ 100 000^{-1}	构成比 Freq. /%	中标率 ASR China/ 100 000^{-1}	世标率 ASR World/ 100 000^{-1}	累积率 Cum. rate 0~74/%	顺位 Rank
合计	合计 Both	274 690	62. 95	21. 44	37. 29	37. 28	4. 57	1
All	男性 Male	181 959	82. 28	25. 57	50. 36	50. 56	6. 25	1
	女性 Female	92 731	43. 09	16. 28	24. 77	24. 54	2. 89	1
城市地区	合计 Both	140 904	66. 08	20. 90	37. 65	37. 67	4. 60	1
Urban areas	男性 Male	91 924	85. 90	25. 17	50. 43	50. 75	6. 30	1
	女性 Female	48 980	46. 11	15. 86	25. 61	25. 34	2. 96	2
农村地区	合计 Both	133 786	59. 97	22. 03	36. 91	36. 84	4. 53	1
Rural areas	男性 Male	90 035	78. 89	25. 99	50. 26	50. 33	6. 21	1
	女性 Female	43 751	40. 15	16. 77	23. 89	23. 69	2. 82	1
东部地区	合计 Both	137 763	69. 61	20. 85	37. 79	37. 64	4. 62	1
Eastern areas	男性 Male	87 382	87. 81	24. 53	49. 17	49. 25	6. 12	1
	女性 Female	50 381	51. 20	16. 54	27. 17	26. 80	3. 17	2
中部地区	合计 Both	64 429	55. 99	21. 38	36. 84	36. 94	4. 54	1
Central areas	男性 Male	44 807	76. 18	26. 82	52. 23	52. 50	6. 51	1
	女性 Female	19 622	34. 88	14. 62	21. 98	21. 88	2. 57	2
西部地区	合计 Both	72 498	58. 78	22. 71	37. 05	37. 18	4. 51	1
Western areas	男性 Male	49 770	79. 24	26. 44	51. 10	51. 49	6. 31	1
	女性 Female	22 728	37. 54	17. 35	23. 07	22. 94	2. 69	1

表 5-10b 2016 年中国肿瘤登记地区肺癌死亡情况
Table 5-10b Mortality of lung cancer in the registration areas of China, 2016

地区 Area	性别 Sex	死亡数 No. deaths	粗率 Crude rate/ 100 000^{-1}	构成比 Freq. /%	中标率 ASR China/ 100 000^{-1}	世标率 ASR World/ 100 000^{-1}	累积率 Cum. rate 0~74/%	顺位 Rank
合计	合计 Both	215 025	49. 28	27. 82	28. 14	28. 08	3. 29	1
All	男性 Male	149 992	67. 83	30. 34	40. 71	40. 76	4. 83	1
	女性 Female	65 033	30. 22	23. 34	16. 16	16. 01	1. 77	1
城市地区	合计 Both	108 521	50. 89	28. 09	27. 64	27. 58	3. 20	1
Urban areas	男性 Male	75 574	70. 62	30. 84	40. 41	40. 49	4. 78	1
	女性 Female	32 947	31. 01	23. 33	15. 68	15. 48	1. 66	1
农村地区	合计 Both	106 504	47. 74	27. 54	28. 59	28. 54	3. 39	1
Rural areas	男性 Male	74 418	65. 21	29. 85	40. 96	40. 97	4. 88	1
	女性 Female	32086	29. 44	23. 35	16. 62	16. 53	1. 88	1
东部地区	合计 Both	105 437	53. 27	27. 59	27. 38	27. 19	3. 18	1
Eastern areas	男性 Male	71 952	72. 31	29. 88	39. 32	39. 22	4. 65	1
	女性 Female	33 485	34. 03	23. 69	16. 28	16. 03	1. 75	1
中部地区	合计 Both	51 802	45. 01	27. 60	28. 89	28. 88	3. 41	1
Central areas	男性 Male	37 234	63. 30	31. 09	42. 85	42. 92	5. 11	1
	女性 Female	14 568	25. 89	21. 44	15. 51	15. 43	1. 71	1
西部地区	合计 Both	57 786	46. 85	28. 45	28. 92	29. 09	3. 42	1
Western areas	男性 Male	40 806	64. 97	30. 51	41. 43	41. 78	4. 95	1
	女性 Female	16 980	28. 05	24. 49	16. 53	16. 54	1. 86	1

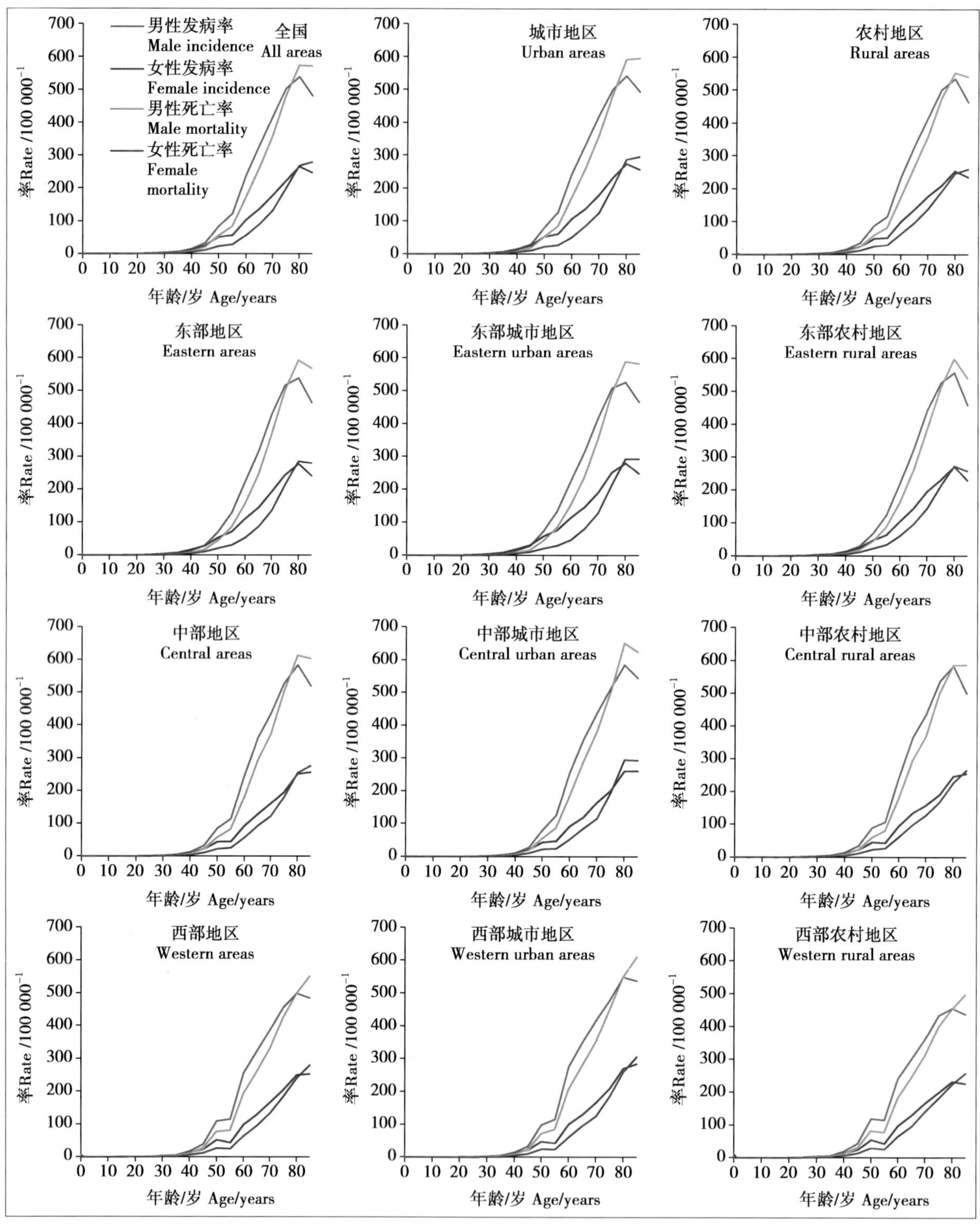

图 5-10a　2016 年中国肿瘤登记地区肺癌年龄别发病率和死亡率

Figure 5-10a　Age-specific incidence and mortality rates of lung cancer in the registration areas of China,2016

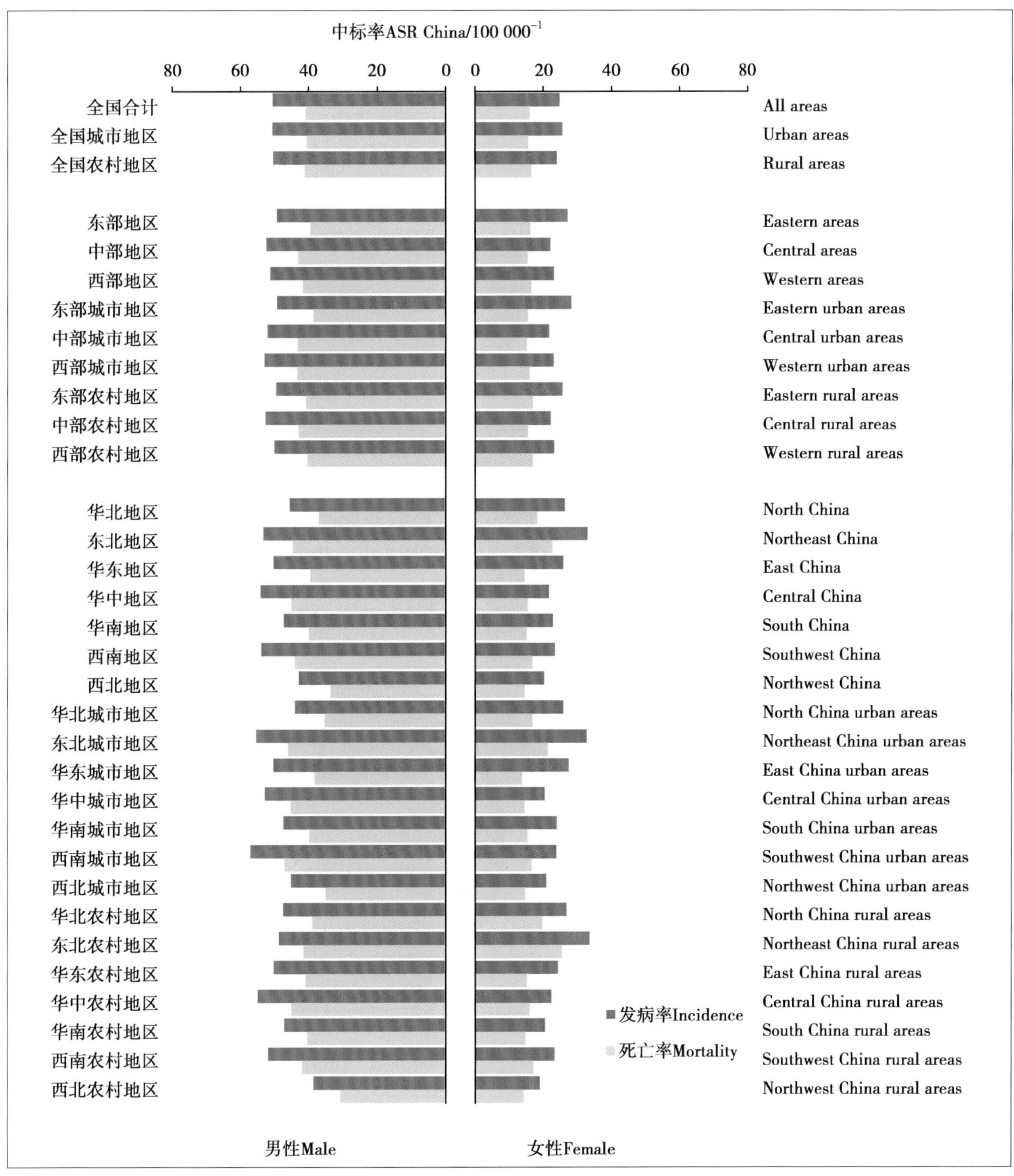

图 5-10b 2016 年中国肿瘤登记不同地区肺癌发病率和死亡率

Figure 5-10b Incidence and mortality rates of lung cancer in the different registration areas of China, 2016

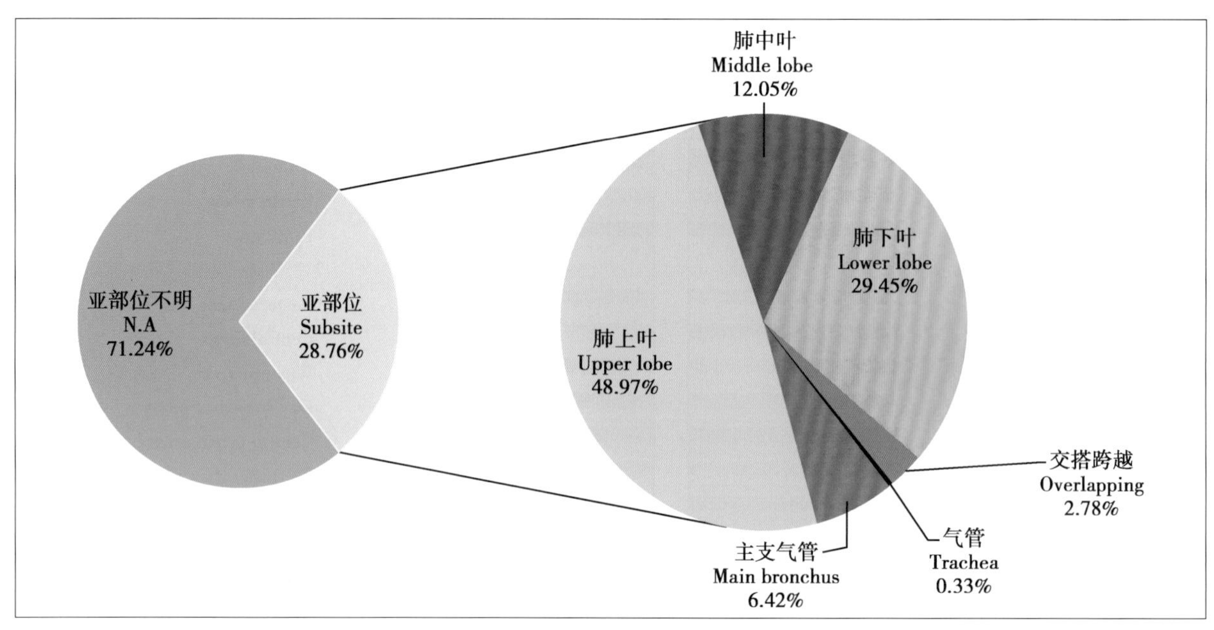

图 5-10c 2016 年中国肿瘤登记地区肺癌亚部位分布情况

Figure 5-10c Subsite distribution of lung cancer in the registration areas of China,2016

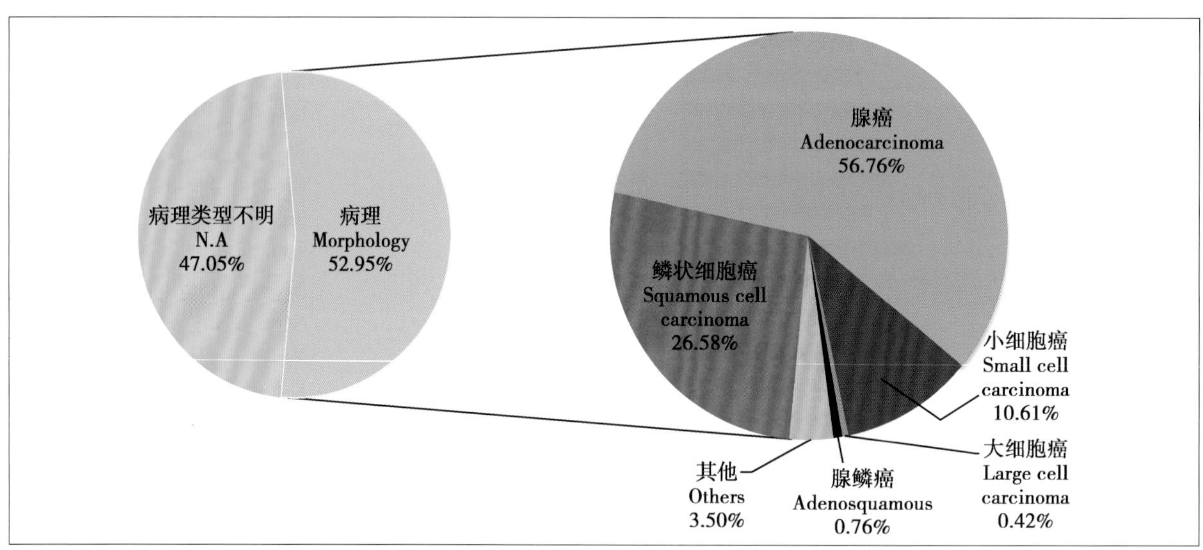

图 5-10d 2016 年中国肿瘤登记地区肺癌病理分型情况

Figure 5-10d Morphological distribution of lung cancer in the registration areas of China,2016

11 骨

2017 年,中国肿瘤登记地区骨癌位居癌症发病谱第 22 位。新发病例数为 7 967 例,占全部癌症发病的 0.62%;其中男性 4 519 例,女性 3 448 例,城市地区 3 592 例,农村地区 4 375 例。骨癌发病率为 1.83/10 万,中标发病率为 1.34/10 万,世标发病率为 1.31/10 万;男性中标发病率为女性的 1.35 倍,农村中标发病率为城市的 1.25 倍。0~74 岁累积发病率为 0.13%(表 5-11a)。

2017 年,中国肿瘤登记地区骨癌位居癌症死亡谱第 20 位。骨癌死亡病例 5 795 例,占全部癌症死亡的 0.75%;其中男性 3 422 例,女性 2 373 例,城市地区 2 634 例,农村地区 3 161 例。骨癌死亡率为 1.33/10 万,中标死亡率为 0.86/10 万,世标死亡率为 0.85/10 万;男性中标死亡率为女性的 1.52 倍,农村中标死亡率为城市的 1.22 倍。0~74 岁累积死亡率为 0.09%(表 5-11b)。

骨癌年龄别发病率和死亡率均在 10~19 岁组出现一个小高峰,但总体看骨癌年龄别发病率和死亡率在 45 岁之前处于较低水平,45 岁之后迅速上升,呈现男性高于女性的分布特征,城乡和不同地区年龄别发病率、死亡率总体趋势基本相同(图 5-11a)。

东、中、西部地区均为农村地区骨癌发病率和死亡率高于城市。中标发病率和死亡率均以西部地区最高,其次是中部地区,东部地区最低。在七大行政区中,发病率和死亡率最高的地区均在西北地区(表 5-11a,表 5-11b,图 5-11b)。

分亚部位比较,39.07%的骨癌发生在四肢的骨、关节和关节软骨,60.93%发生在其他及未特指部位的骨、关节和关节软骨(图 5-11c)。

11 Bone

In 2017, the incidence of bone cancer ranked 22nd among all cancer types in cancer registration areas of China. There were 7 967 new cases diagnosed with bone cancer(4 519 males and 3 448 females, 3 592 in urban areas and 4 375 in rural areas), accounting for 0.62% of all new cancer cases. The crude incidence rate was 1.83 per 100 000, with ASR China 1.34 per 100 000 and ASR World 1.31 per 100 000, respectively. The incidence rate of ASR China in males was 1.35 folds as high as that in females. It was 1.25 folds in rural areas as high as that in urban areas. The cumulative incidence rate for subjects aged 0 to 74 years was 0.13%(Table 5-11a).

In 2017, the mortality of bone cancer ranked 20th among all causes of cancer death in cancer registration areas of China. A total of 5 795 cases died of bone cancer(3 422 males and 2 373 females, 2 634 in urban areas and 3 161 in rural areas), accounting for 0.75% of all cancer deaths. The crude mortality rate was 1.33 per 100 000, with ASR China 0.86 per 100 000 and ASR World 0.85 per 100 000, respectively. The mortality rate of ASR China in males was 1.52 folds as high as that in females, and it was 1.22 folds in rural areas as high as that in urban areas. The cumulative mortality rate for subjects aged 0 to 74 years was 0.09%(Table 5-11b).

Both the age-specific incidence and mortality of bone cancer showed a small peak in the age group of 10-19 years. The age-specific incidence and mortality rate of bone cancer were relatively low before 45 years old, but dramatically increased after then. The incidence and mortality rates in males were higher than those in females across all age groups. The age specific incidence and mortality rates had slight variation among different areas, but showed similar trends(Figure 5-11a).

The incidence and mortality rates of bone cancer were higher in rural areas than those in urban areas. Western areas had the highest incidence and mortality of ASR China, followed by central areas and eastern areas. Among the seven administrative districts, Northwest China had the highest incidence and mortality rate(Table 5-11a, Table 5-11b, Figure 5-11b).

Bysubsite, 39.07% of bone cancer occurred in limbs, whereas others occurred in other unspecific bone and articular cartilage site(Figure 5-11c).

表 5-11a 2017 年中国肿瘤登记地区骨癌发病情况
Table 5-11a Incidence of bone cancer in registration areas of China,2017

地区 Area	性别 Sex	病例数 No. cases	粗率 Crude rate/ 100 000⁻¹	构成比 Freq./%	中标率 ASR China/ 100 000⁻¹	世标率 ASR World/ 100 000⁻¹	累积率 Cum. rate 0~74/%	顺位 Rank
合计	合计 Both	7 967	1.83	0.62	1.34	1.31	0.13	22
All	男性 Male	4 519	2.04	0.64	1.54	1.51	0.15	18
	女性 Female	3 448	1.60	0.61	1.15	1.12	0.11	20
城市地区	合计 Both	3 592	1.68	0.53	1.19	1.16	0.12	22
Urban areas	男性 Male	2 027	1.89	0.56	1.37	1.33	0.13	18
	女性 Female	1 565	1.47	0.51	1.01	0.98	0.10	20
农村地区	合计 Both	4 375	1.96	0.72	1.49	1.46	0.15	21
Rural areas	男性 Male	2 492	2.18	0.72	1.70	1.67	0.17	18
	女性 Female	1 883	1.73	0.72	1.28	1.25	0.13	20
东部地区	合计 Both	3 300	1.67	0.50	1.18	1.15	0.11	22
Eastern areas	男性 Male	1 836	1.85	0.52	1.35	1.31	0.13	18
	女性 Female	1 464	1.49	0.48	1.01	0.99	0.10	20
中部地区	合计 Both	2 137	1.86	0.71	1.49	1.45	0.15	21
Central areas	男性 Male	1 223	2.08	0.73	1.72	1.68	0.17	18
	女性 Female	914	1.62	0.68	1.24	1.22	0.12	20
西部地区	合计 Both	2 530	2.05	0.79	1.52	1.49	0.16	21
Western areas	男性 Male	1 460	2.32	0.78	1.73	1.70	0.18	18
	女性 Female	1 070	1.77	0.82	1.31	1.29	0.13	20

表 5-11b 2017 年中国肿瘤登记地区骨癌死亡情况
Table 5-11b Mortality of laryngeal cancer in registration areas of China,2017

地区 Area	性别 Sex	死亡数 No. deaths	粗率 Crude rate/ 100 000⁻¹	构成比 Freq./%	中标率 ASR China/ 100 000⁻¹	世标率 ASR World/ 100 000⁻¹	累积率 Cum. rate 0~74/%	顺位 Rank
合计	合计 Both	5 795	1.33	0.75	0.86	0.85	0.09	20
All	男性 Male	3 422	1.55	0.69	1.05	1.03	0.11	17
	女性 Female	2 373	1.10	0.85	0.69	0.68	0.07	17
城市地区	合计 Both	2 634	1.24	0.68	0.78	0.76	0.08	20
Urban areas	男性 Male	1 575	1.47	0.64	0.96	0.94	0.10	17
	女性 Female	1 059	1.00	0.75	0.60	0.59	0.06	19
农村地区	合计 Both	3 161	1.42	0.82	0.95	0.94	0.10	19
Rural areas	男性 Male	1 847	1.62	0.74	1.13	1.11	0.12	16
	女性 Female	1 314	1.21	0.96	0.77	0.77	0.09	15
东部地区	合计 Both	2 636	1.33	0.69	0.82	0.80	0.08	20
Eastern areas	男性 Male	1 485	1.49	0.62	0.95	0.93	0.10	17
	女性 Female	1 151	1.17	0.81	0.69	0.67	0.07	18
中部地区	合计 Both	1 375	1.19	0.73	0.85	0.84	0.09	20
Central areas	男性 Male	848	1.44	0.71	1.08	1.05	0.12	17
	女性 Female	527	0.94	0.78	0.63	0.63	0.07	17
西部地区	合计 Both	1 784	1.45	0.88	0.98	0.97	0.11	19
Western areas	男性 Male	1 089	1.73	0.81	1.20	1.19	0.13	15
	女性 Female	695	1.15	1.00	0.76	0.75	0.08	16

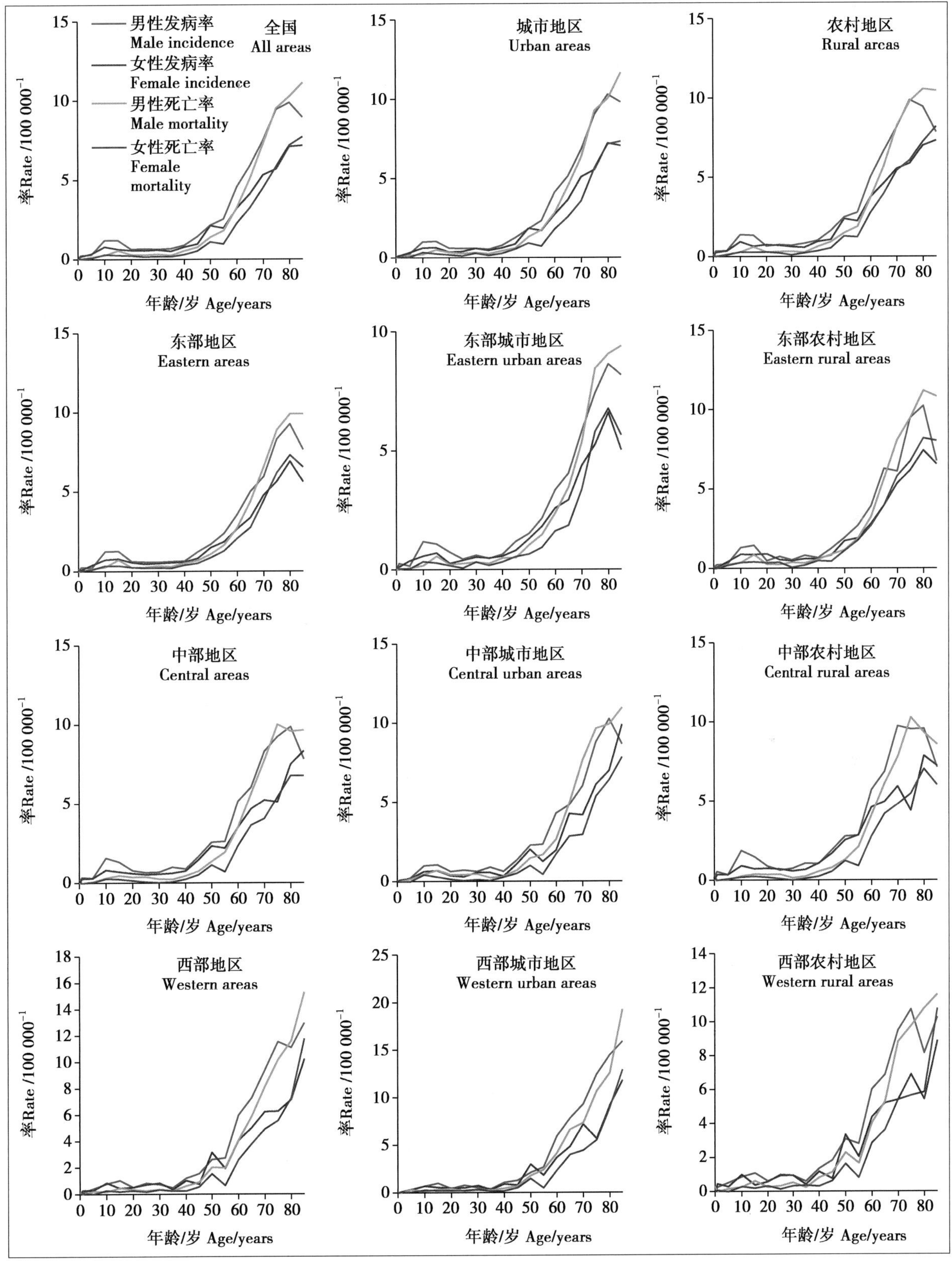

图 5-11a　2017 年中国肿瘤登记地区骨癌年龄别发病率和死亡率

Figure 5-11a　Age-specific incidence and mortality rates of bone cancer in registration areas of China, 2017

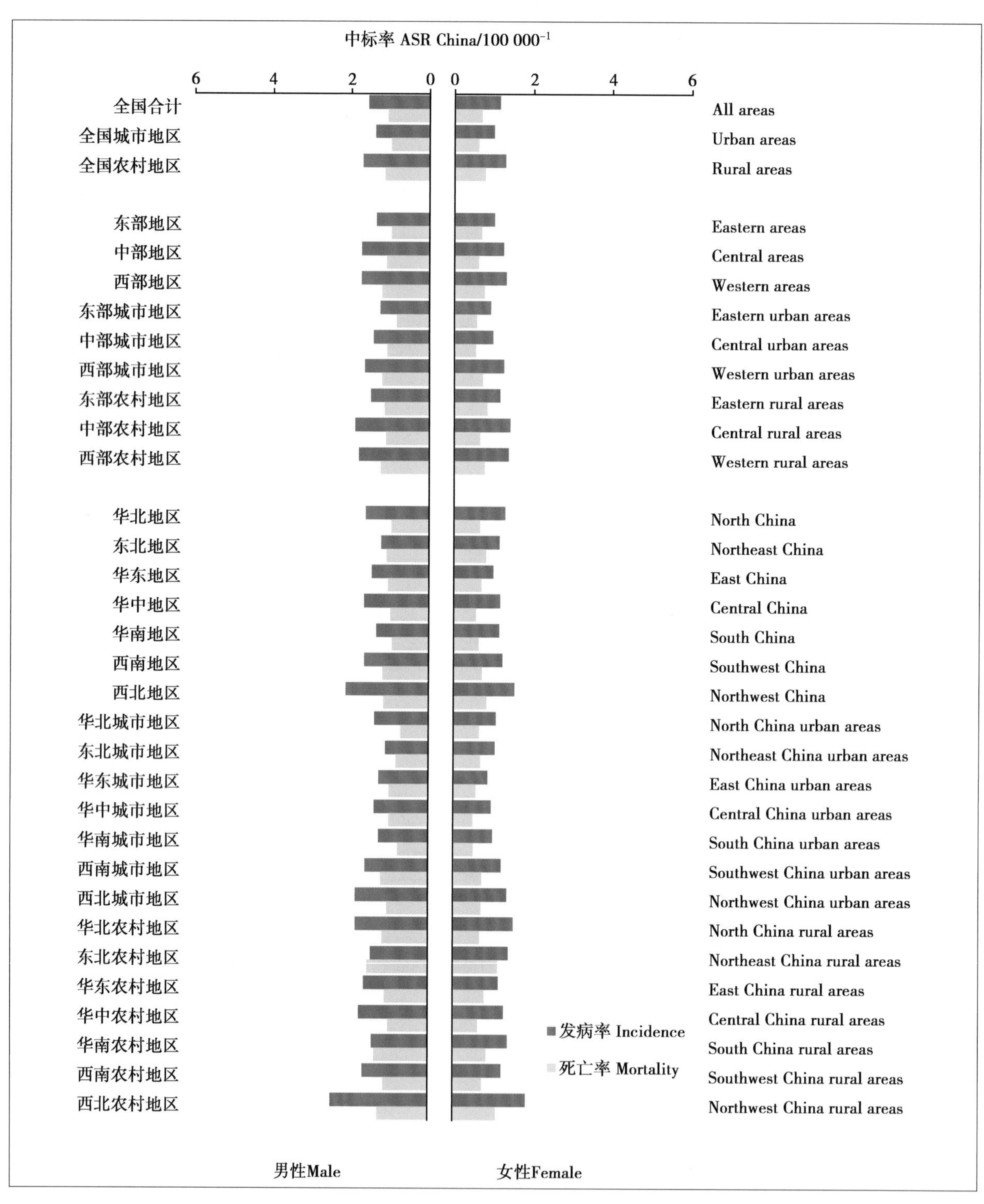

图 5-11b 2017 年中国肿瘤登记不同地区骨癌发病率和死亡率

Figure 5-11b Incidence and mortality rates of bone cancer in different registration areas of China, 2017

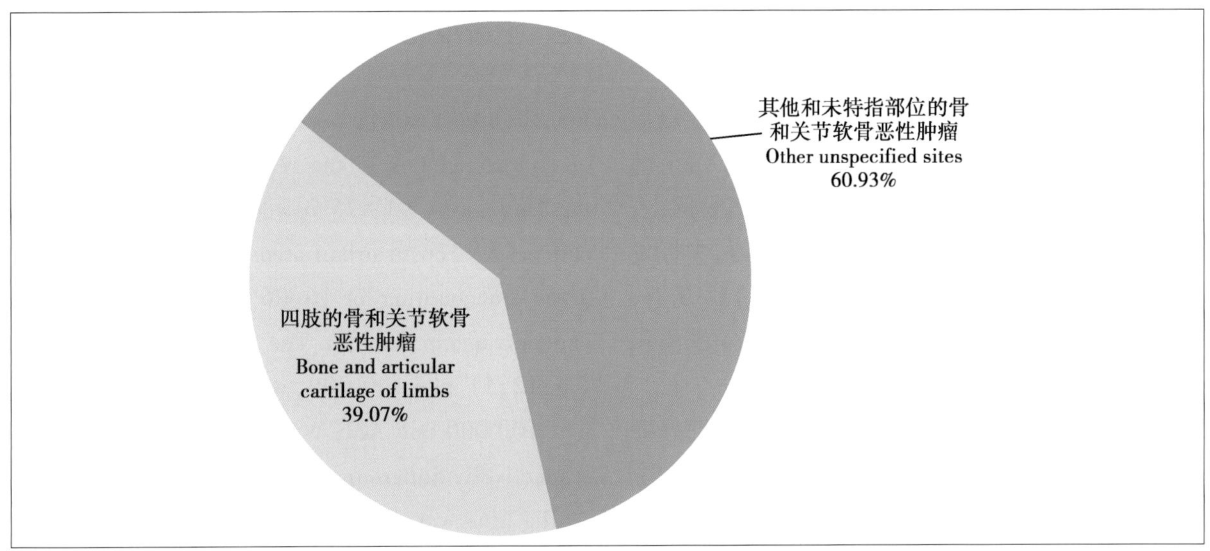

图 5-11c　2017 年中国肿瘤登记地区骨癌亚部位分布情况
Figure 5-11c　Subsite distribution of bone cancer in registration areas of China,2017

12 女性乳腺

中国肿瘤登记地区女性乳腺癌位居女性癌症发病谱第 2 位。新发病例数为 91 475 例,占全部女性癌症发病的 16.06%;城市地区 53 726 例,农村地区 37 749 例。发病率为 42.51/10 万,中标发病率为 30.08/10 万,世标发病率为 28.11/10 万;城市中标发病率为农村的 1.35 倍。0~74 岁累积发病率为 3.01%(表 5-12a)。

中国肿瘤登记地区女性乳腺癌位居女性癌症死亡谱第 5 位。女性乳腺癌死亡 21 000 例,占全部女性癌症死亡的 7.54%;城市地区 11 951 例,农村地区 9 049 例。女性乳腺癌死亡率为 9.76/10 万,中标死亡率 6.17/10 万,世标死亡率 5.98/10 万;城市中标死亡率为农村的 1.21 倍。0~74 岁累积死亡率为 0.66%(表 5-12b)。

城市和农村女性乳腺癌年龄别发病率特征相似。女性乳腺癌发病率均自 20~24 岁组开始快速上升,城市地区至 60~64 岁组达到高峰,而农村地区至 50~54 岁组达到高峰,随后快速下降;女性乳腺癌死亡率从 25~29 岁组开始缓慢上升(图 5-12a)。

12 Female breast

Female breast cancer was the second common cancer among females in the registration areas of China. There were 91 475 new cases of female breast cancer(53 726 in urban areas and 37 749 in rural areas), accounting for 16.06% of new cases of all cancers among females. The crude incidence rate was 42.51 per 100 000, with ASR China 30.08 per 100 000 and ASR World 28.11 per 100 000, respectively. Subgroup analyses showed that the ASR China was 1.35 times in urban areas as that in rural areas. The cumulative incidence rate for subjects aged 0 to 74 years was 3.01% (Table 5-12a).

Female breast cancer was the 5th most common cause of cancer deaths among females in the registration areas of China. A total of 21 000 women died of breast cancer in 2017(11 951 in urban areas and 9 049 in rural areas), accounting for 7.54% of all cancer deaths among females. The crude mortality rate was 9.76 per 100 000, with ASR China 6.17 per 100 000 and ASR World 5.98 per 100 000, respectively. Subgroup analyses showed that the mortality of ASR China was 1.21 times in urban areas as that in rural areas. The cumulative mortality rate for subjects aged 0 to 74 years was 0.66% (Table 5-12b).

Age-specific incidence rates took on almost the same pattern between urban areas and rural areas. The incidence rate increased rapidly from the age group of 20-24 years with the peak occurring in the age group of 60-64 years in urban areas and 50-54 years in rural areas, thereafter began to drop quickly. Age-specific mortality rates increased slowly from the age group of 25-29 years (Figure 5-12a).

城市女性乳腺癌的发病率和死亡率均高于农村。东部地区中标发病率最高，其次是中部地区，西部地区最低；七大行政区中，东北地区、华北地区和华南地区中标发病率依次显著高于全国平均水平，西南地区中标发病率最低；东部地区中标死亡率最高，其次是中部地区，西部地区最低；七大行政区中，华南地区、东北地区和华中地区中标死亡率依次高于全国平均水平，西南地区中标死亡率最低（表 5-12a，表 5-12b，图 5-12b）。

全部女性乳腺癌病例中，26. 50%的病例报告了明确的亚部位，其中上外象限是最主要的亚部位，占 39. 34%；其次是上内象限，占 18. 63%；交搭跨越，占 13. 24%；下外象限，占 8. 53%；下内象限，占 7. 51%；中央部，占 6. 00%；乳头和乳晕，占 4. 11%；腋尾部，占 0. 67%（图 5-12c）。

全部女性乳腺癌病例中有明确组织学类型的病例占 77. 92%，其中导管癌是最主要的病理类型，占 78. 44%；其次是小叶性癌，占 4. 16%；佩吉特病，占 1. 39%；髓样癌，占 0. 30%（图 5-12d）。

Both the incidence and mortality rates of female breast cancer were higher in urban areas than those in rural areas. Eastern areas had the highest incidence rate, followed by Central and Western areas. Among the seven administrative districts, Northeast China, North China and South China had the top three incidence rates, all higher than the national average, and Southwest China had the lowest incidence rate. Eastern areas had the highest mortality rate, followed by Central and Western areas. Among the seven administrative districts, South China, Northeast China and Central China had the top three mortality rates, all higher than the national average, and Southwest China had the lowest mortality rate (Table 5-12a, Table 5-12b, Figure 5-12b).

About 26. 50% female breast cancer cases reported specific subsites. Among them, 39. 34% occurred in upper outer, 18. 63% in upper inner, 13. 24% at overlapping, 8. 53% in lower outer, 7. 51% in lower inner, 6. 00% in central portion, 4. 11% in nipple and areola, and 0. 67% in axillary tail (Figure 5-12c).

About 77. 92% cases of female breast cancer had morphological verification. Among them, ductal cancer was the most common histological type, accounting for 78. 44%, followed by lobular carcinoma (4. 16%), Paget's disease (1. 39%), medullary carcinoma (0. 30%) (Figure 5-12d).

表 5-12a 2017 年中国肿瘤登记地区女性乳腺癌发病情况

Table 5-12a Incidence of female breast cancer in the registration areas of China, 2017

地区 Area	病例数 No. cases	粗率 Crude rate/ 100 000^{-1}	构成比 Freq./%	中标率 ASR China/ 100 000^{-1}	世标率 ASR World/ 100 000^{-1}	累积率 Cum. rate 0~74/%	顺位 Rank
合计 All	91 475	42.51	16.06	30.08	28.11	3.01	2
城市地区 Urban areas	53 726	50.57	17.39	34.49	32.44	3.53	1
农村地区 Rural areas	37 749	34.64	14.47	25.55	23.66	2.49	2
东部地区 Eastern areas	51 902	52.74	17.04	35.61	33.30	3.60	1
中部地区 Central areas	21 613	38.42	16.10	28.91	26.97	2.87	1
西部地区 Western areas	17 960	29.67	13.71	21.77	20.27	2.13	2

表 5-12b 2017 年中国肿瘤登记地区女性乳腺癌死亡情况

Table 5-12b Mortality of female breast cancer in the registration areas of China, 2017

地区 Area	死亡数 No. deaths	粗率 Crude rate/ 100 000^{-1}	构成比 Freq./%	中标率 ASR China/ 100 000^{-1}	世标率 ASR World/ 100 000^{-1}	累积率 Cum. rate 0~74/%	顺位 Rank
合计 All	21 000	9.76	7.54	6.17	5.98	0.66	5
城市地区 Urban areas	11 951	11.25	8.46	6.74	6.55	0.72	5
农村地区 Rural areas	9 049	8.30	6.58	5.56	5.37	0.59	6
东部地区 Eastern areas	11 290	11.47	7.99	6.59	6.41	0.71	5
中部地区 Central areas	5 114	9.09	7.53	6.36	6.14	0.69	5
西部地区 Western areas	4 596	7.59	6.63	5.18	5.00	0.54	5

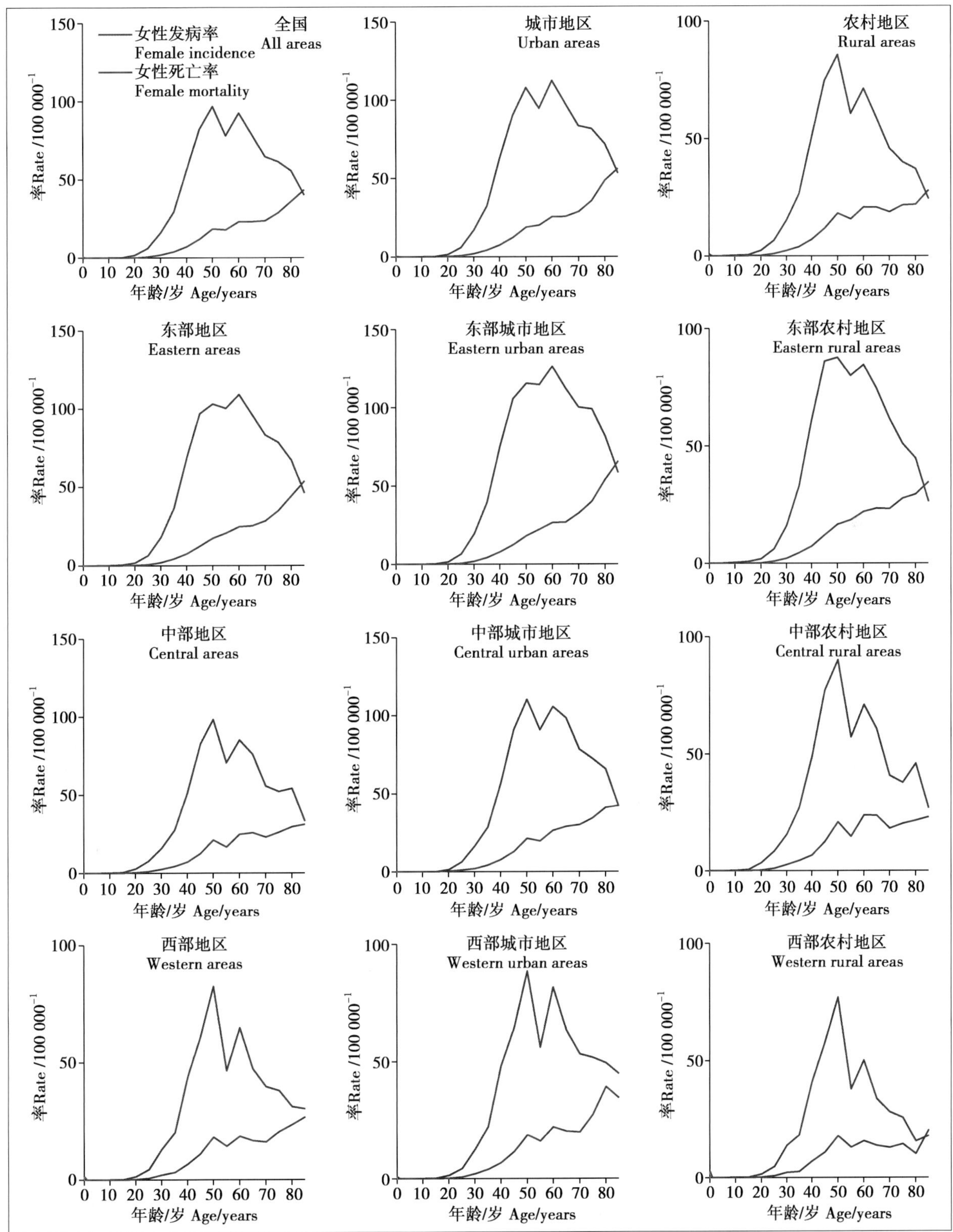

图 5-12a　2017 年中国肿瘤登记地区女性乳腺癌年龄别发病率和死亡率

Figure 5-12a　Age-specific incidence and mortality rates of female breast cancer in the registration areas of China, 2017

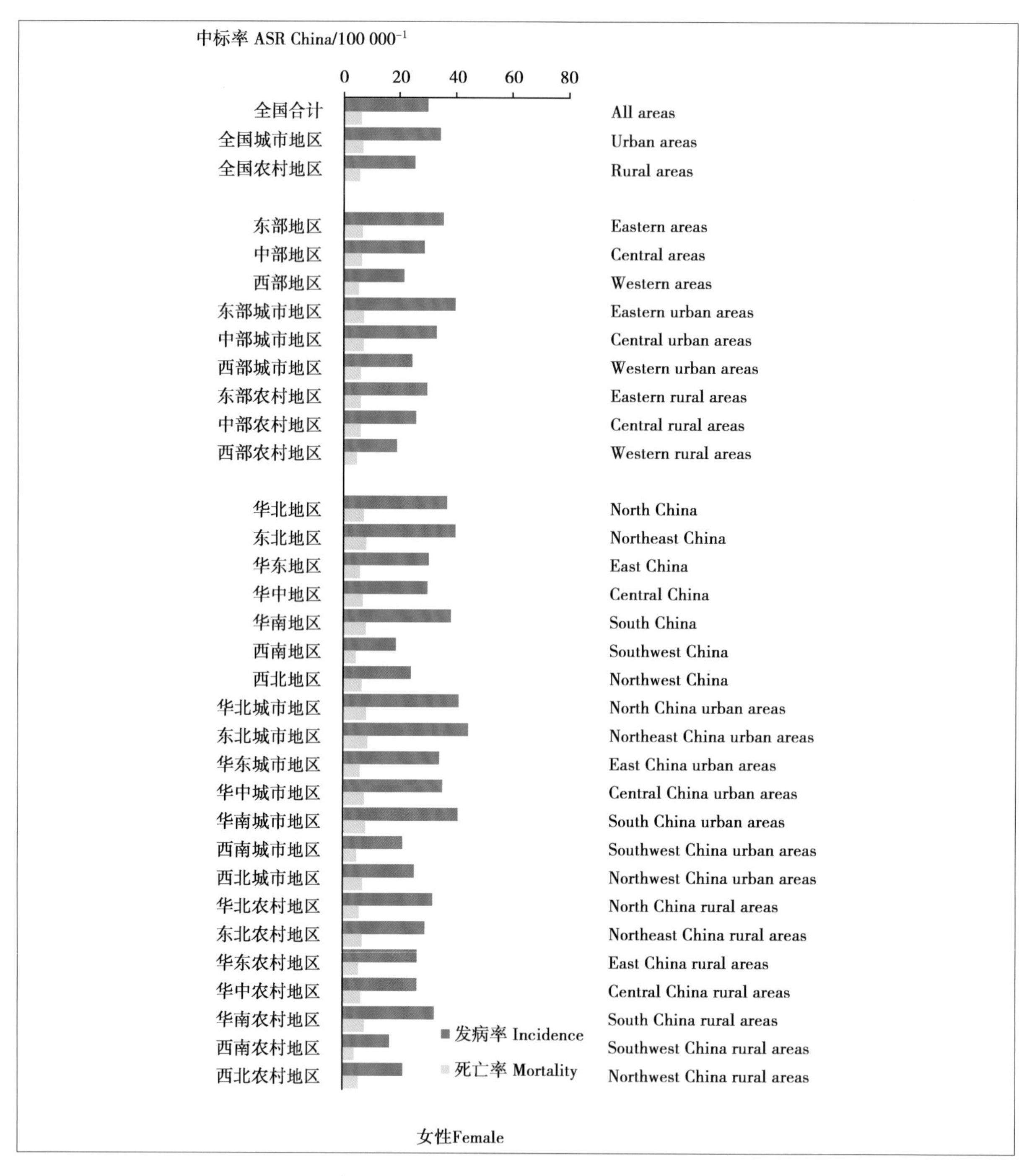

图 5-12b 2017 年中国不同肿瘤登记地区女性乳腺癌发病率和死亡率

Figure 5-12b Incidence and mortality rates of female breast cancer in different registration areas of China,2017

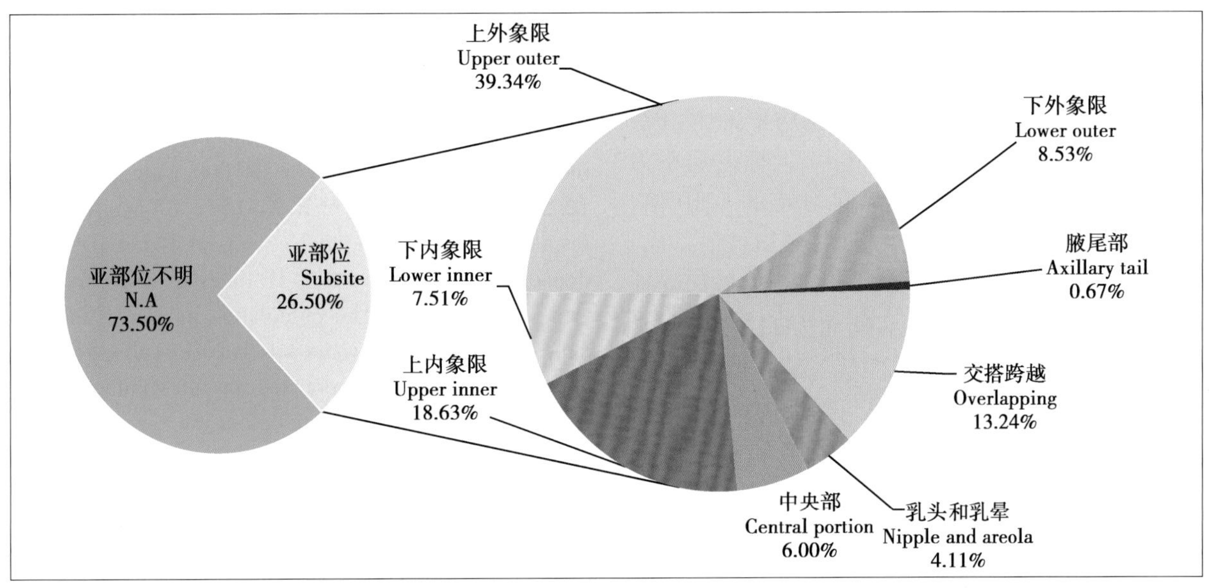

图 5-12c 2017 年中国肿瘤登记地区女性乳腺癌亚部位分布情况
Figure 5-12c Subsite Distribution of female breast cancer in the registration areas of China,2017

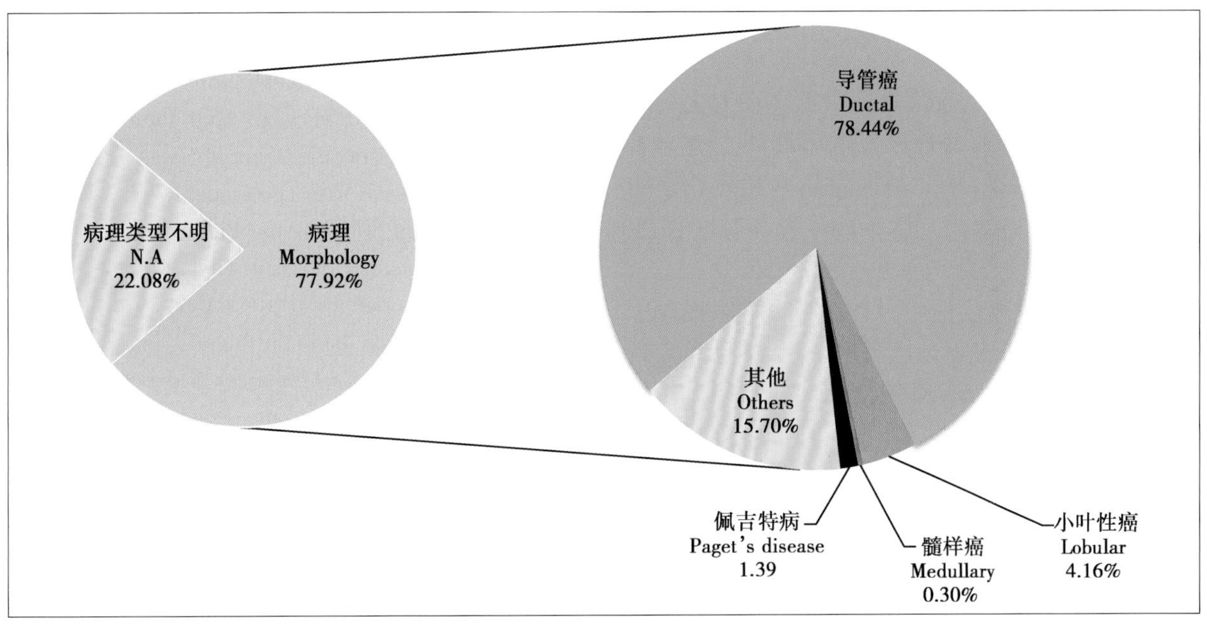

图 5-12d 2017 年中国肿瘤登记地区女性乳腺癌病理分型情况
Figure 5-12d Morphological distribution of female breast cancer in the registration areas of China,2017

13 子宫颈

2017 年中国肿瘤登记地区子宫颈癌位居女性癌症发病谱第 6 位。新发病例数为 36 740 例，占女性全部癌症发病的 6.45%；其中城市地区 17 558 例，农村地区 19 182 例。发病率为 17.07/10 万，中标发病率为 12.28/10 万，世标发病率为 11.35/10 万；农村中标发病率是城市的 1.10 倍。0～74 岁累积发病率为 1.20%（表 5-13a）。

2017 年中国肿瘤登记地区子宫颈癌位居女性癌症死亡谱第 7 位。死亡病例数为 11 936 例，占女性全部癌症死亡的 4.28%。其中城市地区 5 455 例，农村地区 6 481 例。子宫颈癌死亡率为 5.55/10 万，中标死亡率 3.56/10 万，世标死亡率 3.42/10 万；农村中标死亡率为城市的 1.21 倍。0～74 岁累积死亡率为 0.38%（表 5-13b）。

子宫颈癌年龄别发病率在 20 岁之前处于较低水平，自 20 岁以后快速上升，至 50～54 岁年龄组达高峰，之后逐渐下降。年龄别死亡率在 25 岁之前处于较低水平，25 岁以后随年龄增加逐渐升高，在 80～84 岁组达到高峰（图 5-13a）。

农村地区子宫颈癌的发病率和死亡率均高于城市。中标发病率及中标死亡率均以中部地区最高，其次是西部地区，东部地区最低。在七大行政区中，华中地区和西北地区发病率和死亡率显著高于全国平均水平，华北地区发病率和死亡率明显低于全国平均水平（表 5-13a，表 5-13b，图 5-13b）。

全部子宫颈癌病例中，11.13%的病例报告了明确的亚部位，其中宫颈内膜癌、外宫颈癌和宫颈交界部位癌分别占 51.81%、35.27%、12.92%（图 5-13c）。

13 Cervix

In 2017, cervical cancer was the 6th most common female cancer in the registration areas of China. There were 36 740 new cases of cervical cancer (17 558 in urban areas and 19 182 in rural areas), accounting for 6.45% of new cases of all female cancers. The crude incidence rate was 17.07 per 100 000, with ASR China 12.28 per 100 000 and ASR World 11.35 per 100 000, respectively. Subgroup analyses showed that the incidence of ASR China was 1.10 times in rural areas as that in urban areas. The cumulative incidence rate for subjects aged 0 to 74 years was 1.20% (Table 5-13a).

In 2017, cervical cancer was the 7th common cause of cancer deaths among females in the registration areas of China. A total of 11 936 women died of cervical cancer (5 455 in urban areas and 6 481 in rural areas), accounting for 4.28% of all female cancer deaths. The crude mortality rate was 5.55 per 100 000, with ASR China 3.56 per 100 000 and ASR World 3.42 per 100 000, respectively. Subgroup analyses showed that the mortality of ASR China was 1.21 times in rural areas as that in urban areas. The cumulative mortality rate for subjects aged 0 to 74 years was 0.38% (Table 5-13b).

The age-specific incidence rate was low before age 20. It went up rapidly thereafter, with the peak occurring in age group 50-54 years and then decreased gradually. The age-specific mortality was low before age 25 and increased with age gradually, reaching the peak in age group 80-84 years (Figure 5-13a).

Both the incidence and mortality rates of cervical cancer were higher in rural areas than in urban areas. Central areas had both the highest incidence and mortality rates while Eastern areas had both the lowest incidence and mortality rates, leaving Western areas in between. Among the seven administrative districts, both the incidence and mortality rates of cervical cancer in Central China and Northwest China areas were markedly higher than the national average whereas both the incidence and mortality rates in North China were lower than the national average (Table 5-13a, Table 5-13b, Figure 5-13b).

There were 11.13% cases of cervical cancers reported to have occurred in specific subsites, with endocervix, exocervix and overlapping parts comprising 51.81%, 35.27% and 12.92%, respectively (Figure 5-13c).

表 5-13a 2017 年中国肿瘤登记地区子宫颈癌发病情况

Table 5-13a Incidence of cervical cancer in the registration areas of China, 2017

地区 Area	病例数 No. cases	粗率 Crude rate/ $100\ 000^{-1}$	构成比 Freq. /%	中标率 ASR China/ $100\ 000^{-1}$	世标率 ASR World/ $100\ 000^{-1}$	累积率 Cum. rate 0~74/%	顺位 Rank
合计 All	36 740	17.07	6.45	12.28	11.35	1.20	6
城市地区 Urban areas	17 558	16.53	5.68	11.70	10.80	1.14	5
农村地区 Rural areas	19 182	17.60	7.35	12.87	11.91	1.27	5
东部地区 Eastern areas	15 191	15.44	4.99	10.81	9.92	1.04	6
中部地区 Central areas	11 180	19.87	8.33	14.91	13.86	1.49	3
西部地区 Western areas	10 369	17.13	7.92	12.62	11.72	1.25	4

表 5-13b 2017 年中国肿瘤登记地区子宫颈癌死亡情况

Table 5-13b Mortality of cervical cancer in the registration areas of China, 2017

地区 Area	死亡数 No. deaths	粗率 Crude rate/ $100\ 000^{-1}$	构成比 Freq. /%	中标率 ASR China/ $100\ 000^{-1}$	世标率 ASR World/ $100\ 000^{-1}$	累积率 Cum. rate 0~74/%	顺位 Rank
合计 All	11 936	5.55	4.28	3.56	3.42	0.38	7
城市地区 Urban areas	5 455	5.13	3.86	3.23	3.09	0.34	8
农村地区 Rural areas	6 481	5.95	4.72	3.90	3.76	0.43	7
东部地区 Eastern areas	4 636	4.71	3.28	2.83	2.71	0.30	8
中部地区 Central areas	3 652	6.49	5.37	4.45	4.30	0.49	7
西部地区 Western areas	3 648	6.03	5.26	4.09	3.96	0.45	7

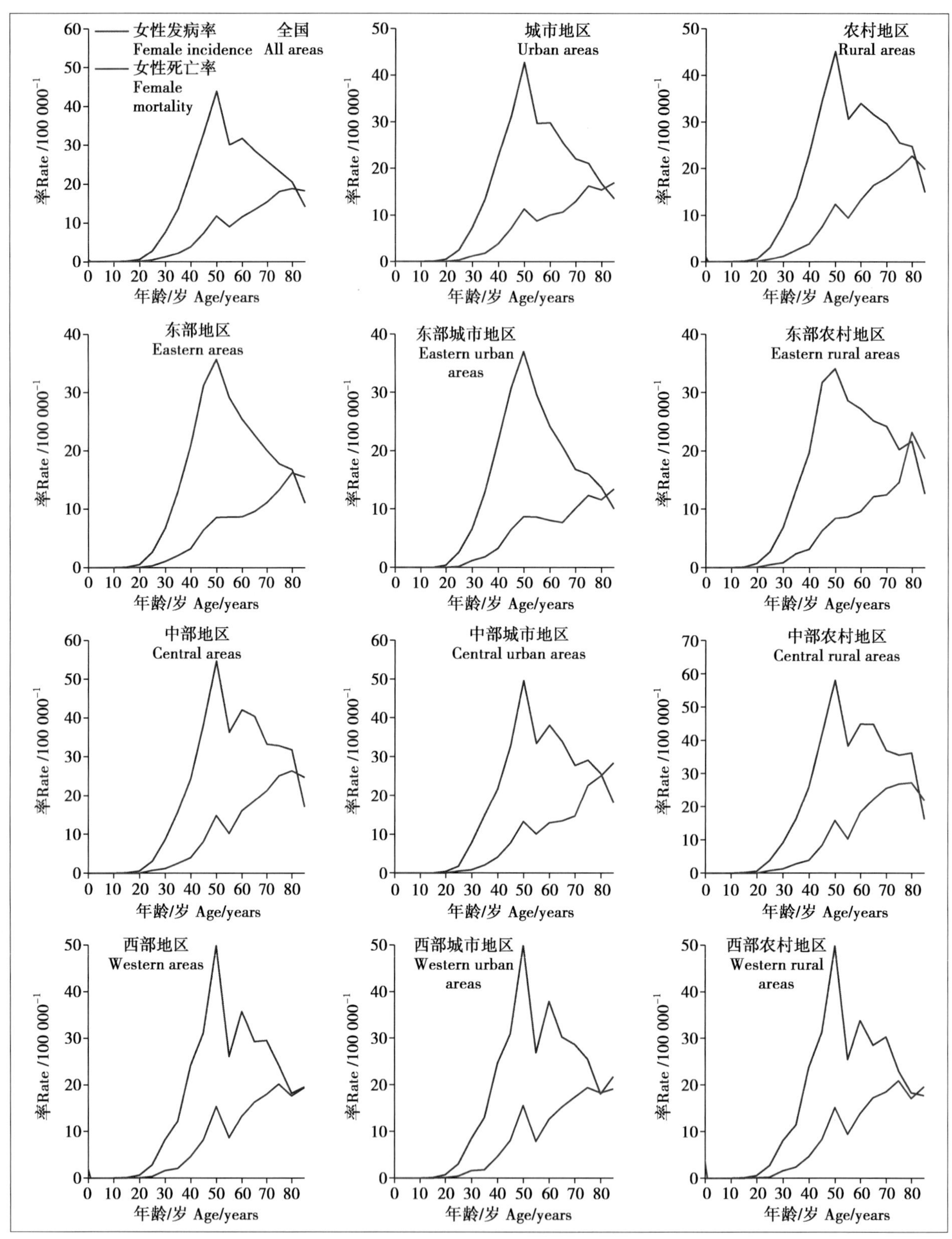

图 5-13a 2017 年中国肿瘤登记地区子宫颈癌年龄别发病率和死亡率
Figure 5-13a Age-specific incidence and mortality rates of cervical cancer in the registration areas of China, 2017

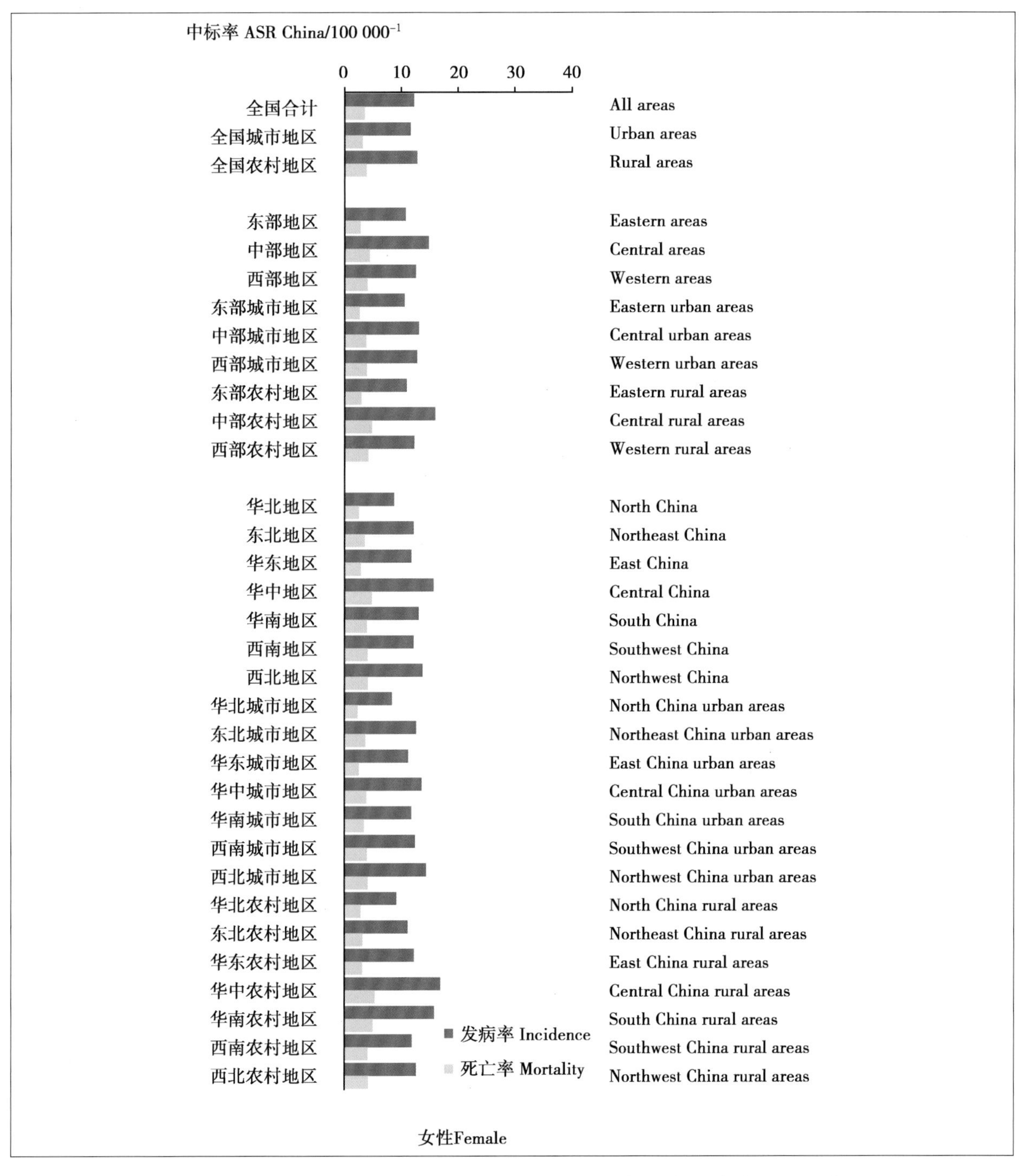

图 5-13b 2017 年中国不同肿瘤登记地区子宫颈癌发病率和死亡率

Figure 5-13b Incidence and mortality rates of cervical cancer in different registration areas of China, 2017

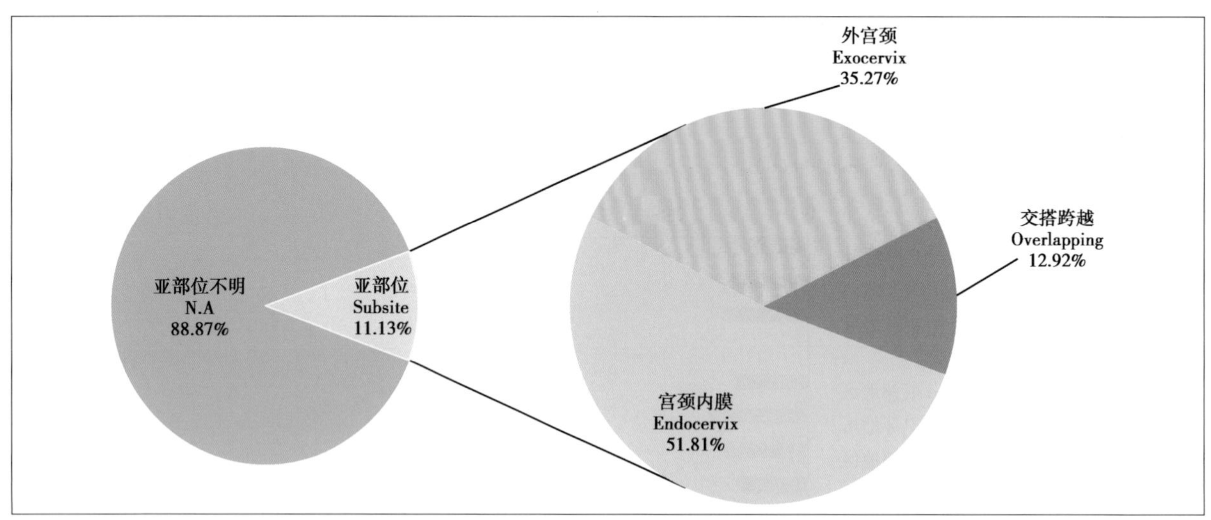

图 5-13c 2017 年中国肿瘤登记地区子宫颈癌亚部位分布情况
Figure 5-13c Subsite distribution of cervical cancer in the registration areas of China,2017

14 子宫体

2017 年中国肿瘤登记地区子宫体癌位居女性癌症发病谱第 9 位。新发病例数为 21 646 例，占女性全部癌症发病的 3.80%；其中城市地区 11 572 例，农村地区 10 074 例。子宫体癌发病率为 10.06/10 万，中标发病率为 6.79/10 万，世标发病率为 6.56/10 万；城市中标发病率为农村的 1.11 倍。0～74 岁累积发病率为 0.74%（表 5-14a）。

2017 年中国肿瘤登记地区子宫体癌位居女性癌症死亡谱第 14 位。子宫体癌死亡病例数为 5 246 例，占女性全部癌症死亡的 1.88%；其中城市地区 2 618 例，农村地区 2 628 例。子宫体癌死亡率为 2.44/10 万，中标死亡率 1.47/10 万，世标死亡率 1.46/10 万；农村中标死亡率为城市的 1.05 倍。0～74 岁累积死亡率为 0.17%（表 5-14b）。

子宫体癌年龄别发病率在 20 岁前处于较低水平，20 岁以后快速上升，至 50～54 岁组达高峰，之后逐渐下降。年龄别死亡率 30 岁前处于较低水平，30 岁以后迅速上升（图 5-14a）。

东部地区中标发病率最高，其次是中部地区，西部地区最低；西部地区中标死亡率最高，其次是中部地区，东部地区最低。在七大行政区中，华南、华北地区子宫体癌发病率明显高于全国平均水平（表 5-14a，表 5-14b，图 5-14b）。

14 Uterus

In 2017, uterus cancer was the 9th most common female cancer in the registration areas of China. There were 21 646 new cases of uterus cancer (11 572 in urban areas and 10 074 in rural areas), accounting for 3.80% of all female cancer cases. The crude incidence rate was 10.06 per 100 000, with ASR China 6.79 per 100 000 and ASR World 6.56 per 100 000, respectively. Subgroup analyses showed that the incidence of ASR China was 1.11 times in urban areas as that in rural areas. The cumulative incidence rate for persons aged 0-74 years was 0.74% (Table 5-14a).

In 2017, uterus cancer was the 14th most common cause of female cancer deaths in the registration areas of China. A total of 5 246 women died of uterus cancer (2 618 in urban areas and 2 628 in rural areas), accounting for 1.88% of all female cancer deaths. The crude mortality rate was 2.44 per 100 000, with ASR China 1.47 per 100 000 and ASR World 1.46 per 100 000, respectively. Subgroup analyses showed that the mortality of ASR China was 1.05 times in rural areas as that in urban areas. The cumulative mortality rate for persons aged 0-74 years was 0.17% (Table 5-14b).

The age-specific incidence rate was low before age 20. It went up rapidly thereafter and reached the peak at age group 50-54, then started to go down gradually from age 55. The age-specific mortality was low before age 30, then gradually went up thereafter (Figure 5-14a).

Eastern areas had the highest incidence rate, followed by Central and Western areas. Western areas had the highest mortality rate, followed by Central and Eastern areas. Among the seven administrative districts, the incidence rates of uterus cancer in South China and North China were obviously higher than the national average (Table 5-14a, Table 5-14b, Figure 5-14b).

表 5-14a 2017 年中国肿瘤登记地区子宫体癌发病情况

Table 5-14a Incidence of uterus cancer in the registration areas of China, 2017

地区 Area	病例数 No. cases	粗率 Crude rate/ 100 000^{-1}	构成比 Freq. /%	中标率 ASR China/ 100 000^{-1}	世标率 ASR World/ 100 000^{-1}	累积率 Cum. rate 0~74/%	顺位 Rank
合计 All	21 646	10. 06	3. 80	6. 79	6. 56	0. 74	9
城市地区 Urban areas	11 572	10. 89	3. 75	7. 14	6. 93	0. 79	8
农村地区 Rural areas	10 074	9. 24	3. 86	6. 43	6. 17	0. 68	9
东部地区 Eastern areas	11 471	11. 66	3. 77	7. 39	7. 16	0. 81	8
中部地区 Central areas	5 187	9. 22	3. 86	6. 73	6. 45	0. 72	9
西部地区 Western areas	4 988	8. 24	3. 81	5. 82	5. 60	0. 62	9

表 5-14b 2017 年中国肿瘤登记地区子宫体癌死亡情况

Table 5-14b Mortality of uterus cancer in the registration areas of China, 2017

地区 Area	死亡数 No. deaths	粗率 Crude rate/ 100 000^{-1}	构成比 Freq. /%	中标率 ASR China/ 100 000^{-1}	世标率 ASR World/ 100 000^{-1}	累积率 Cum. rate 0~74/%	顺位 Rank
合计 All	5 246	2. 44	1. 88	1. 47	1. 46	0. 17	14
城市地区 Urban areas	2 618	2. 46	1. 85	1. 44	1. 42	0. 17	14
农村地区 Rural areas	2 628	2. 41	1. 91	1. 51	1. 49	0. 18	14
东部地区 Eastern areas	2 475	2. 52	1. 75	1. 38	1. 36	0. 16	14
中部地区 Central areas	1 295	2. 30	1. 91	1. 52	1. 51	0. 18	14
西部地区 Western areas	1 476	2. 43	2. 13	1. 60	1. 59	0. 19	13

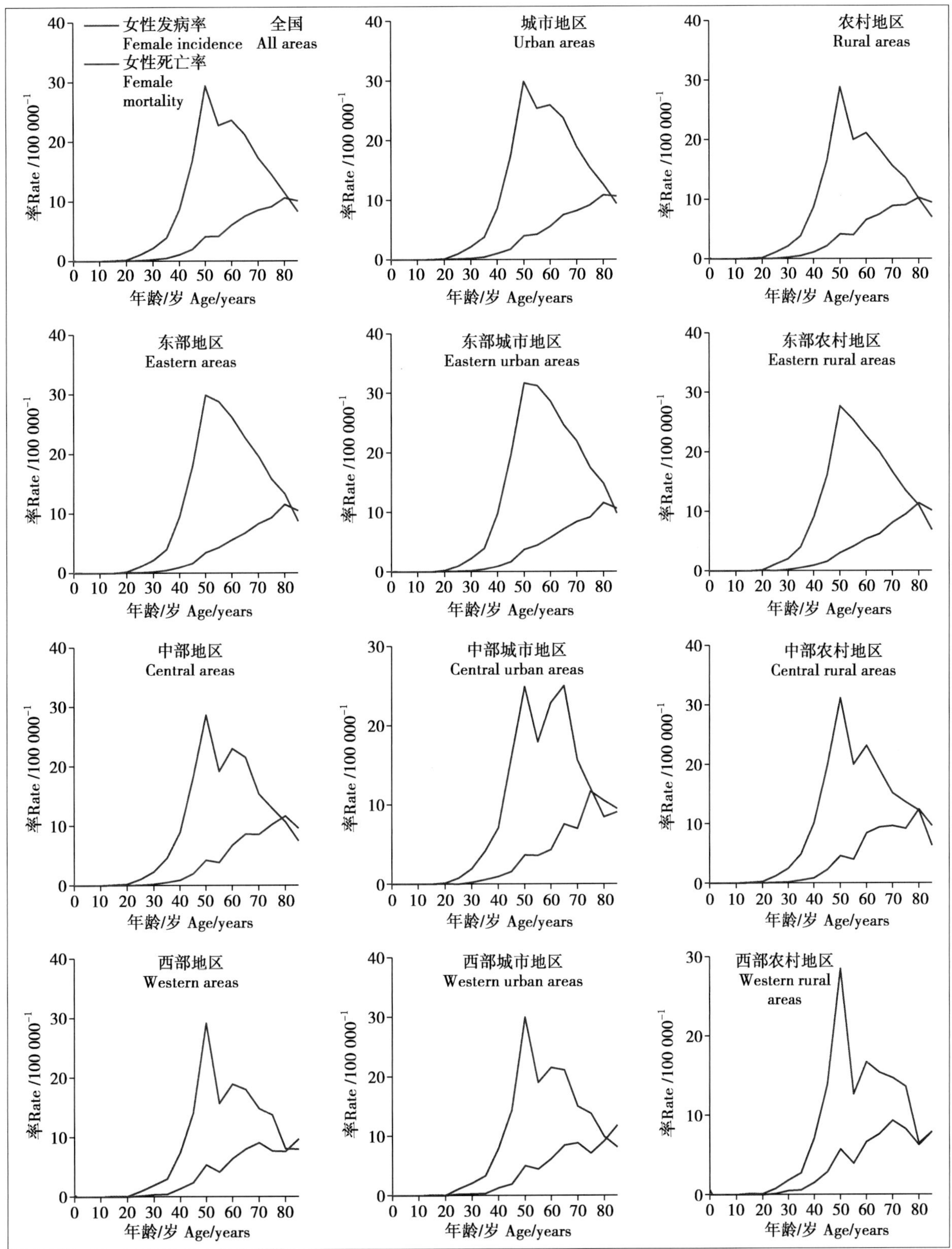

图 5-14a　2017 年中国肿瘤登记地区子宫体癌年龄别发病率和死亡率

Figure 5-14a　Age-specific incidence and mortality rates of uterus cancer in the registration areas of China, 2017

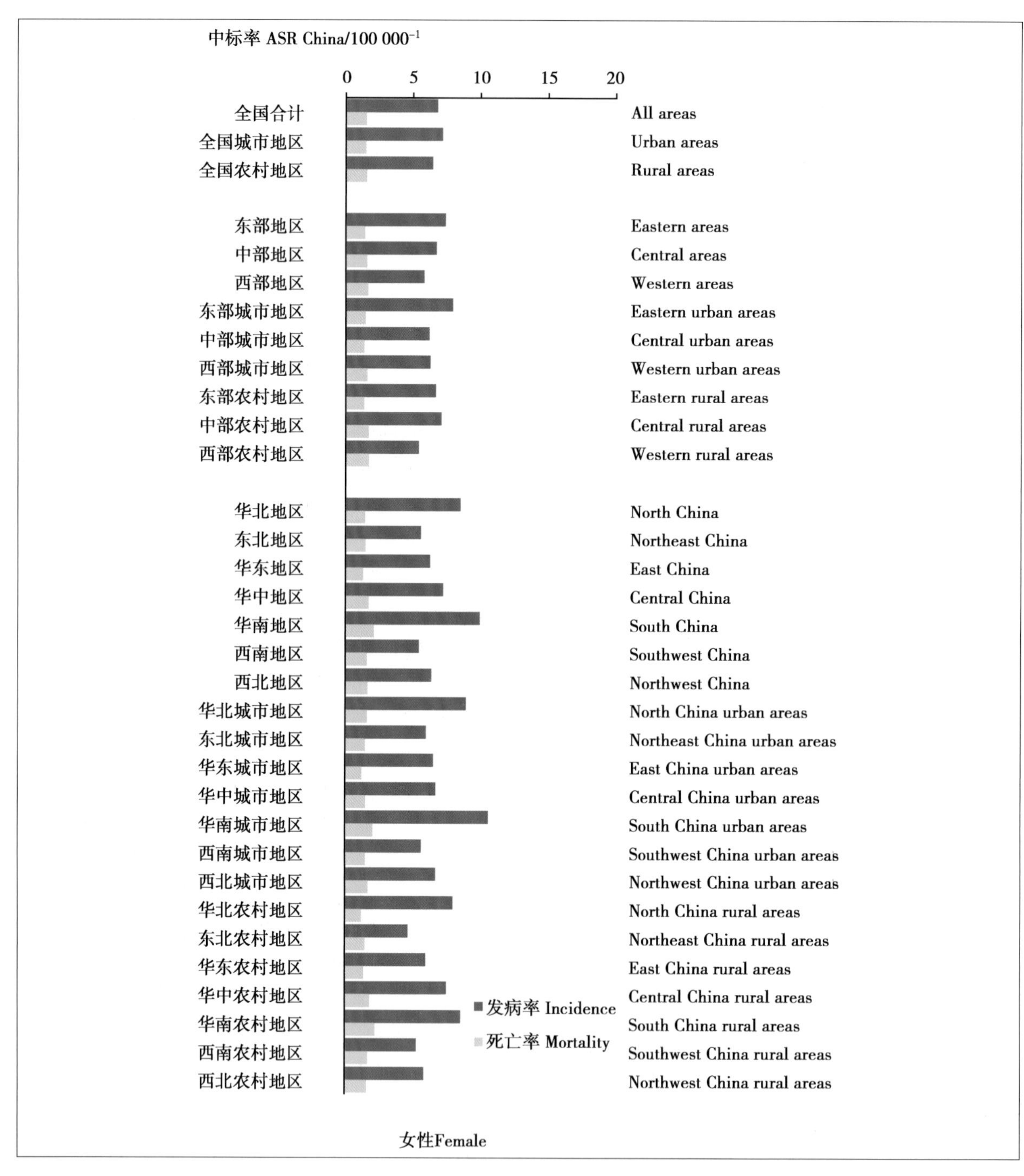

图 5-14b 2017 年中国不同肿瘤登记地区子宫体癌发病率和死亡率

Figure 5-14b Incidence and mortality rates of uterus cancer in different registration areas of China, 2017

15 卵巢

2017 年,中国肿瘤登记地区卵巢癌位居女性癌症发病谱第 11 位。新发病例数为 16 479 例,占女性癌症发病的 2. 89%;其中城市地区 9 185 例,农村地区 7 294 例。发病率为 7. 66/10 万,中标发病率为 5. 43/10 万,世标发病率为 5. 17/10 万;城市中标发病率为农村的 1. 22 倍。0~74 岁累积发病率为 0. 56%(表 5-15a)。

2017 年,中国肿瘤登记地区卵巢癌位居女性癌症死亡谱第 9 位。死亡病例数为 7 751 例,占女性癌症死亡的 2. 78%;其中城市地区 4 531 例,农村地区 3 220 例。死亡率为 3. 60/10 万,中标死亡率为 2. 25/10 万,世标死亡率为 2. 21/10 万;城市中标死亡率为农村的 1. 34 倍。0~74 岁累积死亡率为 0. 26%(表 5-15b)。

卵巢癌年龄别发病率从 35~39 岁组开始快速上升,至 60~64 岁组达高峰。卵巢癌年龄别死亡率从 35~39 岁组开始逐渐上升,至 75~79 岁组达高峰(图 5-15a)。

城市卵巢癌的发病率和死亡率均高于农村。中标发病率和中标死亡率均以东部地区最高,其次是中部地区,西部地区最低。在七大行政区中,中标发病率以华南地区最高,其次是华北地区和东北地区,西南地区最低;中标死亡率以东北地区最高,其次是华北地区和华南地区,西南地区最低(表 5-15a,表 5-15b,图 5-15b)。

15 Ovary

Ovarian cancer was the 11th most common female cancer in the registration areas of China in 2017. There were 16 479 new ovarian cancer cases (9 185 in urban areas and 7 294 in rural areas), accounting for 2. 89% of new female cancer cases of all sites. The crude incidence rate was 7. 66 per 100 000, with ASR China 5. 43 per 100 000 and ASR World 5. 17 per 100 000, respectively. Subgroup analyses showed that the incidence of ASR China was 1. 22 times in urban areas as that in rural areas. The cumulative incidence rate for subjects aged 0 to 74 years was 0. 56% (Table 5-15a).

Ovarian cancer was the9th most common female cause of cancer deaths. A total of 7 751 cases died of ovary cancer in 2017(4 531 in urban areas and 3 220 in rural areas), accounting for 2. 78% of all female cancer deaths. The crude mortality rate was 3. 60 per 100 000, with ASR China 2. 25 per 100 000 and ASR World 2. 21 per 100 000, respectively. Subgroup analyses showed that the mortality of ASR China was 1. 34 times in urban areas as that in rural areas. The cumulative mortality rate for subjects aged 0 to 74 years was 0. 26% (Table 5-15b).

The age-specific incidence rates increased rapidly from the age group of 35-39 years and peaked at the age group of 60-64 years. The age-specific mortality rates increased from the age group of 35-39 years and peaked at the age group of 75-79 years (Figure 5-15a).

The incidence and mortality rates of ovarian cancer were higher in urban areas than in rural areas. Eastern areas had the highest incidence rate and mortality rate (ASR China), followed by Central and Western areas. Among the seven administrative districts, South China had the highest incidence rate (ASR China), followed by North China and Northeast China, while the Southwest China had the lowest incidence rate. Northeast China had the highest mortality rate, followed by North China and South China, Southwest China had the lowest mortality rate (Table 5-15a, Table 5-15b, Figure5-15b).

表 5-15a 2017 年中国肿瘤登记地区卵巢癌发病情况

Table 5-15a Incidence of ovarian cancer in the registration areas of China,2017

地区 Area	病例数 No. cases	粗率 Crude rate/ 100 000^{-1}	构成比 Freq. /%	中标率 ASR China/ 100 000^{-1}	世标率 ASR World/ 100 000^{-1}	累积率 Cum. rate 0~74/%	顺位 Rank
合计 All	16 479	7. 66	2. 89	5. 43	5. 17	0. 56	11
城市地区 Urban areas	9 185	8. 65	2. 97	5. 97	5. 69	0. 62	10
农村地区 Rural areas	7 294	6. 69	2. 80	4. 88	4. 64	0. 50	11
东部地区 Eastern areas	8 311	8. 45	2. 73	5. 69	5. 41	0. 59	11
中部地区 Central areas	3 993	7. 10	2. 97	5. 35	5. 12	0. 56	10
西部地区 Western areas	4 175	6. 90	3. 19	5. 11	4. 84	0. 52	11

表 5-15b 2017 年中国肿瘤登记地区卵巢癌死亡情况

Table 5-15b Mortality of ovarian cancer in the registration areas of China,2017

地区 Area	死亡数 No. deaths	粗率 Crude rate/ 100 000^{-1}	构成比 Freq. /%	中标率 ASR China/ 100 000^{-1}	世标率 ASR world/ 100 000^{-1}	累积率 Cum. rate 0~74/%	顺位 Rank
合计 All	7 751	3. 60	2. 78	2. 25	2. 21	0. 26	9
城市地区 Urban areas	4 531	4. 27	3. 21	2. 57	2. 52	0. 30	9
农村地区 Rural areas	3 220	2. 95	2. 34	1. 92	1. 89	0. 22	11
东部地区 Eastern areas	4 208	4. 28	2. 98	2. 46	2. 42	0. 29	9
中部地区 Central areas	1 816	3. 23	2. 67	2. 20	2. 17	0. 26	10
西部地区 Western areas	1 727	2. 85	2. 49	1. 92	1. 87	0. 21	10

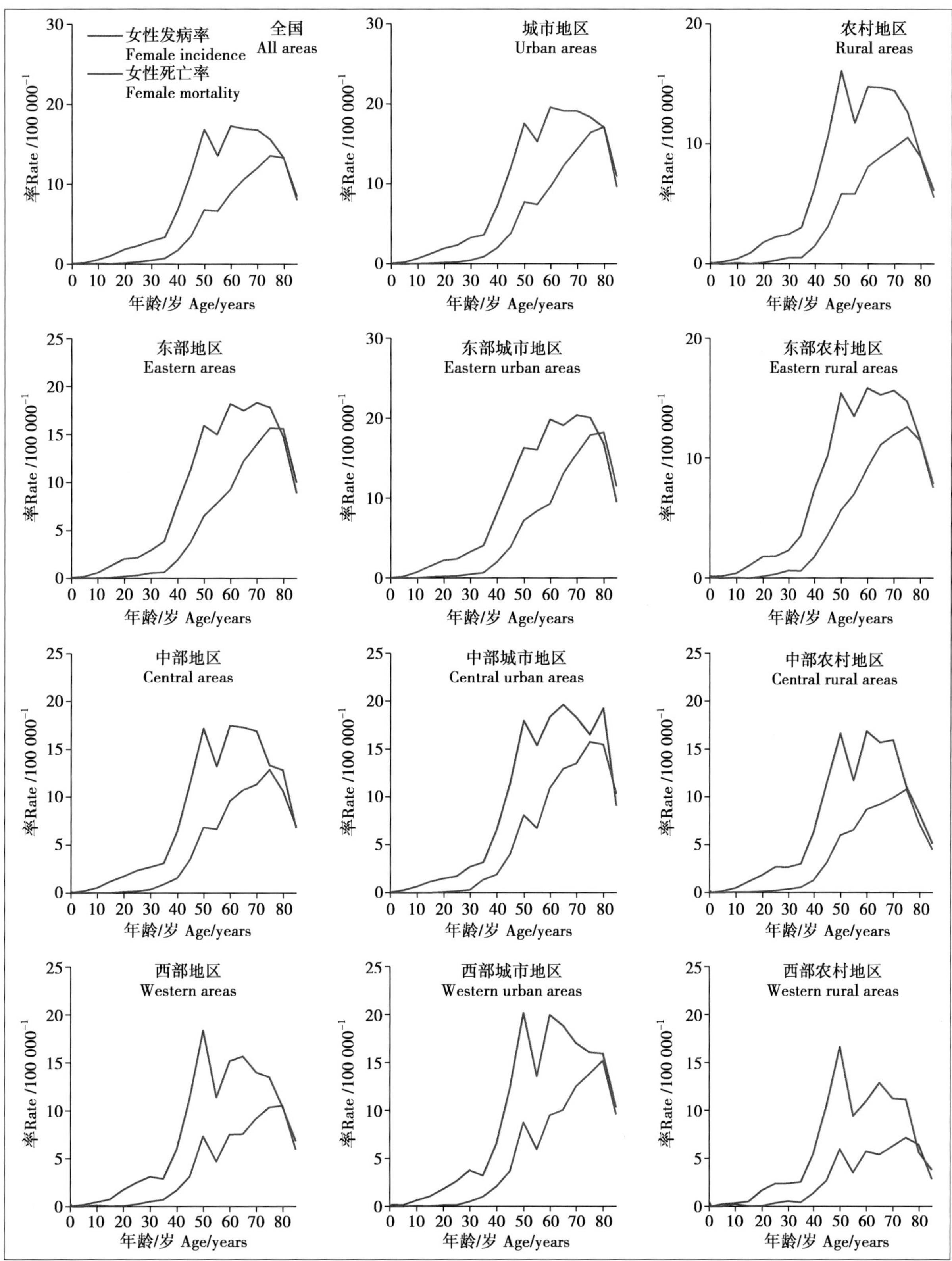

图 5-15a　2017 年中国肿瘤登记地区卵巢癌年龄别发病率和死亡率
Figure 5-15a　Age-specific incidence and mortality rates of ovarian cancer in the registration areas of China, 2017

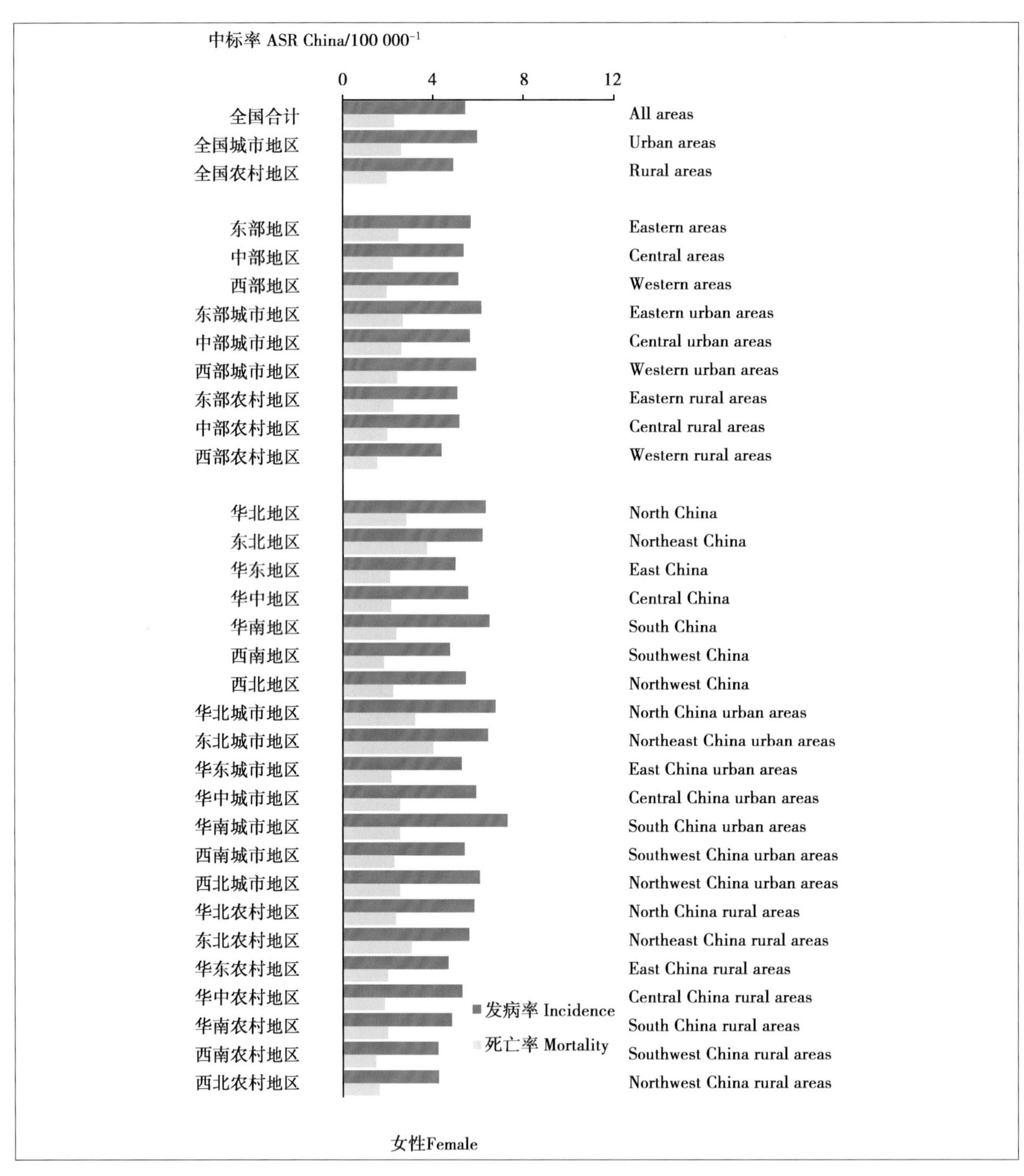

图 5-15b 2017 年中国肿瘤登记不同地区卵巢癌发病率和死亡率

Figure 5-15b Incidence and mortality rates of ovarian cancer in different registration areas of China,2017

16 前列腺

2017 年,中国肿瘤登记地区前列腺癌位居男性癌症发病谱第 6 位。新发病例数为 25 577 例,占全部癌症发病的 3. 59%;其中城市地区 16 543 例,农村地区 9 034 例。发病率为 11. 57/10 万,中标发病率为 6. 64/10 万,世标发病率为 6. 54/10 万;城市中标发病率为农村的 1. 78 倍。0 ~ 74 岁累积发病率为 0. 71%(表 5-16a)。

2017 年,中国肿瘤登记地区前列腺癌位居男性癌症死亡谱第 7 位。死亡病例数为 10 688 例,占全部癌症死亡的 2. 16%;其中城市地区 6 642 例,农村地区 4 046 例。前列腺癌死亡率为 4. 83/10 万,中标死亡率 2. 56/10 万,世标死亡率 2. 61/10 万;城市中标死亡率为农村的 1. 49 倍。0 ~ 74 岁累积死亡率为 0. 19%(表 5-16b)。

前列腺癌年龄别发病率和死亡率在 55 岁之前处于较低水平,55 岁开始呈上升趋势,60 岁以后快速上升,在 85 岁及以上年龄组达到峰值(图 5-16a)。

城市前列腺癌的发病率和死亡率均高于农村。中标发病率和中标死亡率均以东部地区最高,其次是西部地区,中部地区最低。在七大行政区中,华南地区前列腺癌发病率最高,其次是华东地区和华北地区,华中地区最低;死亡率同样是华南地区最高,其次为西北地区和华东地区(表 5-16a,表 5-16b,图 5-16b)。

16 Prostate

Prostate cancer was the 6th most commonmale cancer in the registration areas of China in 2017. There were 25 577 new cases of prostate cancer(16 543 in urban areas and 9 034 in rural areas), accounting for 3. 59% of new cancer cases of all sites. The crude incidence rate was 11. 57 per 100 000, with ASR China 6. 64 per 100 000 and ASR World 6. 54 per 100 000, respectively. Subgroup analyses showed that the incidence of ASR China was 1. 78 times in urban areas as that in rural areas. The cumulative incidence rate for subjects aged 0 to 74 years was 0. 71% (Table 5-16a).

Prostate cancer was the 7th most common male cause of cancer deaths. A total of 10 688 cases died of prostate cancer in 2017 (6 642 in urban areas and 4 046 in rural areas), accounting for 2. 16% of all cancer deaths. The crude mortality rate was 4. 83 per 100 000, with ASR China 2. 56 per 100 000 and ASR World 2. 61 per 100 000, respectively. Subgroup analyses showed that the mortality of ASR China was 1. 49 times in urban areas as that in rural areas. The cumulative mortality rate for subjects aged 0 to 74 years was 0. 19% (Table 5-16b).

The age-specific incidence and mortality rates were low before 55 years old and increased constantly since then. The age-specific incidence and mortality rates dramatically increased over 60 years old. The incidence and mortality rate reached peak atthe age group of 85+ years, respectively (Figure 5-16a).

The prostate cancer incidence rate and mortality rate were higher in urban areas than that in rural areas. Age-standardized incidence and mortality rates were highest in Eastern areas, and followed by Western areas and Central areas. Among the seven administrative districts, the incidence rate was highest in South China, followed by East China and North China, and was lowest in Central China. Mortality rate was also highest in South China, followed by Northwest China and East China (Table 5-16a, Table 5-16b, Figure 5-16b).

表 5-16a 2017 年中国肿瘤登记地区前列腺癌发病情况
Table 5-16a Incidence of prostate cancer in the registration areas of China, 2017

地区 Area	病例数 No. cases	粗率 Crude rate/ 100 000^{-1}	构成比 Freq. /%	中标率 ASR China/ 100 000^{-1}	世标率 ASR World/ 100 000^{-1}	累积率 Cum. rate 0~74/%	顺位 Rank
合计 All	25 577	11. 57	3. 59	6. 64	6. 54	0. 71	6
城市地区 Urban areas	16 543	15. 46	4. 53	8. 49	8. 35	0. 92	6
农村地区 Rural areas	9 034	7. 92	2. 61	4. 77	4. 69	0. 51	6
东部地区 Eastern areas	15 628	15. 71	4. 39	8. 23	8. 09	0. 91	6
中部地区 Central areas	4 411	7. 50	2. 64	4. 91	4. 84	0. 52	6
西部地区 Western areas	5 538	8. 82	2. 94	5. 30	5. 23	0. 53	6

表 5-16b 2017 年中国肿瘤登记地区前列腺癌死亡情况
Table 5-16b Mortality of prostate cancer in the registration areas of China, 2017

地区 Area	死亡数 No. deaths	粗率 Crude rate/ 100 000^{-1}	构成比 Freq. /%	中标率 ASR China/ 100 000^{-1}	世标率 ASR world/ 100 000^{-1}	累积率 Cum. rate 0~74/%	顺位 Rank
合计 All	10 688	4. 83	2. 16	2. 56	2. 61	0. 19	7
城市地区 Urban areas	6 642	6. 21	2. 71	3. 04	3. 10	0. 21	7
农村地区 Rural areas	4 046	3. 55	1. 62	2. 04	2. 06	0. 16	10
东部地区 Eastern areas	6 155	6. 19	2. 56	2. 89	2. 94	0. 21	7
中部地区 Central areas	2 031	3. 45	1. 70	2. 13	2. 16	0. 15	10
西部地区 Western areas	2 502	3. 98	1. 87	2. 31	2. 36	0. 18	8

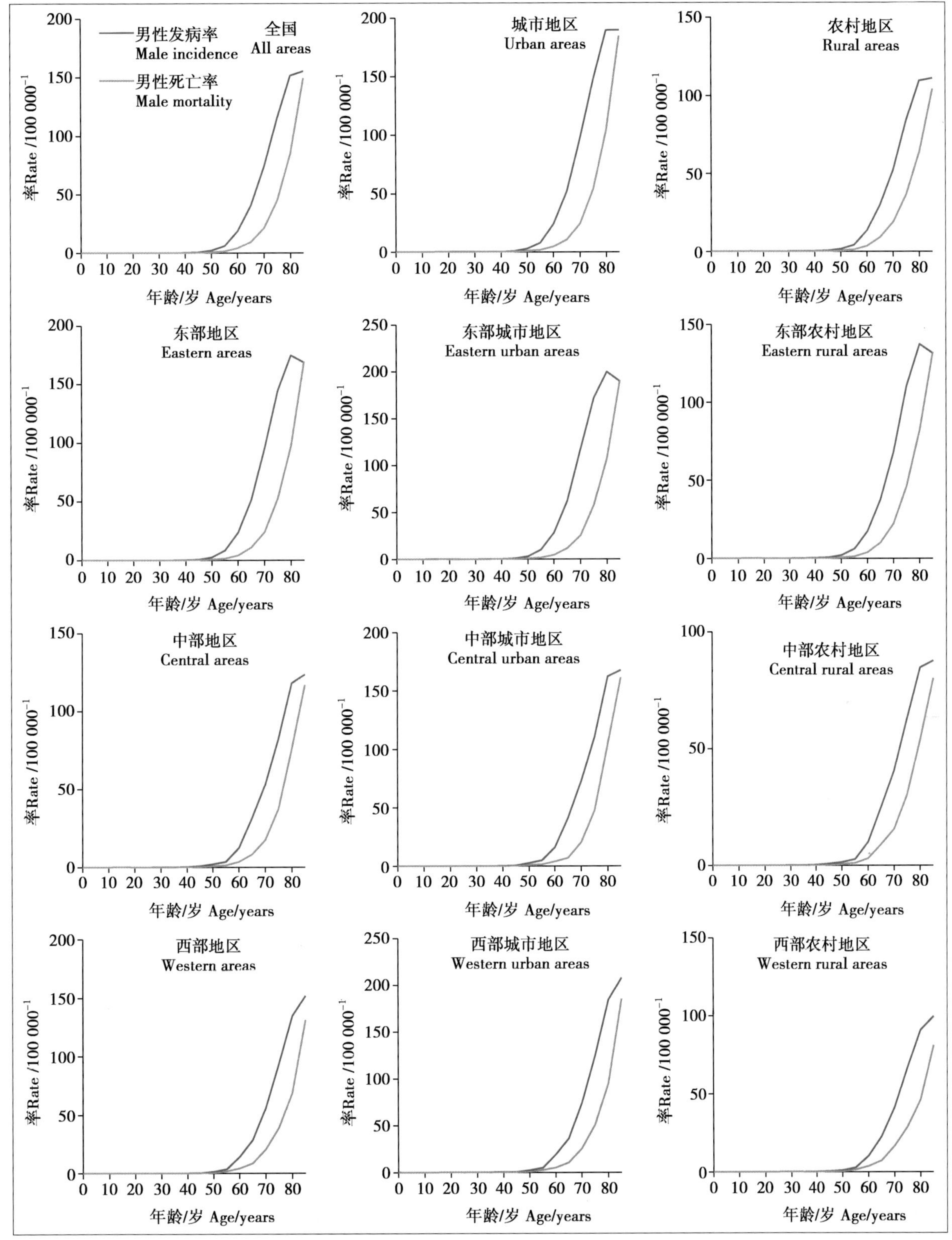

图 5-16a　2017 年中国肿瘤登记地区前列腺癌年龄别发病率和死亡率

Figure 5-16a　Age-specific incidence and mortality rates of prostate cancer in the registration areas of China, 2017

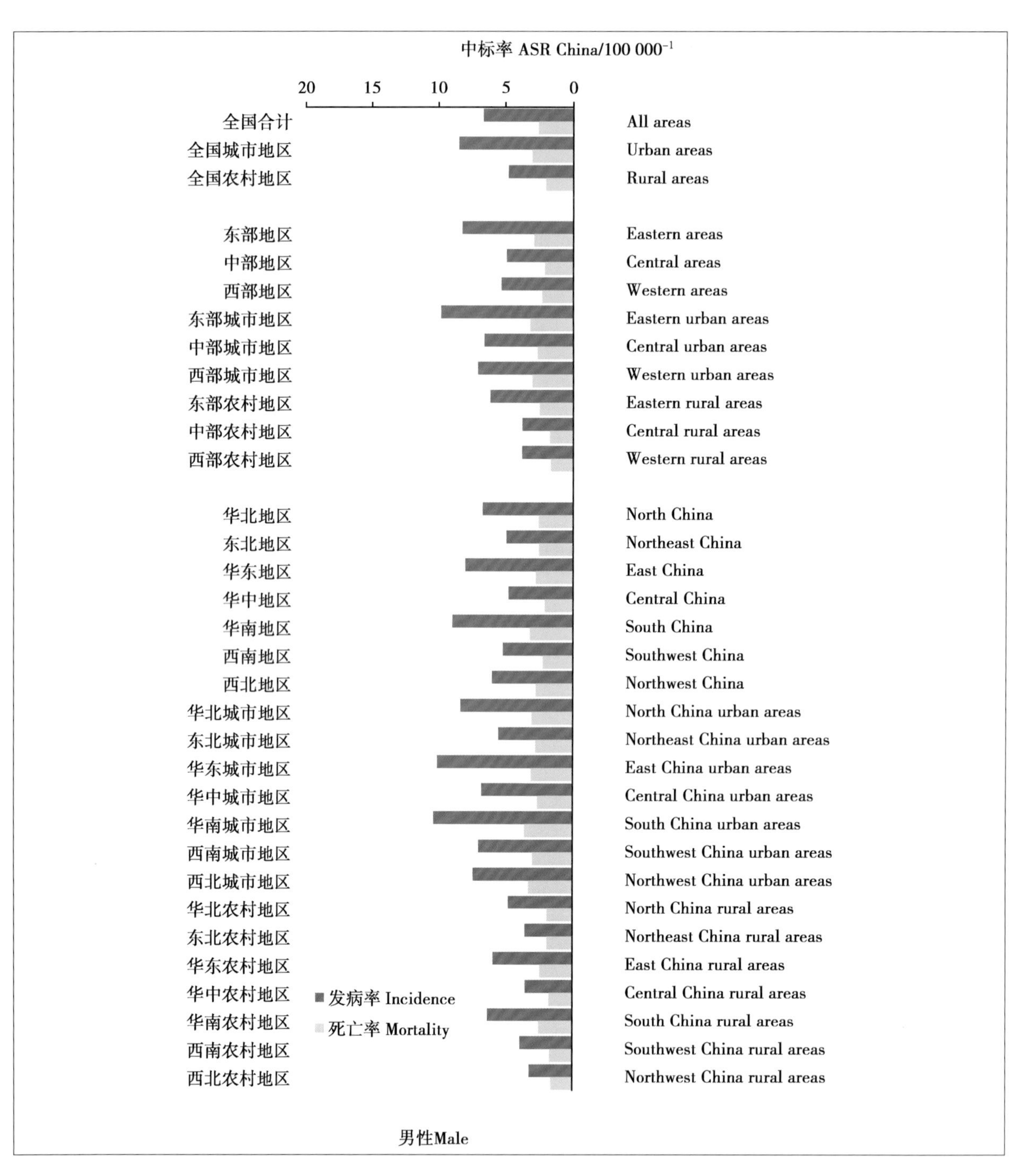

图 5-16b 2017 年中国肿瘤登记地区不同地区前列腺癌发病率和死亡率

Figure 5-16b Incidence and mortality rates of prostate cancer in different registration areas of China,2017

17 肾及泌尿系统不明

2017年,中国肿瘤登记地区肾及泌尿系统不明癌位居癌症发病谱第17位。新发病例数为22 457例,占全部癌症发病的1.75%;其中男性14 093例,女性8 364例,城市地区14 385例,农村地区8 072例。发病率为5.15/10万,中标发病率为3.28/10万,世标发病率3.26/10万;男性中标发病率为女性的1.74倍,城市中标发病率为农村的1.70倍;0~74岁累积发病率为0.38%(表5-17a)。

2017年,中国肿瘤登记地区肾及泌尿系统不明癌位居癌症死亡谱第18位,死亡病例数为8 298例,占全部癌症死亡的1.07%;其中男性5 251例,女性3047例,城市地区5 248例,农村地区3 050例。死亡率为1.90/10万,中标死亡率1.09/10万,世标死亡率1.09/10万;男性中标死亡率为女性的1.91倍,城市中标死亡率为农村的1.56倍。0~74岁累积死亡率为0.12%(表5-17b)。

按部位划分,肾癌发病率为3.99/10万,中标发病率为2.61/10万;肾癌死亡率为1.39/10万,中标死亡率为0.81/10万。肾盂癌的发病率为0.48/10万,中标发病率为0.29/10万;肾盂癌死亡率为0.20/10万,中标死亡率为0.11/10万。输尿管癌的发病率为0.56/10万,中标发病率为0.32/10万;输尿管癌死亡率为0.26/10万,中标死亡率为0.14/10万(表5-17c~表5-17h)。

17 Kidney & unspecified urinary organs

Cancer of the kidney & unspecified urinary organs was the 17th most common cancer in the registration areas of China in 2017. There were 22 457 new cancer cases (14 093 males and 8 364 females, 14 385 in urban areas and 8 072 in rural areas), accounting for 1.75% of new cases of all cancers. The crude incidence rate was 5.15 per 100 000, with ASR China 3.28 per 100 000 and ASR world 3.26 per 100 000, respectively. Subgroup analyses showed that the incidence of ASR China was 1.74 times in males as that in females, and it was 1.70 times in urban areas as that in rural areas. The cumulative incidence rate for subjects aged 0 to 74 years was 0.38% (Table 5-17a).

Cancer of the kidney & unspecified urinary organs was the 18th most common cause of cancer deaths in the registration areas of China. A total of 8 298 cases died of cancer of kidney and unspecified urinary organs in 2017 (5 251 males and 3 047 females, 5 248 in urban areas and 3 050 in rural areas), accounting for 1.07% of all cancer deaths. The crude mortality rate was 1.90 per 100 000, with ASR China 1.09 per 100 000 and ASR world 1.09 per 100 000, respectively. Subgroup analyses showed that the mortality of ASR China was 1.91 times in males as that in females, and it was 1.56 times in urban areas as that in rural areas. The cumulative mortality rate for subjects aged 0 to 74 years was 0.12% (Table 5-17b).

By subsite, the renal cancer incidence was 3.99 per 100 000 with ASR China 2.61 per 100 000; and the mortality was 1.39 per 100 000, with ASR China 0.81 per 100 000. The cancer incidence of renal pelvis was 0.48 per 100 000, with ASR China 0.29 per 100 000; and the mortality was 0.20 per 100 000, with ASR China 0.11 per 100 000. The ureter cancer incidence was 0.56 per 100 000, with ASR China 0.32 per 100 000; and the mortality was 0.26 per 100 000, with ASR China 0.14 per 100 000 (Table 5-17c-Table 5-17h).

肾及泌尿系统不明癌年龄别发病率在 20 岁年龄组之前均处于较低水平，自 20～24 岁组开始快速上升，至 75～79 岁组达高峰，80 岁组以后降低；年龄别死亡率从 40～44 岁组开始迅速上升；男性各年龄别发病率和死亡率均明显高于女性（图 5-17a）。

城市地区肾及泌尿系统不明癌的发病率和死亡率均高于农村地区。中标发病率和中标死亡率均以东部地区最高，其次是中部地区，西部地区最低。在七大行政区中，华北地区发病率最高，东北地区死亡率最高，西南地区发病率和死亡率最低（表 5-17a，表 5-17b，图 5-17b）。

肾（除外肾盂）是肾及泌尿系统不明癌发生的最主要的亚部位，占全部病例的 77. 55%，其次为输尿管，占 10. 85%；肾盂占 9. 39%；其他泌尿器官占 2. 21%（图 5-17c）。

全部肾及泌尿系统不明癌病例中有明确组织学类型的病例占 65. 27%，其中透明细胞腺癌是最主要的病理类型，占 74. 51%；其次是乳头状腺癌，占 3. 34%；肾嫌色细胞癌，占 3. 68%，肾集合管癌占 0. 57%，其他类型癌占 17. 90%（图 5-17d）。

The age-specific incidence of cancer of kidney and unspecified urinary organs was low before 20 years old. It increased rapidly from the age group of 20-24 years and peaked at the age group of 75-79 years, and then it decreased at the age group of 80 years. Age-specific mortality rates increased rapidly from the age group of 40-44 years. Age-specific incidence and mortality rates in males were generally higher than those in females (Figure 5-17a).

The incidence and mortality rates of cancer in kidney & unspecified urinary organs were higher in urban areas than in rural areas. Eastern areas had the highest incidence and mortality rates, followed by the central areas and western areas. Among the seven administrative districts, North China had the highest incidence and Northeast China had the highest mortality. Southwest China had the lowest incidence and mortality (Table 5-17a, Table 5-17b, Figure 5-17b).

Kidney (except for the renal pelvis) was the most commonsubsite of cancer in kidney & unspecified urinary organs, accounting for 77. 55% of total cases, followed by ureter (10. 85%), renal pelvis (9. 39%), and other urinary organs (2. 21%) (Figure 5-17c).

About 65. 27% cases of cancer in kidney and unspecified urinary organs had morphological verification. Among those, clear cell adenocarcinoma was the most common histological type, accounting for 74. 51% of all cases, followed by papillary adenocarcinoma (3. 34%), chromophobe renal cell carcinoma (3. 68%), collecting duct carcinoma (0. 57%), and others (17. 90%) (Figure 5-17d).

表 5-17a 2017 年中国肿瘤登记地区肾及泌尿系统不明癌发病情况

Table 5-17a Incidence of cancer of kidney & unspecified urinary organs in the registration areas of China, 2017

地区 Area	性别 Sex	病例数 No. cases	粗率 Crude rate/ 100 000^{-1}	构成比 Freq. /%	中标率 ASR China/ 100 000^{-1}	世标率 ASR World/ 100 000^{-1}	累积率 Cum. rate 0~74/%	顺位 Rank
合计	合计 Both	22 457	5. 15	1. 75	3. 28	3. 26	0. 38	17
All	男性 Male	14 093	6. 37	1. 98	4. 17	4. 14	0. 48	13
	女性 Female	8 364	3. 89	1. 47	2. 40	2. 39	0. 28	16
城市地区	合计 Both	14 385	6. 75	2. 13	4. 13	4. 09	0. 48	16
Urban areas	男性 Male	9 122	8. 52	2. 50	5. 36	5. 31	0. 62	11
	女性 Female	5 263	4. 95	1. 70	2. 93	2. 91	0. 33	15
农村地区	合计 Both	8 072	3. 62	1. 33	2. 42	2. 41	0. 28	17
Rural areas	男性 Male	4 971	4. 36	1. 43	2. 99	2. 97	0. 35	14
	女性 Female	3 101	2. 85	1. 19	1. 86	1. 86	0. 22	16
东部地区	合计 Both	14 036	7. 09	2. 12	4. 20	4. 17	0. 49	17
Eastern areas	男性 Male	9 018	9. 06	2. 53	5. 54	5. 48	0. 64	11
	女性 Female	5 018	5. 10	1. 65	2. 91	2. 89	0. 33	15
中部地区	合计 Both	4 525	3. 93	1. 50	2. 77	2. 75	0. 32	17
Central areas	男性 Male	2 761	4. 69	1. 65	3. 39	3. 37	0. 40	13
	女性 Female	1 764	3. 14	1. 31	2. 16	2. 14	0. 25	16
西部地区	合计 Both	3 896	3. 16	1. 22	2. 10	2. 09	0. 24	20
Western areas	男性 Male	2 314	3. 68	1. 23	2. 51	2. 49	0. 28	14
	女性 Female	1 582	2. 61	1. 21	1. 69	1. 70	0. 20	17

表 5-17b 2017 年中国肿瘤登记地区肾及泌尿系统不明癌死亡情况

Table 5-17b Mortality of cancer of kidney & unspecified urinary organs in the registration areas of China, 2017

地区 Area	性别 Sex	死亡数 No. deaths	粗率 Crude rate/ 100 000^{-1}	构成比 Freq. /%	中标率 ASR China/ 100 000^{-1}	世标率 ASR World/ 100 000^{-1}	累积率 Cum. rate 0~74/%	顺位 Rank
合计	合计 Both	8 298	1. 90	1. 07	1. 09	1. 09	0. 12	18
All	男性 Male	5 251	2. 37	1. 06	1. 44	1. 45	0. 15	15
	女性 Female	3 047	1. 42	1. 09	0. 75	0. 75	0. 08	15
城市地区	合计 Both	5 248	2. 46	1. 36	1. 32	1. 32	0. 14	17
Urban areas	男性 Male	3 343	3. 12	1. 36	1. 78	1. 79	0. 19	14
	女性 Female	1 905	1. 79	1. 35	0. 88	0. 88	0. 09	15
农村地区	合计 Both	3 050	1. 37	0. 79	0. 84	0. 85	0. 09	20
Rural areas	男性 Male	1 908	1. 67	0. 77	1. 08	1. 10	0. 12	15
	女性 Female	1 142	1. 05	0. 83	0. 61	0. 61	0. 07	17
东部地区	合计 Both	4 984	2. 52	1. 30	1. 29	1. 30	0. 14	16
Eastern areas	男性 Male	3 147	3. 16	1. 31	1. 73	1. 75	0. 19	13
	女性 Female	1 837	1. 87	1. 30	0. 87	0. 87	0. 09	15
中部地区	合计 Both	1 720	1. 49	0. 92	0. 99	0. 98	0. 11	19
Central areas	男性 Male	1 090	1. 85	0. 91	1. 29	1. 29	0. 15	15
	女性 Female	630	1. 12	0. 93	0. 70	0. 69	0. 07	15
西部地区	合计 Both	1 594	1. 29	0. 78	0. 80	0. 80	0. 08	20
Western areas	男性 Male	1 014	1. 61	0. 76	1. 04	1. 05	0. 11	17
	女性 Female	580	0. 96	0. 84	0. 57	0. 57	0. 06	18

表 5-17c 2017 年中国肿瘤登记地区肾癌发病情况
Table 5-17c Incidence of kidney cancer in the registration areas of China, 2017

地区 Area	性别 Sex	病例数 No. cases	粗率 Crude rate/ 100 000^{-1}	构成比 Freq. /%	中标率 ASR China/ 100 000^{-1}	世标率 ASR World/ 100 000^{-1}	累积率 Cum. rate 0~74/%
合计	合计 Both	17 416	4. 00	1. 36	2. 61	2. 59	0. 30
All	男性 Male	11 246	5. 09	1. 58	3. 39	3. 36	0. 39
	女性 Female	6 170	2. 87	1. 08	1. 84	1. 84	0. 21
城市地区	合计 Both	11 172	5. 24	1. 66	3. 30	3. 27	0. 38
Urban areas	男性 Male	7 349	6. 87	2. 01	4. 40	4. 35	0. 51
	女性 Female	3 823	3. 60	1. 24	2. 23	2. 22	0. 25
农村地区	合计 Both	6 244	2. 80	1. 03	1. 91	1. 90	0. 22
Rural areas	男性 Male	3 897	3. 41	1. 12	2. 37	2. 36	0. 27
	女性 Female	2 347	2. 15	0. 90	1. 45	1. 45	0. 17
东部地区	合计 Both	10 991	5. 55	1. 66	3. 40	3. 37	0. 39
Eastern areas	男性 Male	7 260	7. 30	2. 04	4. 56	4. 50	0. 53
	女性 Female	3 731	3. 79	1. 23	2. 27	2. 27	0. 26
中部地区	合计 Both	3 532	3. 07	1. 17	2. 19	2. 18	0. 26
Central areas	男性 Male	2 218	3. 77	1. 33	2. 75	2. 73	0. 32
	女性 Female	1 314	2. 34	0. 98	1. 65	1. 64	0. 19
西部地区	合计 Both	2 893	2. 35	0. 91	1. 59	1. 59	0. 18
Western areas	男性 Male	1 768	2. 81	0. 94	1. 94	1. 93	0. 22
	女性 Female	1 125	1. 86	0. 86	1. 24	1. 25	0. 14

表 5-17d 2017 年中国肿瘤登记地区肾癌死亡情况
Table 5-17d Mortality of kidney cancer in the registration areas of China, 2017

地区 Area	性别 Sex	死亡数 No. deaths	粗率 Crude rate/ 100 000^{-1}	构成比 Freq. /%	中标率 ASR China/ 100 000^{-1}	世标率 ASR World/ 100 000^{-1}	累积率 Cum. rate 0~74/%
合计	合计 Both	6 049	1. 39	0. 78	0. 81	0. 81	0. 09
All	男性 Male	3 998	1. 81	0. 81	1. 11	1. 12	0. 12
	女性 Female	2 051	0. 95	0. 74	0. 52	0. 52	0. 05
城市地区	合计 Both	3 772	1. 77	0. 98	0. 97	0. 98	0. 10
Urban areas	男性 Male	2 546	2. 38	1. 04	1. 37	1. 39	0. 15
	女性 Female	1 226	1. 15	0. 87	0. 59	0. 59	0. 06
农村地区	合计 Both	2 277	1. 02	0. 59	0. 64	0. 64	0. 07
Rural areas	男性 Male	1 452	1. 27	0. 58	0. 83	0. 84	0. 09
	女性 Female	825	0. 76	0. 60	0. 45	0. 45	0. 05
东部地区	合计 Both	3 616	1. 83	0. 95	0. 95	0. 97	0. 10
Eastern areas	男性 Male	2 385	2. 40	0. 99	1. 33	1. 35	0. 14
	女性 Female	1 231	1. 25	0. 87	0. 60	0. 61	0. 06
中部地区	合计 Both	1 275	1. 11	0. 70	0. 74	0. 74	0. 08
Central areas	男性 Male	851	1. 45	0. 71	1. 02	1. 01	0. 12
	女性 Female	424	0. 75	0. 62	0. 48	0. 48	0. 05
西部地区	合计 Both	1 158	0. 94	0. 57	0. 59	0. 59	0. 06
Western areas	男性 Male	762	1. 21	0. 57	0. 79	0. 80	0. 08
	女性 Female	396	0. 65	0. 57	0. 40	0. 39	0. 04

表 5-17e　2017 年中国肿瘤登记地区肾盂癌发病情况
Table 5-17e　Incidence of cancer of renal pelvis in the registration areas of China, 2017

地区 Area	性别 Sex	病例数 No. cases	粗率 Crude rate/100 000^{-1}	构成比 Freq./%	中标率 ASR China/100 000^{-1}	世标率 ASR World/100 000^{-1}	累积率 Cum. rate 0~74/%
合计	合计 Both	2 109	0.48	0.16	0.29	0.28	0.03
All	男性 Male	1 221	0.55	0.17	0.34	0.34	0.04
	女性 Female	888	0.41	0.16	0.23	0.23	0.03
城市地区	合计 Both	1 333	0.63	0.20	0.35	0.35	0.04
Urban areas	男性 Male	751	0.70	0.21	0.41	0.42	0.05
	女性 Female	582	0.55	0.19	0.29	0.28	0.03
农村地区	合计 Both	776	0.35	0.13	0.22	0.22	0.03
Rural areas	男性 Male	470	0.41	0.14	0.27	0.27	0.03
	女性 Female	306	0.28	0.12	0.17	0.17	0.02
东部地区	合计 Both	1 283	0.65	0.19	0.35	0.34	0.04
Eastern areas	男性 Male	757	0.76	0.21	0.43	0.43	0.05
	女性 Female	526	0.53	0.17	0.27	0.26	0.03
中部地区	合计 Both	408	0.35	0.14	0.24	0.24	0.03
Central areas	男性 Male	229	0.39	0.14	0.28	0.28	0.04
	女性 Female	179	0.32	0.13	0.20	0.20	0.02
西部地区	合计 Both	418	0.34	0.13	0.22	0.22	0.03
Western areas	男性 Male	235	0.37	0.12	0.25	0.25	0.03
	女性 Female	183	0.30	0.14	0.18	0.18	0.02

表 5-17f　2017 年中国肿瘤登记地区肾盂癌死亡情况
Table 5-17f　Mortality of cancer of renal pelvis in the registration areas of China, 2017

地区 Area	性别 Sex	死亡数 No. deaths	粗率 Crude rate/100 000^{-1}	构成比 Freq./%	中标率 ASR China/100 000^{-1}	世标率 ASR World/100 000^{-1}	累积率 Cum. rate 0~74/%
All	合计 Both	872	0.20	0.11	0.11	0.11	0.01
合计	男性 Male	494	0.22	0.10	0.13	0.13	0.01
	女性 Female	378	0.18	0.14	0.09	0.09	0.01
城市地区	合计 Both	532	0.25	0.14	0.13	0.13	0.01
Urban areas	男性 Male	293	0.27	0.12	0.15	0.15	0.02
	女性 Female	239	0.22	0.17	0.10	0.10	0.01
农村地区	合计 Both	340	0.15	0.09	0.09	0.09	0.01
Rural areas	男性 Male	201	0.18	0.08	0.11	0.11	0.01
	女性 Female	139	0.13	0.10	0.07	0.07	0.01
东部地区	合计 Both	472	0.24	0.12	0.12	0.11	0.01
Eastern areas	男性 Male	271	0.27	0.11	0.14	0.15	0.02
	女性 Female	201	0.20	0.14	0.09	0.09	0.01
中部地区	合计 Both	202	0.18	0.11	0.12	0.12	0.01
Central areas	男性 Male	109	0.19	0.09	0.13	0.13	0.01
	女性 Female	93	0.17	0.14	0.10	0.10	0.01
西部地区	合计 Both	198	0.16	0.10	0.09	0.10	0.01
Western areas	男性 Male	114	0.18	0.09	0.11	0.12	0.01
	女性 Female	84	0.14	0.12	0.08	0.08	0.01

表 5-17g 2017 年中国肿瘤登记地区输尿管癌发病情况

Table 5-17g Incidence of ureter cancer in the registration areas of China,2017

地区 Area	性别 Sex	病例数 No. cases	粗率 Crude rate/ 100 000^{-1}	构成比 Freq./%	中标率 ASR China/ 100 000^{-1}	世标率 ASR World/ 100 000^{-1}	累积率 Cum. rate 0~74/%
合计	合计 Both	2 436	0. 56	0. 19	0. 32	0. 32	0. 04
All	男性 Male	1 313	0. 59	0. 18	0. 36	0. 36	0. 04
	女性 Female	1 123	0. 52	0. 20	0. 28	0. 28	0. 03
城市地区	合计 Both	1 579	0. 74	0. 23	0. 40	0. 40	0. 05
Urban areas	男性 Male	831	0. 78	0. 23	0. 45	0. 44	0. 05
	女性 Female	748	0. 70	0. 24	0. 36	0. 35	0. 04
农村地区	合计 Both	857	0. 38	0. 14	0. 23	0. 24	0. 03
Rural areas	男性 Male	482	0. 42	0. 14	0. 27	0. 27	0. 03
	女性 Female	375	0. 34	0. 14	0. 20	0. 20	0. 03
东部地区	合计 Both	1 469	0. 74	0. 22	0. 38	0. 38	0. 05
Eastern areas	男性 Male	811	0. 82	0. 23	0. 45	0. 46	0. 06
	女性 Female	658	0. 67	0. 22	0. 32	0. 31	0. 04
中部地区	合计 Both	482	0. 42	0. 16	0. 27	0. 27	0. 03
Central areas	男性 Male	251	0. 43	0. 15	0. 29	0. 29	0. 03
	女性 Female	231	0. 41	0. 17	0. 26	0. 25	0. 03
西部地区	合计 Both	485	0. 39	0. 15	0. 24	0. 23	0. 03
Western areas	男性 Male	251	0. 40	0. 13	0. 25	0. 24	0. 03
	女性 Female	234	0. 39	0. 18	0. 23	0. 22	0. 03

表 5-17h 2017 年中国肿瘤登记地区输尿管癌死亡情况

Table 5-17h Mortality of ureter cancer in the registration areas of China,2017

地区 Area	性别 Sex	死亡数 No. deaths	粗率 Crude rate/ 100 000^{-1}	构成比 Freq./%	中标率 ASR China/ 100 000^{-1}	世标率 ASR World/ 100 000^{-1}	累积率 Cum. rate 0~74/%
合计	合计 Both	1 149	0. 26	0. 14	0. 14	0. 14	0. 01
All	男性 Male	614	0. 28	0. 12	0. 16	0. 16	0. 02
	女性 Female	535	0. 25	0. 19	0. 12	0. 12	0. 01
城市地区	合计 Both	783	0. 37	0. 20	0. 18	0. 18	0. 02
Urban areas	男性 Male	406	0. 38	0. 17	0. 21	0. 20	0. 02
	女性 Female	377	0. 35	0. 27	0. 16	0. 16	0. 01
农村地区	合计 Both	366	0. 16	0. 09	0. 10	0. 10	0. 01
Rural areas	男性 Male	208	0. 18	0. 08	0. 11	0. 12	0. 01
	女性 Female	158	0. 14	0. 11	0. 08	0. 08	0. 01
东部地区	合计 Both	745	0. 38	0. 19	0. 18	0. 18	0. 02
Eastern areas	男性 Male	394	0. 40	0. 16	0. 21	0. 21	0. 02
	女性 Female	351	0. 36	0. 25	0. 16	0. 15	0. 01
中部地区	合计 Both	205	0. 18	0. 11	0. 11	0. 10	0. 01
Central areas	男性 Male	108	0. 18	0. 09	0. 12	0. 12	0. 01
	女性 Female	97	0. 17	0. 14	0. 10	0. 09	0. 01
西部地区	合计 Both	199	0. 16	0. 10	0. 09	0. 09	0. 01
Western areas	男性 Male	112	0. 18	0. 08	0. 11	0. 11	0. 01
	女性 Female	87	0. 14	0. 13	0. 08	0. 08	0. 01

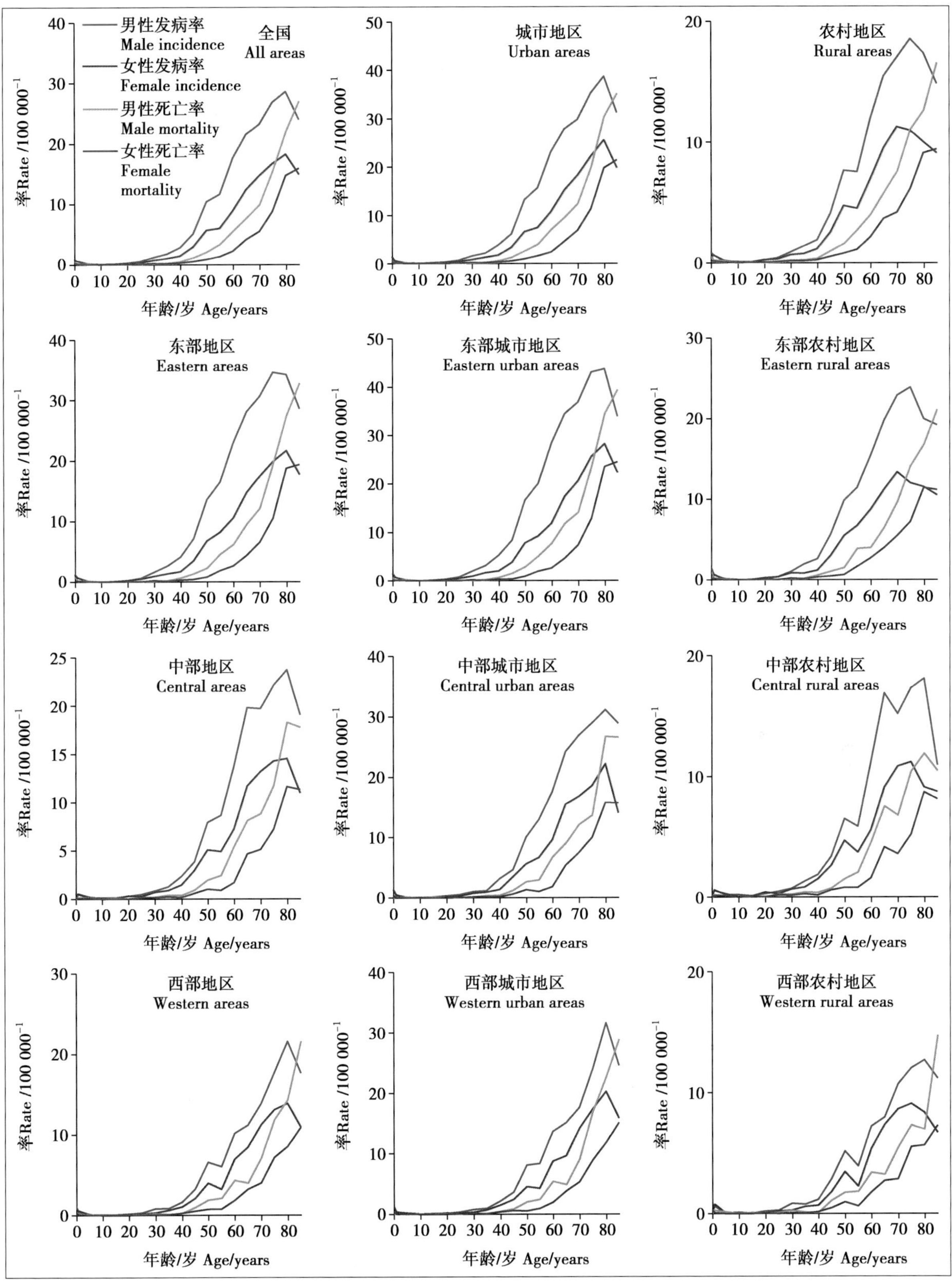

图 5-17a　2017 年中国肿瘤登记地区肾及泌尿系统不明癌年龄别发病率和死亡率

Figure 5-17a　Age-specific incidence and mortality rates of cancer of kidney & unspecified urinary organs in the registration areas of China, 2017

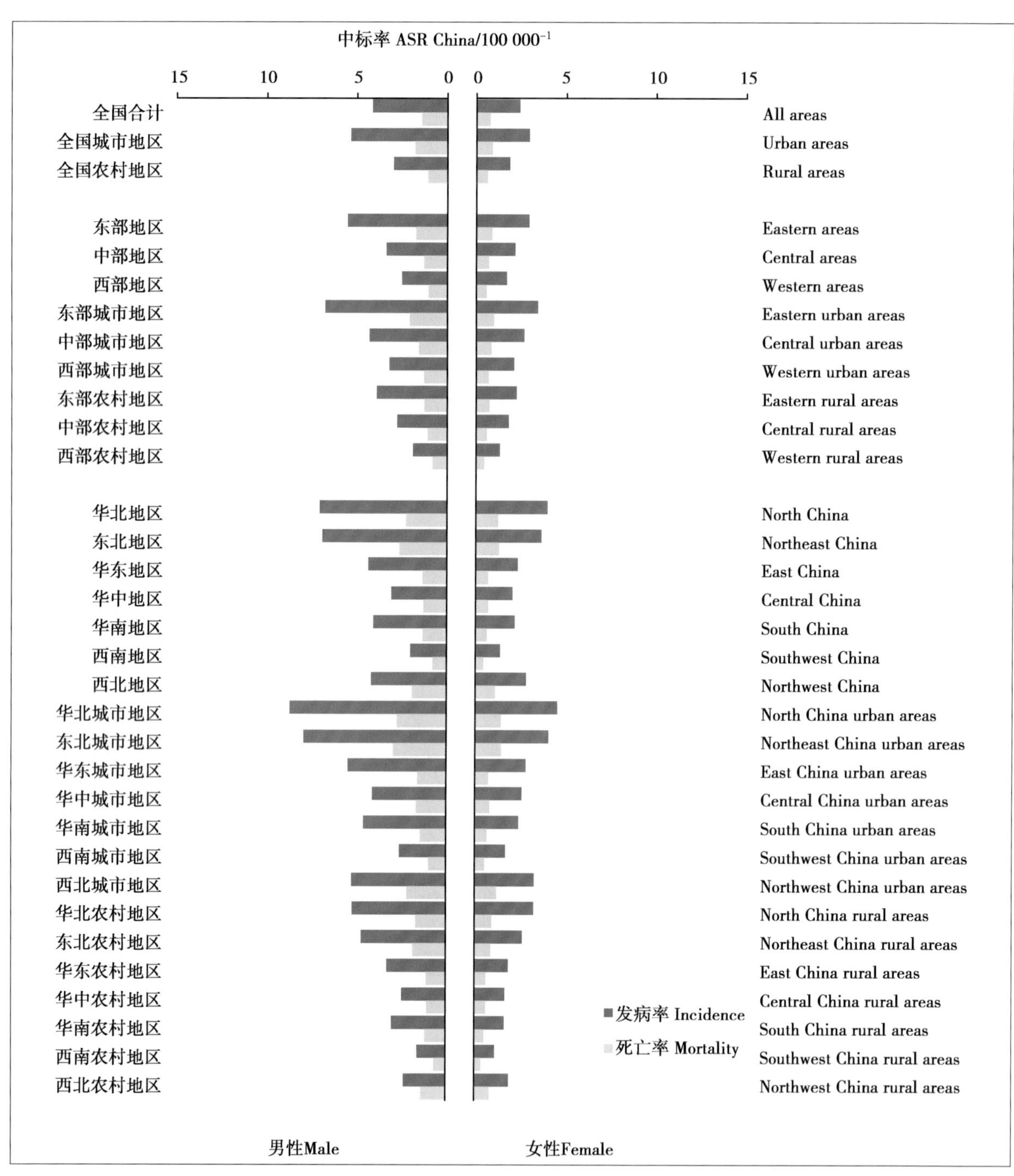

图 5-17b　2017 年中国肿瘤登记地区肾及泌尿系统不明癌不同地区发病率和死亡率
Figure 5-17b　Incidence and mortality rates of cancer of kidney & unspecified urinary organs in different registration areas of China, 2017

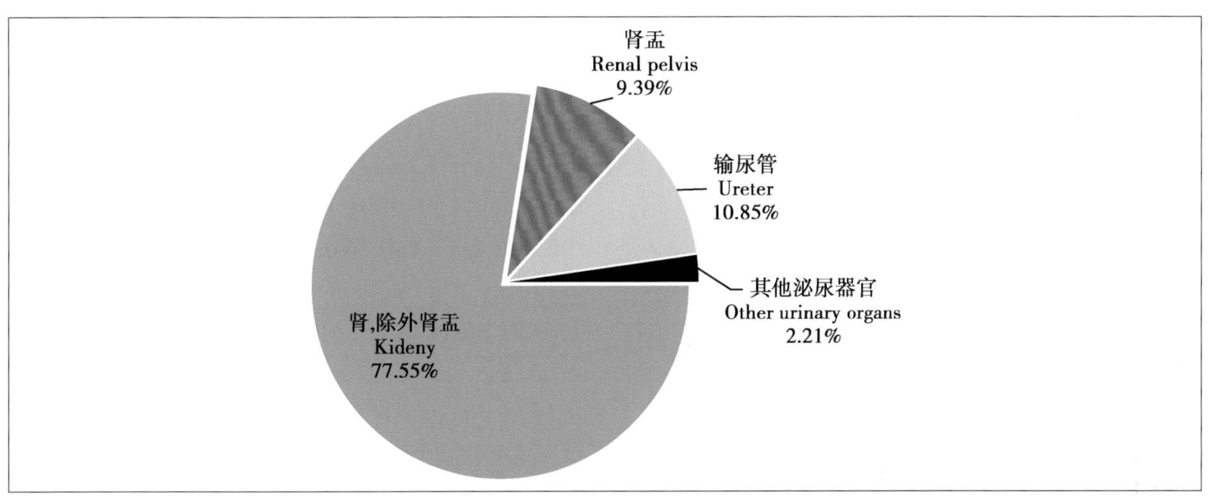

图 5-17c　2017 年中国肿瘤登记地区肾及泌尿系统不明癌亚部位分布情况
Figure 5-17c　Subsite distribution of cancer of kidney & unspecified urinary organs in the registration areas of China,2017

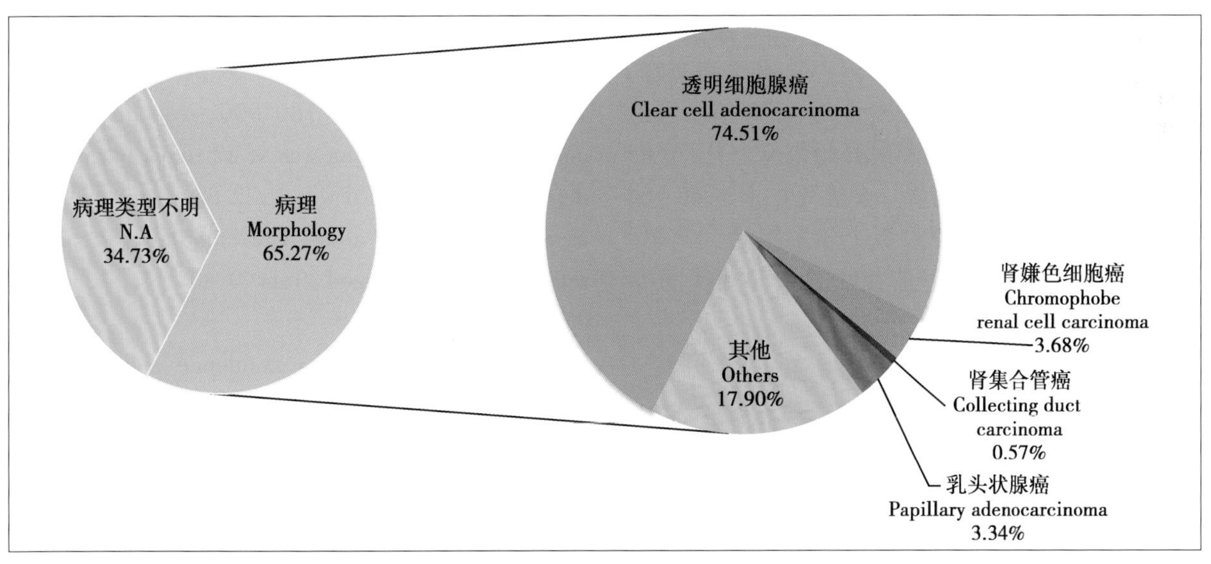

图 5-17d　2017 年中国肿瘤登记地区肾及泌尿系统不明癌病理分型情况
Figure 5-17d　Morphological distribution of cancer of kidney & unspecified urinary organs in the registration areas of China,2017

18 膀胱

2017 年，中国肿瘤登记地区膀胱癌位居癌症发病谱第 16 位。新发病例数为 25 921 例，占全部癌症发病的 2.02%；其中男性 20 485 例，女性 5 436 例，城市地区 15 146 例，农村地区 10 775 例。发病率为 5.94/10 万，中标发病率为 3.43/10 万，世标发病率为 3.40/10 万；男性中标发病率为女性的 4.02 倍，城市中标发病率为农村的 1.33 倍。0~74 岁累积发病率为 0.39%（表 5-18a）。

2017 年，中国肿瘤登记地区膀胱癌位居癌症死亡谱第 15 位。膀胱癌死亡病例 11 072 例，占全部癌症死亡的 1.43%；其中男性 8 695 例，女性 2 377 例，城市地区 6 350 例，农村地区 4 722 例。膀胱癌死亡率为 2.54/10 万，中标死亡率 1.28/10 万，世标死亡率 1.29/10 万；男性中标死亡率为女性的 4.22 倍，城市中标死亡率为农村的 1.22 倍。0~74 岁累积死亡率为 0.11%（表 5-18b）。

膀胱癌的年龄别发病率和死亡率呈明显的性别差异。男性发病率自 40~45 岁组开始快速上升，至 85 岁及以上年龄组达到高峰。女性发病率自 50~54 岁组缓慢上升，至 80~84 岁达到高峰。男性年龄别峰值发病率是女性的 4.73 倍。男性膀胱癌死亡率自 55~59 岁组开始快速上升，至 85 岁及以上年龄组达到高峰。女性死亡率自 60~64 岁组快速上升，至 85 岁及以上年龄组达到高峰。男性年龄别峰值死亡率是女性的 4.71 倍（图 5-18a）。

18 Bladder

Bladder cancer ranked 16th for cancer incidence in the registration areas of China in 2017. There were 25 921 new cases of bladder cancer (20 485 males and 5 436 females, 15 146 in urban areas and 10 775 in rural areas), accounting for 2.02% of all new cancer cases. The crude incidence rate was 5.94 per 100 000, with ASR China 3.43 per 100 000 and ASR World 3.40 per 100 000, respectively. The incidence of ASR China was 4.02 times in males as that in females, and it was 1.33 times in urban areas as that in rural areas. The cumulative incidence rate for subjects aged from 0 to 74 years was 0.39% (Table 5-18a).

Bladder cancer ranked 15th for cancer mortality in the registration areas of China in 2017. A total of 11 072 cases died of bladder cancer (8 695 males and 2 377 females, 6 350 in urban areas and 4 722 in rural areas), accounting for 1.43% of all cancer deaths. The crude mortality rate was 2.54 per 100 000, with ASR China 1.28 per 100 000 and ASR World 1.29 per 100 000, respectively. The mortality of ASR China was 4.22 times in males as that in females, and it was 1.22 times in urban areas as that in rural areas. The cumulative mortality rate for subjects aged from 0 to 74 years was 0.11% (Table 5-18b).

Trends of age-specific incidence and mortality rates showed differences between males and females. The incidence rate in males increased rapidly from the age group of 40-45 years and peaked at the age group of 85+ years. The incidence rate in females increased slowly from the age group of 50-54 years and peaked at the age group of 80-84 years. The peak incidence rate in males was 4.73 times as that in females. The mortality rate in males and females increased rapidly from the age group of 55-59 years and 60-64 years, respectively, and peaked at the age group of 85+ years coincidentally. The peak mortality rate in males was 4.71 times as that in females (Figure 5-18a).

膀胱癌的发病率和死亡率呈现地域差异。东部地区的发病率和死亡率高于中部和西部地区，中部和西部地区发病率和死亡率水平接近。七大行政区中，男性中标发病率和中标死亡率均为东北地区最高，西南地区最低；女性中标发病率和中标死亡率最高的均为东北地区，最低的分别为西南地区和华东地区（表 5-18a，表 5-18b，图 5-18b）。

约 17.90%的膀胱癌新发病例具有明确的亚部位信息，其中膀胱侧壁的比例最高，占 35.84%，其次是膀胱三角区（17.89%）、膀胱后壁（12.29%）、交搭跨越（8.89%）、膀胱前壁（7.11%）、膀胱顶（6.63%）、输尿管口（5.51%）、膀胱颈（4.75%）和脐尿管（1.40%）（图 5-18c）。

全部膀胱癌病例中有明确组织学类型的病例占 65.45%，其中移行细胞癌是最主要的病理类型，占 76.54%；其次是其他类型（7.72%）、鳞状细胞癌（7.54%）和腺癌（6.55%）（图 5-18d）。

The incidence and mortality rates (ASR China) of bladder cancer varied geographically. Eastern areas had the highest incidence and mortality rates, and the incidence and mortality in central areas and western areas were similar. Among seven administrative districts, Northeast China had the highest and Southwest China had the lowest incidence and mortality rate for males. The highest incidence and mortality rates were shown in Northeast China, and the lowest incidence and mortality rates were shown in Southwest China and East China for females (Table 5-18a, Table 5-18b, Figure 5-18b).

About 17.90% of the bladder cancer cases had complete information on subsite. Among them, lateral wall was the most common subsite (35.84%), followed by trigone (17.89%), posterior wall (12.29%), overlapping (8.89%), anterior wall (7.11%), dome (6.63%), ureteric orifice (5.51%), bladder neck (4.75%) and urachus (1.40%) (Figure 5-18c).

About 65.45% of the bladder cancer cases could be morphologically classified. Transitional cell carcinoma was the most common histological type, accounting for 76.54% of all cases, followed by other types (7.72%), squamous cell carcinoma (7.54%) and adenocarcinoma (6.55%) (Figure 5-18d).

表 5-18a 2017 年中国肿瘤登记地区膀胱癌发病情况

Table 5-18a Incidence of bladder cancer in the registration areas of China, 2017

地区 Area	性别 Sex	病例数 No. cases	粗率 Crude rate/ 100 000^{-1}	构成比 Freq./%	中标率 ASR China/ 100 000^{-1}	世标率 ASR World/ 100 000^{-1}	累积率 Cum. rate 0~74/%	顺位 Rank
合计	合计 Both	25 921	5.94	2.02	3.43	3.40	0.39	16
All	男性 Male	20 485	9.26	2.88	5.59	5.56	0.62	7
	女性 Female	5 436	2.53	0.95	1.39	1.37	0.15	17
城市地区	合计 Both	15 146	7.10	2.25	3.91	3.89	0.44	15
Urban areas	男性 Male	11 930	11.15	3.27	6.42	6.40	0.72	7
	女性 Female	3 216	3.03	1.04	1.58	1.56	0.18	17
农村地区	合计 Both	10 775	4.83	1.77	2.93	2.90	0.33	16
Rural areas	男性 Male	8 555	7.50	2.47	4.75	4.71	0.53	7
	女性 Female	2 220	2.04	0.85	1.19	1.17	0.13	19
东部地区	合计 Both	14 555	7.35	2.20	3.86	3.83	0.44	16
Eastern areas	男性 Male	11 484	11.54	3.22	6.36	6.32	0.71	7
	女性 Female	3 071	3.12	1.01	1.55	1.54	0.17	17
中部地区	合计 Both	5 439	4.73	1.81	3.08	3.06	0.35	16
Central areas	男性 Male	4 309	7.33	2.58	5.01	4.99	0.57	7
	女性 Female	1 130	2.01	0.84	1.24	1.22	0.14	18
西部地区	合计 Both	5 927	4.81	1.86	2.96	2.92	0.33	16
Western areas	男性 Male	4 692	7.47	2.49	4.73	4.71	0.52	7
	女性 Female	1 235	2.04	0.94	1.23	1.20	0.13	19

表 5-18b 2017 年中国肿瘤登记地区膀胱癌死亡情况

Table 5-18b Mortality of bladder cancer in the registration areas of China, 2017

地区 Area	性别 Sex	死亡数 No. deaths	粗率 Crude rate/ 100 000^{-1}	构成比 Freq./%	中标率 ASR China/ 100 000^{-1}	世标率 ASR World/ 100 000^{-1}	累积率 Cum. rate 0~74/%	顺位 Rank
合计	合计 Both	11 072	2.54	1.43	1.28	1.29	0.11	15
All	男性 Male	8 695	3.93	1.76	2.15	2.19	0.18	11
	女性 Female	2 377	1.10	0.85	0.51	0.51	0.04	16
城市地区	合计 Both	6 350	2.98	1.64	1.40	1.41	0.12	15
Urban areas	男性 Male	4 958	4.63	2.02	2.36	2.40	0.20	9
	女性 Female	1 392	1.31	0.99	0.56	0.56	0.04	16
农村地区	合计 Both	4 722	2.12	1.22	1.15	1.15	0.10	16
Rural areas	男性 Male	3 737	3.27	1.50	1.93	1.95	0.17	11
	女性 Female	985	0.90	0.72	0.46	0.46	0.04	19
东部地区	合计 Both	6 138	3.10	1.61	1.36	1.36	0.11	15
Eastern areas	男性 Male	4 836	4.86	2.01	2.33	2.37	0.19	9
	女性 Female	1 302	1.32	0.92	0.52	0.52	0.04	16
中部地区	合计 Both	2 359	2.05	1.26	1.21	1.21	0.11	16
Central areas	男性 Male	1 829	3.11	1.53	1.99	2.00	0.18	11
	女性 Female	530	0.94	0.78	0.51	0.50	0.04	16
西部地区	合计 Both	2 575	2.09	1.27	1.18	1.20	0.11	17
Western areas	男性 Male	2 030	3.23	1.52	1.93	1.96	0.17	11
	女性 Female	545	0.90	0.79	0.48	0.49	0.04	19

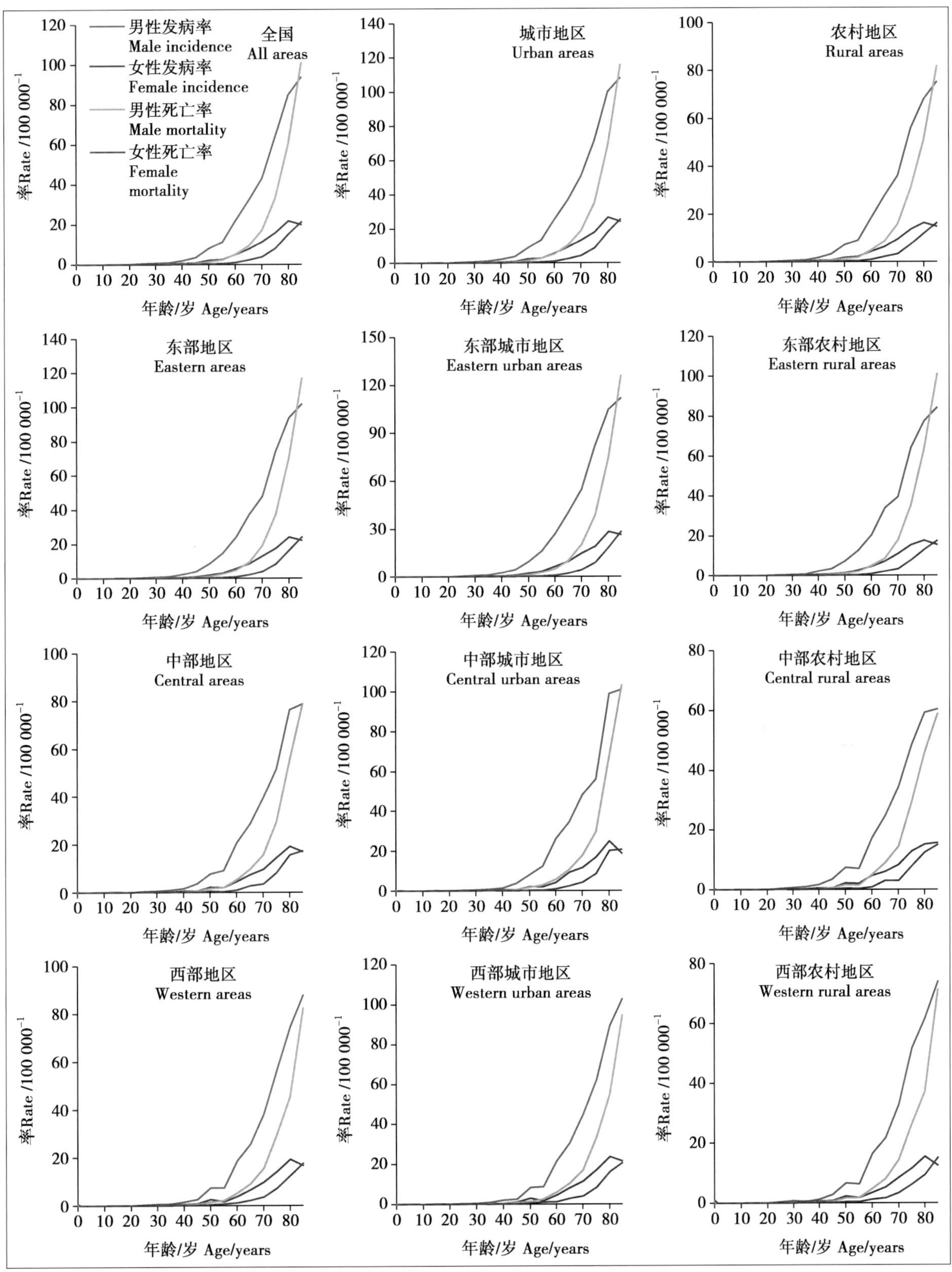

图 5-18a　2017 年中国肿瘤登记地区膀胱癌年龄别发病率和死亡率

Figure 5-18a　Age-specific incidence and mortality rates of bladder cancer in the registration areas of China, 2017

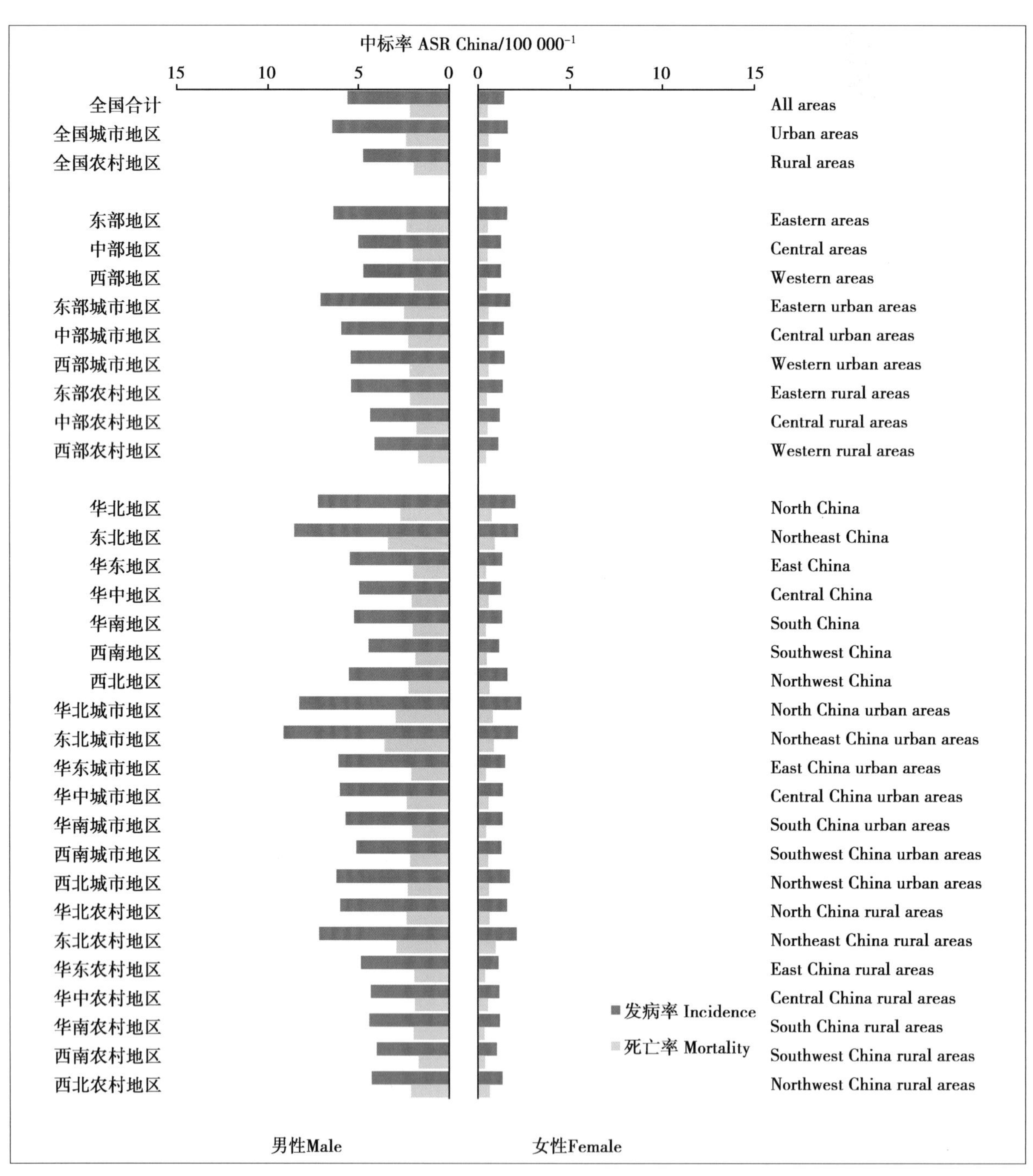

图 5-18b　2017 年中国肿瘤登记不同地区膀胱癌发病率和死亡率

Figure 5-18b　Incidence and mortality rates of bladder cancer in different registration areas of China,2017

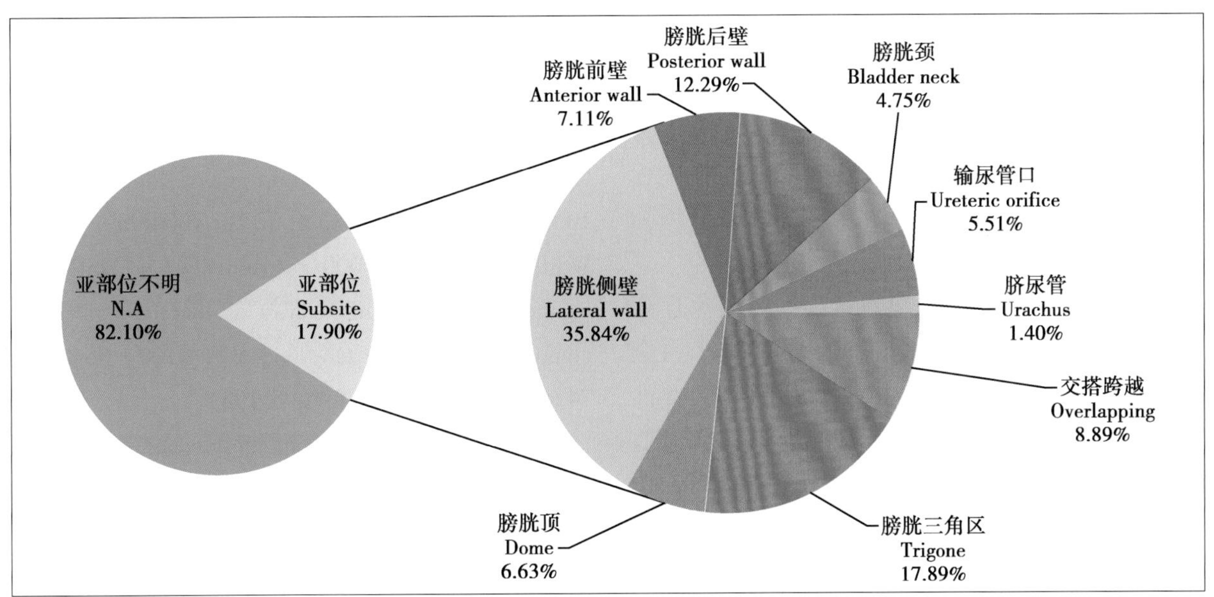

图 5-18c 2017 年中国肿瘤登记地区膀胱癌亚部位分布情况

Figure 5-18c Subsite distribution of bladder cancer in the registration areas of China,2017

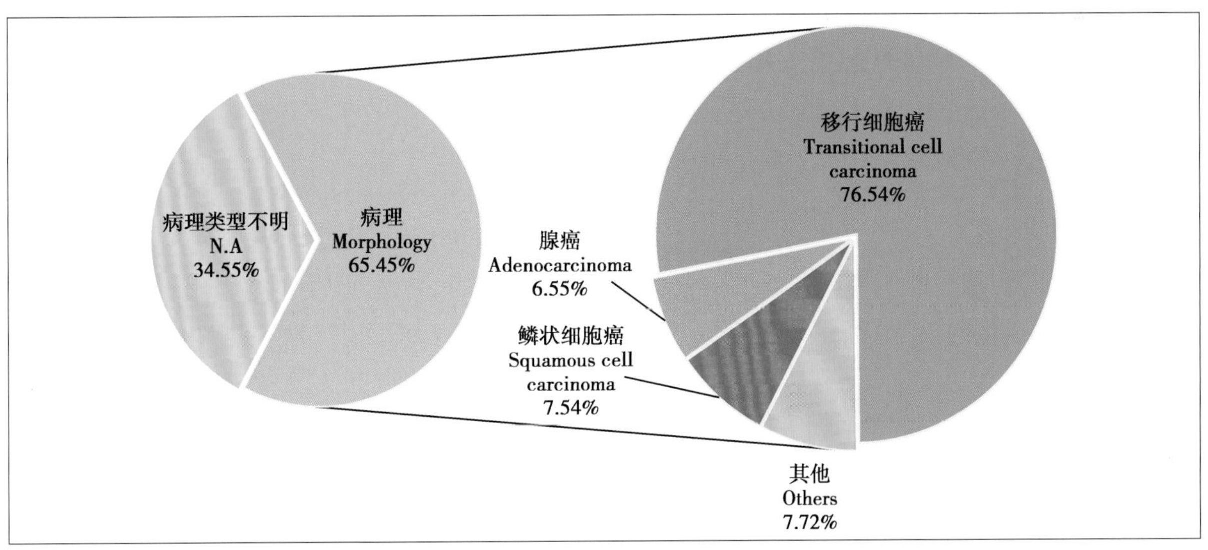

图 5-18d 2017 年中国肿瘤登记地区膀胱癌病理分型情况

Figure 5-18d Morphological distribution of bladder cancer in the registration areas of China,2017

19 脑

2017 年,中国肿瘤登记地区脑瘤位居癌症发病谱的第 11 位。新发病例数为 33 969 例,占全部癌症发病的 2.65%;其中男性 15 790 例,女性 18 179 例,城市地区 17 426 例,农村地区 16 543 例。脑瘤发病率为 7.79/10 万,中标发病率为 5.62/10 万,世标发病率为 5.51/10 万;女性中标发病率为男性的 1.09 倍。0~74 岁累积发病率为 0.57%(表 5-19a)。

2017 年,中国肿瘤登记地区脑瘤位居癌症死亡谱的第 10 位。脑瘤死亡病例为 17 255 例,占全部癌症死亡的 2.23%;其中男性 9 656 例,女性 7 599 例,城市地区 8 292 例,农村地区 8 963 例。脑瘤死亡率为 3.95/10 万,中标死亡率 2.72/10 万,世标死亡率 2.70/10 万;男性中标死亡率为女性的 1.34 倍。0~74 岁累积死亡率为 0.28%(表 5-19b)。

脑瘤年龄别发病率 20 岁前处于较低水平,之后均随年龄增长而升高,男性在 85 岁及以上年龄组达高峰,女性在 80~84 岁组达高峰。脑瘤年龄别死亡率 40 岁前处于较低水平,之后均随年龄增长而升高,并在 80~84 岁组达到高峰(图 5-19a)。

19 Brain

Brain tumor ranked 11th for cancer incidence in the registration areas of China in 2017. There were 33 969 new cases of brain tumor(15 790 males and 18 179 females, 17 426 in urban areas and 16 543 in rural areas), accounting for 2.65% of all cancer cases. The crude incidence rate of brain tumor was 7.79 per 100 000, with ASR China 5.62 per 100 000 and ASR World 5.51 per 100 000, respectively. The ASR China was 1.09 times in females as that in males. The cumulative incidence rate for subjects aged from 0 to 74 years was 0.57%(Table 5-19a).

Brain tumor was the 10th most common cause of cancer deaths in the registration areas of China in 2017. The number of deaths due to brain tumor was 17 255(9 656 males and 7 599 females, 8 292 in urban areas and 8 963 in rural areas), accounting for 2.23% of all cancer deaths. The crude mortality rate of brain tumor was 3.95 per 100 000, with ASR China 2.72 per 100 000 and ASR World 2.70 per 100 000, respectively. The ASR China was 1.34 times in males as that in females. The cumulative mortality rate for subjects aged from 0 to 74 years was 0.28%(Table 5-19b).

The age-specific incidence rate of brain tumor was relatively low before 20 years old and increased with age after that. It reached peak at the age group of 85+ years in males and at the age group of 80-84 years in females. The age-specific mortality rate of brain tumor was relatively low before 40 years old and increased with age after that. It reached peak at the age group of 80-84 years(Figure 5-19a).

脑瘤的发病率城市地区高于农村地区，而死亡率城市地区低于农村地区。中标发病率以东部地区最高，中部和西部地区发病率水平接近。中标死亡率以西部地区最高，其次为中部地区，东部地区最低。在七大行政区中，华南地区男性和女性的中标发病率最高，东北地区男性和西南地区女性中标发病率最低；西北地区男性和女性的中标死亡率最高，华北地区男性和华南地区女性的中标死亡率最低（表 5-19a，表 5-19b，图 5-19b）。

约 36.28%的脑瘤新发病例具有明确的亚部位信息，其中大脑占 23.65%，额叶占 21.37%，颞叶占 13.47%，小脑占 10.96%，交搭跨越占 8.30%，脑室占 6.86%，脑干占 6.05%，顶叶占 5.52%，枕叶占 2.90%（图 5-19c）。

The incidence rate of brain tumor in urban areas was higher than that in rural areas, while the mortality rate in urban areas was lower than that in rural areas. The incidence rate (ASR China) was highest in eastern areas, and the incidence rates in central areas and western areas were similar. Western areas had the highest mortality rate (ASR China), followed by central and eastern areas. Among the seven administrative districts, the highest incidence rates (ASR China) were shown in South China for both sexes, while Northeast China and Southwest China had the lowest incidence rates (ASR China) for males and females, respectively. The highest mortality rates (ASR China) were found in Northwest China for both sexes, while North China and South China had the lowest mortality rates (ASR China) for males and females, respectively (Table 5-19a, Table 5-19b, Figure 5-19b).

About 36.28% of brain tumor cases had specified subcategorical information. Among those, 23.65% of cases occurred in cerebrum, followed by frontal lobe of brain (21.37%), temporal lobe (13.47%), cerebellum (10.96%), overlapping (8.30%), cerebral ventricle (6.86%), brain stem (6.05%), parietal lobe (5.52%) and occipital lobe (2.90%) (Figure 5-19c).

表 5-19a 2017 年中国肿瘤登记地区脑瘤发病情况
Table 5-19a Incidence of brain tumor in the registration areas of China, 2017

地区 Area	性别 Sex	病例数 No. cases	粗率 Crude rate/ 100 000⁻¹	构成比 Freq./%	中标率 ASR China/ 100 000⁻¹	世标率 ASR World/ 100 000⁻¹	累积率 Cum. rate 0~74/%	顺位 Rank
合计	合计 Both	33 969	7.79	2.65	5.62	5.51	0.57	11
All	男性 Male	15 790	7.14	2.22	5.37	5.26	0.54	10
	女性 Female	18 179	8.45	3.19	5.87	5.75	0.61	10
城市地区	合计 Both	17 426	8.17	2.59	5.72	5.63	0.58	12
Urban areas	男性 Male	7 819	7.31	2.14	5.32	5.25	0.54	13
	女性 Female	9 607	9.04	3.11	6.11	5.99	0.63	9
农村地区	合计 Both	16 543	7.42	2.72	5.52	5.39	0.56	11
Rural areas	男性 Male	7 971	6.98	2.30	5.41	5.27	0.54	8
	女性 Female	8 572	7.87	3.29	5.63	5.51	0.59	10
东部地区	合计 Both	17 693	8.94	2.68	6.13	6.01	0.62	11
Eastern areas	男性 Male	7 835	7.87	2.20	5.65	5.54	0.56	13
	女性 Female	9 858	10.02	3.24	6.59	6.46	0.68	10
中部地区	合计 Both	7 770	6.75	2.58	5.20	5.11	0.54	12
Central areas	男性 Male	3 812	6.48	2.28	5.15	5.08	0.53	8
	女性 Female	3 958	7.04	2.95	5.24	5.13	0.55	11
西部地区	合计 Both	8 506	6.90	2.66	5.20	5.07	0.53	11
Western areas	男性 Male	4 143	6.60	2.20	5.15	5.01	0.51	9
	女性 Female	4 363	7.21	3.33	5.25	5.13	0.55	10

表 5-19b 2017 年中国肿瘤登记地区脑瘤死亡情况
Table 5-19b Mortality of brain tumor in the registration areas of China, 2017

地区 Area	性别 Sex	死亡数 No. deaths	粗率 Crude rate/ 100 000⁻¹	构成比 Freq./%	中标率 ASR China/ 100 000⁻¹	世标率 ASR World/ 100 000⁻¹	累积率 Cum. rate 0~74/%	顺位 Rank
合计	合计 Both	17 255	3.95	2.23	2.72	2.70	0.28	10
All	男性 Male	9 656	4.37	1.95	3.11	3.09	0.32	9
	女性 Female	7 599	3.53	2.73	2.32	2.31	0.24	10
城市地区	合计 Both	8 292	3.89	2.15	2.58	2.57	0.26	12
Urban areas	男性 Male	4 587	4.29	1.87	2.94	2.93	0.31	11
	女性 Female	3 705	3.49	2.62	2.23	2.22	0.22	11
农村地区	合计 Both	8 963	4.02	2.32	2.85	2.83	0.30	9
Rural areas	男性 Male	5 069	4.44	2.03	3.27	3.24	0.34	7
	女性 Female	3 894	3.57	2.83	2.42	2.40	0.25	9
东部地区	合计 Both	8 086	4.09	2.12	2.60	2.58	0.27	13
Eastern areas	男性 Male	4 402	4.42	1.83	2.94	2.92	0.31	11
	女性 Female	3 684	3.74	2.61	2.26	2.23	0.23	11
中部地区	合计 Both	4 288	3.73	2.28	2.77	2.76	0.29	9
Central areas	男性 Male	2 411	4.10	2.01	3.14	3.13	0.33	7
	女性 Female	1 877	3.34	2.76	2.40	2.39	0.25	9
西部地区	合计 Both	4 881	3.96	2.40	2.88	2.86	0.29	10
Western areas	男性 Male	2 843	4.53	2.13	3.38	3.35	0.34	7
	女性 Female	2 038	3.37	2.94	2.37	2.37	0.24	9

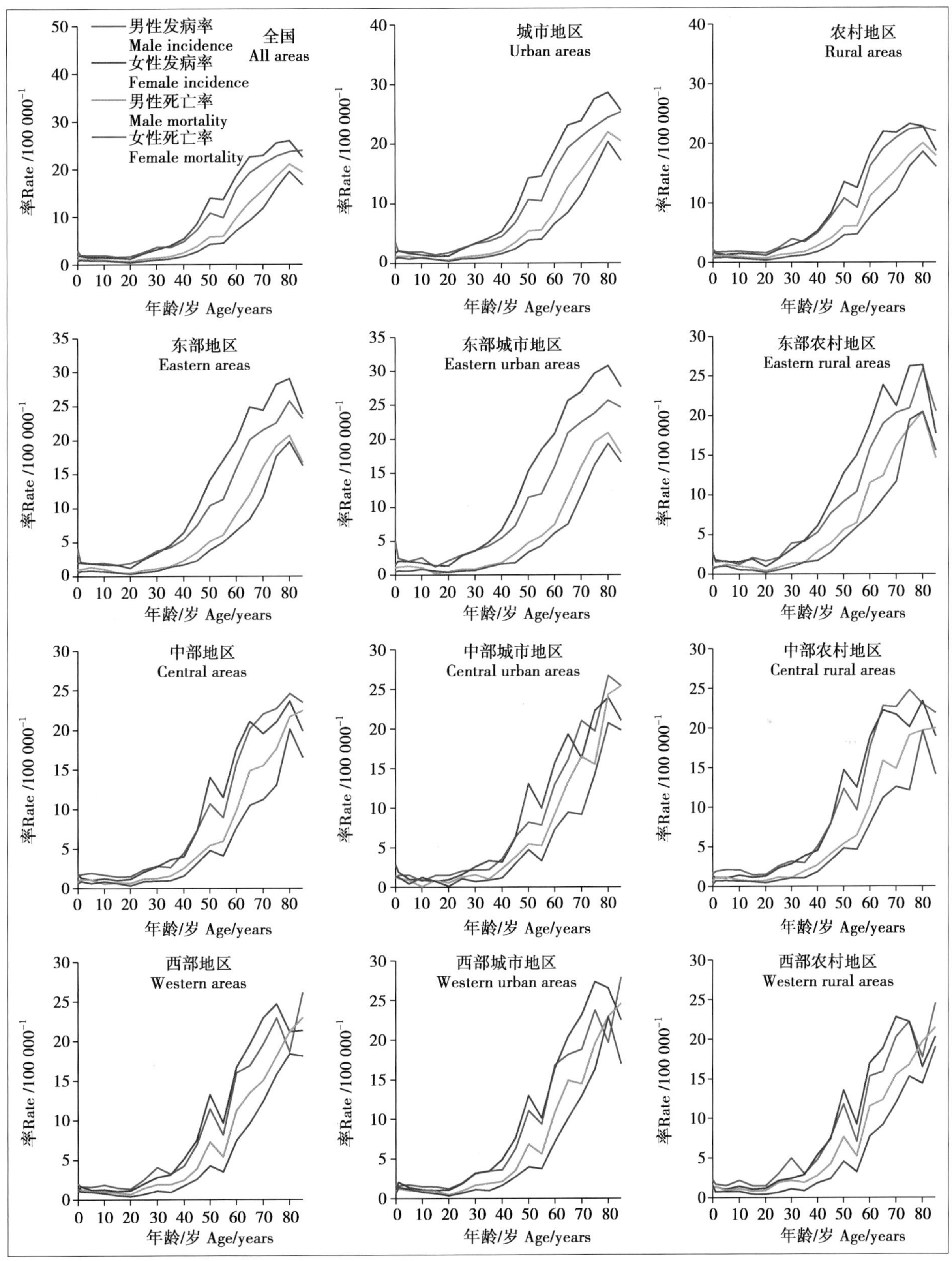

图 5-19a　2017 年中国肿瘤登记地区脑瘤年龄别发病率和死亡率

Figure 5-19a　Age-specific incidence and mortality rates of brain tumor in the registration areas of China,2017

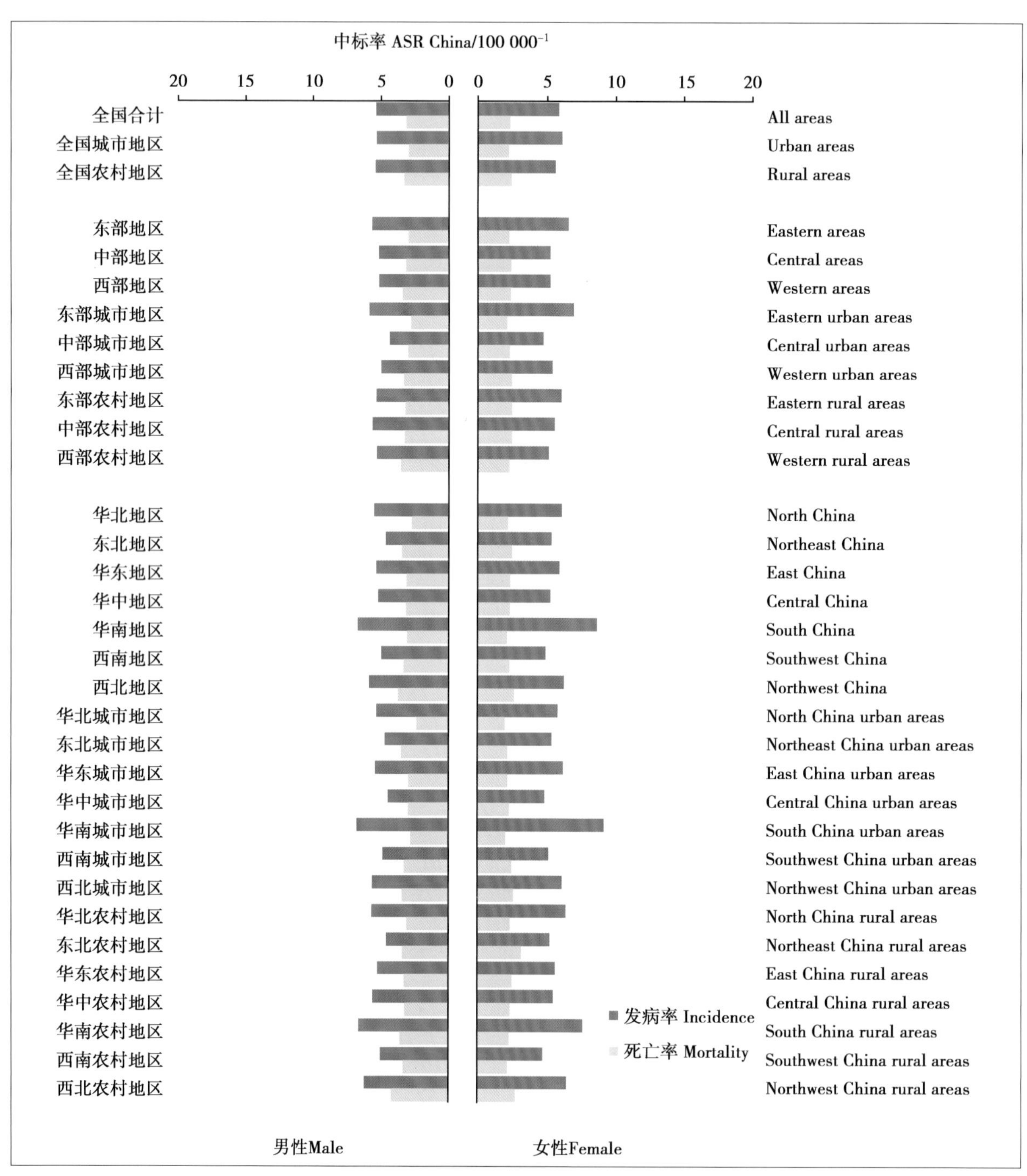

图 5-19b　2017 年中国肿瘤登记不同地区脑瘤发病率和死亡率

Figure 5-19b　Incidence and mortality rates of brain tumor in different registration areas of China, 2017

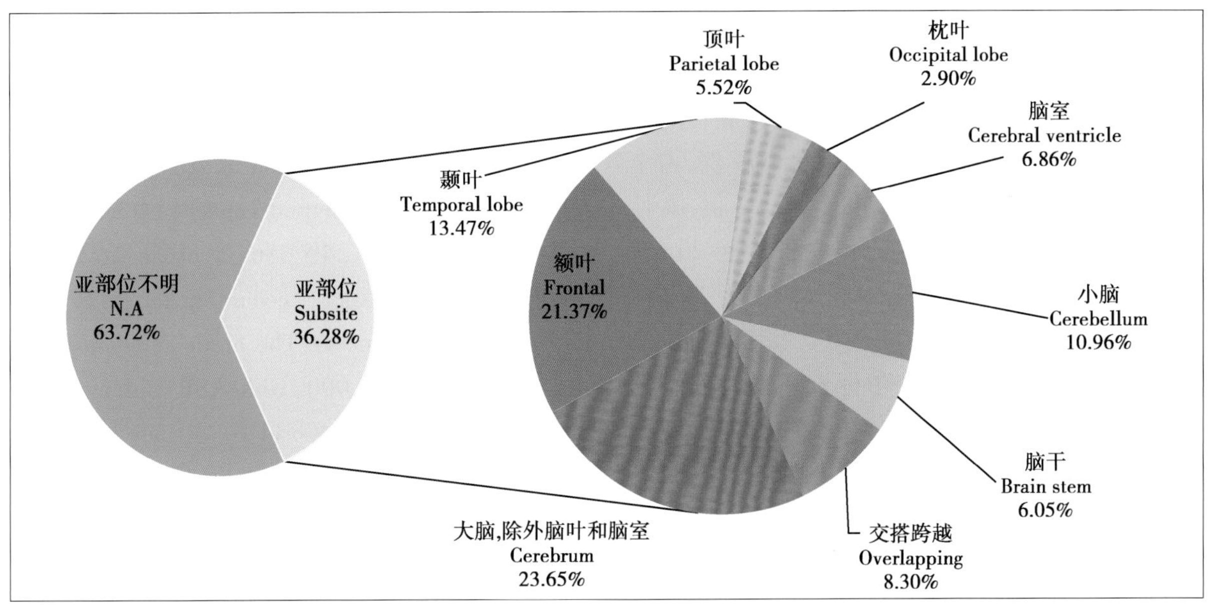

图 5-19c　2017 年中国肿瘤登记地区脑瘤亚部位分布情况
Figure 5-19c　Subsite distribution of brain tumor in the registration areas of China, 2017

20 甲状腺

2017年,中国肿瘤登记地区甲状腺癌位居癌症发病谱第8位。新发病例数为60 693例,占全部癌症发病的4.74%;其中男性14 572例,女性46 121例,城市地区40 656例,农村地区20 037例。发病率为13.91/10万,中标发病率为11.94/10万,世标发病率为10.30/10万。女性中标发病率为男性的3.08倍,城市中标发病率为农村的2.10倍。0~74岁累积发病率为0.98%(表5-20a)。

2017年,中国肿瘤登记地区甲状腺癌位居癌症死亡谱第22位。因甲状腺癌死亡病例2 551例,占全部癌症死亡的0.33%;其中男性979例,女性1 572例,城市地区1 471例,农村地区1 080例。甲状腺癌死亡率为0.58/10万,中标死亡率为0.36/10万,世标死亡率为0.35/10万;女性中标死亡率为男性的1.54倍,城市中标死亡率为农村的1.26倍。0~74岁累积死亡率为0.04%(表5-20b)。

甲状腺癌年龄别发病率呈明显的性别差异。女性自15~19岁组开始快速上升,至50~54岁组达高峰;而男性从20~24岁组开始呈缓慢上升趋势。女性各年龄别发病率均明显高于男性。甲状腺癌年龄别死亡率从40~44岁组开始缓慢上升,至85岁及以上组到达高峰(图5-20a)。

20 Thyroid

Thyroid cancer was the 8th most common cancer in the registration areas of China in 2017. There were 60 693 new cases of thyroid cancer (14 572 males and 46 121 females, 40 656 in urban areas and 20 037 in rural areas), accounting for 4.74% of new cases of all cancers. The crude incidence rate was 13.91 per 100 000, with ASR China 11.94 per 100 000 and ASR World 10.30 per 100 000, respectively. The incidence of ASR China was 3.08 times in females as that in males, and it was 2.10 times in urban areas as that in rural areas. The cumulative incidence rate for subjects aged from 0 to 74 years was 0.98% (Table 5-20a).

Thyroid cancer ranked 22nd for cancer mortality in the registration areas of China in 2017. A total of 2 551 cases died of thyroid cancer (979 males and 1 572 females, 1 471 in urban areas and 1 080 in rural areas), accounting for 0.33% of all cancer deaths. The crude mortality rate was 0.58 per 100 000, with ASR China 0.36 per 100 000 and ASR World 0.35 per 100 000, respectively. The mortality of ASR China was 1.54 times in females as that in males, and it was 1.26 times in urban areas as that in rural areas. The cumulative mortality rate for subjects aged from 0 to 74 years was 0.04% (Table 5-20b).

The age-specific incidence rate of thyroid cancer showed differences between males and females. The incidence rate in females increased rapidly from the age group of 15-19 years and peaked at the age group of 50-54 years, while the incidence rate in males increased from the age group of 20-24 years with a slower speed. The age-specific incidence rates in females were generally higher than those in males. The age-specific mortality rate of thyroid cancer increased slowly from the age group of 40-44 years, and peaked at the age group of 85+ years (Figure 5-20a).

城市地区的甲状腺癌发病率和死亡率均高于农村地区。中标发病率以东部地区最高，其次是中部地区，西部地区最低；中标死亡率以中部地区最高，其次是东部地区，西部地区最低。七大行政区中，华北地区男性和东北地区女性中标发病率最高，西南地区男性和女性的中标发病率最低；东北地区男性和华中地区女性中标死亡率最高，西南地区男性和女性的中标发病率最低（表 5-20a，表 5-20b，图 5-20b）。

全部甲状腺癌病例中有明确组织学类型的病例占 86.02%，其中乳头状腺癌是最主要的病理类型，占 92.41%；其次是其他类型、滤泡性腺癌和髓样癌，分别占 6.11%、1.17% 和 0.31%（图 5-20c）。

The incidence and mortality rates of thyroid cancer were higher in urban areas than those in rural areas. Eastern areas had the highest incidence rate (ASR China), followed by central and western areas. Central areas had the highest mortality rate (ASR China), followed by eastern and western areas. Among the seven administrative districts, the highest incidence rates (ASR China) were shown in North China and Northeast China for males and females, respectively, while the lowest incidence rates were shown in Southwest China for both sexes. The highest mortality rates (ASR China) were shown in Northeast China and in Central China for males and females, respectively, while the lowest mortality rates (ASR China) were shown in Southwest China for both sexes (Table 5-20a, Table 5-20b, Figure 5-20b).

About 86.02% cases of thyroid cancer had morphological verification. Among those, papillary thyroid cancer was the most common histological type, accounting for 92.41% of all cases, followed by other types (6.11%), follicular adenoma (1.17%) and medullary thyroid cancer (0.31%) (Figure 5-20c).

表 5-20a 2017 年中国肿瘤登记地区甲状腺癌发病情况

Table 5-20a Incidence of thyroid cancer in the registration areas of China, 2017

地区 Area	性别 Sex	病例数 No. cases	粗率 Crude rate/ 100 000^{-1}	构成比 Freq. /%	中标率 ASR China/ 100 000^{-1}	世标率 ASR World/ 100 000^{-1}	累积率 Cum. rate 0~74/%	顺位 Rank
合计	合计 Both	60 693	13.91	4.74	11.94	10.30	0.98	8
All	男性 Male	14 572	6.59	2.05	5.88	4.97	0.47	12
	女性 Female	46 121	21.43	8.10	18.10	15.71	1.49	4
城市地区	合计 Both	40 656	19.07	6.03	16.18	13.88	1.31	6
Urban areas	男性 Male	10 047	9.39	2.75	8.30	6.96	0.65	8
	女性 Female	30 609	28.81	9.91	24.02	20.78	1.97	3
农村地区	合计 Both	20 037	8.98	3.30	7.70	6.73	0.64	9
Rural areas	男性 Male	4 525	3.97	1.31	3.49	3.02	0.29	15
	女性 Female	15 512	14.24	5.95	12.04	10.56	1.01	7
东部地区	合计 Both	40 993	20.71	6.20	17.64	15.14	1.42	6
Eastern areas	男性 Male	9 967	10.02	2.80	8.95	7.52	0.70	9
	女性 Female	31 026	31.53	10.19	26.32	22.76	2.15	3
中部地区	合计 Both	11 727	10.19	3.89	8.78	7.70	0.74	8
Central areas	男性 Male	2 715	4.62	1.62	4.08	3.53	0.34	14
	女性 Female	9 012	16.02	6.71	13.60	11.98	1.15	7
西部地区	合计 Both	7 973	6.46	2.50	5.61	4.85	0.45	12
Western areas	男性 Male	1 890	3.01	1.00	2.64	2.27	0.21	15
	女性 Female	6 083	10.05	4.64	8.67	7.51	0.70	7

表 5-20b 2017 年中国肿瘤登记地区甲状腺癌死亡情况

Table 5-20b Mortality of thyroid cancer in the registration areas of China, 2017

地区 Area	性别 Sex	死亡数 No. deaths	粗率 Crude rate/ 100 000^{-1}	构成比 Freq. /%	中标率 ASR China/ 100 000^{-1}	世标率 ASR World/ 100 000^{-1}	累积率 Cum. rate 0~74/%	顺位 Rank
合计	合计 Both	2 551	0.58	0.33	0.36	0.35	0.04	22
All	男性 Male	979	0.44	0.20	0.28	0.27	0.03	19
	女性 Female	1 572	0.73	0.56	0.43	0.42	0.05	20
城市地区	合计 Both	1 471	0.69	0.38	0.39	0.38	0.04	22
Urban areas	男性 Male	590	0.55	0.24	0.32	0.32	0.03	19
	女性 Female	881	0.83	0.62	0.46	0.45	0.05	20
农村地区	合计 Both	1 080	0.48	0.28	0.31	0.31	0.03	22
Rural areas	男性 Male	389	0.34	0.16	0.23	0.22	0.02	20
	女性 Female	691	0.63	0.50	0.40	0.39	0.04	20
东部地区	合计 Both	1 311	0.66	0.34	0.36	0.35	0.04	22
Eastern areas	男性 Male	512	0.51	0.21	0.29	0.28	0.03	19
	女性 Female	799	0.81	0.57	0.42	0.41	0.05	20
中部地区	合计 Both	684	0.59	0.36	0.41	0.40	0.04	22
Central areas	男性 Male	250	0.43	0.21	0.30	0.30	0.03	20
	女性 Female	434	0.77	0.64	0.52	0.49	0.05	20
西部地区	合计 Both	556	0.45	0.27	0.30	0.29	0.03	23
Western areas	男性 Male	217	0.35	0.16	0.23	0.22	0.02	19
	女性 Female	339	0.56	0.49	0.37	0.36	0.04	20

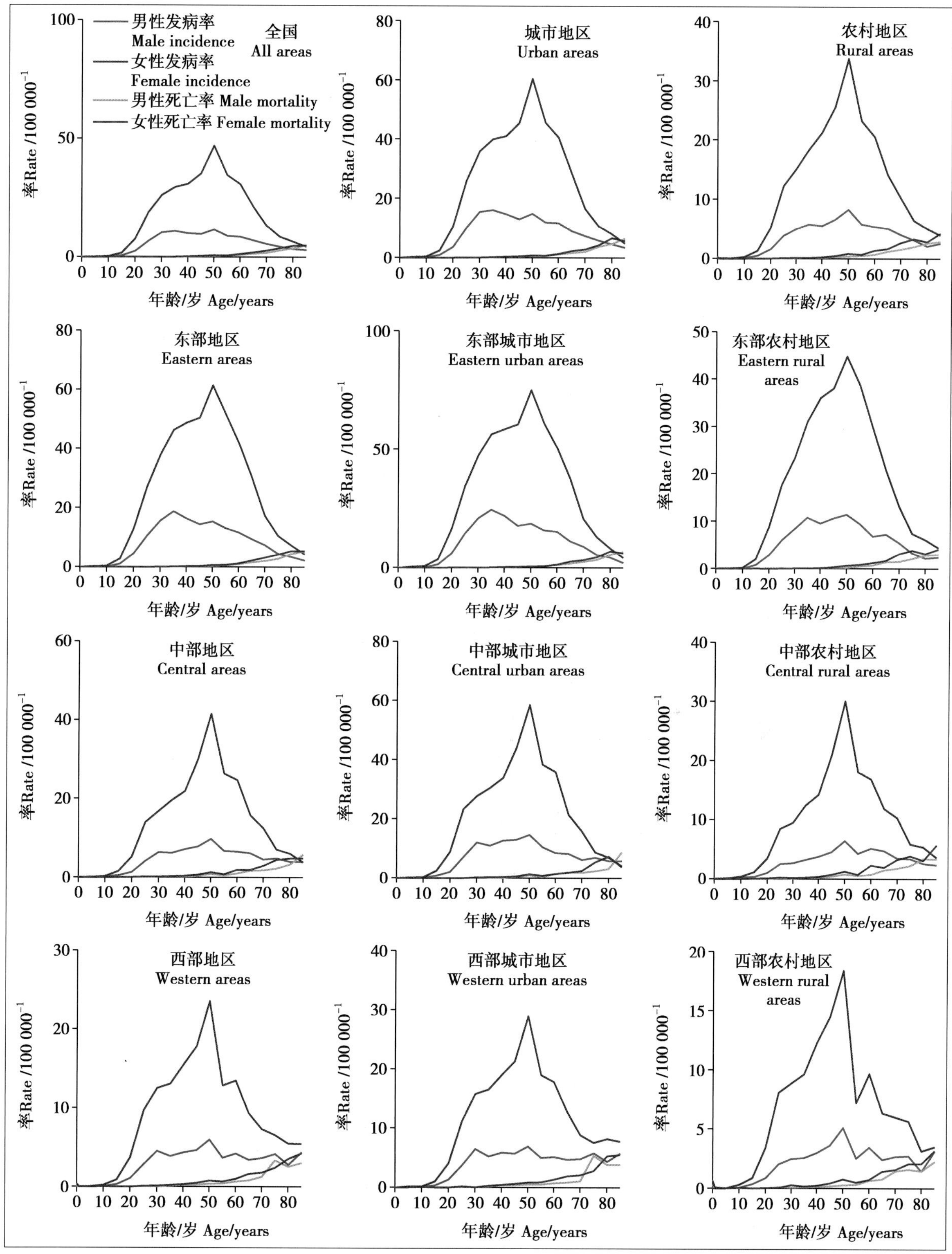

图 5-20a　2017 年中国肿瘤登记地区甲状腺癌年龄别发病率和死亡率

Figure 5-20a　Age-specific incidence and mortality rates of thyroid cancer in the registration areas of China,2017

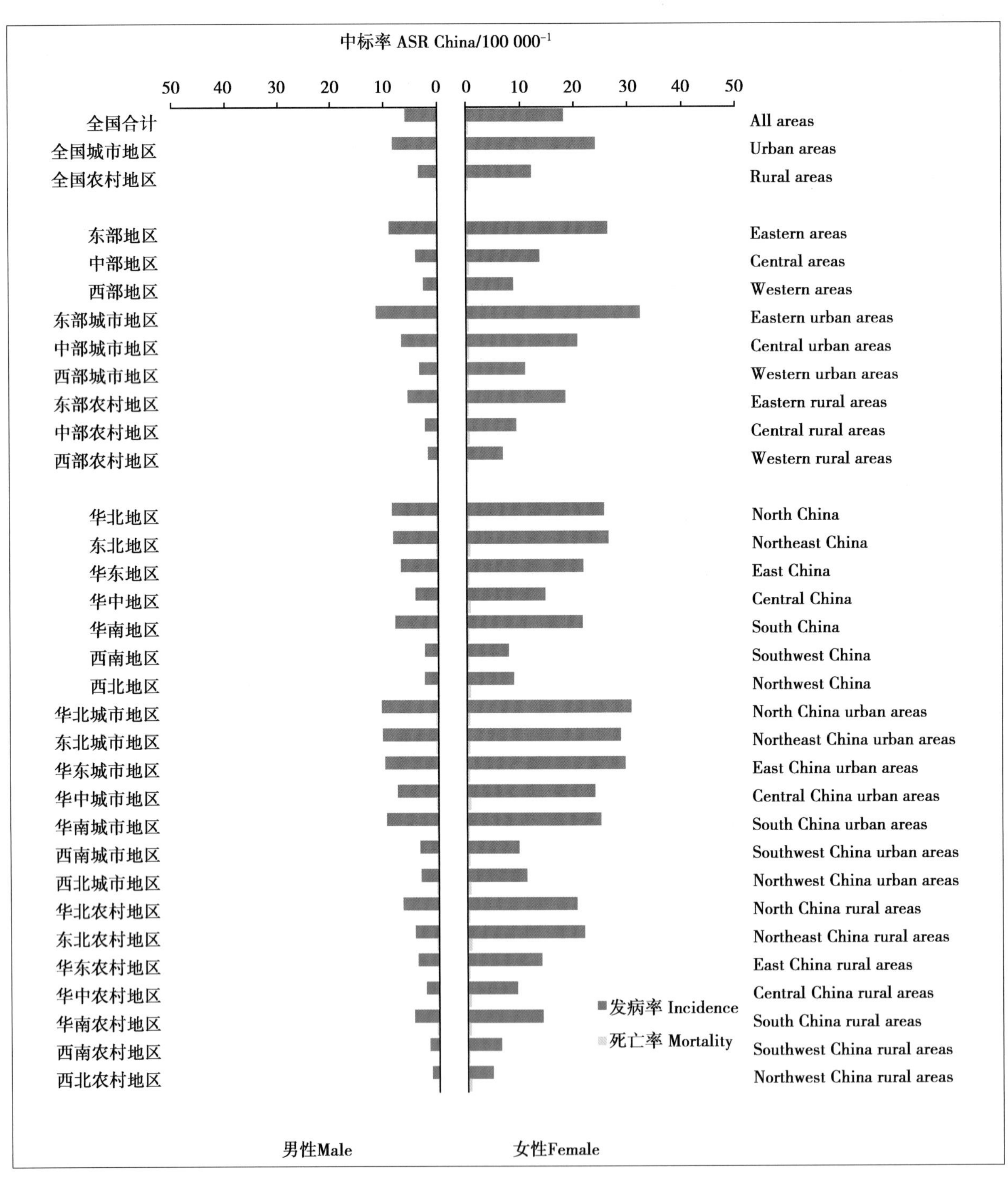

图 5-20b 2017 年中国肿瘤登记不同地区甲状腺癌发病率和死亡率

Figure 5-20b Incidence and mortality rates of thyroid cancer in different registration areas of China,2017

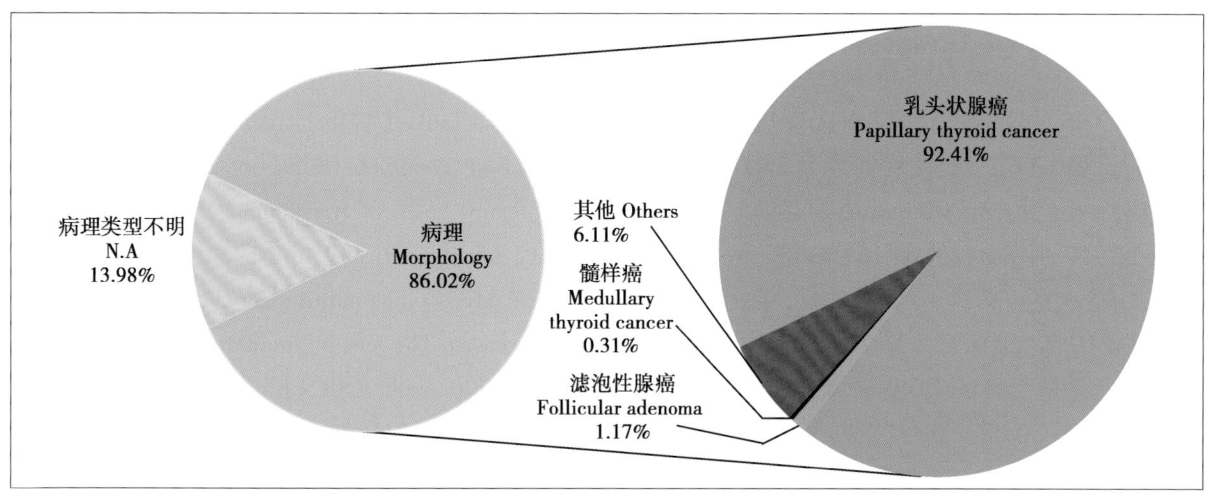

图 5-20c　2017 年中国肿瘤登记地区甲状腺癌病理分型情况
Figure 5-20c　Morphological distribution of thyroid cancer in the registration areas of China, 2017

21 淋巴瘤

2017 年,中国肿瘤登记地区淋巴瘤位居癌症发病谱第 14 位。新发病例数为 28 180 例,占全部癌症发病的 2.20%;其中男性 16 268 例,女性 11 912 例;城市地区 16 099 例,农村地区 12 081 例。发病率为 6.46/10 万,中标发病率为 4.34/10 万,世标发病率为 4.26/10 万;男性中标发病率是女性的 1.40 倍,城市中标发病率是农村的 1.30 倍。0~74 岁累积发病率为 0.48%(表 5-21a)。

2017 年,中国肿瘤登记地区淋巴瘤位居癌症死亡谱第 12 位。因淋巴瘤死亡病例 15 951 例,占全部癌症死亡的 2.06%;其中男性 9 690 例,女性 6 261 例,城市地区 8 892 例,农村地区 7 059 例。淋巴瘤死亡率为 3.66/10 万,中标死亡率 2.24/10 万,世标死亡率 2.21/10 万;男性中标死亡率为女性的 1.65 倍,城市中标死亡率为农村的 1.19 倍。0~74 岁累积死亡率为 0.25%(表 5-21b)。

淋巴瘤年龄别发病率在 35 岁以前处于较低水平,自 35~39 岁组开始快速上升,于 80~84 岁组达到高峰。淋巴瘤年龄别死亡率从 40~44 岁组开始快速上升,男性死亡率至 85 岁及以上年龄组达到高峰,女性死亡率至 80~84 岁组达到高峰。总体上,男性年龄别发病率和死亡率均高于女性(图 5-21a)。

21 Lymphoma

Lymphoma ranked 14th for cancer incidence in the registration areas of China in 2017. There were 28 180 new cases of lymphoma (16 268 males and 11 912 females, 16 099 in urban areas and 12 081 in rural areas), accounting for 2.20% of all new cancer cases. The crude incidence rate was 6.46 per 100 000, with ASR China 4.34 per 100 000 and ASR World 4.26 per 100 000, respectively. The incidence of the ASR China was 1.40 times in males as that in females, and it was 1.30 times in urban areas as that in rural areas. The cumulative incidence rate for subjects aged from 0 to 74 years was 0.48% (Table 5-21a).

Lymphoma ranked 12th for cancer mortality in the registration areas of China in 2017. A total of 15 951 cases died of lymphoma (9 690 males and 6 261 females, 8 892 in urban areas and 7 059 in rural areas), accounting for 2.06% of all cancer deaths. The crude mortality rate was 3.66 per 100 000, with ASR China 2.24 per 100 000 and ASR World 2.21 per 100 000, respectively. The mortality rate of the ASR China was 1.65 times in males as that in females, and it was 1.19 times in the urban areas as that in rural areas. The cumulative mortality rate for subjects aged from 0 to 74 years was 0.25% (Table 5-21b).

The age-specific incidence rate of lymphoma was relatively low before 35 years old and increased rapidly from the age group of 35-39 years and then peaked at the age group of 80-84 years. The age-specific mortality rate of lymphoma increased rapidly from the age group of 40-44 years, and peaked at the age group of 85 years and above and 80-84 years for males and females, respectively. The age-specific incidence and mortality rates of lymphoma were generally higher in males than those in females (Figure 5-21a).

城市地区淋巴瘤的发病率和死亡率均高于农村地区。中标发病率和死亡率均为东部地区最高，其次是中部地区，西部地区最低。七大行政区中，华南地区的中标发病率和中标死亡率最高，西北地区的中标发病率和中标死亡率最低（表5-21a，表5-21b，图5-21b）。

全部淋巴瘤病例中，非霍奇金淋巴瘤的其他和未特指类型（ICD-10：C85）是最主要的病理类型，占43.49%；其次是多发性骨髓瘤和恶性浆细胞性肿瘤（C90），占23.81%；弥漫性非霍奇金淋巴瘤（C83），占17.62%；霍奇金淋巴瘤（C81），占4.86%；周围和皮的T细胞淋巴瘤（C84），占4.15%；滤泡性非霍奇金淋巴瘤（C82），占3.78%；其他和未特指的淋巴、造血和有关组织的恶性肿瘤（C96），占1.35%；以及恶性免疫增生性疾病（C88），占0.93%（图5-21c）。

The incidence and mortality rates of lymphoma were higher in urban areas than those in rural areas. Eastern areas had the highest incidence rate and mortality rate (ASR China), followed by the central areas and western areas. Among the seven administrative districts, the highest incidence and mortality rates (ASR China) were shown in South China, while the lowest incidence and mortality rates (ASR China) rates were shown in Northwest China (Table 5-21a, Table 5-21b, Figure 5-21b).

Among all lymphoma cases, other and unspecified types of non-Hodgkin lymphoma (ICD-10: C85) was the most common histological type, accounting for 43.49% of all cases, followed by multiple myeloma & malignant plasma cell neoplasms (C90, 23.81%), diffuse non-Hodgkin lymphoma (C83, 17.62%), Hodgkin lymphoma (C81, 4.86%), peripheral & cutaneous T-cell lymphoma (C84, 4.15%), follicular non-Hodgkin lymphoma (C82, 3.78%), other and unspecified malignant neoplasms of lymphoid, hematopoietic and related tissue (C96 1.35%), and malignant immunoproliferative disease (C88, 0.93%) (Figure 5-21c).

表 5-21a 2017 年中国肿瘤登记地区淋巴瘤发病情况

Table 5-21a Incidence of lymphoma in the registration areas of China,2017

地区 Area	性别 Sex	病例数 No. cases	粗率 Crude rate/ 100 000^{-1}	构成比 Freq./%	中标率 ASR China/ 100 000^{-1}	世标率 ASR World/ 100 000^{-1}	累积率 Cum. rate 0~74/%	顺位 Rank
合计	合计 Both	28 180	6.46	2.20	4.34	4.26	0.48	14
All	男性 Male	16 268	7.36	2.29	5.07	4.99	0.56	9
	女性 Female	11 912	5.54	2.09	3.63	3.54	0.41	13
城市地区	合计 Both	16 099	7.55	2.39	4.91	4.81	0.54	14
Urban areas	男性 Male	9 205	8.60	2.52	5.74	5.64	0.63	10
	女性 Female	6 894	6.49	2.23	4.11	4.00	0.46	13
农村地区	合计 Both	12 081	5.42	1.99	3.78	3.71	0.42	15
Rural areas	男性 Male	7 063	6.19	2.04	4.41	4.35	0.49	11
	女性 Female	5 018	4.60	1.92	3.14	3.07	0.35	14
东部地区	合计 Both	15 947	8.06	2.41	5.03	4.92	0.56	14
Eastern areas	男性 Male	9 135	9.18	2.56	5.88	5.77	0.65	10
	女性 Female	6 812	6.92	2.24	4.23	4.10	0.47	13
中部地区	合计 Both	6 189	5.38	2.05	3.97	3.91	0.44	13
Central areas	男性 Male	3 558	6.05	2.13	4.59	4.53	0.51	9
	女性 Female	2 631	4.68	1.96	3.35	3.30	0.37	13
西部地区	合计 Both	6 044	4.90	1.89	3.48	3.42	0.38	15
Western areas	男性 Male	3 575	5.69	1.90	4.13	4.07	0.44	12
	女性 Female	2 469	4.08	1.88	2.82	2.77	0.32	14

表 5-21b 2017 年中国肿瘤登记地区淋巴瘤死亡情况

Table 5-21b Mortality of lymphoma in the registration areas of China,2017

地区 Area	性别 Sex	死亡数 No. deaths	粗率 Crude rate/ 100 000^{-1}	构成比 Freq./%	中标率 ASR China/ 100 000^{-1}	世标率 ASR World/ 100 000^{-1}	累积率 Cum. rate 0~74/%	顺位 Rank
合计	合计 Both	15 951	3.66	2.06	2.24	2.21	0.25	12
All	男性 Male	9 690	4.38	1.96	2.81	2.78	0.32	8
	女性 Female	6 261	2.91	2.25	1.70	1.67	0.19	13
城市地区	合计 Both	8 892	4.17	2.30	2.43	2.39	0.27	11
Urban areas	男性 Male	5 336	4.99	2.18	3.04	3.00	0.33	8
	女性 Female	3 556	3.35	2.52	1.86	1.82	0.20	12
农村地区	合计 Both	7 059	3.16	1.83	2.05	2.03	0.24	12
Rural areas	男性 Male	4 354	3.82	1.75	2.57	2.55	0.30	9
	女性 Female	2 705	2.48	1.97	1.53	1.51	0.17	13
东部地区	合计 Both	8 952	4.52	2.34	2.50	2.46	0.28	10
Eastern areas	男性 Male	5 332	5.36	2.21	3.11	3.08	0.35	8
	女性 Female	3 620	3.68	2.56	1.92	1.87	0.21	12
中部地区	合计 Both	3 654	3.18	1.95	2.19	2.17	0.25	13
Central areas	男性 Male	2 232	3.79	1.86	2.73	2.70	0.31	8
	女性 Female	1 422	2.53	2.09	1.66	1.65	0.19	13
西部地区	合计 Both	3 345	2.71	1.65	1.82	1.80	0.21	13
Western areas	男性 Male	2 126	3.38	1.59	2.34	2.31	0.26	10
	女性 Female	1 219	2.01	1.76	1.29	1.29	0.15	14

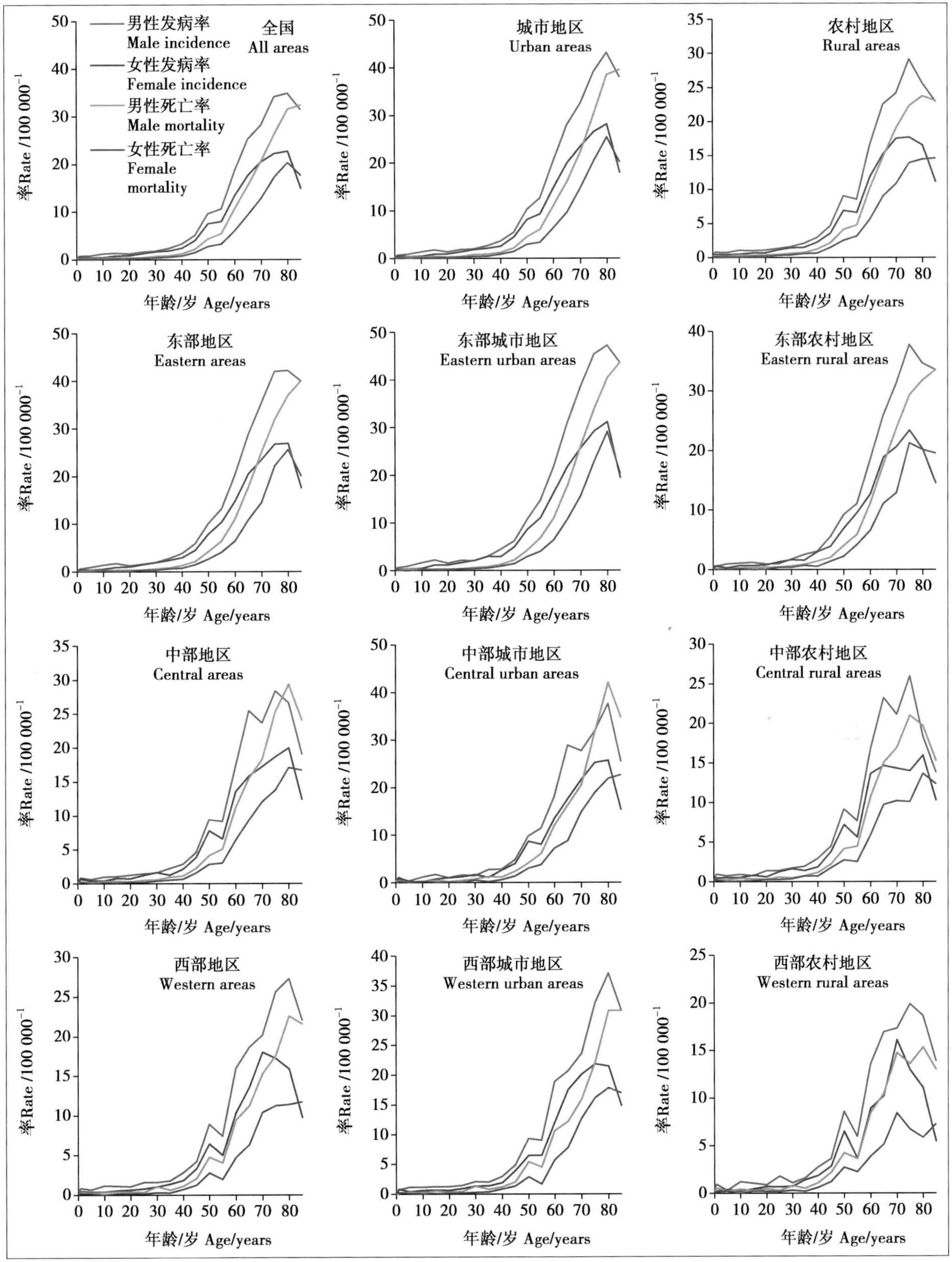

图 5-21a　2017 年中国肿瘤登记地区淋巴瘤年龄别发病率和死亡率
Figure 5-21a　Age-specific incidence and mortality rates of lymphoma in the registration areas of China,2017

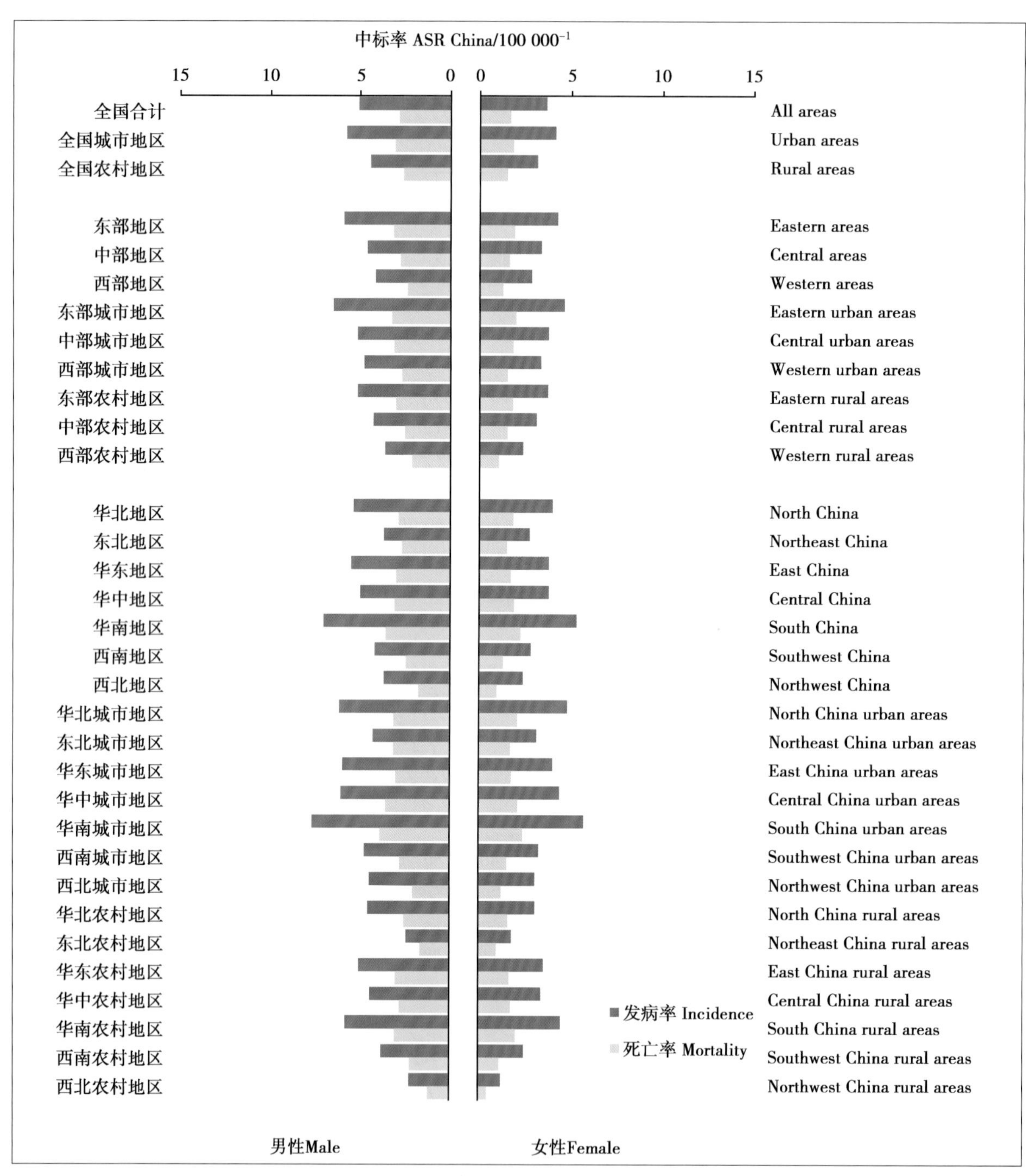

图 5-21b 2017 年中国肿瘤登记不同地区淋巴瘤发病率和死亡率

Figure 5-21b Incidence and mortality rates of lymphoma in different registration areas of China, 2017

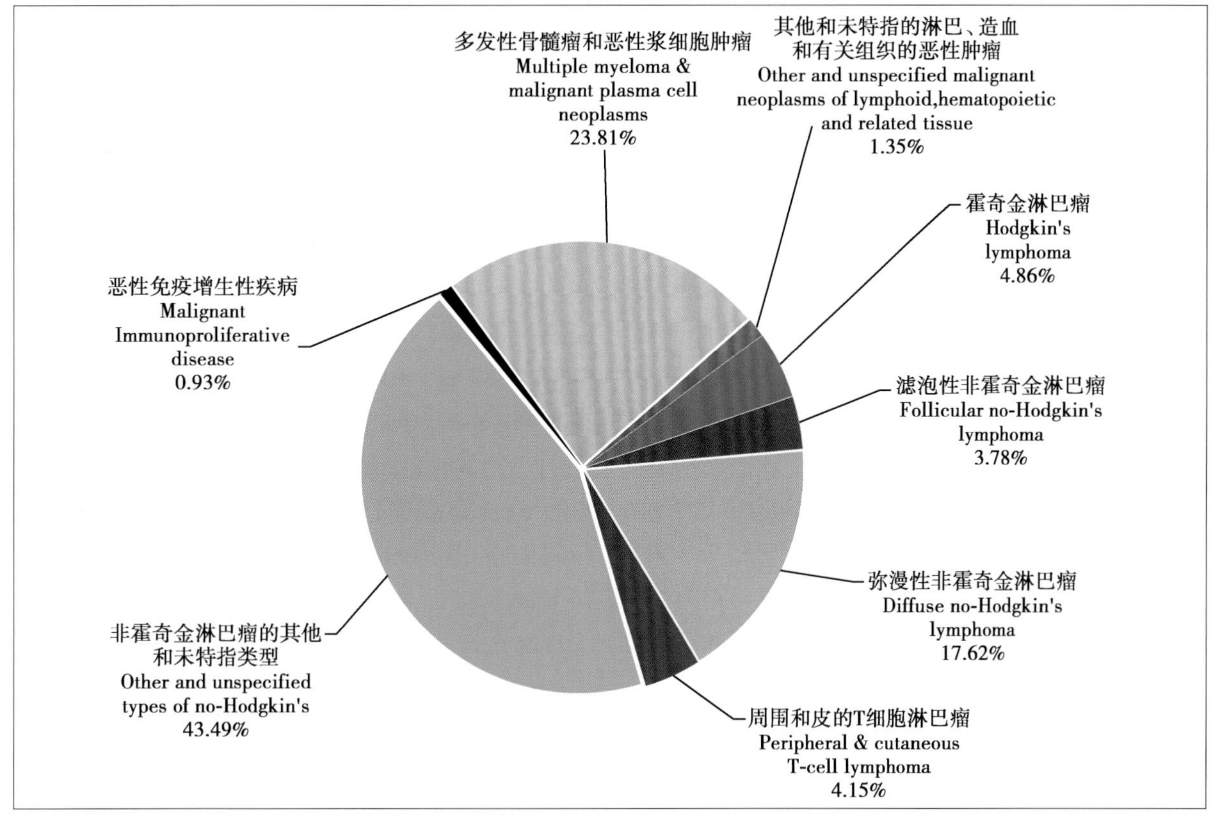

图 5-21c 2017 年中国肿瘤登记地区淋巴瘤病理分型情况
Figure 5-21c Morphological distribution of lymphoma in the registration areas of China,2017

22 白血病

2017 年,中国肿瘤登记地区白血病位居癌症发病谱第 15 位。新发病例数为 27 160 例,占全部癌症发病的 2.12%;其中男性 15 467 例,女性 11 693 例;城市地区 14 363 例,农村地区 12 797 例。白血病发病率为 6.22/10 万,中标发病率为 4.83/10 万,世标发病率为 4.98/10 万;男性中标发病率为女性的 1.32 倍,城市地区中标发病率为农村地区的 1.09 倍。0~74 岁累积率为 0.46%(表 5-22a)。

2017 年,中国肿瘤登记地区白血病位居癌症死亡谱第 11 位。因白血病死亡病例为 15 989 例,占全部癌症死亡的 2.07%;其中男性 9 274 例,女性 6 715 例;城市地区 8 166 例,农村地区 7 823 例。白血病死亡率为 3.66/10 万,中标死亡率为 2.65/10 万,世标死亡率为 2.67/10 万;男性中标死亡率为女性的 1.41 倍。0~74 岁累积死亡率为 0.26%(表 5-22b)。

白血病年龄别发病率和死亡率在 0~4 岁年龄组出现一个小高峰,在 5 岁以后趋于平缓,40 岁后开始快速上升,至 80~84 岁年龄组达到高峰(图 5-22a)。

城市地区白血病发病率和死亡率与农村地区接近。东部地区的中标发病率和死亡率较中部和西部高。七大行政区中,华南地区中标发病率和中标死亡率最高,西北地区中标发病率和中标死亡率最低(表 5-22a,表 5-22b,图 5-22b)。

22 Leukemia

Leukemia ranked 15th for cancer incidence in the registration areas of China in 2017. There were 27 160 new cases of leukemia(15 467 males and 11 693 females,14 363 in urban areas and 12 797 in rural areas), accounting for 2.12% of all cancer cases. The crude incidence rate was 6.22 per 100 000, with ASR China 4.83 per 100 000 and ASR World 4.98 per 100 000, respectively. The incidence of ASR China was 1.32 times in males as that in females, and it was 1.09 times in urban areas as that in rural areas. The cumulative incidence rate for subjects aged from 0 to 74 years was 0.46% (Table 5-22a).

Leukemia ranked 11th for cancer mortality in the registration areas of China in 2017. A total of 15 989 cases died of leukemia (9 274 males and 6 715 females, 8 166 in urban areas and 7 823 in rural areas), accounting for 2.07% of all cancer deaths. The crude mortality rate was 3.66 per 100 000, with ASR China 2.65 per 100 000 and ASR World 2.67 per 100 000, respectively. The mortality of ASR China was 1.41 times in males as that in females. The cumulative mortality rate for subjects aged from 0 to 74 years was 0.26% (Table 5-22b).

The first peak of the age-specific incidence rate and mortality rate occurred in the age group of 0-4 years. Age-specific incidence and mortality rates were relatively stable at 5-39 years and dramatically increased after the age of 40, and peaked at the age group of 80-84 years (Figure 5-22a).

The incidence and mortality rates of leukemia in urban areas were close to those in rural areas. Eastern areas had the highest incidence rate (ASR China), followed by central areas and western areas. Among the seven administrative districts, South China had the highest incidence and mortality rates (ASR China) while Northwest China had the lowest incidence and mortality rates (ASR China) (Table 5-22a, Table 5-22b, Figure 5-22b).

全部白血病新发病例中，髓样白血病（ICD-10：C92）是最主要的病理类型，占 35.61%；其次是未特指细胞类型的白血病（C95），占 35.43%；淋巴样白血病（C91），占 22.12%；单核细胞白血病（C93），占 3.77%；以及特指细胞类型的其他白血病（C94），占 3.06%（图 5-22c）。

2017 年，中国肿瘤登记地区淋巴样白血病新发病例为 5 240 例，发病率为 1.20/10 万（中标率为 1.04/10 万，世标率为 1.20/10 万），占全部癌症发病的 0.41%。淋巴样白血病死亡病例为 3 551 例，死亡率为 0.81/10 万（中标率为 0.63/10 万，世标率为 0.65/10 万），占全部癌症死亡的 0.46%（表 5-22c，表 5-22d）。

2017 年，中国肿瘤登记地区髓样白血病新发病例为 13 526 例，发病率为 3.10/10 万（中标率为 2.30/10 万，世标率为 2.24/10 万），占全部癌症发病的 1.06%。髓样白血病死亡病例为 5 293 例，死亡率为 1.21/10 万（中标率为 0.84/10 万，世标率为 0.83/10 万），占全部癌症死亡的 0.68%（表 5-22e，表 5-22f）。

Among all leukemia cases, myeloid leukemia (ICD-10: C92) was the most common histological type, accounting for 35.61% of all cases, followed by leukemia of unspecified cell type (C95, 35.43%), lymphoid leukemia (C91, 22.12%), monocytic leukemia (C93, 3.77%), and other leukemias (C94, 3.06%) (Figure 5-22c).

There were 5 240 new cases diagnosed as lymphoid leukemia in the registration areas of China in 2017, accounting for 0.41% of all cancer cases. The crude incidence rate was 1.20 per 100 000, with ASR China 1.04 per 100 000 and ASR World 1.20 per 100 000, respectively. A total of 3 551 cases died of lymphoid leukemia, accounting for 0.46% of all cancer deaths. The crude mortality rate was 0.81 per 100 000, with ASR China 0.63 per 100 000 and ASR World 0.65 per 100 000, respectively (Table 5-22c, Table 5-22d).

There were 13 526 new cases diagnosed as myeloid leukemia in the registration areas of China in 2017, accounting for 1.06% of all cancer cases. The crude incidence rate was 3.10 per 100 000, with ASR China 2.30 per 100 000 and ASR World 2.24 per 100 000, respectively. A total of 5 293 cases died of myeloid leukemia, accounting for 0.68% of all cancer deaths. The crude mortality rate of myeloid leukemia was 1.21 per 100 000, with ASR China 0.84 per 100 000 and ASR World 0.83 per 100 000, respectively (Table 5-22e, Table 5-22f).

表 5-22a 2017 年中国肿瘤登记地区白血病发病情况
Table 5-22a Incidence of leukemia in the registration areas of China, 2017

地区 Area	性别 Sex	病例数 No. cases	粗率 Crude rate/ 100 000^{-1}	构成比 Freq./%	中标率 ASR China/ 100 000^{-1}	世标率 ASR World/ 100 000^{-1}	累积率 Cum. rate 0~74/%	顺位 Rank
合计	合计 Both	27 160	6.22	2.12	4.83	4.98	0.46	15
All	男性 Male	15 467	6.99	2.17	5.51	5.67	0.52	11
	女性 Female	11 693	5.43	2.05	4.16	4.28	0.40	14
城市地区	合计 Both	14 363	6.74	2.13	5.05	5.20	0.48	17
Urban areas	男性 Male	8 159	7.62	2.23	5.77	5.94	0.54	12
	女性 Female	6 204	5.84	2.01	4.35	4.48	0.42	14
农村地区	合计 Both	12 797	5.74	2.11	4.62	4.75	0.44	14
Rural areas	男性 Male	7 308	6.40	2.11	5.25	5.40	0.49	10
	女性 Female	5 489	5.04	2.10	3.98	4.08	0.38	13
东部地区	合计 Both	14 721	7.44	2.23	5.44	5.62	0.52	15
Eastern areas	男性 Male	8 408	8.45	2.36	6.26	6.47	0.59	12
	女性 Female	6 313	6.42	2.07	4.63	4.77	0.44	14
中部地区	合计 Both	6 129	5.33	2.03	4.46	4.57	0.42	14
Central areas	男性 Male	3 441	5.85	2.06	4.97	5.10	0.46	11
	女性 Female	2 688	4.78	2.00	3.93	4.02	0.38	12
西部地区	合计 Both	6 310	5.12	1.98	4.16	4.27	0.39	14
Western areas	男性 Male	3 618	5.76	1.92	4.73	4.86	0.44	11
	女性 Female	2 692	4.45	2.06	3.58	3.67	0.35	13

表 5-22b 2017 年中国肿瘤登记地区白血病死亡情况
Table 5-22b Mortality of leukemia in the registration areas of China, 2017

地区 Area	性别 Sex	死亡数 No. deaths	粗率 Crude rate/ 100 000^{-1}	构成比 Freq./%	中标率 ASR China/ 100 000^{-1}	世标率 ASR World/ 100 000^{-1}	累积率 Cum. rate 0~74/%	顺位 Rank
合计	合计 Both	15 989	3.66	2.07	2.65	2.67	0.26	11
All	男性 Male	9 274	4.19	1.88	3.11	3.13	0.30	10
	女性 Female	6 715	3.12	2.41	2.20	2.23	0.22	12
城市地区	合计 Both	8 166	3.83	2.11	2.62	2.65	0.26	13
Urban areas	男性 Male	4 724	4.41	1.93	3.10	3.13	0.30	10
	女性 Female	3 442	3.24	2.44	2.16	2.19	0.21	13
农村地区	合计 Both	7 823	3.51	2.02	2.67	2.68	0.26	11
Rural areas	男性 Male	4 550	3.99	1.83	3.12	3.11	0.30	8
	女性 Female	3 273	3.00	2.38	2.23	2.25	0.22	10
东部地区	合计 Both	8 171	4.13	2.14	2.72	2.74	0.27	12
Eastern areas	男性 Male	4 711	4.73	1.96	3.22	3.23	0.32	10
	女性 Female	3 460	3.52	2.45	2.25	2.27	0.22	13
中部地区	合计 Both	3 784	3.29	2.02	2.60	2.61	0.26	11
Central areas	男性 Male	2 211	3.76	1.85	3.05	3.05	0.30	9
	女性 Female	1 573	2.80	2.32	2.15	2.17	0.21	12
西部地区	合计 Both	4 034	3.27	1.99	2.55	2.58	0.25	11
Western areas	男性 Male	2 352	3.74	1.76	2.97	3.00	0.28	9
	女性 Female	1 682	2.78	2.43	2.13	2.16	0.21	11

表 5-22c 2017 年中国肿瘤登记地区淋巴样白血病发病情况
Table 5-22c Incidence of lymphoid leukemia in the registration areas of China,2017

地区 Area	性别 Sex	病例数 No. cases	粗率 Crude rate/ 100 000^{-1}	构成比 Freq./%	中标率 ASR China/ 100 000^{-1}	世标率 ASR World/ 100 000^{-1}	累积率 Cum. rate 0~74/%
合计	合计 Both	5 240	1.20	0.41	1.04	1.20	0.09
All	男性 Male	3 042	1.38	0.43	1.20	1.38	0.10
	女性 Female	2 198	1.02	0.39	0.88	1.01	0.08
城市地区	合计 Both	2 947	1.38	0.44	1.19	1.38	0.10
Urban areas	男性 Male	1 694	1.58	0.46	1.37	1.59	0.12
	女性 Female	1 253	1.18	0.41	1.01	1.17	0.09
农村地区	合计 Both	2 293	1.03	0.38	0.90	1.03	0.08
Rural areas	男性 Male	1 348	1.18	0.39	1.04	1.18	0.09
	女性 Female	945	0.87	0.36	0.76	0.86	0.07
东部地区	合计 Both	2 992	1.51	0.45	1.30	1.53	0.11
Eastern areas	男性 Male	1 750	1.76	0.49	1.52	1.77	0.13
	女性 Female	1 242	1.26	0.41	1.07	1.28	0.09
中部地区	合计 Both	1 105	0.96	0.37	0.85	0.95	0.08
Central areas	男性 Male	613	1.04	0.37	0.92	1.05	0.08
	女性 Female	492	0.87	0.37	0.78	0.85	0.07
西部地区	合计 Both	1 143	0.93	0.36	0.82	0.91	0.07
Western areas	男性 Male	679	1.08	0.36	0.96	1.06	0.08
	女性 Female	464	0.77	0.35	0.68	0.75	0.06

表 5-22d 2017 年中国肿瘤登记地区淋巴样白血病死亡情况
Table 5-22d Mortality of lymphoid leukemia in the registration areas of China,2017

地区 Area	性别 Sex	死亡数 No. deaths	粗率 Crude rate/ 100 000^{-1}	构成比 Freq./%	中标率 ASR China/ 100 000^{-1}	世标率 ASR World/ 100 000^{-1}	累积率 Cum. rate 0~74/%
合计	合计 Both	3 551	0.81	0.46	0.63	0.65	0.06
All	男性 Male	2 081	0.94	0.42	0.74	0.77	0.07
	女性 Female	1 470	0.68	0.53	0.51	0.52	0.05
城市地区	合计 Both	1 873	0.88	0.48	0.66	0.68	0.06
Urban areas	男性 Male	1 096	1.02	0.45	0.79	0.82	0.07
	女性 Female	777	0.73	0.55	0.53	0.55	0.05
农村地区	合计 Both	1 678	0.75	0.43	0.59	0.61	0.06
Rural areas	男性 Male	985	0.86	0.40	0.70	0.72	0.07
	女性 Female	693	0.64	0.50	0.49	0.50	0.05
东部地区	合计 Both	1 809	0.91	0.47	0.67	0.69	0.06
Eastern areas	男性 Male	1 046	1.05	0.43	0.79	0.82	0.07
	女性 Female	763	0.78	0.54	0.54	0.55	0.05
中部地区	合计 Both	839	0.73	0.45	0.59	0.61	0.06
Central areas	男性 Male	494	0.84	0.41	0.70	0.72	0.07
	女性 Female	345	0.61	0.51	0.49	0.50	0.05
西部地区	合计 Both	903	0.73	0.44	0.59	0.62	0.06
Western areas	男性 Male	541	0.86	0.40	0.72	0.74	0.06
	女性 Female	362	0.60	0.52	0.47	0.49	0.05

表 5-22e 2017 年中国肿瘤登记地区髓样白血病发病情况
Table 5-22e Incidence of myeloid leukemia in the registration areas of China,2017

地区 Area	性别 Sex	病例数 No. cases	粗率 Crude rate/ 100 000^{-1}	构成比 Freq./%	中标率 ASR China/ 100 000^{-1}	世标率 ASR World/ 100 000^{-1}	累积率 Cum. rate 0~74/%
合计	合计 Both	13 526	3. 10	1. 06	2. 30	2. 24	0. 23
All	男性 Male	7 580	3. 43	1. 07	2. 58	2. 51	0. 25
	女性 Female	5 946	2. 76	1. 04	2. 03	1. 98	0. 20
城市地区	合计 Both	7 917	3. 71	1. 17	2. 65	2. 57	0. 26
Urban areas	男性 Male	4 432	4. 14	1. 21	2. 99	2. 90	0. 29
	女性 Female	3 485	3. 28	1. 13	2. 32	2. 26	0. 23
农村地区	合计 Both	5 609	2. 51	0. 92	1. 96	1. 91	0. 19
Rural areas	男性 Male	3 148	2. 76	0. 91	2. 18	2. 13	0. 21
	女性 Female	2 461	2. 26	0. 94	1. 74	1. 69	0. 17
东部地区	合计 Both	8 570	4. 33	1. 30	3. 03	2. 93	0. 30
Eastern areas	男性 Male	4 833	4. 86	1. 36	3. 44	3. 34	0. 34
	女性 Female	3 737	3. 80	1. 23	2. 63	2. 54	0. 26
中部地区	合计 Both	2 429	2. 11	0. 81	1. 71	1. 66	0. 17
Central areas	男性 Male	1 331	2. 26	0. 80	1. 86	1. 80	0. 18
	女性 Female	1 098	1. 95	0. 82	1. 55	1. 53	0. 15
西部地区	合计 Both	2 527	2. 05	0. 79	1. 63	1. 59	0. 16
Western areas	男性 Male	1 416	2. 25	0. 75	1. 80	1. 76	0. 17
	女性 Female	1 111	1. 84	0. 85	1. 46	1. 42	0. 14

表 5-22f 2017 年中国肿瘤登记地区髓样白血病死亡情况
Table 5-22f Mortality of myeloid leukemia in the registration areas of China,2017

地区 Area	性别 Sex	死亡数 No. deaths	粗率 Crude rate/ 100 000^{-1}	构成比 Freq./%	中标率 ASR China/ 100 000^{-1}	世标率 ASR World/ 100 000^{-1}	累积率 Cum. rate 0~74/%
合计	合计 Both	5 293	1. 21	0. 68	0. 84	0. 83	0. 09
All	男性 Male	3 015	1. 36	0. 61	0. 97	0. 95	0. 10
	女性 Female	2 278	1. 06	0. 82	0. 71	0. 71	0. 07
城市地区	合计 Both	3 114	1. 46	0. 81	0. 94	0. 93	0. 10
Urban areas	男性 Male	1 742	1. 63	0. 71	1. 07	1. 06	0. 11
	女性 Female	1 372	1. 29	0. 97	0. 81	0. 80	0. 08
农村地区	合计 Both	2 179	0. 98	0. 56	0. 73	0. 72	0. 08
Rural areas	男性 Male	1 273	1. 12	0. 51	0. 86	0. 83	0. 09
	女性 Female	906	0. 83	0. 66	0. 61	0. 60	0. 06
东部地区	合计 Both	3 125	1. 58	0. 82	1. 00	0. 98	0. 10
Eastern areas	男性 Male	1 783	1. 79	0. 74	1. 15	1. 13	0. 12
	女性 Female	1 342	1. 36	0. 95	0. 86	0. 84	0. 09
中部地区	合计 Both	1 016	0. 88	0. 54	0. 68	0. 67	0. 07
Central areas	男性 Male	565	0. 96	0. 47	0. 76	0. 75	0. 08
	女性 Female	451	0. 80	0. 66	0. 59	0. 58	0. 06
西部地区	合计 Both	1 152	0. 93	0. 57	0. 70	0. 69	0. 07
Western areas	男性 Male	667	1. 06	0. 50	0. 82	0. 80	0. 08
	女性 Female	485	0. 80	0. 70	0. 58	0. 58	0. 06

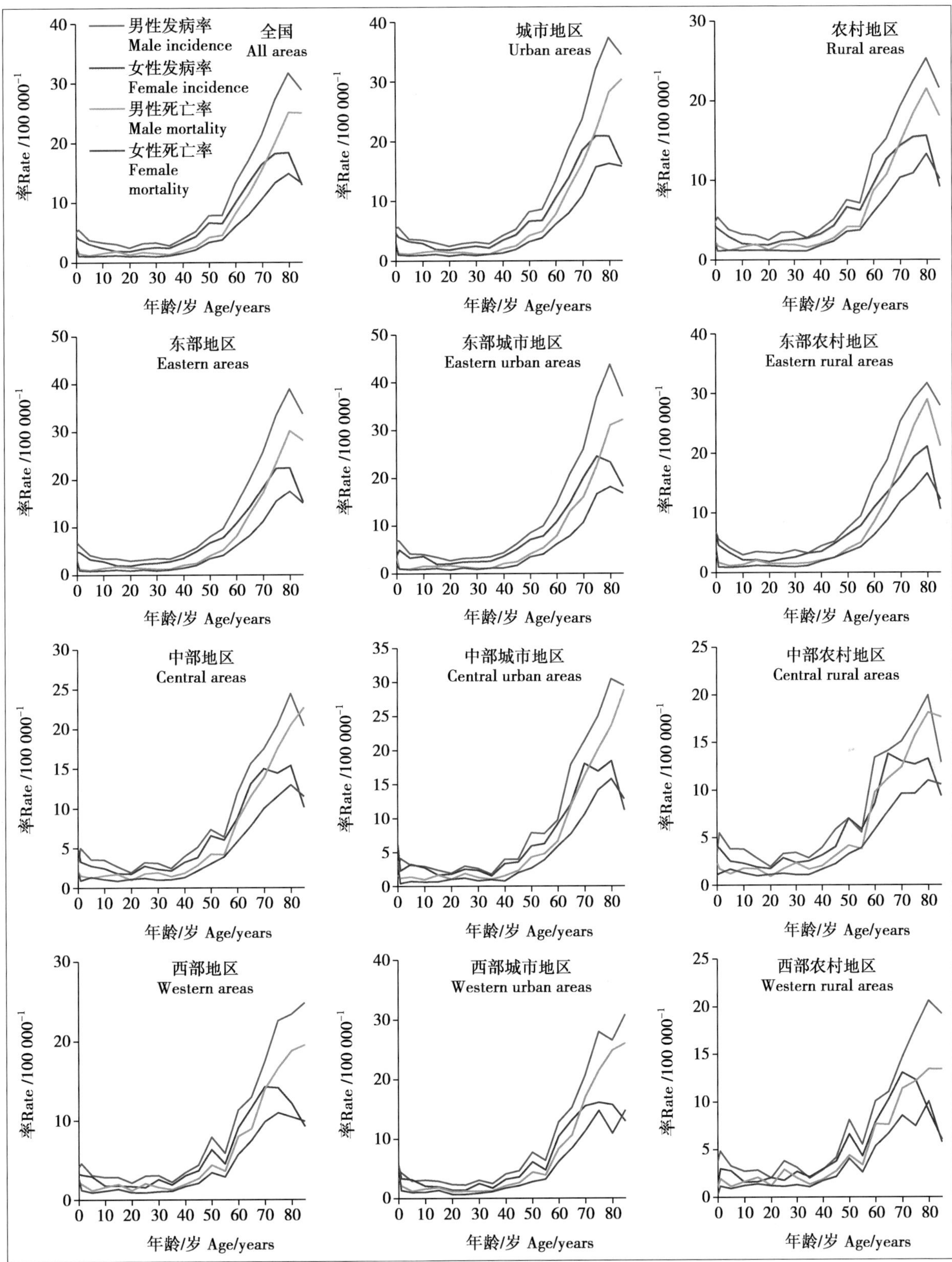

图 5-22a 2017 年中国肿瘤登记地区白血病年龄别发病率和死亡率
Figure 5-22a Age-specific incidence and mortality rates of leukemia in the registration areas of China, 2017

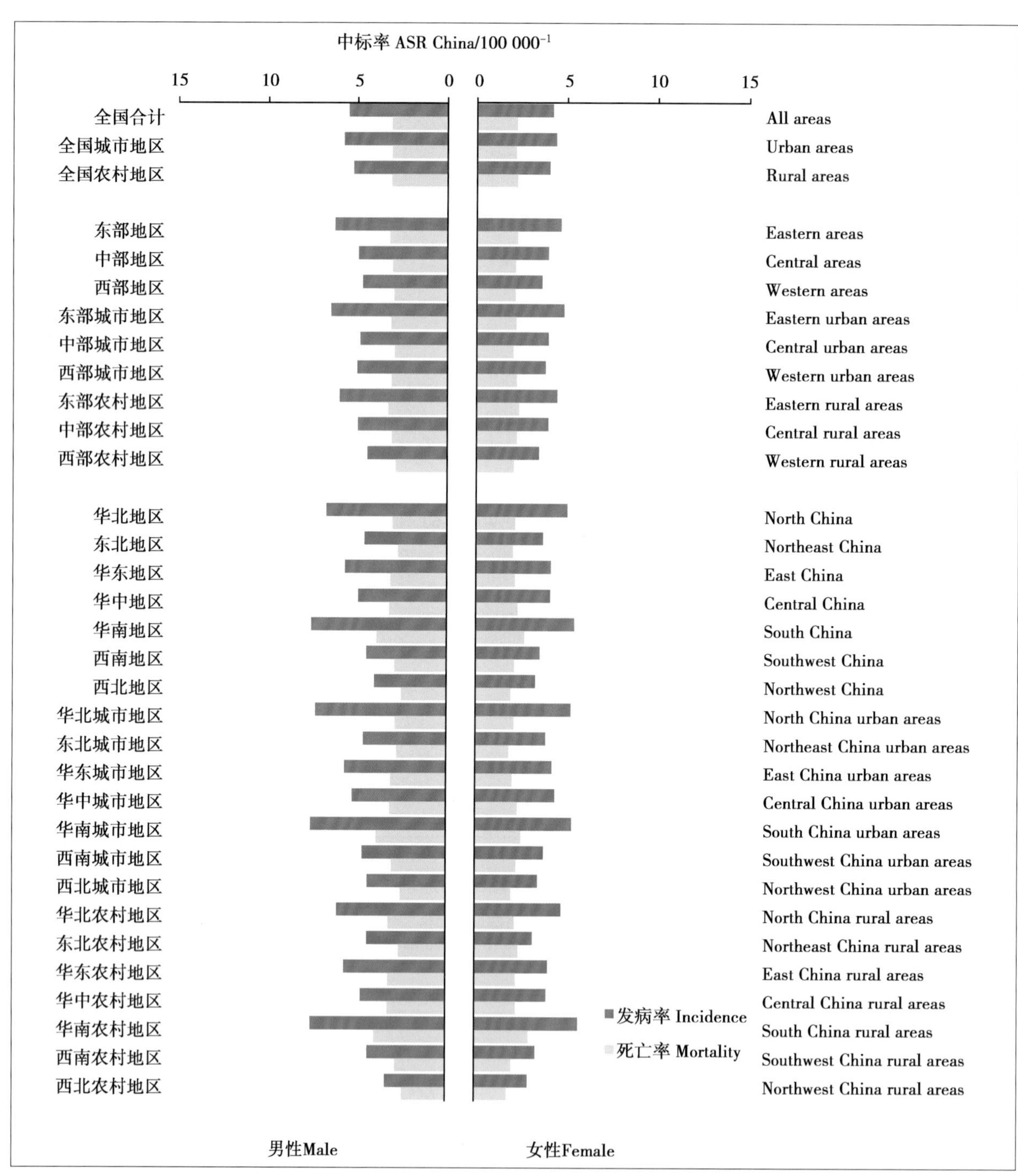

图 5-22b 2017 年中国肿瘤登记不同地区白血病发病率和死亡率

Figure 5-22b Incidence and mortality rates of leukemia in different registration areas of China,2017

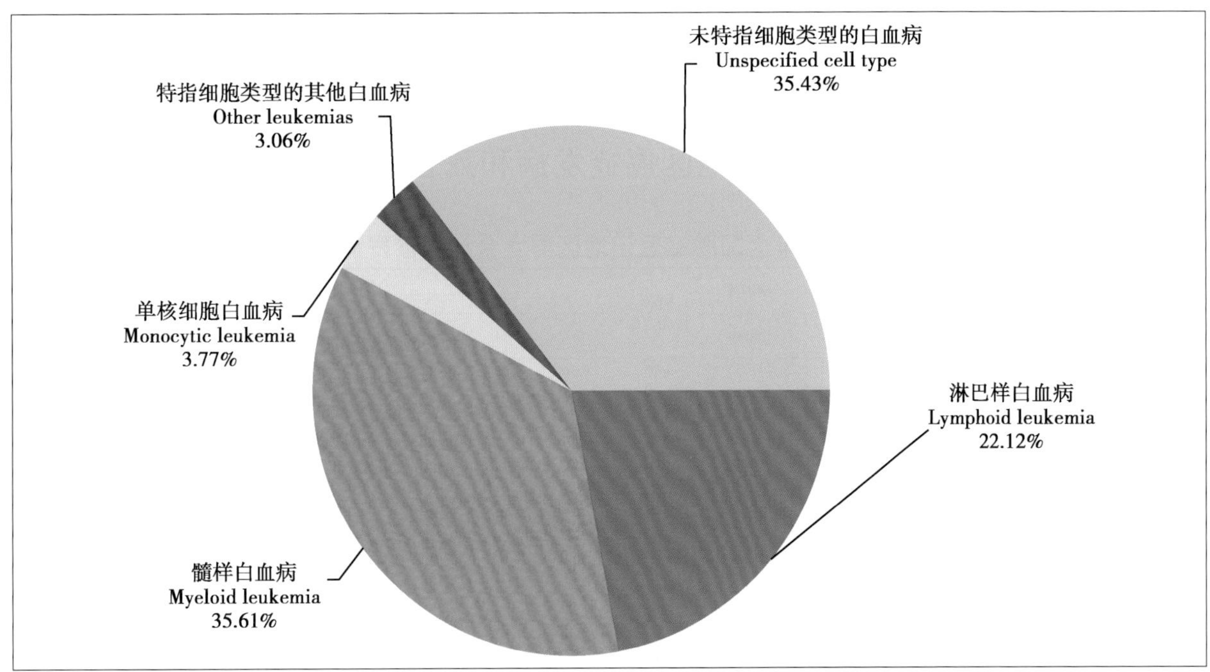

图 5-22c 2017 年中国肿瘤登记地区白血病病理分型情况
Figure 5-22c Morphological distribution of leukemia in the registration areas of China,2017

附录

附录 1　2017 年全国肿瘤登记地区癌症发病和死亡结果

附表 1-1　2017 年全国肿瘤登记地区男女合计癌症发病主要指标

	部位 Site	病例数 No. cases	构成 Freq. /%	年龄组								
				0～	1～4	5～9	10～14	15～19	20～24	25～29	30～34	35～39
唇	Lip	754	0. 06	0. 02	0. 02	0. 01	0. 01	0. 01	0. 01	0. 01	0. 02	0. 03
舌	Tongue	3 497	0. 27	0. 00	0. 02	0. 01	0. 01	0. 01	0. 03	0. 09	0. 20	0. 30
口	Mouth	4 655	0. 36	0. 02	0. 01	0. 03	0. 05	0. 06	0. 06	0. 10	0. 17	0. 23
唾液腺	Salivary glands	2 599	0. 20	0. 02	0. 01	0. 01	0. 09	0. 09	0. 19	0. 26	0. 25	0. 43
扁桃腺	Tonsil	718	0. 06	0. 00	0. 01	0. 00	0. 00	0. 00	0. 02	0. 01	0. 03	0. 04
其他口咽	Other oropharynx	1 178	0. 09	0. 00	0. 01	0. 02	0. 01	0. 01	0. 01	0. 02	0. 03	0. 08
鼻咽	Nasopharynx	15 838	1. 24	0. 04	0. 01	0. 04	0. 11	0. 28	0. 39	0. 92	1. 84	2. 56
下咽	Hypopharynx	2 139	0. 17	0. 02	0. 00	0. 01	0. 00	0. 02	0. 01	0. 02	0. 01	0. 04
咽,部位不明	Pharynx unspecified	1 057	0. 08	0. 00	0. 01	0. 01	0. 01	0. 01	0. 01	0. 02	0. 01	0. 03
食管	Esophagus	83 901	6. 55	0. 09	0. 02	0. 01	0. 01	0. 01	0. 07	0. 16	0. 18	0. 46
胃	Stomach	123 200	9. 61	0. 06	0. 02	0. 02	0. 06	0. 17	0. 40	1. 19	2. 24	3. 30
小肠	Small intestine	5 115	0. 40	0. 00	0. 00	0. 00	0. 01	0. 00	0. 04	0. 07	0. 15	0. 27
结肠	Colon	61 613	4. 81	0. 00	0. 01	0. 01	0. 06	0. 12	0. 32	1. 00	1. 78	2. 72
直肠	Rectum	63 185	4. 93	0. 06	0. 01	0. 02	0. 03	0. 07	0. 18	0. 76	1. 34	2. 12
肛门	Anus	1 558	0. 12	0. 00	0. 00	0. 00	0. 00	0. 00	0. 02	0. 02	0. 02	0. 09
肝脏	Liver	122 898	9. 59	1. 16	0. 36	0. 11	0. 17	0. 37	0. 58	1. 94	3. 99	7. 51
胆囊及其他	Gallbladder etc.	17 442	1. 36	0. 04	0. 02	0. 00	0. 00	0. 01	0. 03	0. 06	0. 17	0. 33
胰腺	Pancreas	30 869	2. 41	0. 06	0. 02	0. 02	0. 04	0. 04	0. 08	0. 17	0. 36	0. 76
鼻、鼻窦及其他	Nose, sinuses etc.	2 029	0. 16	0. 02	0. 05	0. 02	0. 03	0. 04	0. 07	0. 09	0. 15	0. 17
喉	Larynx	8 016	0. 63	0. 04	0. 02	0. 01	0. 00	0. 03	0. 02	0. 04	0. 04	0. 12
气管、支气管、肺	Trachea, bronchus & lung	274 690	21. 44	0. 04	0. 06	0. 05	0. 10	0. 21	0. 52	1. 40	3. 25	5. 82
其他胸腔器官	Other thoracic organs	4 145	0. 32	0. 32	0. 12	0. 04	0. 06	0. 24	0. 18	0. 26	0. 33	0. 37
骨	Bone	7 967	0. 62	0. 04	0. 23	0. 32	1. 02	0. 95	0. 61	0. 62	0. 63	0. 60
皮肤黑色素瘤	Melanoma of skin	2 225	0. 17	0. 00	0. 06	0. 05	0. 04	0. 02	0. 05	0. 09	0. 15	0. 20
皮肤其他	Other skin	11 280	0. 88	0. 06	0. 09	0. 09	0. 12	0. 21	0. 21	0. 28	0. 45	0. 55
间皮瘤	Mesothelioma	629	0. 05	0. 00	0. 00	0. 00	0. 00	0. 01	0. 01	0. 03	0. 02	0. 07
卡波氏肉瘤	Kaposi sarcoma	107	0. 01	0. 02	0. 01	0. 00	0. 00	0. 02	0. 02	0. 01	0. 01	0. 01
结缔组织、软组织	Connective & soft tissue	4 008	0. 31	0. 62	0. 29	0. 18	0. 28	0. 26	0. 32	0. 45	0. 54	0. 50
乳腺	Breast	91 475	7. 23	0. 09	0. 00	0. 00	0. 14	0. 32	1. 86	6. 16	16. 20	29. 40
外阴	Vulva	1 056	0. 08	0. 05	0. 01	0. 00	0. 00	0. 02	0. 05	0. 04	0. 08	0. 20
阴道	Vagina	590	0. 05	0. 05	0. 01	0. 00	0. 00	0. 01	0. 01	0. 00	0. 04	0. 11
子宫颈	Cervix uteri	36 740	2. 87	0. 00	0. 00	0. 00	0. 00	0. 09	0. 57	2. 82	7. 58	13. 57
子宫体	Corpus uteri	18 167	1. 42	0. 00	0. 00	0. 00	0. 00	0. 05	0. 13	0. 84	1. 76	3. 22
子宫,部位不明	Uterus unspecified	3 479	0. 27	0. 00	0. 00	0. 00	0. 00	0. 03	0. 05	0. 21	0. 41	0. 66
卵巢	Ovary	16 479	1. 29	0. 09	0. 10	0. 20	0. 55	1. 10	1. 87	2. 30	2. 91	3. 39
其他女性生殖器	Other female genital organs	1 254	0. 10	0. 05	0. 02	0. 00	0. 01	0. 05	0. 08	0. 13	0. 14	0. 23
胎盘	Placenta	202	0. 02	0. 00	0. 00	0. 01	0. 01	0. 03	0. 12	0. 28	0. 24	0. 15
阴茎	Penis	1 698	0. 13	0. 00	0. 00	0. 01	0. 01	0. 03	0. 02	0. 04	0. 12	0. 21
前列腺	Prostate	25 577	2. 00	0. 04	0. 00	0. 00	0. 00	0. 05	0. 03	0. 04	0. 09	0. 08
睾丸	Testis	1 024	0. 08	0. 53	0. 31	0. 05	0. 04	0. 16	0. 35	0. 65	0. 79	0. 65
其他男性生殖器	Other male genital organs	391	0. 03	0. 00	0. 03	0. 01	0. 03	0. 03	0. 01	0. 04	0. 07	0. 05
肾	Kidney	17 416	1. 36	0. 75	0. 59	0. 14	0. 06	0. 09	0. 22	0. 41	0. 88	1. 30
肾盂	Renal pelvis	2 109	0. 16	0. 00	0. 01	0. 01	0. 00	0. 01	0. 01	0. 01	0. 06	0. 05
输尿管	Ureter	2 436	0. 19	0. 09	0. 00	0. 00	0. 00	0. 00	0. 00	0. 01	0. 03	0. 01
膀胱	Bladder	25 921	2. 02	0. 09	0. 02	0. 00	0. 01	0. 09	0. 09	0. 30	0. 40	0. 63
其他泌尿器官	Other urinary organs	496	0. 04	0. 00	0. 00	0. 00	0. 00	0. 00	0. 01	0. 00	0. 00	0. 01
眼	Eye	727	0. 06	0. 95	0. 52	0. 07	0. 02	0. 02	0. 01	0. 03	0. 02	0. 03
脑、神经系统	Brain, nervous system	33 969	2. 65	2. 32	1. 84	1. 66	1. 68	1. 43	1. 42	2. 39	3. 35	3. 74
甲状腺	Thyroid	60 693	4. 74	0. 00	0. 02	0. 08	0. 20	1. 19	5. 04	12. 88	18. 28	20. 26
肾上腺	Adrenal gland	1 033	0. 08	0. 43	0. 20	0. 06	0. 02	0. 03	0. 01	0. 07	0. 10	0. 11
其他内分泌腺	Other endocrine	1 449	0. 11	0. 04	0. 06	0. 08	0. 20	0. 12	0. 14	0. 16	0. 19	0. 26
霍奇金淋巴瘤	Hodgkin lymphoma	1 365	0. 11	0. 00	0. 04	0. 07	0. 17	0. 21	0. 22	0. 27	0. 26	0. 20
非霍奇金淋巴瘤	Non-Hodgkin lymphoma	19 866	1. 55	0. 19	0. 55	0. 51	0. 66	0. 78	0. 74	1. 07	1. 34	1. 70
免疫增生性疾病	Immunoproliferative diseases	261	0. 02	0. 02	0. 01	0. 01	0. 01	0. 02	0. 00	0. 01	0. 01	0. 01
多发性骨髓瘤	Multiple myeloma	6 688	0. 52	0. 00	0. 05	0. 02	0. 04	0. 06	0. 06	0. 08	0. 11	0. 16
淋巴样白血病	Lymphoid leukemia	5 240	0. 41	1. 50	2. 62	1. 78	0. 94	0. 67	0. 44	0. 54	0. 52	0. 44
髓样白血病	Myeloid leukemia	13 526	1. 06	1. 10	0. 73	0. 62	1. 03	0. 94	1. 03	1. 34	1. 45	1. 44
白血病,未特指	Leukemia unspecified	8 394	0. 66	2. 19	1. 40	0. 98	0. 91	0. 86	0. 64	0. 81	0. 89	0. 70
其他或未指明部位	Other and unspecified	23 108	1. 80	1. 85	1. 09	0. 60	0. 50	0. 61	0. 63	1. 05	1. 21	1. 49
所有部位合计	All sites	1 281 357	100. 00	14. 76	11. 44	7. 94	9. 16	11. 35	17. 72	38. 21	62. 72	88. 19
所有部位除外 C44	All sites except C44	1 270 077	99. 12	14. 70	11. 35	7. 86	9. 04	11. 14	17. 50	37. 93	62. 27	87. 64

Appendix

Appendix 1 Cancer incidence and mortality in registration areas of China,2017

Appendix Table 1-1 Cancer incidence in registration areas of China,both sexes in 2017

Age group										粗率 Crude rate/ 100 000^{-1}	中标率 ASR China/ 100 000^{-1}	世标率 ASR world/ 100 000^{-1}	累积率 Cum. rate/%		ICD10
40~44	45~49	50~54	55~59	60~64	65~69	70~74	75~79	80~84	85+				0~64	0~74	
0.05	0.08	0.18	0.19	0.32	0.52	0.72	1.14	1.34	1.55	0.17	0.10	0.10	0.00	0.01	C00
0.48	0.83	1.44	1.58	2.00	2.14	2.62	2.64	3.00	2.64	0.80	0.52	0.51	0.03	0.06	C01-02
0.39	0.67	1.43	1.52	2.90	3.58	4.10	5.21	5.35	5.55	1.07	0.67	0.66	0.04	0.08	C03-06
0.40	0.65	0.95	0.96	1.41	1.47	1.77	1.73	1.37	1.18	0.60	0.44	0.41	0.03	0.04	C07-08
0.10	0.23	0.41	0.35	0.36	0.46	0.44	0.40	0.46	0.35	0.16	0.11	0.11	0.01	0.01	C09
0.11	0.16	0.44	0.49	0.79	0.89	1.03	1.09	0.97	1.00	0.27	0.17	0.17	0.01	0.02	C10
4.36	5.66	7.85	5.90	8.01	8.25	7.23	6.30	5.93	4.34	3.63	2.64	2.47	0.19	0.27	C11
0.11	0.36	0.98	1.19	1.67	1.74	1.53	1.55	1.40	1.00	0.49	0.30	0.31	0.02	0.04	C12-13
0.07	0.15	0.34	0.39	0.73	0.77	1.08	1.02	1.10	1.31	0.24	0.15	0.15	0.01	0.02	C14
1.62	5.48	16.35	24.55	52.94	81.28	103.09	116.71	124.39	110.13	19.23	11.14	11.25	0.51	1.43	C15
6.86	13.14	29.37	38.09	74.57	106.92	134.89	162.80	171.51	144.95	28.24	16.88	16.78	0.85	2.06	C16
0.44	0.82	1.56	1.77	3.04	3.99	4.85	5.63	6.27	5.41	1.17	0.72	0.71	0.04	0.09	C17
4.53	7.94	15.62	20.15	34.65	47.70	60.45	76.26	93.52	82.92	14.12	8.54	8.40	0.44	0.99	C18
4.79	8.96	17.87	21.27	38.71	51.73	62.09	73.46	82.95	70.24	14.48	8.78	8.71	0.48	1.05	C19-20
0.13	0.22	0.46	0.42	0.82	1.18	1.55	2.07	2.20	2.18	0.36	0.22	0.21	0.01	0.02	C21
16.29	27.16	45.54	47.09	71.22	86.06	96.52	114.05	123.14	120.39	28.17	17.82	17.50	1.11	2.03	C22
0.70	1.65	3.51	5.10	9.48	14.11	18.78	25.03	31.19	30.94	4.00	2.30	2.30	0.11	0.27	C23-24
1.59	3.23	6.83	9.16	17.18	24.25	32.69	43.11	52.85	49.80	7.07	4.13	4.11	0.20	0.48	C25
0.28	0.49	0.73	0.81	1.07	1.25	1.56	1.60	1.90	1.51	0.47	0.31	0.30	0.02	0.03	C30-31
0.36	0.87	2.68	3.46	6.06	6.96	7.79	8.47	8.07	5.24	1.84	1.11	1.13	0.07	0.14	C32
14.30	28.90	67.86	89.70	171.29	233.30	296.43	354.54	388.25	339.78	62.95	37.29	37.28	1.92	4.57	C33-34
0.58	0.91	1.51	1.56	2.28	2.70	3.13	2.88	3.02	2.95	0.95	0.66	0.65	0.04	0.07	C37-38
0.84	1.21	2.13	2.25	3.88	4.99	6.38	7.47	8.35	7.88	1.83	1.34	1.31	0.08	0.13	C40-41
0.22	0.40	0.63	0.64	1.12	1.50	1.97	2.34	2.77	3.08	0.51	0.33	0.32	0.02	0.04	C43
0.85	1.34	2.31	2.56	4.94	7.13	10.39	14.21	22.21	30.31	2.59	1.54	1.52	0.07	0.16	C44
0.04	0.09	0.21	0.28	0.44	0.44	0.49	0.53	0.68	0.50	0.14	0.09	0.09	0.01	0.01	C45
0.01	0.01	0.04	0.04	0.03	0.06	0.10	0.09	0.16	0.11	0.02	0.02	0.02	0.00	0.00	C46
0.70	0.85	1.17	1.23	1.94	2.14	2.30	2.84	3.12	2.97	0.92	0.70	0.68	0.04	0.07	C47;C49
56.40	82.18	96.59	77.90	92.45	78.44	64.52	61.22	55.47	39.81	42.51	30.08	28.11	2.30	3.01	C50
0.25	0.39	0.59	0.61	1.07	1.46	1.87	2.00	2.68	2.91	0.49	0.30	0.29	0.02	0.03	C51
0.18	0.29	0.44	0.38	0.66	0.89	1.10	0.95	0.92	0.55	0.27	0.17	0.17	0.01	0.02	C52
22.86	33.02	43.89	30.10	31.81	28.47	25.84	23.23	20.52	14.13	17.07	12.28	11.35	0.93	1.20	C53
7.23	14.07	25.71	20.02	20.23	17.45	13.80	10.81	8.03	4.77	8.44	5.71	5.52	0.47	0.62	C54
1.48	2.80	3.70	2.78	3.43	3.75	3.50	3.74	3.43	3.53	1.62	1.08	1.03	0.08	0.11	C55
6.84	11.40	16.85	13.56	17.29	16.96	16.78	15.58	13.30	8.01	7.66	5.43	5.17	0.39	0.56	C56
0.45	0.78	1.36	1.10	1.56	1.28	1.26	1.03	1.30	1.06	0.58	0.39	0.38	0.03	0.04	C57
0.11	0.12	0.11	0.03	0.02	0.02	0.00	0.02	0.00	0.00	0.09	0.10	0.08	0.01	0.01	C58
0.31	0.67	1.05	1.25	1.84	2.50	3.40	3.49	4.16	4.80	0.77	0.50	0.49	0.03	0.06	C60
0.21	0.59	2.16	5.91	18.72	40.57	73.83	115.20	151.48	155.09	11.57	6.64	6.54	0.14	0.71	C61
0.62	0.47	0.40	0.34	0.42	0.67	0.51	0.74	0.76	1.31	0.46	0.43	0.40	0.03	0.03	C62
0.02	0.10	0.12	0.28	0.39	0.71	0.84	0.74	1.39	0.98	0.18	0.12	0.12	0.01	0.01	C63
1.96	3.60	7.11	7.33	10.56	12.81	13.14	13.56	13.63	11.09	3.99	2.61	2.59	0.17	0.30	C64
0.06	0.21	0.48	0.63	1.22	1.75	2.25	2.99	3.40	2.88	0.48	0.29	0.28	0.01	0.03	C65
0.08	0.15	0.34	0.74	1.21	2.02	2.90	4.22	4.71	3.69	0.56	0.32	0.32	0.01	0.04	C66
1.21	2.16	5.15	6.89	13.50	19.91	26.97	38.56	50.19	49.50	5.94	3.43	3.40	0.15	0.39	C67
0.02	0.05	0.11	0.12	0.23	0.35	0.57	0.71	1.11	0.85	0.11	0.07	0.06	0.00	0.01	C68
0.08	0.08	0.19	0.14	0.35	0.46	0.37	0.52	0.70	0.70	0.17	0.12	0.16	0.01	0.01	C69
5.08	7.88	12.31	11.72	17.25	20.92	21.99	24.16	24.90	23.06	7.79	5.62	5.51	0.36	0.57	C70-72,D32-33,D42-43
20.41	22.47	29.06	21.71	19.74	14.29	9.60	6.70	5.20	3.93	13.91	11.94	10.30	0.86	0.98	C73
0.15	0.21	0.37	0.39	0.46	0.58	0.68	0.69	0.79	0.83	0.24	0.17	0.18	0.01	0.02	C74
0.29	0.35	0.51	0.52	0.70	0.76	0.64	0.65	0.62	0.66	0.33	0.27	0.25	0.02	0.02	C75
0.20	0.22	0.36	0.36	0.51	0.78	0.75	0.84	0.94	0.87	0.31	0.26	0.25	0.02	0.02	C81
2.22	3.50	6.27	6.45	10.88	14.24	16.11	19.06	19.77	15.26	4.55	3.10	3.03	0.18	0.33	C82-C86;C96
0.02	0.03	0.05	0.08	0.14	0.26	0.26	0.33	0.25	0.11	0.06	0.04	0.04	0.00	0.00	C88
0.40	0.75	1.88	2.39	4.45	6.12	7.15	7.63	7.20	5.15	1.53	0.94	0.94	0.05	0.12	C90
0.51	0.68	1.20	1.07	2.08	2.32	2.78	3.80	3.51	2.75	1.20	1.04	1.20	0.07	0.09	C91
1.99	2.63	3.90	3.96	6.08	8.17	9.96	11.53	12.44	9.34	3.10	2.30	2.24	0.14	0.23	C92-C94,D45-47
1.12	1.39	2.09	2.10	3.38	4.61	6.05	7.10	8.35	7.14	1.92	1.49	1.54	0.09	0.14	C95
2.48	3.84	6.34	7.13	11.58	15.15	19.01	24.05	30.34	34.08	5.30	3.45	3.45	0.19	0.36	O&U
147.78	235.99	403.66	433.43	713.41	920.62	1 112.03	1 322.67	1 465.77	1 313.11	293.66	188.10	183.68	10.91	21.07	C00-96, D32-33, D42-43,D45-47
146.93	234.65	401.35	430.87	708.47	913.50	1 101.63	1 308.46	1 443.56	1 282.80	291.08	186.56	182.16	10.84	20.91	C00-96, D32-33, D42-43,D45-47 exc. C44

附表 1-2　2017 年全国肿瘤登记地区男性癌症发病主要指标

部位 Site		病例数 No. cases	构成 Freq. /%	年龄组								
				0~	1~4	5~9	10~14	15~19	20~24	25~29	30~34	35~39
唇	Lip	427	0. 06	0. 00	0. 03	0. 02	0. 02	0. 02	0. 01	0. 01	0. 02	0. 04
舌	Tongue	2 309	0. 32	0. 00	0. 02	0. 00	0. 02	0. 02	0. 04	0. 11	0. 23	0. 39
口	Mouth	2 995	0. 42	0. 00	0. 01	0. 03	0. 07	0. 04	0. 07	0. 11	0. 22	0. 23
唾液腺	Salivary glands	1 475	0. 21	0. 00	0. 01	0. 01	0. 10	0. 07	0. 20	0. 26	0. 26	0. 42
扁桃腺	Tonsil	515	0. 07	0. 00	0. 01	0. 01	0. 01	0. 00	0. 02	0. 01	0. 02	0. 04
其他口咽	Other oropharynx	991	0. 14	0. 00	0. 00	0. 02	0. 02	0. 02	0. 01	0. 02	0. 04	0. 12
鼻咽	Nasopharynx	11 185	1. 57	0. 04	0. 01	0. 04	0. 13	0. 36	0. 49	1. 22	2. 49	3. 52
下咽	Hypopharynx	1 990	0. 28	0. 00	0. 00	0. 02	0. 01	0. 04	0. 01	0. 01	0. 01	0. 05
咽,部位不明	Pharynx unspecified	822	0. 12	0. 00	0. 00	0. 02	0. 00	0. 02	0. 01	0. 02	0. 01	0. 04
食管	Esophagus	61 585	8. 65	0. 04	0. 01	0. 00	0. 01	0. 01	0. 10	0. 18	0. 25	0. 61
胃	Stomach	86 224	12. 12	0. 04	0. 03	0. 02	0. 08	0. 16	0. 37	0. 91	1. 99	3. 25
小肠	Small intestine	2 925	0. 41	0. 00	0. 00	0. 01	0. 01	0. 00	0. 03	0. 08	0. 17	0. 31
结肠	Colon	34 556	4. 86	0. 00	0. 01	0. 01	0. 08	0. 11	0. 34	1. 06	1. 87	3. 09
直肠	Rectum	38 503	5. 41	0. 08	0. 00	0. 03	0. 03	0. 11	0. 22	0. 79	1. 46	2. 44
肛门	Anus	915	0. 13	0. 00	0. 00	0. 01	0. 00	0. 00	0. 03	0. 02	0. 03	0. 08
肝脏	Liver	90 767	12. 76	1. 22	0. 46	0. 11	0. 19	0. 43	0. 79	2. 95	6. 67	12. 58
胆囊及其他	Gallbladder etc.	8 206	1. 15	0. 04	0. 01	0. 00	0. 00	0. 02	0. 02	0. 07	0. 19	0. 29
胰腺	Pancreas	17 732	2. 49	0. 04	0. 02	0. 01	0. 02	0. 03	0. 06	0. 15	0. 42	0. 90
鼻、鼻窦及其他	Nose, sinuses etc.	1 270	0. 18	0. 04	0. 06	0. 02	0. 04	0. 07	0. 09	0. 10	0. 16	0. 21
喉	Larynx	7 290	1. 02	0. 00	0. 03	0. 02	0. 00	0. 03	0. 02	0. 02	0. 06	0. 20
气管、支气管、肺	Trachea, bronchus & lung	181 959	25. 57	0. 04	0. 07	0. 09	0. 10	0. 30	0. 52	1. 36	3. 17	5. 61
其他胸腔器官	Other thoracic organs	2 511	0. 35	0. 24	0. 15	0. 04	0. 08	0. 34	0. 23	0. 39	0. 39	0. 42
骨	Bone	4 519	0. 64	0. 04	0. 26	0. 31	1. 21	1. 21	0. 64	0. 68	0. 65	0. 69
皮肤黑色素瘤	Melanoma of skin	1 166	0. 16	0. 00	0. 08	0. 06	0. 06	0. 01	0. 04	0. 06	0. 16	0. 18
皮肤其他	Other skin	5 712	0. 80	0. 00	0. 10	0. 09	0. 10	0. 25	0. 20	0. 30	0. 47	0. 51
间皮瘤	Mesothelioma	345	0. 05	0. 00	0. 00	0. 00	0. 00	0. 00	0. 01	0. 01	0. 02	0. 07
卡波氏肉瘤	Kaposi sarcoma	66	0. 01	0. 04	0. 01	0. 01	0. 00	0. 01	0. 02	0. 01	0. 00	0. 01
结缔组织、软组织	Connective & soft tissue	2 135	0. 30	0. 61	0. 35	0. 20	0. 23	0. 21	0. 34	0. 45	0. 51	0. 50
乳腺	Breast	1 216	0. 17	0. 00	0. 00	0. 00	0. 00	0. 02	0. 05	0. 07	0. 16	0. 25
外阴	Vulva	—	—	—	—	—	—	—	—	—	—	—
阴道	Vagina	—	—	—	—	—	—	—	—	—	—	—
子宫颈	Cervix uteri	—	—	—	—	—	—	—	—	—	—	—
子宫体	Corpus uteri	—	—	—	—	—	—	—	—	—	—	—
子宫,部位不明	Uterus unspecified	—	—	—	—	—	—	—	—	—	—	—
卵巢	Ovary	—	—	—	—	—	—	—	—	—	—	—
其他女性生殖器	Other female genital organs	—	—	—	—	—	—	—	—	—	—	—
胎盘	Placenta	—	—	—	—	—	—	—	—	—	—	—
阴茎	Penis	1 698	0. 24	0. 00	0. 00	0. 01	0. 01	0. 03	0. 02	0. 04	0. 12	0. 21
前列腺	Prostate	25 577	3. 59	0. 04	0. 00	0. 00	0. 00	0. 05	0. 03	0. 04	0. 09	0. 08
睾丸	Testis	1 024	0. 14	0. 53	0. 31	0. 05	0. 04	0. 16	0. 35	0. 65	0. 79	0. 65
其他男性生殖器	Other male genital organs	391	0. 05	0. 00	0. 03	0. 01	0. 03	0. 03	0. 01	0. 04	0. 07	0. 05
肾	Kidney	11 246	1. 58	0. 69	0. 57	0. 12	0. 08	0. 10	0. 22	0. 46	1. 10	1. 62
肾盂	Renal pelvis	1 221	0. 17	0. 00	0. 01	0. 01	0. 00	0. 02	0. 00	0. 01	0. 07	0. 08
输尿管	Ureter	1 313	0. 18	0. 12	0. 00	0. 00	0. 00	0. 00	0. 01	0. 02	0. 02	0. 02
膀胱	Bladder	20 485	2. 88	0. 04	0. 02	0. 00	0. 02	0. 12	0. 08	0. 39	0. 66	0. 91
其他泌尿器官	Other urinary organs	313	0. 04	0. 00	0. 00	0. 01	0. 00	0. 00	0. 02	0. 01	0. 01	0. 01
眼	Eye	381	0. 05	0. 93	0. 55	0. 07	0. 03	0. 03	0. 01	0. 04	0. 02	0. 03
脑、神经系统	Brain, nervous system	15 790	2. 22	2. 84	1. 92	1. 84	1. 87	1. 56	1. 65	2. 52	3. 59	3. 53
甲状腺	Thyroid	14 572	2. 05	0. 00	0. 00	0. 04	0. 09	0. 65	2. 52	6. 85	10. 40	10. 99
肾上腺	Adrenal gland	575	0. 08	0. 45	0. 17	0. 07	0. 02	0. 04	0. 00	0. 05	0. 11	0. 11
其他内分泌腺	Other endocrine	737	0. 10	0. 04	0. 07	0. 09	0. 30	0. 14	0. 13	0. 12	0. 18	0. 17
霍奇金淋巴瘤	Hodgkin lymphoma	833	0. 12	0. 00	0. 05	0. 13	0. 23	0. 25	0. 23	0. 30	0. 24	0. 21
非霍奇金淋巴瘤	Non-Hodgkin lymphoma	11 442	1. 61	0. 20	0. 62	0. 63	0. 94	0. 99	0. 90	1. 18	1. 36	1. 91
免疫增生性疾病	Immunoproliferative diseases	170	0. 02	0. 04	0. 02	0. 01	0. 01	0. 03	0. 00	0. 01	0. 01	0. 01
多发性骨髓瘤	Multiple myeloma	3 823	0. 54	0. 00	0. 06	0. 02	0. 04	0. 07	0. 08	0. 10	0. 16	0. 21
淋巴样白血病	Lymphoid leukemia	3 042	0. 43	1. 62	2. 94	2. 05	1. 03	0. 91	0. 55	0. 60	0. 59	0. 50
髓样白血病	Myeloid leukemia	7 580	1. 07	1. 10	0. 86	0. 61	1. 14	1. 06	1. 11	1. 56	1. 61	1. 52
白血病,未特指	Leukemia unspecified	4 845	0. 68	2. 39	1. 66	1. 04	1. 13	1. 05	0. 75	0. 98	1. 07	0. 75
其他或未指明部位	Other and unspecified	12 249	1. 72	1. 42	1. 11	0. 61	0. 57	0. 52	0. 60	0. 91	1. 17	1. 40
所有部位合计	All sites	711 618	100. 00	14. 97	12. 68	8. 59	10. 17	11. 70	14. 24	28. 30	45. 55	62. 00
所有部位除外 C44	All sites except C44	705 906	99. 20	14. 97	12. 58	8. 51	10. 06	11. 45	14. 05	28. 00	45. 08	61. 49

Appendix Table 1-2 Cancer incidence in registration areas of China, male in 2017

Age group										粗率 Crude rate/ 100 000^{-1}	中标率 ASR China/ 100 000^{-1}	世标率 ASR world/ 100 000^{-1}	累积率 Cum. rate/%		ICD10
40~44	45~49	50~54	55~59	60~64	65~69	70~74	75~79	80~84	85+				0~64	0~74	
0.05	0.12	0.19	0.24	0.42	0.65	0.86	1.14	1.62	1.64	0.19	0.12	0.12	0.01	0.01	C00
0.67	1.20	2.07	2.29	2.64	3.02	2.96	3.15	3.67	3.33	1.04	0.70	0.68	0.05	0.08	C01-02
0.49	0.93	2.14	2.18	3.96	4.75	5.12	5.86	6.71	7.69	1.35	0.87	0.87	0.05	0.10	C03-06
0.43	0.68	1.01	1.08	1.79	1.71	2.22	2.12	1.98	1.64	0.67	0.48	0.46	0.03	0.05	C07-08
0.11	0.26	0.65	0.56	0.49	0.79	0.60	0.57	0.83	0.33	0.23	0.15	0.15	0.01	0.02	C09
0.18	0.26	0.77	0.86	1.40	1.64	1.65	1.90	1.62	1.53	0.45	0.29	0.29	0.02	0.04	C10
5.96	8.08	11.33	8.68	11.40	11.47	10.20	9.63	8.46	5.40	5.06	3.72	3.47	0.27	0.38	C11
0.18	0.66	1.81	2.26	3.17	3.36	2.84	2.90	2.81	1.96	0.90	0.57	0.58	0.04	0.07	C12-13
0.11	0.25	0.58	0.65	1.18	1.20	1.73	1.65	1.78	1.69	0.37	0.23	0.24	0.01	0.03	C14
2.58	9.11	27.10	40.90	84.17	123.79	150.52	164.99	170.08	155.63	27.85	16.91	17.14	0.83	2.20	C15
7.76	16.68	39.96	56.14	113.32	158.70	199.66	237.49	244.16	203.28	38.99	24.04	24.05	1.20	3.00	C16
0.59	1.02	1.76	2.12	3.43	4.71	5.50	6.43	7.43	6.98	1.32	0.85	0.83	0.05	0.10	C17
4.92	8.53	17.47	23.43	40.34	55.95	71.20	88.66	105.50	102.92	15.63	9.81	9.69	0.51	1.14	C18
5.20	10.31	21.30	26.77	49.50	66.96	79.30	91.75	103.52	90.98	17.41	10.91	10.86	0.59	1.32	C19-20
0.14	0.27	0.47	0.57	1.06	1.53	2.07	2.31	2.58	2.07	0.41	0.26	0.26	0.01	0.03	C21
27.44	45.35	73.74	74.90	108.90	125.25	133.19	152.76	157.89	158.69	41.05	27.08	26.53	1.77	3.07	C22
0.64	1.56	3.21	5.48	9.75	14.42	18.00	23.32	28.04	30.31	3.71	2.25	2.26	0.11	0.27	C23-24
1.96	4.18	8.68	11.76	20.92	28.67	37.93	48.65	58.50	58.76	8.02	4.92	4.91	0.25	0.58	C25
0.32	0.60	0.87	1.09	1.46	1.58	2.00	1.97	2.77	1.69	0.57	0.39	0.38	0.03	0.04	C30~31
0.62	1.56	4.99	6.51	11.28	12.94	14.25	15.38	15.39	10.52	3.30	2.04	2.07	0.13	0.26	C32
14.87	32.72	84.34	121.85	237.82	329.68	418.52	502.17	538.66	479.39	82.28	50.36	50.56	2.51	6.25	C33-34
0.60	1.03	1.71	1.95	2.94	3.40	3.97	3.49	3.96	3.87	1.14	0.81	0.79	0.05	0.09	C37-38
0.90	1.45	2.15	2.54	4.55	5.88	7.50	9.44	9.88	8.94	2.04	1.54	1.51	0.09	0.15	C40-41
0.19	0.37	0.63	0.66	1.27	1.54	2.16	2.67	3.70	3.65	0.53	0.35	0.34	0.02	0.04	C43
0.86	1.35	2.40	2.74	5.60	7.86	11.59	14.09	23.58	30.25	2.58	1.63	1.61	0.07	0.17	C44
0.04	0.09	0.26	0.32	0.46	0.56	0.53	0.55	0.86	0.71	0.16	0.10	0.10	0.01	0.01	C45
0.01	0.01	0.05	0.06	0.02	0.09	0.11	0.17	0.23	0.16	0.03	0.02	0.02	0.00	0.00	C46
0.71	0.80	1.22	1.34	2.17	2.37	2.66	3.41	3.96	3.60	0.97	0.73	0.72	0.05	0.07	C47;C49
0.43	0.56	0.87	0.97	1.15	1.68	1.73	2.24	2.41	3.00	0.55	0.37	0.36	0.02	0.04	C50
—	—	—	—	—	—	—	—	—	—	—	—	—	—	—	C51
—	—	—	—	—	—	—	—	—	—	—	—	—	—	—	C52
—	—	—	—	—	—	—	—	—	—	—	—	—	—	—	C53
—	—	—	—	—	—	—	—	—	—	—	—	—	—	—	C54
—	—	—	—	—	—	—	—	—	—	—	—	—	—	—	C55
—	—	—	—	—	—	—	—	—	—	—	—	—	—	—	C56
—	—	—	—	—	—	—	—	—	—	—	—	—	—	—	C57
—	—	—	—	—	—	—	—	—	—	—	—	—	—	—	C58
0.31	0.67	1.05	1.25	1.84	2.50	3.40	3.49	4.16	4.80	0.77	0.50	0.49	0.03	0.06	C60
0.21	0.59	2.16	5.91	18.72	40.57	73.83	115.20	151.48	155.09	11.57	6.64	6.54	0.14	0.71	C61
0.62	0.47	0.40	0.34	0.42	0.67	0.51	0.74	0.76	1.31	0.46	0.43	0.40	0.03	0.03	C62
0.02	0.10	0.12	0.28	0.39	0.71	0.84	0.74	1.39	0.98	0.18	0.12	0.12	0.01	0.01	C63
2.63	4.60	9.18	9.69	14.14	16.74	16.91	18.39	18.37	15.43	5.09	3.39	3.36	0.22	0.39	C64
0.07	0.25	0.66	0.83	1.59	2.12	2.55	3.05	3.67	3.33	0.55	0.34	0.34	0.02	0.04	C65
0.10	0.17	0.40	0.96	1.54	2.24	2.99	4.38	4.89	3.87	0.59	0.36	0.36	0.02	0.04	C66
1.90	3.50	8.08	11.28	21.96	32.15	43.10	63.72	84.86	93.87	9.26	5.59	5.56	0.24	0.62	C67
0.02	0.06	0.13	0.14	0.28	0.43	0.72	0.99	1.65	1.36	0.14	0.09	0.08	0.00	0.01	C68
0.07	0.08	0.20	0.18	0.36	0.48	0.44	0.53	0.63	0.60	0.17	0.13	0.17	0.01	0.01	C69
4.79	7.28	10.75	9.85	15.88	19.24	21.10	22.68	23.65	23.93	7.14	5.37	5.26	0.34	0.54	C70-72,D32-33,D42-43
9.98	9.73	11.59	8.95	8.63	7.07	5.65	4.51	3.44	3.11	6.59	5.88	4.97	0.40	0.47	C73
0.13	0.21	0.41	0.49	0.56	0.65	0.69	0.97	1.12	1.09	0.26	0.19	0.19	0.01	0.02	C74
0.29	0.30	0.49	0.53	0.72	0.87	0.80	0.76	0.76	0.60	0.33	0.27	0.26	0.02	0.03	C75
0.26	0.28	0.47	0.49	0.68	1.00	0.86	1.06	1.26	1.04	0.38	0.31	0.30	0.02	0.03	C81
2.51	3.87	7.00	7.28	12.75	16.91	18.69	23.70	23.82	21.53	5.17	3.61	3.54	0.21	0.39	C82-C86;C96
0.02	0.03	0.07	0.10	0.18	0.40	0.36	0.40	0.40	0.27	0.08	0.05	0.05	0.00	0.01	C88
0.48	0.86	2.07	2.72	4.93	6.90	8.27	8.95	9.38	8.50	1.73	1.09	1.10	0.06	0.13	C90
0.55	0.77	1.17	1.15	2.40	2.77	3.02	4.74	4.56	4.69	1.38	1.20	1.38	0.07	0.10	C91
2.15	2.75	4.34	4.34	6.76	8.99	11.41	14.09	16.35	13.63	3.43	2.58	2.51	0.15	0.25	C92-C94,D45-47
1.25	1.62	2.28	2.32	4.01	5.23	6.88	8.34	10.70	10.47	2.19	1.73	1.79	0.10	0.16	C95
2.22	3.60	6.37	7.69	12.95	17.91	21.94	28.21	33.76	39.79	5.54	3.68	3.69	0.20	0.40	O&U
109.53	191.75	383.11	477.67	858.26	1 162.71	1 435.54	1 730.51	1 913.60	1 789.88	321.80	206.07	204.34	11.07	24.06	C00-96, D32-33, D42-43,D45-47
108.66	190.40	380.72	474.92	852.66	1 154.85	1 423.95	1 716.41	1 890.02	1 759.62	319.22	204.44	202.73	11.00	23.89	C00-96, D32-33, D42-43,D45-47 exc. C44

附表 1-3 2017 年全国肿瘤登记地区女性癌症发病主要指标

部位 Site		病例数 No. cases	构成 Freq. /%	年龄组								
				0~	1~4	5~9	10~14	15~19	20~24	25~29	30~34	35~39
唇	Lip	327	0.06	0.05	0.01	0.00	0.01	0.00	0.01	0.01	0.02	0.01
舌	Tongue	1 188	0.21	0.00	0.01	0.02	0.00	0.01	0.02	0.07	0.17	0.21
口	Mouth	1 660	0.29	0.05	0.01	0.04	0.02	0.09	0.06	0.09	0.12	0.22
唾液腺	Salivary glands	1 124	0.20	0.05	0.00	0.01	0.08	0.10	0.18	0.27	0.25	0.44
扁桃腺	Tonsil	203	0.04	0.00	0.00	0.00	0.00	0.00	0.02	0.01	0.03	0.03
其他口咽	Other oropharynx	187	0.03	0.00	0.02	0.02	0.00	0.00	0.01	0.01	0.03	0.04
鼻咽	Nasopharynx	4 653	0.82	0.05	0.00	0.04	0.09	0.20	0.29	0.62	1.18	1.60
下咽	Hypopharynx	149	0.03	0.05	0.00	0.01	0.00	0.00	0.00	0.02	0.01	0.03
咽,部位不明	Pharynx unspecified	235	0.04	0.00	0.01	0.01	0.02	0.01	0.01	0.01	0.01	0.02
食管	Esophagus	22 316	3.92	0.14	0.03	0.02	0.01	0.02	0.03	0.13	0.11	0.31
胃	Stomach	36 976	6.49	0.09	0.01	0.01	0.04	0.18	0.43	1.46	2.50	3.36
小肠	Small intestine	2 190	0.38	0.00	0.00	0.00	0.01	0.00	0.05	0.06	0.13	0.22
结肠	Colon	27 057	4.75	0.00	0.00	0.01	0.05	0.14	0.30	0.94	1.69	2.35
直肠	Rectum	24 682	4.33	0.05	0.01	0.01	0.04	0.04	0.14	0.73	1.23	1.79
肛门	Anus	643	0.11	0.00	0.00	0.00	0.00	0.01	0.01	0.01	0.01	0.10
肝脏	Liver	32 131	5.64	1.10	0.25	0.12	0.15	0.31	0.35	0.92	1.29	2.39
胆囊及其他	Gallbladder etc.	9 236	1.62	0.05	0.02	0.00	0.00	0.01	0.04	0.05	0.15	0.36
胰腺	Pancreas	13 137	2.31	0.09	0.02	0.04	0.06	0.05	0.11	0.18	0.30	0.61
鼻、鼻窦及其他	Nose, sinuses etc.	759	0.13	0.00	0.04	0.02	0.02	0.02	0.06	0.08	0.14	0.13
喉	Larynx	726	0.13	0.09	0.01	0.01	0.01	0.02	0.03	0.05	0.02	0.04
气管、支气管、肺	Trachea, bronchus & lung	92 731	16.28	0.05	0.05	0.01	0.10	0.11	0.53	1.44	3.34	6.02
其他胸腔器官	Other thoracic organs	1 634	0.29	0.41	0.09	0.04	0.05	0.13	0.12	0.14	0.27	0.32
骨	Bone	3 448	0.61	0.05	0.20	0.35	0.80	0.65	0.57	0.56	0.61	0.52
皮肤黑色素瘤	Melanoma of skin	1 059	0.19	0.00	0.04	0.04	0.02	0.03	0.06	0.12	0.13	0.22
皮肤其他	Other skin	5 568	0.98	0.14	0.08	0.09	0.13	0.16	0.23	0.27	0.43	0.59
间皮瘤	Mesothelioma	284	0.05	0.00	0.00	0.00	0.00	0.02	0.01	0.04	0.01	0.08
卡波氏肉瘤	Kaposi sarcoma	41	0.01	0.00	0.01	0.00	0.01	0.04	0.01	0.01	0.01	0.00
结缔组织、软组织	Connective & soft tissue	1 873	0.33	0.64	0.23	0.16	0.33	0.32	0.30	0.45	0.56	0.51
乳腺	Breast	91 475	16.06	0.09	0.00	0.00	0.14	0.32	1.86	6.16	16.20	29.40
外阴	Vulva	1 056	0.19	0.05	0.01	0.00	0.00	0.02	0.05	0.04	0.08	0.20
阴道	Vagina	590	0.10	0.05	0.01	0.00	0.00	0.01	0.01	0.00	0.04	0.11
子宫颈	Cervix uteri	36 740	6.45	0.00	0.00	0.00	0.00	0.09	0.57	2.82	7.58	13.57
子宫体	Corpus uteri	18 167	3.19	0.00	0.00	0.00	0.00	0.05	0.13	0.84	1.76	3.22
子宫,部位不明	Uterus unspecified	3 479	0.61	0.00	0.00	0.00	0.00	0.03	0.05	0.21	0.41	0.66
卵巢	Ovary	16 479	2.89	0.09	0.10	0.20	0.55	1.10	1.87	2.30	2.91	3.39
其他女性生殖器	Other female genital organs	1 254	0.22	0.05	0.02	0.00	0.01	0.05	0.08	0.13	0.14	0.23
胎盘	Placenta	202	0.04	0.00	0.00	0.01	0.01	0.03	0.12	0.28	0.24	0.15
阴茎	Penis	—	—	—	—	—	—	—	—	—	—	—
前列腺	Prostate	—	—	—	—	—	—	—	—	—	—	—
睾丸	Testis	—	—	—	—	—	—	—	—	—	—	—
其他男性生殖器	Other male genital organs	—	—	—	—	—	—	—	—	—	—	—
肾	Kidney	6 170	1.08	0.82	0.62	0.16	0.03	0.07	0.22	0.35	0.65	0.98
肾盂	Renal pelvis	888	0.16	0.00	0.01	0.01	0.01	0.00	0.02	0.00	0.04	0.02
输尿管	Ureter	1 123	0.20	0.05	0.00	0.00	0.00	0.00	0.00	0.00	0.03	0.01
膀胱	Bladder	5 436	0.95	0.14	0.01	0.01	0.01	0.05	0.10	0.21	0.14	0.34
其他泌尿器官	Other urinary organs	183	0.03	0.00	0.00	0.00	0.00	0.00	0.00	0.00	0.00	0.01
眼	Eye	346	0.06	0.96	0.48	0.06	0.01	0.00	0.00	0.02	0.03	0.03
脑、神经系统	Brain, nervous system	18 179	3.19	1.74	1.75	1.45	1.46	1.29	1.18	2.26	3.11	3.94
甲状腺	Thyroid	46 121	8.10	0.00	0.03	0.13	0.33	1.79	7.67	19.03	26.18	29.64
肾上腺	Adrenal gland	458	0.08	0.41	0.23	0.05	0.02	0.01	0.02	0.08	0.09	0.11
其他内分泌腺	Other endocrine	712	0.12	0.05	0.04	0.06	0.08	0.09	0.15	0.19	0.20	0.35
霍奇金淋巴瘤	Hodgkin lymphoma	532	0.09	0.00	0.02	0.01	0.11	0.17	0.22	0.24	0.28	0.19
非霍奇金淋巴瘤	Non-Hodgkin lymphoma	8 424	1.48	0.18	0.47	0.37	0.34	0.55	0.57	0.95	1.32	1.49
免疫增生性疾病	Immunoproliferative diseases	91	0.02	0.00	0.00	0.01	0.01	0.00	0.01	0.01	0.00	0.02
多发性骨髓瘤	Multiple myeloma	2 865	0.50	0.00	0.03	0.01	0.03	0.05	0.03	0.06	0.06	0.11
淋巴样白血病	Lymphoid leukemia	2 198	0.39	1.37	2.25	1.48	0.83	0.40	0.32	0.47	0.45	0.37
髓样白血病	Myeloid leukemia	5 946	1.04	1.10	0.59	0.62	0.91	0.81	0.95	1.12	1.29	1.35
白血病,未特指	Leukemia unspecified	3 549	0.62	1.97	1.10	0.92	0.67	0.66	0.53	0.64	0.72	0.64
其他或未指明部位	Other and unspecified	10 859	1.91	2.33	1.07	0.59	0.41	0.70	0.66	1.19	1.26	1.58
所有部位合计	All sites	569 739	100.00	14.53	10.01	7.21	8.00	10.96	21.35	48.34	79.95	114.66
所有部位除外 C44	All sites except C44	564 171	99.02	14.39	9.93	7.12	7.87	10.80	21.11	48.07	79.53	114.06

Appendix Table 1-3 Cancer incidence in registration areas of China, female in 2017

Age group										粗率 Crude rate/ 100 000^{-1}	中标率 ASR China/ 100 000^{-1}	世标率 ASR world/ 100 000^{-1}	累积率 Cum. rate/%		ICD10
40~44	45~49	50~54	55~59	60~64	65~69	70~74	75~79	80~84	85+				0~64	0~74	
0. 05	0. 05	0. 16	0. 15	0. 22	0. 40	0. 58	1. 15	1. 11	1. 49	0. 15	0. 08	0. 08	0. 00	0. 01	C00
0. 29	0. 46	0. 80	0. 86	1. 35	1. 26	2. 28	2. 18	2. 46	2. 19	0. 55	0. 35	0. 33	0. 02	0. 04	C01-02
0. 29	0. 42	0. 70	0. 83	1. 83	2. 42	3. 11	4. 62	4. 24	4. 12	0. 77	0. 47	0. 46	0. 02	0. 05	C03-06
0. 38	0. 61	0. 89	0. 83	1. 03	1. 23	1. 32	1. 37	0. 87	0. 87	0. 52	0. 39	0. 36	0. 03	0. 04	C07-08
0. 09	0. 19	0. 16	0. 13	0. 23	0. 13	0. 29	0. 25	0. 16	0. 36	0. 09	0. 06	0. 06	0. 00	0. 01	C09
0. 03	0. 05	0. 10	0. 11	0. 17	0. 15	0. 44	0. 36	0. 43	0. 66	0. 09	0. 05	0. 05	0. 00	0. 01	C10
2. 73	3. 21	4. 26	3. 07	4. 59	5. 07	4. 34	3. 30	3. 87	3. 64	2. 16	1. 57	1. 45	0. 11	0. 16	C11
0. 05	0. 05	0. 11	0. 10	0. 16	0. 12	0. 26	0. 32	0. 24	0. 36	0. 07	0. 04	0. 04	0. 00	0. 00	C12-13
0. 03	0. 05	0. 10	0. 12	0. 28	0. 35	0. 45	0. 46	0. 54	1. 06	0. 11	0. 06	0. 07	0. 00	0. 01	C14
0. 63	1. 80	5. 26	7. 91	21. 46	39. 13	57. 22	73. 16	86. 99	79. 73	10. 37	5. 54	5. 52	0. 19	0. 67	C15
5. 94	9. 56	18. 46	19. 72	35. 50	55. 57	72. 26	95. 42	112. 05	105. 99	17. 18	9. 99	9. 75	0. 49	1. 13	C16
0. 29	0. 62	1. 35	1. 41	2. 64	3. 28	4. 21	4. 91	5. 33	4. 37	1. 02	0. 61	0. 60	0. 03	0. 07	C17
4. 14	7. 36	13. 71	16. 80	28. 91	39. 53	50. 05	65. 06	83. 72	69. 57	12. 57	7. 31	7. 17	0. 38	0. 83	C18
4. 37	7. 61	14. 34	15. 66	27. 83	36. 63	45. 44	56. 95	66. 12	56. 38	11. 47	6. 73	6. 63	0. 37	0. 78	C19-20
0. 12	0. 17	0. 46	0. 27	0. 57	0. 83	1. 05	1. 85	1. 89	2. 26	0. 30	0. 17	0. 17	0. 01	0. 02	C21
4. 94	8. 74	16. 48	18. 79	33. 23	47. 20	61. 06	79. 13	94. 70	94. 81	14. 93	8. 61	8. 53	0. 44	0. 98	C22
0. 76	1. 74	3. 83	4. 70	9. 21	13. 79	19. 53	26. 57	33. 77	31. 36	4. 29	2. 35	2. 34	0. 10	0. 27	C23-24
1. 22	2. 26	4. 93	6. 51	13. 41	19. 86	27. 62	38. 11	48. 23	43. 82	6. 10	3. 37	3. 34	0. 15	0. 39	C25
0. 24	0. 37	0. 59	0. 52	0. 68	0. 93	1. 13	1. 26	1. 19	1. 38	0. 35	0. 23	0. 23	0. 01	0. 02	C30-31
0. 09	0. 16	0. 30	0. 36	0. 80	1. 02	1. 54	2. 23	2. 08	1. 71	0. 34	0. 20	0. 20	0. 01	0. 02	C32
13. 73	25. 05	50. 87	56. 99	104. 22	137. 74	178. 38	221. 36	265. 15	246. 50	43. 09	24. 77	24. 54	1. 31	2. 89	C33-34
0. 55	0. 80	1. 30	1. 17	1. 63	1. 99	2. 32	2. 33	2. 24	2. 33	0. 76	0. 52	0. 50	0. 03	0. 05	C37-38
0. 78	0. 97	2. 12	1. 96	3. 21	4. 11	5. 30	5. 69	7. 11	7. 18	1. 60	1. 15	1. 12	0. 07	0. 11	C40-41
0. 24	0. 44	0. 62	0. 61	0. 97	1. 46	1. 79	2. 04	2. 00	2. 70	0. 49	0. 32	0. 31	0. 02	0. 03	C43
0. 83	1. 34	2. 22	2. 38	4. 28	6. 40	9. 24	14. 32	21. 09	30. 34	2. 59	1. 45	1. 43	0. 07	0. 14	C44
0. 05	0. 09	0. 17	0. 24	0. 41	0. 33	0. 45	0. 52	0. 54	0. 36	0. 13	0. 08	0. 08	0. 01	0. 01	C45
0. 01	0. 00	0. 02	0. 02	0. 05	0. 03	0. 09	0. 02	0. 11	0. 07	0. 02	0. 02	0. 02	0. 00	0. 00	C46
0. 70	0. 91	1. 12	1. 12	1. 71	1. 90	1. 95	2. 33	2. 43	2. 55	0. 87	0. 67	0. 65	0. 04	0. 06	C47;C49
56. 40	82. 18	96. 59	77. 90	92. 45	78. 44	64. 52	61. 22	55. 47	39. 81	42. 51	30. 08	28. 11	2. 30	3. 01	C50
0. 25	0. 39	0. 59	0. 61	1. 07	1. 46	1. 87	2. 00	2. 68	2. 91	0. 49	0. 30	0. 29	0. 02	0. 03	C51
0. 18	0. 29	0. 44	0. 38	0. 66	0. 89	1. 10	0. 95	0. 92	0. 55	0. 27	0. 17	0. 17	0. 01	0. 02	C52
22. 86	33. 02	43. 89	30. 10	31. 81	28. 47	25. 84	23. 23	20. 52	14. 13	17. 07	12. 28	11. 35	0. 93	1. 20	C53
7. 23	14. 07	25. 71	20. 02	20. 23	17. 45	13. 80	10. 81	8. 03	4. 77	8. 44	5. 71	5. 52	0. 47	0. 62	C54
1. 48	2. 80	3. 70	2. 78	3. 43	3. 75	3. 50	3. 74	3. 43	3. 53	1. 62	1. 08	1. 03	0. 08	0. 11	C55
6. 84	11. 40	16. 85	13. 56	17. 29	16. 96	16. 78	15. 58	13. 30	8. 01	7. 66	5. 43	5. 17	0. 39	0. 56	C56
0. 45	0. 78	1. 36	1. 10	1. 56	1. 28	1. 26	1. 03	1. 30	1. 06	0. 58	0. 39	0. 38	0. 03	0. 04	C57
0. 11	0. 12	0. 11	0. 03	0. 02	0. 02	0. 00	0. 02	0. 00	0. 00	0. 09	0. 10	0. 08	0. 01	0. 01	C58
—	—	—	—	—	—	—	—	—	—	—	—	—	—	—	C60
—	—	—	—	—	—	—	—	—	—	—	—	—	—	—	C61
—	—	—	—	—	—	—	—	—	—	—	—	—	—	—	C62
—	—	—	—	—	—	—	—	—	—	—	—	—	—	—	C63
1. 29	2. 58	4. 99	4. 93	6. 95	8. 91	9. 49	9. 20	9. 76	8. 19	2. 87	1. 84	1. 84	0. 12	0. 21	C64
0. 06	0. 17	0. 29	0. 43	0. 85	1. 37	1. 96	2. 94	3. 19	2. 59	0. 41	0. 23	0. 23	0. 01	0. 03	C65
0. 06	0. 13	0. 27	0. 52	0. 87	1. 81	2. 82	4. 07	4. 57	3. 57	0. 52	0. 28	0. 28	0. 01	0. 03	C66
0. 52	0. 80	2. 12	2. 42	4. 97	7. 77	11. 36	15. 86	21. 82	19. 85	2. 53	1. 39	1. 37	0. 06	0. 15	C67
0. 02	0. 04	0. 09	0. 10	0. 19	0. 27	0. 42	0. 46	0. 68	0. 51	0. 09	0. 05	0. 05	0. 00	0. 01	C68
0. 09	0. 09	0. 19	0. 09	0. 34	0. 44	0. 31	0. 52	0. 76	0. 76	0. 16	0. 11	0. 15	0. 01	0. 01	C69
5. 38	8. 50	13. 92	13. 62	18. 62	22. 58	22. 86	25. 49	25. 93	22. 47	8. 45	5. 87	5. 75	0. 38	0. 61	C70-72,D32-33,D42-43
31. 03	35. 36	47. 06	34. 70	30. 95	21. 44	13. 43	8. 69	6. 65	4. 48	21. 43	18. 10	15. 71	1. 32	1. 49	C73
0. 17	0. 21	0. 34	0. 29	0. 36	0. 51	0. 67	0. 44	0. 51	0. 66	0. 21	0. 16	0. 17	0. 01	0. 02	C74
0. 29	0. 40	0. 54	0. 51	0. 68	0. 65	0. 48	0. 55	0. 51	0. 69	0. 33	0. 26	0. 24	0. 02	0. 02	C75
0. 14	0. 17	0. 24	0. 24	0. 34	0. 55	0. 65	0. 65	0. 68	0. 76	0. 25	0. 21	0. 19	0. 01	0. 02	C81
1. 92	3. 13	5. 51	5. 61	9. 00	11. 58	13. 60	14. 87	16. 46	11. 07	3. 91	2. 60	2. 53	0. 16	0. 28	C82-C86;C96
0. 03	0. 04	0. 04	0. 07	0. 10	0. 12	0. 16	0. 27	0. 14	0. 00	0. 04	0. 03	0. 03	0. 00	0. 00	C88
0. 31	0. 64	1. 70	2. 05	3. 96	5. 35	6. 07	6. 43	5. 41	2. 91	1. 33	0. 79	0. 80	0. 05	0. 10	C90
0. 48	0. 59	1. 22	0. 98	1. 75	1. 86	2. 54	2. 96	2. 65	1. 46	1. 02	0. 88	1. 01	0. 06	0. 08	C91
1. 82	2. 50	3. 44	3. 57	5. 40	7. 35	8. 56	9. 22	9. 25	6. 48	2. 76	2. 03	1. 98	0. 12	0. 20	C92-C94,D45-47
0. 98	1. 16	1. 90	1. 88	2. 75	4. 00	5. 25	5. 98	6. 43	4. 92	1. 65	1. 25	1. 29	0. 07	0. 12	C95
2. 76	4. 08	6. 31	6. 57	10. 20	12. 41	16. 17	20. 29	27. 55	30. 27	5. 05	3. 23	3. 22	0. 19	0. 33	O&U
186. 72	280. 75	424. 84	388. 41	567. 40	680. 57	799. 21	954. 73	1 099. 24	994. 57	264. 75	172. 02	164. 93	10. 75	18. 15	C00-96, D32-33, D42-43,D45-47
185. 90	279. 42	422. 62	386. 03	563. 12	674. 17	789. 97	940. 41	1 078. 16	964. 23	262. 16	170. 57	163. 50	10. 68	18. 00	C00-96, D32-33, D42-43,D45-47 exc. C44

附表 1-4　2017 年全国城市肿瘤登记地区男女合计癌症发病主要指标

部位 Site		病例数 No. cases	构成 Freq. /%	年龄组								
				0~	1~4	5~9	10~14	15~19	20~24	25~29	30~34	35~39
唇	Lip	391	0.06	0.00	0.02	0.01	0.01	0.01	0.00	0.01	0.03	0.02
舌	Tongue	2 065	0.31	0.00	0.01	0.01	0.02	0.01	0.06	0.09	0.21	0.33
口	Mouth	2 518	0.37	0.00	0.01	0.02	0.01	0.05	0.08	0.08	0.16	0.23
唾液腺	Salivary glands	1 381	0.20	0.04	0.00	0.01	0.08	0.15	0.22	0.27	0.26	0.45
扁桃腺	Tonsil	420	0.06	0.00	0.00	0.00	0.00	0.00	0.01	0.02	0.03	0.03
其他口咽	Other oropharynx	646	0.10	0.00	0.02	0.03	0.01	0.01	0.01	0.01	0.02	0.08
鼻咽	Nasopharynx	7 940	1.18	0.04	0.00	0.04	0.11	0.28	0.37	1.03	1.99	2.53
下咽	Hypopharynx	1 230	0.18	0.00	0.00	0.00	0.00	0.00	0.01	0.01	0.01	0.04
咽,部位不明	Pharynx unspecified	495	0.07	0.00	0.01	0.01	0.01	0.03	0.00	0.01	0.01	0.02
食管	Esophagus	31 690	4.70	0.04	0.02	0.00	0.00	0.03	0.03	0.12	0.16	0.30
胃	Stomach	56 101	8.32	0.13	0.00	0.01	0.01	0.12	0.32	1.12	2.07	3.27
小肠	Small intestine	2 924	0.43	0.00	0.00	0.01	0.01	0.00	0.06	0.11	0.13	0.28
结肠	Colon	39 317	5.83	0.00	0.00	0.02	0.08	0.12	0.39	1.16	1.98	3.05
直肠	Rectum	33 852	5.02	0.04	0.00	0.03	0.01	0.07	0.19	0.78	1.36	2.05
肛门	Anus	727	0.11	0.00	0.00	0.01	0.00	0.01	0.01	0.01	0.02	0.06
肝脏	Liver	56 889	8.44	1.55	0.46	0.11	0.13	0.26	0.54	1.53	3.25	6.48
胆囊及其他	Gallbladder etc.	9 760	1.45	0.04	0.02	0.00	0.00	0.01	0.01	0.09	0.17	0.35
胰腺	Pancreas	17 284	2.56	0.09	0.01	0.03	0.06	0.05	0.05	0.18	0.34	0.72
鼻、鼻窦及其他	Nose, sinuses etc.	1 005	0.15	0.00	0.06	0.03	0.04	0.05	0.07	0.08	0.14	0.18
喉	Larynx	4 541	0.67	0.04	0.02	0.03	0.00	0.03	0.04	0.04	0.02	0.13
气管、支气管、肺	Trachea, bronchus & lung	140 904	20.90	0.09	0.04	0.03	0.08	0.21	0.51	1.31	3.22	6.03
其他胸腔器官	Other thoracic organs	2 360	0.35	0.58	0.18	0.03	0.07	0.24	0.24	0.27	0.38	0.43
骨	Bone	3 592	0.53	0.04	0.13	0.27	0.82	0.85	0.49	0.50	0.59	0.50
皮肤黑色素瘤	Melanoma of skin	1 221	0.18	0.00	0.04	0.05	0.02	0.02	0.02	0.09	0.16	0.15
皮肤其他	Other skin	6 309	0.94	0.04	0.13	0.06	0.13	0.24	0.23	0.28	0.52	0.62
间皮瘤	Mesothelioma	379	0.06	0.00	0.00	0.00	0.00	0.02	0.01	0.04	0.01	0.06
卡波氏肉瘤	Kaposi sarcoma	56	0.01	0.04	0.01	0.01	0.00	0.02	0.02	0.01	0.01	0.01
结缔组织、软组织	Connective & soft tissue	2 325	0.34	0.84	0.27	0.17	0.38	0.27	0.36	0.54	0.64	0.58
乳腺	Breast	53 726	8.07	0.19	0.00	0.00	0.04	0.16	1.40	5.84	17.06	32.30
外阴	Vulva	560	0.08	0.09	0.00	0.00	0.00	0.02	0.05	0.02	0.07	0.16
阴道	Vagina	328	0.05	0.00	0.00	0.00	0.00	0.00	0.02	0.00	0.01	0.13
子宫颈	Cervix uteri	17 558	2.60	0.00	0.00	0.00	0.00	0.04	0.50	2.53	7.28	13.39
子宫体	Corpus uteri	10 010	1.49	0.00	0.00	0.00	0.00	0.00	0.09	0.78	1.80	3.19
子宫,部位不明	Uterus unspecified	1 562	0.23	0.00	0.00	0.00	0.00	0.04	0.08	0.20	0.39	0.65
卵巢	Ovary	9 185	1.36	0.00	0.11	0.21	0.70	1.29	1.94	2.33	3.30	3.67
其他女性生殖器	Other female genital organs	698	0.10	0.09	0.02	0.00	0.00	0.02	0.06	0.07	0.12	0.16
胎盘	Placenta	95	0.01	0.00	0.00	0.00	0.00	0.04	0.09	0.23	0.14	0.20
阴茎	Penis	837	0.12	0.00	0.00	0.00	0.00	0.00	0.04	0.02	0.12	0.20
前列腺	Prostate	16 543	2.45	0.08	0.00	0.00	0.00	0.06	0.04	0.07	0.12	0.09
睾丸	Testis	602	0.09	0.93	0.42	0.02	0.02	0.24	0.38	0.86	0.99	0.79
其他男性生殖器	Other male genital organs	262	0.04	0.00	0.04	0.02	0.02	0.04	0.01	0.01	0.07	0.02
肾	Kidney	11 172	1.66	1.07	0.55	0.14	0.04	0.11	0.24	0.49	1.06	1.60
肾盂	Renal pelvis	1 333	0.20	0.00	0.00	0.01	0.00	0.01	0.01	0.01	0.05	0.05
输尿管	Ureter	1 579	0.23	0.00	0.00	0.00	0.00	0.00	0.00	0.01	0.02	0.01
膀胱	Bladder	15 146	2.25	0.09	0.03	0.00	0.00	0.14	0.09	0.30	0.40	0.69
其他泌尿器官	Other urinary organs	301	0.04	0.00	0.00	0.00	0.00	0.00	0.01	0.00	0.00	0.00
眼	Eye	340	0.05	0.98	0.51	0.03	0.03	0.02	0.01	0.03	0.03	0.02
脑、神经系统	Brain, nervous system	17 426	2.59	2.62	2.08	1.77	1.66	1.27	1.47	2.44	3.28	3.90
甲状腺	Thyroid	40 656	6.03	0.00	0.00	0.14	0.23	1.60	6.99	18.06	25.90	28.17
肾上腺	Adrenal gland	527	0.08	0.40	0.26	0.06	0.01	0.03	0.01	0.06	0.09	0.09
其他内分泌腺	Other endocrine	740	0.11	0.00	0.06	0.07	0.24	0.17	0.18	0.13	0.19	0.23
霍奇金淋巴瘤	Hodgkin lymphoma	726	0.11	0.00	0.03	0.10	0.24	0.33	0.28	0.36	0.27	0.25
非霍奇金淋巴瘤	Non-Hodgkin lymphoma	11 339	1.68	0.22	0.52	0.51	0.69	0.92	0.83	1.18	1.52	1.94
免疫增生性疾病	Immunoproliferative diseases	182	0.03	0.04	0.01	0.02	0.02	0.04	0.01	0.01	0.01	0.02
多发性骨髓瘤	Multiple myeloma	3 852	0.57	0.00	0.05	0.01	0.01	0.07	0.05	0.07	0.10	0.17
淋巴样白血病	Lymphoid leukemia	2 947	0.44	1.60	3.23	2.13	1.13	0.79	0.48	0.53	0.58	0.41
髓样白血病	Myeloid leukemia	7 917	1.17	1.38	0.64	0.67	1.27	0.99	1.09	1.35	1.58	1.56
白血病,未特指	Leukemia unspecified	3 499	0.52	2.13	0.98	0.61	0.80	0.68	0.51	0.63	0.58	0.48
其他或未指明部位	Other and unspecified	13 390	1.99	2.17	1.43	0.49	0.46	0.57	0.62	1.07	1.18	1.62
所有部位合计	All sites	674 037	100.00	17.08	12.19	7.89	9.33	11.86	19.58	43.02	70.78	98.10
所有部位除外 C44	All sites except C44	667 728	99.06	17.04	12.06	7.83	9.20	11.61	19.35	42.73	70.26	97.48

Appendix Table 1-4 Cancer incidence in urban registration areas of China, both sexes in 2017

Age group										粗率 Crude rate/ 100 000⁻¹	中标率 ASR China/ 100 000⁻¹	世标率 ASR world/ 100 000⁻¹	累积率 Cum. rate/%		ICD10
40~44	45~49	50~54	55~59	60~64	65~69	70~74	75~79	80~84	85+				0~64	0~74	
0.07	0.07	0.21	0.15	0.30	0.54	0.66	1.33	1.35	1.71	0.18	0.11	0.10	0.00	0.01	C00
0.50	0.93	1.75	1.90	2.28	2.56	3.11	2.96	4.00	3.06	0.97	0.61	0.59	0.04	0.07	C01-02
0.40	0.69	1.53	1.81	2.96	3.83	4.01	5.72	6.11	6.67	1.18	0.70	0.69	0.04	0.08	C03-06
0.39	0.66	1.01	1.02	1.40	1.65	1.91	1.99	1.55	1.23	0.65	0.46	0.44	0.03	0.05	C07-08
0.11	0.30	0.55	0.42	0.41	0.49	0.45	0.46	0.51	0.32	0.20	0.13	0.12	0.01	0.01	C09
0.12	0.20	0.54	0.52	0.86	0.98	0.99	1.27	0.98	0.99	0.30	0.19	0.19	0.01	0.02	C10
4.44	5.47	7.68	6.16	7.89	8.43	7.44	6.00	5.94	4.01	3.72	2.66	2.48	0.19	0.27	C11
0.12	0.37	1.23	1.43	1.87	1.91	1.68	1.73	1.83	0.99	0.58	0.34	0.35	0.03	0.04	C12-13
0.08	0.16	0.31	0.43	0.69	0.65	0.90	0.83	1.10	1.19	0.23	0.14	0.14	0.01	0.02	C14
1.38	4.51	13.71	20.74	39.21	57.06	75.20	84.09	89.80	82.46	14.86	8.31	8.40	0.40	1.06	C15
6.68	11.84	26.47	36.53	66.00	92.75	119.59	144.79	157.07	133.58	26.31	15.17	15.06	0.77	1.83	C16
0.48	0.77	1.75	2.00	3.36	4.40	5.41	6.78	7.85	6.83	1.37	0.81	0.80	0.04	0.09	C17
5.08	8.99	17.69	26.07	42.32	60.36	78.55	100.36	124.35	111.24	18.44	10.63	10.47	0.53	1.23	C18
4.89	9.08	18.03	24.27	41.44	54.08	65.74	76.34	90.40	76.19	15.87	9.25	9.20	0.51	1.11	C19-20
0.14	0.19	0.42	0.40	0.75	1.07	1.46	1.85	2.11	2.14	0.34	0.20	0.20	0.01	0.02	C21
14.42	24.27	40.94	45.18	64.89	77.37	89.53	106.52	116.79	116.43	26.68	16.23	15.99	1.01	1.85	C22
0.77	1.84	3.68	5.54	10.08	15.53	19.83	29.05	35.00	35.56	4.58	2.52	2.51	0.11	0.29	C23-24
1.52	3.38	7.22	10.52	18.76	26.10	35.70	47.63	61.22	58.53	8.11	4.51	4.50	0.21	0.52	C25
0.27	0.43	0.72	0.76	1.08	1.24	1.40	1.79	1.91	1.55	0.47	0.31	0.30	0.02	0.03	C30-31
0.37	0.85	3.08	4.24	6.67	7.89	8.44	9.44	8.81	6.23	2.13	1.24	1.26	0.08	0.16	C32
14.39	27.73	67.07	94.91	174.75	233.44	297.25	358.11	395.06	353.31	66.08	37.65	37.67	1.95	4.60	C33-34
0.64	0.94	1.59	2.02	2.55	2.97	3.56	3.14	3.69	3.61	1.11	0.75	0.74	0.05	0.08	C37-38
0.70	1.06	1.83	2.02	3.41	4.37	5.91	7.15	8.58	8.18	1.68	1.19	1.16	0.07	0.12	C40-41
0.25	0.44	0.67	0.68	1.17	1.73	2.30	2.56	3.21	3.45	0.57	0.35	0.34	0.02	0.04	C43
0.96	1.43	2.47	3.12	5.45	8.14	11.50	15.52	23.94	31.07	2.96	1.70	1.68	0.08	0.18	C44
0.06	0.06	0.24	0.36	0.51	0.62	0.51	0.76	0.73	0.71	0.18	0.11	0.11	0.01	0.01	C45
0.00	0.00	0.04	0.05	0.03	0.05	0.12	0.14	0.17	0.08	0.03	0.02	0.02	0.00	0.00	C46
0.73	0.81	1.26	1.50	2.19	2.50	2.75	3.81	4.22	3.85	1.09	0.80	0.78	0.05	0.08	C47;C49
62.71	90.05	107.76	94.61	112.32	97.77	83.51	81.68	72.00	53.05	50.57	34.49	32.44	2.62	3.53	C50
0.28	0.41	0.58	0.58	1.18	1.54	1.93	2.09	2.50	3.76	0.53	0.30	0.30	0.02	0.03	C51
0.20	0.28	0.53	0.35	0.75	1.05	1.26	1.04	0.92	0.81	0.31	0.19	0.18	0.01	0.02	C52
22.63	31.27	42.68	29.63	29.81	25.49	22.02	21.04	16.71	13.50	16.53	11.70	10.80	0.90	1.14	C53
7.43	14.90	27.08	22.67	22.98	20.30	15.91	12.43	9.04	5.64	9.42	6.18	6.01	0.50	0.69	C54
1.21	2.37	2.86	2.79	3.03	3.59	3.07	3.06	3.63	3.76	1.47	0.96	0.91	0.07	0.10	C55
7.29	12.11	17.60	15.29	19.62	19.16	19.13	18.36	17.07	9.60	8.65	5.97	5.69	0.43	0.62	C56
0.44	0.76	1.52	1.30	1.88	1.54	1.61	1.27	1.12	1.54	0.66	0.42	0.41	0.03	0.05	C57
0.11	0.15	0.11	0.03	0.04	0.04	0.00	0.00	0.00	0.00	0.09	0.09	0.07	0.01	0.01	C58
0.27	0.60	1.08	1.30	1.80	2.44	3.41	2.85	4.51	5.53	0.78	0.48	0.48	0.03	0.06	C60
0.21	0.62	2.82	7.76	23.98	51.66	97.19	146.84	189.18	189.48	15.46	8.49	8.35	0.18	0.92	C61
0.81	0.57	0.40	0.40	0.46	0.73	0.62	0.77	0.63	1.26	0.56	0.53	0.48	0.03	0.04	C62
0.02	0.14	0.13	0.34	0.58	0.92	1.21	1.19	2.07	1.26	0.24	0.15	0.15	0.01	0.02	C63
2.57	4.29	8.79	9.75	13.70	16.26	16.54	17.78	18.68	14.17	5.24	3.30	3.27	0.22	0.38	C64
0.06	0.20	0.58	0.79	1.44	2.13	3.01	3.80	4.53	4.17	0.63	0.35	0.35	0.02	0.04	C65
0.12	0.18	0.42	0.84	1.42	2.56	3.59	5.70	6.86	4.80	0.74	0.40	0.40	0.02	0.05	C66
1.27	2.32	5.75	8.08	15.45	22.75	31.41	43.08	59.64	58.61	7.10	3.91	3.89	0.17	0.44	C67
0.02	0.05	0.12	0.14	0.27	0.42	0.65	0.95	1.32	1.27	0.14	0.08	0.08	0.00	0.01	C68
0.08	0.10	0.16	0.14	0.37	0.36	0.38	0.40	0.70	0.56	0.16	0.12	0.15	0.01	0.01	C69
4.93	7.73	12.47	12.54	17.23	21.30	22.60	25.41	26.78	25.56	8.17	5.72	5.63	0.36	0.58	C70-72,D32-33,D42-43
27.95	29.21	37.39	28.74	26.27	18.95	12.12	8.48	6.50	4.33	19.07	16.18	13.88	1.15	1.31	C73
0.13	0.23	0.32	0.45	0.44	0.68	0.65	0.83	0.65	1.03	0.25	0.17	0.18	0.01	0.02	C74
0.29	0.29	0.42	0.56	0.76	0.85	0.71	0.91	0.70	0.56	0.35	0.28	0.26	0.02	0.03	C75
0.21	0.21	0.37	0.38	0.40	0.77	0.68	0.85	1.04	1.11	0.34	0.30	0.28	0.02	0.02	C81
2.44	3.90	6.81	7.77	12.02	16.01	18.47	21.38	24.22	18.73	5.32	3.50	3.41	0.21	0.38	C82-C86;C96
0.03	0.05	0.06	0.10	0.21	0.35	0.45	0.40	0.31	0.12	0.09	0.06	0.06	0.00	0.01	C88
0.41	0.79	1.93	2.69	4.98	6.80	8.27	9.82	9.31	6.11	1.81	1.06	1.06	0.06	0.13	C90
0.63	0.69	1.29	1.25	2.08	2.57	3.38	4.89	4.36	3.53	1.38	1.19	1.38	0.07	0.10	C91
2.31	2.92	4.40	4.58	6.87	9.86	12.24	14.35	15.87	13.25	3.71	2.65	2.57	0.15	0.26	C92-C94,D45-47
0.83	1.15	1.67	1.79	2.82	3.88	5.32	6.84	7.99	6.79	1.64	1.21	1.25	0.07	0.11	C95
2.80	4.10	6.70	8.34	13.02	17.00	22.45	29.19	38.21	42.30	6.28	3.88	3.89	0.21	0.41	O&U
159.21	243.16	415.05	472.35	733.41	930.97	1 135.76	1 364.38	1 543.03	1 398.40	316.08	196.53	191.54	11.48	21.82	C00-96, D32-33, D42-43,D45-47
158.25	241.73	412.58	469.23	727.97	922.84	1 124.25	1 348.86	1 519.08	1 367.33	313.13	194.83	189.86	11.41	21.64	C00-96, D32-33, D42-43,D45-47 exc. C44

附表 1-5　2017 年全国城市肿瘤登记地区男性癌症发病主要指标

部位 Site		病例数 No. cases	构成 Freq. /%	年龄组								
				0～	1～4	5～9	10～14	15～19	20～24	25～29	30～34	35～39
唇	Lip	208	0.06	0.00	0.02	0.02	0.00	0.02	0.00	0.01	0.04	0.02
舌	Tongue	1 317	0.36	0.00	0.02	0.00	0.04	0.02	0.07	0.11	0.22	0.39
口	Mouth	1 620	0.44	0.00	0.02	0.02	0.00	0.04	0.10	0.11	0.22	0.21
唾液腺	Salivary glands	812	0.22	0.00	0.00	0.00	0.08	0.17	0.20	0.29	0.33	0.42
扁桃腺	Tonsil	299	0.08	0.00	0.00	0.00	0.00	0.00	0.00	0.01	0.02	0.02
其他口咽	Other oropharynx	542	0.15	0.00	0.00	0.02	0.02	0.02	0.00	0.00	0.02	0.12
鼻咽	Nasopharynx	5 651	1.55	0.08	0.00	0.03	0.14	0.37	0.42	1.39	2.85	3.50
下咽	Hypopharynx	1 167	0.32	0.00	0.00	0.00	0.00	0.00	0.01	0.00	0.01	0.07
咽，部位不明	Pharynx unspecified	396	0.11	0.00	0.00	0.00	0.00	0.04	0.00	0.01	0.00	0.04
食管	Esophagus	24 082	6.60	0.08	0.02	0.00	0.00	0.02	0.06	0.11	0.17	0.46
胃	Stomach	38 907	10.66	0.08	0.00	0.00	0.00	0.11	0.31	0.74	1.73	3.23
小肠	Small intestine	1 661	0.45	0.00	0.00	0.02	0.00	0.00	0.06	0.12	0.13	0.35
结肠	Colon	22 051	6.04	0.00	0.00	0.02	0.12	0.07	0.41	1.23	1.98	3.39
直肠	Rectum	20 902	5.72	0.08	0.00	0.03	0.02	0.07	0.23	0.82	1.46	2.37
肛门	Anus	423	0.12	0.00	0.00	0.02	0.00	0.00	0.03	0.01	0.04	0.04
肝脏	Liver	42 010	11.50	1.52	0.59	0.14	0.20	0.34	0.67	2.32	5.49	10.95
胆囊及其他	Gallbladder etc.	4 632	1.27	0.08	0.02	0.00	0.00	0.02	0.00	0.09	0.22	0.34
胰腺	Pancreas	9 789	2.68	0.08	0.00	0.02	0.04	0.07	0.03	0.16	0.37	0.88
鼻、鼻窦及其他	Nose, sinuses etc.	631	0.17	0.00	0.10	0.02	0.06	0.07	0.07	0.10	0.15	0.20
喉	Larynx	4 178	1.14	0.00	0.02	0.03	0.00	0.06	0.03	0.02	0.04	0.24
气管、支气管、肺	Trachea, bronchus & lung	91 924	25.17	0.08	0.04	0.03	0.08	0.35	0.48	1.22	2.92	5.39
其他胸腔器官	Other thoracic organs	1 451	0.40	0.34	0.22	0.02	0.08	0.35	0.31	0.38	0.41	0.49
骨	Bone	2 027	0.56	0.00	0.14	0.23	1.00	1.05	0.61	0.60	0.60	0.54
皮肤黑色素瘤	Melanoma of skin	629	0.17	0.00	0.04	0.05	0.02	0.00	0.01	0.07	0.21	0.07
皮肤其他	Other skin	3 243	0.89	0.00	0.18	0.09	0.10	0.32	0.23	0.29	0.51	0.55
间皮瘤	Mesothelioma	216	0.06	0.00	0.00	0.00	0.00	0.00	0.03	0.02	0.01	0.05
卡波氏肉瘤	Kaposi sarcoma	38	0.01	0.08	0.00	0.02	0.00	0.02	0.04	0.01	0.00	0.01
结缔组织、软组织	Connective & soft tissue	1 246	0.34	0.59	0.30	0.19	0.32	0.17	0.38	0.55	0.63	0.53
乳腺	Breast	677	0.19	0.00	0.00	0.00	0.00	0.04	0.06	0.09	0.19	0.34
外阴	Vulva	—	—	—	—	—	—	—	—	—	—	—
阴道	Vagina	—	—	—	—	—	—	—	—	—	—	—
子宫颈	Cervix uteri	—	—	—	—	—	—	—	—	—	—	—
子宫体	Corpus uteri	—	—	—	—	—	—	—	—	—	—	—
子宫，部位不明	Uterus unspecified	—	—	—	—	—	—	—	—	—	—	—
卵巢	Ovary	—	—	—	—	—	—	—	—	—	—	—
其他女性生殖器	Other female genital organs	—	—	—	—	—	—	—	—	—	—	—
胎盘	Placenta	—	—	—	—	—	—	—	—	—	—	—
阴茎	Penis	837	0.23	0.00	0.00	0.00	0.00	0.00	0.04	0.02	0.12	0.20
前列腺	Prostate	16 543	4.53	0.08	0.00	0.00	0.00	0.06	0.04	0.07	0.12	0.09
睾丸	Testis	602	0.16	0.93	0.42	0.02	0.02	0.24	0.38	0.86	0.99	0.79
其他男性生殖器	Other male genital organs	262	0.07	0.00	0.04	0.02	0.02	0.04	0.01	0.01	0.07	0.02
肾	Kidney	7 349	2.01	0.76	0.49	0.14	0.04	0.13	0.26	0.60	1.40	1.99
肾盂	Renal pelvis	751	0.21	0.00	0.00	0.02	0.00	0.02	0.00	0.01	0.07	0.07
输尿管	Ureter	831	0.23	0.00	0.00	0.00	0.00	0.00	0.00	0.01	0.02	0.02
膀胱	Bladder	11 930	3.27	0.08	0.04	0.00	0.00	0.19	0.09	0.46	0.67	1.05
其他泌尿器官	Other urinary organs	191	0.05	0.00	0.00	0.00	0.00	0.00	0.01	0.00	0.00	0.00
眼	Eye	184	0.05	1.10	0.55	0.02	0.06	0.04	0.03	0.04	0.02	0.04
脑、神经系统	Brain, nervous system	7 819	2.14	3.46	2.10	1.87	1.87	1.38	1.72	2.53	3.25	3.64
甲状腺	Thyroid	10 047	2.75	0.00	0.00	0.03	0.08	0.88	3.59	10.09	15.52	16.10
肾上腺	Adrenal gland	297	0.08	0.42	0.20	0.07	0.00	0.06	0.00	0.05	0.11	0.12
其他内分泌腺	Other endocrine	375	0.10	0.00	0.08	0.07	0.40	0.22	0.20	0.10	0.19	0.12
霍奇金淋巴瘤	Hodgkin lymphoma	452	0.12	0.00	0.02	0.17	0.30	0.41	0.23	0.37	0.28	0.26
非霍奇金淋巴瘤	Non-Hodgkin lymphoma	6 427	1.76	0.25	0.57	0.68	1.06	1.18	1.07	1.38	1.51	2.14
免疫增生性疾病	Immunoproliferative diseases	115	0.03	0.08	0.02	0.02	0.02	0.07	0.00	0.00	0.02	0.01
多发性骨髓瘤	Multiple myeloma	2 211	0.61	0.00	0.06	0.02	0.02	0.11	0.06	0.10	0.15	0.21
淋巴样白血病	Lymphoid leukemia	1 694	0.46	1.69	3.74	2.37	1.17	1.10	0.61	0.58	0.69	0.51
髓样白血病	Myeloid leukemia	4 432	1.21	1.35	0.69	0.69	1.39	1.08	1.14	1.54	1.70	1.80
白血病，未特指	Leukemia unspecified	2 033	0.56	2.45	1.19	0.54	0.90	0.80	0.64	0.76	0.67	0.52
其他或未指明部位	Other and unspecified	7 039	1.93	1.77	1.52	0.47	0.48	0.47	0.64	0.95	1.05	1.52
所有部位合计	All sites	365 150	100.00	17.54	13.46	8.21	10.14	12.29	15.67	31.42	49.63	66.43
所有部位除外 C44	All sites except C44	361 907	99.11	17.54	13.28	8.12	10.04	11.97	15.43	31.14	49.12	65.88

Appendix Table 1-5 Cancer incidence in urban registration areas of China, male in 2017

Age group										粗率 Crude rate/ 100 000⁻¹	中标率 ASR China/ 100 000⁻¹	世标率 ASR world/ 100 000⁻¹	累积率 Cum. rate/%		ICD10
40~44	45~49	50~54	55~59	60~64	65~69	70~74	75~79	80~84	85+				0~64	0~74	
0.06	0.11	0.24	0.17	0.34	0.62	0.84	1.28	1.50	1.65	0.19	0.12	0.12	0.01	0.01	C00
0.65	1.38	2.43	2.71	3.06	3.52	3.29	3.36	4.57	3.59	1.23	0.79	0.78	0.06	0.09	C01-02
0.46	0.96	2.41	2.71	4.15	5.08	4.68	6.38	7.82	9.31	1.51	0.92	0.92	0.06	0.11	C03-06
0.46	0.69	1.16	1.29	1.80	1.89	2.48	2.34	2.50	2.04	0.76	0.54	0.51	0.03	0.06	C07-08
0.16	0.35	0.82	0.64	0.54	0.92	0.68	0.64	0.81	0.29	0.28	0.18	0.18	0.01	0.02	C09
0.21	0.33	0.95	0.87	1.59	1.81	1.55	2.25	1.50	1.55	0.51	0.32	0.32	0.02	0.04	C10
6.05	7.96	11.24	9.12	11.39	12.06	10.63	9.52	8.64	5.04	5.28	3.80	3.54	0.27	0.39	C11
0.21	0.70	2.32	2.75	3.61	3.77	3.29	3.40	3.69	2.04	1.09	0.66	0.67	0.05	0.08	C12-13
0.14	0.29	0.52	0.76	1.20	1.12	1.49	1.36	1.56	1.36	0.37	0.23	0.23	0.02	0.03	C14
2.27	7.76	23.90	36.62	65.20	89.61	115.04	122.79	125.45	121.18	22.50	13.18	13.38	0.68	1.71	C15
7.32	14.49	35.37	53.37	100.26	137.90	179.37	213.57	224.11	192.00	36.36	21.55	21.56	1.08	2.67	C16
0.66	0.92	1.97	2.51	3.79	5.12	6.14	7.65	9.52	8.93	1.55	0.95	0.94	0.05	0.11	C17
5.39	9.57	19.82	30.64	50.06	72.13	93.93	119.30	139.66	136.31	20.61	12.33	12.21	0.61	1.44	C18
5.23	10.38	22.29	31.32	55.00	72.07	85.13	96.22	115.06	97.99	19.53	11.73	11.72	0.65	1.43	C19-20
0.20	0.22	0.36	0.52	0.98	1.44	1.86	2.17	2.38	2.43	0.40	0.24	0.24	0.01	0.03	C21
24.70	41.11	67.50	73.00	101.23	114.45	125.15	140.81	148.17	151.15	39.26	24.92	24.51	1.64	2.84	C22
0.68	1.77	3.64	5.77	10.59	16.49	19.16	27.20	32.05	35.80	4.33	2.51	2.52	0.12	0.29	C23-24
1.84	4.34	9.03	13.72	23.36	30.78	41.17	52.70	66.36	68.40	9.15	5.35	5.36	0.27	0.63	C25
0.32	0.50	0.89	1.06	1.49	1.56	1.95	2.21	2.82	1.75	0.59	0.39	0.38	0.03	0.04	C30-31
0.66	1.58	5.78	8.05	12.77	14.89	15.93	17.51	16.90	12.32	3.90	2.33	2.37	0.15	0.30	C32
14.08	29.63	81.02	127.42	242.69	331.70	421.95	502.20	542.24	492.95	85.90	50.43	50.75	2.53	6.30	C33-34
0.59	1.08	1.95	2.59	3.42	4.02	4.71	3.83	4.63	4.75	1.36	0.93	0.92	0.06	0.10	C37-38
0.78	1.25	1.81	2.32	4.10	5.12	6.79	9.01	10.27	9.80	1.89	1.37	1.33	0.07	0.13	C40-41
0.19	0.36	0.69	0.72	1.29	1.79	2.45	3.15	4.07	4.27	0.59	0.37	0.36	0.02	0.04	C43
1.03	1.36	2.59	3.51	6.20	9.27	13.24	15.56	25.29	33.18	3.03	1.83	1.82	0.08	0.20	C44
0.07	0.06	0.30	0.46	0.59	0.77	0.59	0.77	0.88	0.97	0.20	0.12	0.12	0.01	0.01	C45
0.00	0.00	0.05	0.06	0.03	0.06	0.16	0.26	0.31	0.10	0.04	0.03	0.03	0.00	0.00	C46
0.80	0.81	1.38	1.80	2.41	2.73	3.22	4.42	5.13	5.04	1.16	0.85	0.83	0.05	0.08	C47;C49
0.58	0.49	0.98	1.10	1.34	1.81	1.67	2.68	2.44	3.10	0.63	0.42	0.40	0.03	0.04	C50
—	—	—	—	—	—	—	—	—	—	—	—	—	—	—	C51
—	—	—	—	—	—	—	—	—	—	—	—	—	—	—	C52
—	—	—	—	—	—	—	—	—	—	—	—	—	—	—	C53
—	—	—	—	—	—	—	—	—	—	—	—	—	—	—	C54
—	—	—	—	—	—	—	—	—	—	—	—	—	—	—	C55
—	—	—	—	—	—	—	—	—	—	—	—	—	—	—	C56
—	—	—	—	—	—	—	—	—	—	—	—	—	—	—	C57
—	—	—	—	—	—	—	—	—	—	—	—	—	—	—	C58
0.27	0.60	1.08	1.30	1.80	2.44	3.41	2.85	4.51	5.53	0.78	0.48	0.48	0.03	0.06	C60
0.21	0.62	2.82	7.76	23.98	51.66	97.19	146.84	189.18	189.48	15.46	8.49	8.35	0.18	0.92	C61
0.81	0.57	0.40	0.40	0.46	0.73	0.62	0.77	0.63	1.26	0.56	0.53	0.48	0.03	0.04	C62
0.02	0.14	0.13	0.34	0.58	0.92	1.21	1.19	2.07	1.26	0.24	0.15	0.15	0.01	0.02	C63
3.56	5.63	11.74	13.20	18.99	21.93	21.89	24.48	25.04	19.40	6.87	4.40	4.35	0.29	0.51	C64
0.05	0.25	0.80	1.02	1.89	2.60	3.32	3.70	4.82	4.66	0.70	0.41	0.42	0.02	0.05	C65
0.18	0.21	0.47	1.19	1.84	2.71	3.75	5.61	6.89	5.04	0.78	0.45	0.44	0.02	0.05	C66
2.09	3.74	9.01	13.48	25.44	36.69	50.69	71.57	100.03	108.37	11.15	6.42	6.40	0.28	0.72	C67
0.04	0.03	0.16	0.20	0.33	0.52	0.81	1.40	1.88	2.04	0.18	0.10	0.10	0.00	0.01	C68
0.05	0.10	0.17	0.20	0.40	0.46	0.50	0.21	0.69	0.49	0.17	0.13	0.17	0.01	0.01	C69
4.47	6.77	10.70	10.47	15.57	19.35	21.20	22.95	24.48	25.42	7.31	5.32	5.25	0.33	0.54	C70-72,D32-33,D42-43
14.79	13.03	14.93	11.97	11.75	9.06	7.35	5.87	4.63	3.49	9.39	8.30	6.96	0.56	0.65	C73
0.12	0.26	0.37	0.53	0.54	0.73	0.65	1.32	0.81	1.26	0.28	0.19	0.20	0.01	0.02	C74
0.27	0.20	0.41	0.59	0.82	0.94	0.90	1.02	0.75	0.49	0.35	0.29	0.28	0.02	0.03	C75
0.23	0.27	0.53	0.57	0.55	1.04	0.81	1.32	1.50	1.46	0.42	0.36	0.34	0.02	0.03	C81
2.88	4.21	7.46	8.71	14.04	18.80	21.45	25.71	29.05	26.10	6.01	4.06	3.98	0.23	0.44	C82-C86;C96
0.02	0.03	0.06	0.11	0.28	0.54	0.62	0.43	0.50	0.29	0.11	0.07	0.08	0.00	0.01	C88
0.49	0.96	2.15	3.21	5.58	7.60	9.61	11.69	12.08	10.09	2.07	1.25	1.25	0.07	0.15	C90
0.69	0.78	1.34	1.36	2.27	2.94	3.69	6.16	5.45	5.82	1.58	1.37	1.59	0.08	0.12	C91
2.54	3.05	4.93	5.16	7.60	11.41	13.76	17.77	20.66	18.53	4.14	2.99	2.90	0.17	0.29	C92-C94,D45-47
0.93	1.41	1.87	2.02	3.32	4.50	6.17	8.12	11.21	10.09	1.90	1.41	1.46	0.08	0.13	C95
2.49	3.91	6.81	8.72	14.71	20.39	25.61	34.60	41.00	49.29	6.58	4.15	4.18	0.22	0.45	O&U
112.96	187.24	381.73	510.08	867.20	1 162.45	1 463.71	1 770.08	1 998.19	1 899.12	341.22	210.69	208.81	11.34	24.47	C00-96, D32-33, D42-43,D45-47
111.92	185.87	379.14	506.57	861.00	1 153.19	1 450.48	1 754.52	1 972.90	1 865.94	338.19	208.86	206.99	11.25	24.27	C00-96, D32-33, D42-43,D45-47 exc. C44

附表 1-6 2017 年全国城市肿瘤登记地区女性癌症发病主要指标

部位 Site		病例数 No. cases	构成 Freq. /%	年龄组								
				0~	1~4	5~9	10~14	15~19	20~24	25~29	30~34	35~39
唇	Lip	183	0. 06	0. 00	0. 02	0. 00	0. 02	0. 00	0. 00	0. 01	0. 02	0. 02
舌	Tongue	748	0. 24	0. 00	0. 00	0. 02	0. 00	0. 00	0. 05	0. 06	0. 20	0. 28
口	Mouth	898	0. 29	0. 00	0. 00	0. 02	0. 02	0. 06	0. 06	0. 05	0. 11	0. 25
唾液腺	Salivary glands	569	0. 18	0. 09	0. 00	0. 02	0. 09	0. 12	0. 24	0. 25	0. 20	0. 47
扁桃腺	Tonsil	121	0. 04	0. 00	0. 00	0. 00	0. 00	0. 00	0. 02	0. 02	0. 04	0. 03
其他口咽	Other oropharynx	104	0. 03	0. 00	0. 05	0. 04	0. 00	0. 00	0. 02	0. 01	0. 01	0. 05
鼻咽	Nasopharynx	2 289	0. 74	0. 00	0. 00	0. 04	0. 07	0. 18	0. 32	0. 67	1. 16	1. 57
下咽	Hypopharynx	63	0. 02	0. 00	0. 00	0. 00	0. 00	0. 00	0. 00	0. 02	0. 00	0. 01
咽,部位不明	Pharynx unspecified	99	0. 03	0. 00	0. 02	0. 02	0. 02	0. 02	0. 00	0. 00	0. 02	0. 01
食管	Esophagus	7 608	2. 46	0. 00	0. 02	0. 00	0. 00	0. 04	0. 00	0. 12	0. 14	0. 15
胃	Stomach	17 194	5. 57	0. 19	0. 00	0. 02	0. 02	0. 12	0. 33	1. 48	2. 40	3. 32
小肠	Small intestine	1 263	0. 41	0. 00	0. 00	0. 00	0. 02	0. 00	0. 06	0. 10	0. 12	0. 21
结肠	Colon	17 266	5. 59	0. 00	0. 00	0. 02	0. 04	0. 16	0. 36	1. 09	1. 98	2. 72
直肠	Rectum	12 950	4. 19	0. 00	0. 00	0. 02	0. 00	0. 06	0. 15	0. 75	1. 27	1. 74
肛门	Anus	304	0. 10	0. 00	0. 00	0. 00	0. 00	0. 02	0. 00	0. 00	0. 01	0. 08
肝脏	Liver	14 879	4. 82	1. 59	0. 32	0. 08	0. 04	0. 18	0. 39	0. 75	1. 07	2. 09
胆囊及其他	Gallbladder etc.	5 128	1. 66	0. 00	0. 02	0. 00	0. 00	0. 00	0. 03	0. 09	0. 12	0. 36
胰腺	Pancreas	7 495	2. 43	0. 09	0. 02	0. 04	0. 09	0. 02	0. 08	0. 21	0. 32	0. 57
鼻、鼻窦及其他	Nose, sinuses etc.	374	0. 12	0. 00	0. 02	0. 04	0. 02	0. 02	0. 08	0. 06	0. 14	0. 16
喉	Larynx	363	0. 12	0. 09	0. 02	0. 02	0. 00	0. 00	0. 05	0. 05	0. 01	0. 02
气管、支气管、肺	Trachea, bronchus & lung	48 980	15. 86	0. 09	0. 05	0. 02	0. 09	0. 06	0. 55	1. 40	3. 51	6. 66
其他胸腔器官	Other thoracic organs	909	0. 29	0. 84	0. 14	0. 04	0. 07	0. 12	0. 17	0. 15	0. 36	0. 36
骨	Bone	1 565	0. 51	0. 09	0. 11	0. 33	0. 63	0. 65	0. 36	0. 40	0. 59	0. 46
皮肤黑色素瘤	Melanoma of skin	592	0. 19	0. 00	0. 05	0. 04	0. 02	0. 04	0. 03	0. 11	0. 12	0. 22
皮肤其他	Other skin	3 066	0. 99	0. 09	0. 07	0. 04	0. 16	0. 16	0. 23	0. 28	0. 52	0. 69
间皮瘤	Mesothelioma	163	0. 05	0. 00	0. 00	0. 00	0. 00	0. 04	0. 00	0. 05	0. 01	0. 07
卡波氏肉瘤	Kaposi sarcoma	18	0. 01	0. 00	0. 02	0. 00	0. 00	0. 02	0. 00	0. 00	0. 01	0. 00
结缔组织、软组织	Connective & soft tissue	1 079	0. 35	1. 12	0. 23	0. 16	0. 45	0. 38	0. 35	0. 53	0. 65	0. 64
乳腺	Breast	53 726	17. 39	0. 19	0. 00	0. 00	0. 04	0. 16	1. 40	5. 84	17. 06	32. 30
外阴	Vulva	560	0. 18	0. 09	0. 00	0. 00	0. 00	0. 02	0. 05	0. 02	0. 07	0. 16
阴道	Vagina	328	0. 11	0. 00	0. 00	0. 00	0. 00	0. 00	0. 02	0. 00	0. 01	0. 13
子宫颈	Cervix uteri	17 558	5. 68	0. 00	0. 00	0. 00	0. 00	0. 04	0. 50	2. 53	7. 28	13. 39
子宫体	Corpus uteri	10 010	3. 24	0. 00	0. 00	0. 00	0. 00	0. 00	0. 09	0. 78	1. 80	3. 19
子宫,部位不明	Uterus unspecified	1 562	0. 51	0. 00	0. 00	0. 00	0. 00	0. 04	0. 08	0. 20	0. 39	0. 65
卵巢	Ovary	9 185	2. 97	0. 00	0. 11	0. 21	0. 70	1. 29	1. 94	2. 33	3. 30	3. 67
其他女性生殖器	Other female genital organs	698	0. 23	0. 09	0. 02	0. 00	0. 00	0. 02	0. 06	0. 07	0. 12	0. 16
胎盘	Placenta	95	0. 03	0. 00	0. 00	0. 00	0. 00	0. 04	0. 09	0. 23	0. 14	0. 20
阴茎	Penis	—	—	—	—	—	—	—	—	—	—	—
前列腺	Prostate	—	—	—	—	—	—	—	—	—	—	—
睾丸	Testis	—	—	—	—	—	—	—	—	—	—	—
其他男性生殖器	Other male genital organs	—	—	—	—	—	—	—	—	—	—	—
肾	Kidney	3 823	1. 24	1. 40	0. 61	0. 14	0. 04	0. 08	0. 21	0. 38	0. 72	1. 23
肾盂	Renal pelvis	582	0. 19	0. 00	0. 00	0. 00	0. 00	0. 00	0. 02	0. 00	0. 02	0. 02
输尿管	Ureter	748	0. 24	0. 00	0. 00	0. 00	0. 00	0. 00	0. 00	0. 00	0. 02	0. 00
膀胱	Bladder	3 216	1. 04	0. 09	0. 02	0. 00	0. 00	0. 08	0. 09	0. 13	0. 13	0. 34
其他泌尿器官	Other urinary organs	110	0. 04	0. 00	0. 00	0. 00	0. 00	0. 00	0. 00	0. 00	0. 00	0. 00
眼	Eye	156	0. 05	0. 84	0. 48	0. 04	0. 00	0. 00	0. 00	0. 02	0. 04	0. 00
脑、神经系统	Brain, nervous system	9 607	3. 11	1. 69	2. 06	1. 65	1. 42	1. 15	1. 20	2. 34	3. 30	4. 15
甲状腺	Thyroid	30 609	9. 91	0. 00	0. 00	0. 25	0. 40	2. 39	10. 51	25. 94	35. 98	40. 05
肾上腺	Adrenal gland	230	0. 07	0. 37	0. 32	0. 06	0. 02	0. 00	0. 02	0. 06	0. 07	0. 07
其他内分泌腺	Other endocrine	365	0. 12	0. 00	0. 05	0. 08	0. 07	0. 10	0. 15	0. 16	0. 18	0. 35
霍奇金淋巴瘤	Hodgkin lymphoma	274	0. 09	0. 00	0. 05	0. 02	0. 18	0. 24	0. 32	0. 36	0. 26	0. 23
非霍奇金淋巴瘤	Non-Hodgkin lymphoma	4 912	1. 59	0. 19	0. 48	0. 33	0. 27	0. 65	0. 58	0. 98	1. 54	1. 75
免疫增生性疾病	Immunoproliferative diseases	67	0. 02	0. 00	0. 00	0. 02	0. 02	0. 00	0. 02	0. 01	0. 00	0. 02
多发性骨髓瘤	Multiple myeloma	1 641	0. 53	0. 00	0. 05	0. 00	0. 00	0. 02	0. 05	0. 04	0. 06	0. 13
淋巴样白血病	Lymphoid leukemia	1 253	0. 41	1. 50	2. 65	1. 86	1. 08	0. 45	0. 35	0. 48	0. 46	0. 32
髓样白血病	Myeloid leukemia	3 485	1. 13	1. 40	0. 59	0. 64	1. 12	0. 89	1. 05	1. 16	1. 46	1. 33
白血病,未特指	Leukemia unspecified	1 466	0. 47	1. 78	0. 75	0. 70	0. 70	0. 55	0. 36	0. 50	0. 50	0. 45
其他或未指明部位	Other and unspecified	6 351	2. 06	2. 62	1. 34	0. 52	0. 45	0. 69	0. 59	1. 19	1. 31	1. 71
所有部位合计	All sites	308 887	100. 00	16. 58	10. 75	7. 53	8. 41	11. 39	23. 64	54. 48	91. 34	129. 23
所有部位除外 C44	All sites except C44	305 821	99. 01	16. 49	10. 69	7. 49	8. 26	11. 23	23. 41	54. 20	90. 81	128. 54

Appendix Table 1-6 Cancer incidence in urban registration areas of China, female in 2017

Age group										粗率 Crude rate/ 100 000⁻¹	中标率 ASR China/ 100 000⁻¹	世标率 ASR world/ 100 000⁻¹	累积率 Cum. rate/%		ICD10
40~44	45~49	50~54	55~59	60~64	65~69	70~74	75~79	80~84	85+				0~64	0~74	
0.08	0.02	0.17	0.13	0.25	0.47	0.50	1.38	1.23	1.75	0.17	0.09	0.09	0.00	0.01	C00
0.35	0.48	1.04	1.09	1.51	1.62	2.95	2.61	3.53	2.69	0.70	0.43	0.41	0.03	0.05	C01-02
0.35	0.43	0.63	0.91	1.79	2.62	3.39	5.15	4.70	4.84	0.85	0.48	0.47	0.02	0.05	C03-06
0.32	0.63	0.86	0.75	1.00	1.42	1.37	1.68	0.77	0.67	0.54	0.39	0.37	0.02	0.04	C07-08
0.05	0.24	0.26	0.20	0.29	0.08	0.23	0.30	0.26	0.34	0.11	0.07	0.07	0.01	0.01	C09
0.04	0.06	0.11	0.16	0.13	0.16	0.47	0.41	0.56	0.60	0.10	0.06	0.06	0.00	0.01	C10
2.83	2.96	4.02	3.17	4.44	4.91	4.44	2.91	3.73	3.29	2.15	1.53	1.42	0.11	0.15	C11
0.04	0.04	0.10	0.10	0.15	0.10	0.18	0.26	0.31	0.27	0.06	0.03	0.03	0.00	0.00	C12-13
0.02	0.02	0.09	0.10	0.19	0.18	0.35	0.37	0.72	1.07	0.09	0.05	0.05	0.00	0.01	C14
0.49	1.26	3.24	4.69	13.53	25.36	37.67	50.11	60.71	55.67	7.16	3.65	3.63	0.12	0.43	C15
6.05	9.18	17.33	19.50	32.13	48.80	63.28	84.40	102.35	93.14	16.19	9.14	8.90	0.46	1.02	C16
0.30	0.62	1.53	1.49	2.92	3.69	4.73	6.01	6.49	5.37	1.19	0.68	0.67	0.04	0.08	C17
4.77	8.41	15.50	21.45	34.66	48.90	64.07	83.73	111.86	93.88	16.25	9.02	8.84	0.46	1.02	C18
4.55	7.78	13.65	17.15	28.04	36.56	47.48	58.88	70.26	61.11	12.19	6.88	6.78	0.38	0.80	C19-20
0.08	0.16	0.47	0.28	0.53	0.71	1.08	1.57	1.89	1.95	0.29	0.16	0.16	0.01	0.02	C21
4.18	7.39	13.65	17.05	28.99	41.26	55.98	76.42	91.16	92.40	14.01	7.71	7.64	0.38	0.87	C22
0.87	1.91	3.71	5.31	9.58	14.60	20.47	30.67	37.41	35.39	4.83	2.53	2.51	0.11	0.29	C23-24
1.19	2.41	5.37	7.28	14.22	21.55	30.54	43.17	57.03	51.71	7.06	3.71	3.67	0.16	0.42	C25
0.22	0.35	0.55	0.46	0.68	0.93	0.88	1.42	1.18	1.41	0.35	0.23	0.22	0.01	0.02	C30-31
0.08	0.13	0.30	0.39	0.65	1.07	1.37	2.35	2.20	2.01	0.34	0.19	0.19	0.01	0.02	C32
14.69	25.82	52.73	62.04	107.62	137.77	179.79	231.60	274.92	256.66	46.11	25.61	25.34	1.38	2.96	C33-34
0.70	0.80	1.23	1.45	1.69	1.95	2.48	2.54	2.91	2.82	0.86	0.57	0.56	0.04	0.06	C37-38
0.62	0.87	1.85	1.71	2.72	3.63	5.08	5.52	7.21	7.05	1.47	1.01	0.98	0.06	0.10	C40-41
0.30	0.51	0.65	0.64	1.04	1.66	2.16	2.05	2.50	2.89	0.56	0.34	0.33	0.02	0.04	C43
0.88	1.49	2.35	2.72	4.70	7.04	9.87	15.49	22.84	29.61	2.89	1.57	1.54	0.07	0.16	C44
0.06	0.06	0.17	0.26	0.43	0.47	0.44	0.75	0.61	0.54	0.15	0.09	0.09	0.01	0.01	C45
0.00	0.00	0.02	0.04	0.03	0.04	0.09	0.04	0.05	0.07	0.02	0.01	0.01	0.00	0.00	C46
0.66	0.80	1.14	1.20	1.97	2.27	2.31	3.28	3.47	3.02	1.02	0.76	0.74	0.05	0.07	C47;C49
62.71	90.05	107.76	94.61	112.32	97.77	83.51	81.68	72.00	53.05	50.57	34.49	32.44	2.62	3.53	C50
0.28	0.41	0.58	0.58	1.18	1.54	1.93	2.09	2.50	3.76	0.53	0.30	0.30	0.02	0.03	C51
0.20	0.28	0.53	0.35	0.75	1.05	1.26	1.04	0.92	0.81	0.31	0.19	0.18	0.01	0.02	C52
22.63	31.27	42.68	29.63	29.81	25.49	22.02	21.04	16.71	13.50	16.53	11.70	10.80	0.90	1.14	C53
7.43	14.90	27.08	22.67	22.98	20.30	15.91	12.43	9.04	5.64	9.42	6.18	6.01	0.50	0.69	C54
1.21	2.37	2.86	2.79	3.03	3.59	3.07	3.06	3.63	3.76	1.47	0.96	0.91	0.07	0.10	C55
7.29	12.11	17.60	15.29	19.62	19.16	19.13	18.36	17.07	9.60	8.65	5.97	5.69	0.43	0.62	C56
0.44	0.76	1.52	1.30	1.88	1.54	1.61	1.27	1.12	1.54	0.66	0.42	0.41	0.03	0.05	C57
0.11	0.15	0.11	0.03	0.04	0.04	0.00	0.00	0.00	0.00	0.09	0.09	0.07	0.01	0.01	C58
—	—	—	—	—	—	—	—	—	—	—	—	—	—	—	C60
—	—	—	—	—	—	—	—	—	—	—	—	—	—	—	C61
—	—	—	—	—	—	—	—	—	—	—	—	—	—	—	C62
—	—	—	—	—	—	—	—	—	—	—	—	—	—	—	C63
1.58	2.95	5.76	6.27	8.48	10.75	11.51	11.90	13.49	10.54	3.60	2.23	2.22	0.14	0.25	C64
0.07	0.16	0.36	0.56	1.00	1.66	2.72	3.88	4.29	3.83	0.55	0.29	0.28	0.01	0.03	C65
0.06	0.16	0.36	0.49	1.00	2.41	3.45	5.78	6.85	4.63	0.70	0.36	0.35	0.01	0.04	C66
0.46	0.90	2.40	2.63	5.58	9.18	13.26	18.06	26.67	24.18	3.03	1.58	1.56	0.06	0.18	C67
0.01	0.06	0.07	0.09	0.22	0.32	0.50	0.56	0.87	0.74	0.10	0.05	0.05	0.00	0.01	C68
0.11	0.10	0.15	0.07	0.34	0.26	0.26	0.56	0.72	0.60	0.15	0.10	0.14	0.01	0.01	C69
5.38	8.71	14.30	14.63	18.87	23.19	23.92	27.57	28.67	25.65	9.04	6.11	5.99	0.40	0.63	C70-72,D32-33,D42-43
41.06	45.44	60.48	45.68	40.61	28.59	16.62	10.78	8.02	4.90	28.81	24.02	20.78	1.74	1.97	C73
0.15	0.20	0.27	0.36	0.35	0.63	0.64	0.41	0.51	0.87	0.22	0.15	0.17	0.01	0.02	C74
0.30	0.39	0.43	0.54	0.71	0.77	0.53	0.82	0.66	0.60	0.34	0.26	0.24	0.02	0.02	C75
0.18	0.16	0.21	0.19	0.25	0.51	0.55	0.45	0.66	0.87	0.26	0.23	0.21	0.01	0.02	C81
2.01	3.60	6.15	6.83	10.04	13.28	15.65	17.57	20.29	13.63	4.62	2.95	2.86	0.18	0.32	C82-C86;C96
0.04	0.07	0.05	0.09	0.15	0.16	0.29	0.37	0.15	0.00	0.06	0.04	0.04	0.00	0.00	C88
0.33	0.62	1.70	2.16	4.39	6.02	7.01	8.17	7.05	3.36	1.54	0.88	0.88	0.05	0.11	C90
0.57	0.59	1.24	1.13	1.88	2.21	3.10	3.77	3.47	1.95	1.18	1.01	1.17	0.06	0.09	C91
2.08	2.80	3.86	4.00	6.16	8.35	10.80	11.34	11.96	9.60	3.28	2.32	2.26	0.14	0.23	C92-C94,D45-47
0.74	0.90	1.45	1.55	2.34	3.28	4.53	5.71	5.37	4.50	1.38	1.01	1.04	0.06	0.10	C95
3.10	4.29	6.58	7.96	11.36	13.71	19.48	24.44	35.92	37.47	5.98	3.63	3.63	0.21	0.37	O&U
205.29	299.22	449.29	434.21	601.20	705.60	826.84	1 008.21	1 171.48	1 051.82	290.77	184.56	176.50	11.64	19.30	C00-96, D32-33, D42-43,D45-47
204.41	297.73	446.95	431.49	596.50	698.56	816.97	992.73	1 148.63	1 022.20	287.88	182.99	174.97	11.56	19.14	C00-96, D32-33, D42-43,D45-47 exc. C44

附表 1-7 2017 年全国农村肿瘤登记地区男女合计癌症发病主要指标

	部位 Site	病例数 No. cases	构成 Freq./%	年龄组								
				0~	1~4	5~9	10~14	15~19	20~24	25~29	30~34	35~39
唇	Lip	363	0.06	0.04	0.02	0.01	0.02	0.01	0.02	0.01	0.01	0.03
舌	Tongue	1 432	0.24	0.00	0.02	0.01	0.00	0.02	0.01	0.09	0.19	0.26
口	Mouth	2 137	0.35	0.04	0.01	0.05	0.07	0.08	0.04	0.12	0.18	0.22
唾液腺	Salivary glands	1 218	0.20	0.00	0.01	0.01	0.10	0.04	0.16	0.26	0.24	0.41
扁桃腺	Tonsil	298	0.05	0.00	0.01	0.01	0.01	0.00	0.03	0.01	0.02	0.04
其他口咽	Other oropharynx	532	0.09	0.00	0.00	0.02	0.01	0.01	0.02	0.02	0.05	0.08
鼻咽	Nasopharynx	7 898	1.30	0.04	0.01	0.04	0.12	0.29	0.40	0.82	1.67	2.60
下咽	Hypopharynx	909	0.15	0.04	0.00	0.02	0.01	0.04	0.01	0.02	0.01	0.04
咽,部位不明	Pharynx unspecified	562	0.09	0.00	0.00	0.02	0.01	0.00	0.02	0.02	0.01	0.03
食管	Esophagus	52 211	8.60	0.12	0.02	0.02	0.02	0.00	0.10	0.19	0.21	0.62
胃	Stomach	67 099	11.05	0.00	0.04	0.02	0.10	0.22	0.47	1.25	2.43	3.34
小肠	Small intestine	2 191	0.36	0.00	0.00	0.00	0.01	0.00	0.02	0.03	0.18	0.25
结肠	Colon	22 296	3.67	0.00	0.01	0.00	0.05	0.12	0.27	0.85	1.56	2.38
直肠	Rectum	29 333	4.83	0.08	0.01	0.02	0.05	0.08	0.17	0.74	1.32	2.19
肛门	Anus	831	0.14	0.00	0.00	0.00	0.00	0.00	0.02	0.02	0.02	0.12
肝脏	Liver	66 009	10.87	0.79	0.28	0.11	0.21	0.45	0.61	2.33	4.79	8.59
胆囊及其他	Gallbladder etc.	7 682	1.26	0.04	0.01	0.00	0.00	0.02	0.04	0.04	0.17	0.30
胰腺	Pancreas	13 585	2.24	0.04	0.03	0.02	0.02	0.04	0.11	0.15	0.39	0.79
鼻、鼻窦及其他	Nose, sinuses etc.	1 024	0.17	0.04	0.04	0.01	0.02	0.04	0.07	0.09	0.16	0.15
喉	Larynx	3 475	0.57	0.04	0.02	0.00	0.01	0.02	0.01	0.04	0.06	0.10
气管、支气管、肺	Trachea, bronchus & lung	133 786	22.03	0.00	0.08	0.07	0.11	0.21	0.53	1.49	3.29	5.59
其他胸腔器官	Other thoracic organs	1 785	0.29	0.08	0.07	0.05	0.06	0.23	0.12	0.26	0.27	0.31
骨	Bone	4 375	0.72	0.04	0.32	0.37	1.17	1.02	0.71	0.73	0.67	0.71
皮肤黑色素瘤	Melanoma of skin	1 004	0.17	0.00	0.08	0.05	0.06	0.02	0.07	0.09	0.13	0.26
皮肤其他	Other skin	4 971	0.82	0.08	0.06	0.11	0.11	0.18	0.20	0.28	0.38	0.48
间皮瘤	Mesothelioma	250	0.04	0.00	0.00	0.00	0.00	0.00	0.01	0.02	0.03	0.09
卡波氏肉瘤	Kaposi sarcoma	51	0.01	0.00	0.01	0.00	0.01	0.02	0.01	0.01	0.01	0.01
结缔组织、软组织	Connective & soft tissue	1 683	0.28	0.42	0.32	0.19	0.20	0.25	0.28	0.37	0.42	0.42
乳腺	Breast	37 749	6.30	0.00	0.00	0.00	0.21	0.44	2.26	6.48	15.24	26.27
外阴	Vulva	496	0.08	0.00	0.02	0.00	0.00	0.02	0.05	0.05	0.08	0.24
阴道	Vagina	262	0.04	0.09	0.02	0.00	0.00	0.02	0.00	0.00	0.07	0.10
子宫颈	Cervix uteri	19 182	3.16	0.00	0.00	0.00	0.00	0.13	0.63	3.11	7.92	13.77
子宫体	Corpus uteri	8 157	1.34	0.00	0.00	0.00	0.00	0.08	0.16	0.89	1.72	3.24
子宫,部位不明	Uterus unspecified	1 917	0.32	0.00	0.00	0.00	0.00	0.02	0.03	0.22	0.44	0.67
卵巢	Ovary	7 294	1.20	0.18	0.08	0.20	0.43	0.93	1.80	2.27	2.48	3.08
其他女性生殖器	Other female genital organs	556	0.09	0.00	0.02	0.00	0.02	0.08	0.09	0.19	0.16	0.31
胎盘	Placenta	107	0.02	0.00	0.00	0.02	0.02	0.02	0.14	0.32	0.35	0.10
阴茎	Penis	861	0.14	0.00	0.00	0.01	0.02	0.06	0.00	0.06	0.13	0.23
前列腺	Prostate	9 034	1.49	0.00	0.00	0.00	0.00	0.04	0.01	0.01	0.05	0.06
睾丸	Testis	422	0.07	0.16	0.21	0.07	0.06	0.09	0.33	0.47	0.59	0.50
其他男性生殖器	Other male genital organs	129	0.02	0.00	0.02	0.00	0.03	0.03	0.00	0.06	0.06	0.07
肾	Kidney	6 244	1.03	0.46	0.64	0.14	0.07	0.07	0.21	0.33	0.68	0.99
肾盂	Renal pelvis	776	0.13	0.00	0.02	0.01	0.01	0.01	0.01	0.01	0.07	0.06
输尿管	Ureter	857	0.14	0.17	0.00	0.00	0.00	0.00	0.01	0.02	0.03	0.02
膀胱	Bladder	10 775	1.77	0.08	0.00	0.01	0.02	0.05	0.09	0.30	0.41	0.56
其他泌尿器官	Other urinary organs	195	0.03	0.00	0.00	0.01	0.00	0.00	0.01	0.01	0.01	0.02
眼	Eye	387	0.06	0.92	0.52	0.10	0.01	0.02	0.00	0.04	0.01	0.04
脑、神经系统	Brain, nervous system	16 543	2.72	2.04	1.62	1.57	1.70	1.56	1.38	2.35	3.43	3.57
甲状腺	Thyroid	20 037	3.30	0.00	0.03	0.04	0.17	0.87	3.36	7.96	9.98	11.97
肾上腺	Adrenal gland	506	0.08	0.46	0.14	0.06	0.02	0.02	0.01	0.08	0.12	0.13
其他内分泌腺	Other endocrine	709	0.12	0.08	0.05	0.08	0.17	0.08	0.11	0.19	0.20	0.28
霍奇金淋巴瘤	Hodgkin lymphoma	639	0.11	0.00	0.04	0.05	0.12	0.12	0.18	0.18	0.24	0.15
非霍奇金淋巴瘤	Non-Hodgkin lymphoma	8 527	1.40	0.17	0.57	0.50	0.64	0.67	0.67	0.96	1.14	1.45
免疫增生性疾病	Immunoproliferative diseases	79	0.01	0.00	0.01	0.00	0.00	0.00	0.00	0.01	0.00	0.01
多发性骨髓瘤	Multiple myeloma	2 836	0.47	0.00	0.04	0.02	0.06	0.05	0.06	0.09	0.12	0.16
淋巴样白血病	Lymphoid leukemia	2 293	0.38	1.42	2.07	1.49	0.78	0.57	0.40	0.54	0.45	0.46
髓样白血病	Myeloid leukemia	5 609	0.92	0.83	0.82	0.57	0.85	0.90	0.98	1.33	1.30	1.30
白血病,未特指	Leukemia unspecified	4 895	0.81	2.25	1.77	1.29	1.00	1.01	0.76	0.99	1.24	0.92
其他或未指明部位	Other and unspecified	9 718	1.60	1.54	0.78	0.69	0.52	0.63	0.64	1.03	1.25	1.36
所有部位合计	All sites	607 320	100.00	12.58	10.76	7.99	9.03	10.94	16.12	33.66	53.95	77.80
所有部位除外 C44	All sites except C44	602 349	99.18	12.50	10.70	7.88	8.92	10.77	15.92	33.38	53.57	77.33

Appendix Table 1-7 Cancer incidence in rural registration areas of China, both sexes in 2017

Age group										粗率 Crude rate/ 100 000^{-1}	中标率 ASR China/ 100 000^{-1}	世标率 ASR world/ 100 000^{-1}	累积率 Cum. rate/%		ICD10
40~44	45~49	50~54	55~59	60~64	65~69	70~74	75~79	80~84	85+				0~64	0~74	
0.03	0.10	0.14	0.24	0.34	0.50	0.77	0.95	1.32	1.36	0.16	0.10	0.10	0.00	0.01	C00
0.47	0.74	1.14	1.24	1.70	1.71	2.13	2.31	1.89	2.14	0.64	0.44	0.42	0.03	0.05	C01-02
0.38	0.66	1.33	1.21	2.84	3.33	4.18	4.68	4.51	4.17	0.96	0.63	0.62	0.04	0.07	C03-06
0.42	0.64	0.89	0.89	1.43	1.28	1.63	1.46	1.17	1.12	0.55	0.41	0.39	0.03	0.04	C07-08
0.09	0.16	0.27	0.27	0.30	0.43	0.44	0.34	0.41	0.39	0.13	0.09	0.09	0.01	0.01	C09
0.09	0.12	0.35	0.45	0.72	0.81	1.07	0.91	0.95	1.02	0.24	0.16	0.16	0.01	0.02	C10
4.29	5.84	8.01	5.62	8.13	8.08	7.01	6.61	5.93	4.76	3.54	2.63	2.46	0.19	0.26	C11
0.10	0.35	0.73	0.94	1.46	1.56	1.38	1.36	0.91	1.02	0.41	0.26	0.27	0.02	0.03	C12-13
0.06	0.15	0.38	0.34	0.77	0.89	1.25	1.22	1.10	1.46	0.25	0.16	0.16	0.01	0.02	C14
1.84	6.39	18.95	28.49	67.39	105.48	130.02	150.01	163.14	143.97	23.40	14.02	14.16	0.62	1.80	C15
7.03	14.39	32.23	39.71	83.58	121.07	149.67	181.18	187.69	158.87	30.08	18.62	18.52	0.92	2.28	C16
0.41	0.88	1.37	1.53	2.71	3.59	4.30	4.46	4.51	3.69	0.98	0.64	0.62	0.04	0.08	C17
4.01	6.95	13.58	14.02	26.58	35.05	42.96	51.65	58.98	48.30	9.99	6.40	6.27	0.35	0.74	C18
4.70	8.85	17.72	18.16	35.84	49.39	58.56	70.51	74.62	62.96	13.15	8.30	8.20	0.45	0.99	C19-20
0.12	0.26	0.51	0.45	0.89	1.28	1.64	2.29	2.30	2.23	0.37	0.24	0.23	0.01	0.03	C21
18.07	29.90	50.08	49.07	77.87	94.75	103.27	121.74	130.26	125.23	29.59	19.41	19.02	1.21	2.20	C22
0.63	1.47	3.36	4.63	8.85	12.68	17.76	20.93	26.92	25.29	3.44	2.08	2.08	0.10	0.25	C23-24
1.67	3.08	6.45	7.75	15.52	22.39	29.79	38.49	43.47	39.12	6.09	3.74	3.71	0.18	0.44	C25
0.28	0.54	0.74	0.85	1.06	1.26	1.71	1.40	1.89	1.46	0.46	0.32	0.31	0.02	0.04	C30-31
0.35	0.88	2.29	2.66	5.41	6.02	7.16	7.48	7.25	4.03	1.56	0.98	0.99	0.06	0.13	C32
14.22	30.02	68.64	84.32	167.65	233.16	295.64	350.90	380.62	323.23	59.97	36.91	36.84	1.88	4.53	C33-34
0.51	0.88	1.42	1.08	2.01	2.42	2.72	2.62	2.27	2.14	0.80	0.57	0.56	0.04	0.06	C37-38
0.98	1.36	2.43	2.50	4.38	5.61	6.84	7.79	8.10	7.52	1.96	1.49	1.46	0.09	0.15	C40-41
0.19	0.37	0.59	0.60	1.07	1.27	1.66	2.11	2.27	2.62	0.45	0.31	0.30	0.02	0.03	C43
0.74	1.26	2.15	1.99	4.41	6.12	9.32	12.88	20.27	29.37	2.23	1.38	1.36	0.06	0.14	C44
0.02	0.11	0.19	0.20	0.36	0.27	0.46	0.30	0.63	0.24	0.11	0.08	0.07	0.01	0.01	C45
0.01	0.01	0.04	0.03	0.03	0.07	0.07	0.04	0.16	0.15	0.02	0.02	0.02	0.00	0.00	C46
0.68	0.90	1.08	0.95	1.69	1.78	1.86	1.85	1.89	1.89	0.75	0.59	0.58	0.04	0.06	C47;C49
50.29	74.60	85.55	60.50	71.12	58.78	45.70	39.79	36.91	24.11	34.64	25.55	23.66	1.96	2.49	C50
0.23	0.37	0.60	0.63	0.95	1.38	1.82	1.92	2.87	1.91	0.46	0.29	0.28	0.02	0.03	C51
0.17	0.30	0.36	0.41	0.57	0.72	0.95	0.86	0.92	0.24	0.24	0.16	0.16	0.01	0.02	C52
23.08	34.70	45.08	30.60	33.95	31.51	29.62	25.53	24.80	14.88	17.60	12.87	11.91	0.96	1.27	C53
7.04	13.27	24.35	17.27	17.28	14.56	11.71	9.11	6.89	3.74	7.49	5.22	5.02	0.43	0.56	C54
1.74	3.21	4.54	2.76	3.87	3.92	3.93	4.46	3.21	3.26	1.76	1.21	1.15	0.09	0.13	C55
6.41	10.72	16.11	11.76	14.80	14.73	14.46	12.67	9.07	6.13	6.69	4.88	4.64	0.36	0.50	C56
0.46	0.80	1.22	0.89	1.21	1.01	0.93	0.78	1.49	0.48	0.51	0.37	0.35	0.03	0.04	C57
0.11	0.10	0.11	0.03	0.00	0.00	0.00	0.04	0.00	0.00	0.10	0.11	0.09	0.01	0.01	C58
0.35	0.73	1.03	1.19	1.89	2.55	3.38	4.13	3.78	3.86	0.75	0.51	0.50	0.03	0.06	C60
0.21	0.56	1.51	4.02	13.29	29.69	51.86	83.82	109.37	110.99	7.92	4.77	4.69	0.10	0.51	C61
0.44	0.36	0.39	0.28	0.37	0.61	0.41	0.72	0.91	1.37	0.37	0.34	0.31	0.02	0.03	C62
0.02	0.07	0.11	0.21	0.20	0.51	0.50	0.29	0.63	0.62	0.11	0.08	0.08	0.00	0.01	C63
1.39	2.93	5.46	4.83	7.26	9.36	9.85	9.25	7.98	7.33	2.80	1.91	1.90	0.12	0.22	C64
0.07	0.21	0.38	0.47	1.00	1.36	1.52	2.17	2.14	1.31	0.35	0.22	0.22	0.01	0.03	C65
0.05	0.12	0.26	0.63	0.99	1.49	2.24	2.70	2.30	2.33	0.38	0.23	0.24	0.01	0.03	C66
1.16	2.01	4.56	5.65	11.44	17.06	22.67	33.95	39.59	38.35	4.83	2.93	2.90	0.13	0.33	C67
0.02	0.05	0.10	0.10	0.19	0.28	0.49	0.47	0.88	0.34	0.09	0.05	0.05	0.00	0.01	C68
0.09	0.06	0.23	0.13	0.33	0.56	0.36	0.65	0.69	0.87	0.17	0.13	0.17	0.01	0.01	C69
5.23	8.02	12.14	10.87	17.27	20.54	21.41	22.88	22.79	20.00	7.42	5.52	5.39	0.35	0.56	C70-72,D32-33,D42-43
13.26	16.03	20.84	14.44	12.88	9.63	7.17	4.89	3.75	3.45	8.98	7.70	6.73	0.56	0.64	C73
0.17	0.20	0.42	0.34	0.47	0.48	0.71	0.55	0.95	0.58	0.23	0.17	0.17	0.01	0.02	C74
0.29	0.41	0.60	0.48	0.64	0.67	0.57	0.39	0.54	0.78	0.32	0.26	0.25	0.02	0.02	C75
0.19	0.23	0.34	0.34	0.63	0.78	0.83	0.83	0.82	0.58	0.29	0.23	0.22	0.01	0.02	C81
2.01	3.12	5.73	5.09	9.69	12.47	13.83	16.69	14.78	11.02	3.82	2.70	2.64	0.16	0.29	C82-C86;C96
0.02	0.01	0.05	0.07	0.06	0.17	0.07	0.26	0.19	0.10	0.04	0.02	0.02	0.00	0.00	C88
0.38	0.72	1.84	2.08	3.89	5.44	6.07	5.39	4.82	3.98	1.27	0.82	0.82	0.05	0.11	C90
0.40	0.68	1.10	0.89	2.08	2.06	2.19	2.70	2.55	1.80	1.03	0.90	1.03	0.06	0.08	C91
1.68	2.34	3.40	3.31	5.26	6.48	7.76	8.66	8.61	4.56	2.51	1.96	1.91	0.12	0.19	C92-C94,D45-47
1.39	1.62	2.51	2.42	3.96	5.34	6.75	7.36	8.76	7.57	2.19	1.76	1.81	0.10	0.17	C95
2.19	3.59	5.99	5.88	10.07	13.30	15.68	18.80	21.53	24.03	4.36	3.01	2.99	0.17	0.32	O&U
136.94	229.16	392.43	393.16	692.37	910.29	1 089.11	1 280.09	1 379.20	1 208.78	272.23	179.48	175.66	10.32	20.32	C00-96, D32-33, D42-43,D45-47
136.20	227.90	390.29	391.17	687.96	904.17	1 079.78	1 267.22	1 358.93	1 179.42	270.00	178.10	174.29	10.26	20.18	C00-96, D32-33, D42-43,D45-47 exc. C44

附表 1-8 2017 年全国农村肿瘤登记地区男性癌症发病主要指标

部位 Site		病例数 No. cases	构成 Freq. /%	年龄组								
				0~	1~4	5~9	10~14	15~19	20~24	25~29	30~34	35~39
唇	Lip	219	0.06	0.00	0.04	0.01	0.03	0.01	0.01	0.01	0.00	0.06
舌	Tongue	992	0.29	0.00	0.02	0.00	0.00	0.01	0.01	0.10	0.24	0.38
口	Mouth	1 375	0.40	0.00	0.00	0.04	0.12	0.04	0.04	0.10	0.22	0.25
唾液腺	Salivary glands	663	0.19	0.00	0.02	0.01	0.12	0.00	0.19	0.23	0.18	0.41
扁桃腺	Tonsil	216	0.06	0.00	0.02	0.01	0.02	0.00	0.04	0.01	0.03	0.06
其他口咽	Other oropharynx	449	0.13	0.00	0.00	0.03	0.02	0.01	0.03	0.03	0.06	0.13
鼻咽	Nasopharynx	5 534	1.60	0.00	0.02	0.04	0.12	0.35	0.54	1.06	2.12	3.55
下咽	Hypopharynx	823	0.24	0.00	0.00	0.03	0.02	0.07	0.01	0.01	0.01	0.02
咽,部位不明	Pharynx unspecified	426	0.12	0.00	0.00	0.03	0.00	0.00	0.01	0.03	0.01	0.04
食管	Esophagus	37 503	10.82	0.00	0.00	0.00	0.02	0.00	0.14	0.25	0.33	0.75
胃	Stomach	47 317	13.66	0.00	0.05	0.04	0.14	0.20	0.43	1.07	2.26	3.27
小肠	Small intestine	1 264	0.36	0.00	0.00	0.00	0.02	0.00	0.00	0.03	0.21	0.26
结肠	Colon	12 505	3.61	0.00	0.02	0.00	0.05	0.13	0.29	0.91	1.76	2.78
直肠	Rectum	17 601	5.08	0.08	0.00	0.03	0.03	0.13	0.21	0.76	1.45	2.52
肛门	Anus	492	0.14	0.00	0.00	0.00	0.00	0.00	0.03	0.03	0.03	0.12
肝脏	Liver	48 757	14.07	0.94	0.36	0.09	0.18	0.50	0.89	3.52	7.92	14.24
胆囊及其他	Gallbladder etc.	3 574	1.03	0.00	0.00	0.00	0.00	0.01	0.04	0.05	0.15	0.24
胰腺	Pancreas	7 943	2.29	0.00	0.04	0.00	0.00	0.00	0.09	0.15	0.49	0.91
鼻、鼻窦及其他	Nose, sinuses etc.	639	0.18	0.08	0.02	0.01	0.03	0.06	0.10	0.09	0.18	0.22
喉	Larynx	3 112	0.90	0.00	0.04	0.00	0.00	0.01	0.01	0.01	0.09	0.16
气管、支气管、肺	Trachea, bronchus & lung	90 035	25.99	0.00	0.09	0.13	0.11	0.26	0.55	1.49	3.43	5.84
其他胸腔器官	Other thoracic organs	1 060	0.31	0.16	0.09	0.06	0.08	0.32	0.16	0.39	0.36	0.34
骨	Bone	2 492	0.72	0.08	0.36	0.37	1.38	1.34	0.67	0.75	0.71	0.84
皮肤黑色素瘤	Melanoma of skin	537	0.15	0.00	0.11	0.07	0.09	0.01	0.06	0.05	0.12	0.30
皮肤其他	Other skin	2 469	0.71	0.00	0.04	0.09	0.11	0.19	0.16	0.31	0.44	0.47
间皮瘤	Mesothelioma	129	0.04	0.00	0.00	0.00	0.00	0.00	0.00	0.00	0.04	0.08
卡波氏肉瘤	Kaposi sarcoma	28	0.01	0.00	0.02	0.00	0.00	0.00	0.00	0.01	0.00	0.01
结缔组织、软组织	Connective & soft tissue	889	0.26	0.63	0.39	0.22	0.17	0.25	0.30	0.36	0.37	0.47
乳腺	Breast	539	0.16	0.00	0.00	0.00	0.00	0.00	0.04	0.05	0.12	0.16
外阴	Vulva	—	—	—	—	—	—	—	—	—	—	—
阴道	Vagina	—	—	—	—	—	—	—	—	—	—	—
子宫颈	Cervix uteri	—	—	—	—	—	—	—	—	—	—	—
子宫体	Corpus uteri	—	—	—	—	—	—	—	—	—	—	—
子宫,部位不明	Uterus unspecified	—	—	—	—	—	—	—	—	—	—	—
卵巢	Ovary	—	—	—	—	—	—	—	—	—	—	—
其他女性生殖器	Other female genital organs	—	—	—	—	—	—	—	—	—	—	—
胎盘	Placenta	—	—	—	—	—	—	—	—	—	—	—
阴茎	Penis	861	0.25	0.00	0.00	0.01	0.02	0.06	0.00	0.06	0.13	0.23
前列腺	Prostate	9 034	2.61	0.00	0.00	0.00	0.00	0.04	0.01	0.01	0.05	0.06
睾丸	Testis	422	0.12	0.16	0.21	0.07	0.06	0.09	0.33	0.47	0.59	0.50
其他男性生殖器	Other male genital organs	129	0.04	0.00	0.02	0.00	0.03	0.03	0.00	0.06	0.06	0.07
肾	Kidney	3 897	1.12	0.63	0.64	0.10	0.11	0.07	0.19	0.34	0.78	1.25
肾盂	Renal pelvis	470	0.14	0.00	0.02	0.00	0.00	0.01	0.00	0.01	0.06	0.10
输尿管	Ureter	482	0.14	0.23	0.00	0.00	0.00	0.00	0.01	0.03	0.03	0.02
膀胱	Bladder	8 555	2.47	0.00	0.00	0.00	0.03	0.07	0.08	0.33	0.64	0.77
其他泌尿器官	Other urinary organs	122	0.04	0.00	0.00	0.01	0.00	0.00	0.03	0.01	0.01	0.02
眼	Eye	197	0.06	0.78	0.55	0.11	0.00	0.03	0.00	0.05	0.01	0.02
脑、神经系统	Brain, nervous system	7 971	2.30	2.27	1.75	1.82	1.87	1.71	1.58	2.52	3.95	3.43
甲状腺	Thyroid	4 525	1.31	0.00	0.00	0.04	0.09	0.48	1.59	3.86	5.00	5.79
肾上腺	Adrenal gland	278	0.08	0.47	0.14	0.07	0.03	0.03	0.00	0.06	0.12	0.11
其他内分泌腺	Other endocrine	362	0.10	0.08	0.05	0.11	0.23	0.07	0.08	0.15	0.17	0.22
霍奇金淋巴瘤	Hodgkin lymphoma	381	0.11	0.00	0.07	0.10	0.17	0.12	0.23	0.23	0.19	0.16
非霍奇金淋巴瘤	Non-Hodgkin lymphoma	5 015	1.45	0.16	0.66	0.59	0.84	0.85	0.77	1.00	1.21	1.68
免疫增生性疾病	Immunoproliferative diseases	55	0.02	0.00	0.02	0.00	0.00	0.00	0.00	0.01	0.00	0.01
多发性骨髓瘤	Multiple myeloma	1 612	0.47	0.00	0.05	0.03	0.06	0.04	0.10	0.09	0.18	0.22
淋巴样白血病	Lymphoid leukemia	1 348	0.39	1.56	2.23	1.78	0.92	0.76	0.50	0.62	0.47	0.49
髓样白血病	Myeloid leukemia	3 148	0.91	0.86	1.02	0.55	0.95	1.03	1.08	1.57	1.50	1.23
白血病,未特指	Leukemia unspecified	2 812	0.81	2.34	2.07	1.45	1.30	1.24	0.84	1.19	1.49	0.99
其他或未指明部位	Other and unspecified	5 210	1.50	1.09	0.75	0.73	0.64	0.57	0.56	0.88	1.30	1.27
所有部位合计	All sites	346 468	100.00	12.58	11.99	8.91	10.19	11.24	13.02	25.42	41.26	57.50
所有部位除外 C44	All sites except C44	343 999	99.29	12.58	11.95	8.82	10.09	11.05	12.85	25.12	40.82	57.03

Appendix Table 1-8 Cancer incidence in rural registration areas of China, male in 2017

Age group										粗率 Crude rate/ $100\ 000^{-1}$	中标率 ASR China/ $100\ 000^{-1}$	世标率 ASR world/ $100\ 000^{-1}$	累积率 Cum. rate/%		ICD10
40~44	45~49	50~54	55~59	60~64	65~69	70~74	75~79	80~84	85+				0~64	0~74	
0.04	0.12	0.14	0.31	0.49	0.67	0.88	1.01	1.75	1.62	0.19	0.13	0.13	0.01	0.01	C00
0.70	1.02	1.71	1.85	2.21	2.53	2.65	2.95	2.66	2.99	0.87	0.61	0.59	0.04	0.07	C01-02
0.51	0.90	1.88	1.65	3.77	4.43	5.54	5.35	5.45	5.60	1.20	0.81	0.81	0.05	0.10	C03-06
0.40	0.68	0.85	0.87	1.78	1.53	1.98	1.90	1.40	1.12	0.58	0.43	0.41	0.03	0.05	C07-08
0.07	0.17	0.47	0.47	0.44	0.67	0.53	0.51	0.84	0.37	0.19	0.13	0.13	0.01	0.02	C09
0.14	0.20	0.59	0.84	1.20	1.47	1.75	1.56	1.75	1.49	0.39	0.27	0.26	0.02	0.03	C10
5.88	8.18	11.41	8.23	11.42	10.89	9.80	9.73	8.25	5.85	4.85	3.64	3.41	0.26	0.37	C11
0.14	0.63	1.32	1.75	2.71	2.96	2.42	2.40	1.82	1.87	0.72	0.47	0.49	0.03	0.06	C12-13
0.08	0.22	0.64	0.54	1.15	1.27	1.95	1.94	2.03	2.12	0.37	0.24	0.24	0.01	0.03	C14
2.88	10.39	30.26	45.29	103.73	157.32	183.90	206.84	219.92	199.83	32.86	20.65	20.93	0.97	2.68	C15
8.17	18.75	44.47	59.00	126.78	179.11	218.76	261.20	266.57	217.75	41.46	26.51	26.54	1.32	3.31	C16
0.52	1.12	1.56	1.72	3.07	4.31	4.90	5.23	5.10	4.48	1.11	0.74	0.73	0.04	0.09	C17
4.48	7.54	15.16	16.03	30.32	40.07	49.82	58.28	67.34	60.10	10.96	7.27	7.14	0.40	0.85	C18
5.18	10.24	20.33	22.10	43.83	61.94	73.82	87.32	90.63	82.00	15.42	10.07	9.99	0.53	1.21	C19-20
0.09	0.32	0.57	0.63	1.15	1.61	2.28	2.44	2.80	1.62	0.43	0.28	0.28	0.01	0.03	C21
29.99	49.37	79.88	76.85	116.82	135.85	140.76	164.61	168.74	168.35	42.72	29.21	28.53	1.90	3.29	C22
0.61	1.36	2.79	5.18	8.89	12.40	16.92	19.47	23.57	23.27	3.13	1.98	1.99	0.10	0.24	C23-24
2.07	4.03	8.34	9.76	18.41	26.61	34.88	44.63	49.72	46.41	6.96	4.48	4.44	0.22	0.53	C25
0.32	0.70	0.85	1.12	1.43	1.59	2.04	1.73	2.73	1.62	0.56	0.40	0.39	0.03	0.04	C30-31
0.59	1.55	4.22	4.93	9.73	11.03	12.66	13.27	13.71	8.21	2.73	1.75	1.77	0.11	0.23	C32
15.59	35.64	87.61	116.12	232.81	327.69	415.29	502.13	534.67	462.00	78.89	50.26	50.33	2.50	6.21	C33-34
0.62	0.97	1.48	1.28	2.44	2.80	3.27	3.16	3.22	2.74	0.93	0.69	0.67	0.04	0.07	C37-38
1.01	1.63	2.48	2.77	5.01	6.62	8.17	9.86	9.44	7.84	2.18	1.70	1.67	0.10	0.17	C40-41
0.20	0.37	0.57	0.60	1.24	1.29	1.90	2.19	3.29	2.86	0.47	0.33	0.33	0.02	0.03	C43
0.71	1.33	2.21	1.96	4.98	6.47	10.03	12.64	21.68	26.50	2.16	1.43	1.40	0.06	0.15	C44
0.01	0.11	0.21	0.18	0.32	0.35	0.47	0.34	0.84	0.37	0.11	0.08	0.07	0.00	0.01	C45
0.01	0.02	0.05	0.06	0.00	0.12	0.06	0.08	0.14	0.25	0.02	0.02	0.02	0.00	0.00	C46
0.62	0.79	1.06	0.87	1.93	2.02	2.13	2.40	2.66	1.74	0.78	0.61	0.61	0.04	0.06	C47;C49
0.29	0.62	0.77	0.82	0.95	1.55	1.78	1.81	2.38	2.86	0.47	0.32	0.31	0.02	0.04	C50
—	—	—	—	—	—	—	—	—	—	—	—	—	—	—	C51
—	—	—	—	—	—	—	—	—	—	—	—	—	—	—	C52
—	—	—	—	—	—	—	—	—	—	—	—	—	—	—	C53
—	—	—	—	—	—	—	—	—	—	—	—	—	—	—	C54
—	—	—	—	—	—	—	—	—	—	—	—	—	—	—	C55
—	—	—	—	—	—	—	—	—	—	—	—	—	—	—	C56
—	—	—	—	—	—	—	—	—	—	—	—	—	—	—	C57
—	—	—	—	—	—	—	—	—	—	—	—	—	—	—	C58
0.35	0.73	1.03	1.19	1.89	2.55	3.38	4.13	3.78	3.86	0.75	0.51	0.50	0.03	0.06	C60
0.21	0.56	1.51	4.02	13.29	29.69	51.86	83.82	109.37	110.99	7.92	4.77	4.69	0.10	0.51	C61
0.44	0.36	0.39	0.28	0.37	0.61	0.41	0.72	0.91	1.37	0.37	0.34	0.31	0.02	0.03	C62
0.02	0.07	0.11	0.21	0.20	0.51	0.50	0.29	0.63	0.62	0.11	0.08	0.08	0.00	0.01	C63
1.77	3.63	6.66	6.08	9.15	11.66	12.22	12.35	10.91	10.33	3.41	2.37	2.36	0.15	0.27	C64
0.09	0.25	0.53	0.65	1.29	1.65	1.84	2.40	2.38	1.62	0.41	0.27	0.27	0.02	0.03	C65
0.03	0.14	0.33	0.72	1.23	1.78	2.28	3.16	2.66	2.36	0.42	0.27	0.27	0.01	0.03	C66
1.72	3.28	7.17	9.02	18.38	27.69	35.96	55.92	67.90	75.28	7.50	4.75	4.71	0.21	0.53	C67
0.01	0.09	0.09	0.07	0.23	0.35	0.64	0.59	1.40	0.50	0.11	0.07	0.07	0.00	0.01	C68
0.10	0.06	0.24	0.16	0.32	0.51	0.38	0.84	0.56	0.75	0.17	0.13	0.17	0.01	0.01	C69
5.08	7.76	10.79	9.21	16.20	19.14	21.00	22.42	22.73	22.02	6.98	5.41	5.27	0.34	0.54	C70-72,D32-33,D42-43
5.53	6.61	8.31	5.84	5.41	5.13	4.05	3.16	2.10	2.61	3.97	3.49	3.02	0.24	0.29	C73
0.14	0.17	0.44	0.46	0.58	0.57	0.73	0.63	1.47	0.87	0.24	0.18	0.19	0.01	0.02	C74
0.31	0.39	0.56	0.47	0.63	0.80	0.70	0.51	0.77	0.75	0.32	0.26	0.25	0.02	0.02	C75
0.28	0.29	0.42	0.40	0.81	0.96	0.90	0.80	0.98	0.50	0.33	0.27	0.27	0.02	0.03	C81
2.17	3.54	6.55	5.81	11.43	15.05	16.10	21.70	17.97	15.68	4.39	3.17	3.11	0.19	0.34	C82-C86;C96
0.01	0.02	0.07	0.09	0.08	0.27	0.12	0.38	0.28	0.25	0.05	0.03	0.03	0.00	0.00	C88
0.47	0.77	1.98	2.22	4.26	6.21	7.00	6.24	6.36	6.47	1.41	0.94	0.94	0.05	0.12	C90
0.41	0.76	1.01	0.94	2.53	2.61	2.39	3.33	3.57	3.24	1.18	1.04	1.18	0.07	0.09	C91
1.79	2.46	3.76	3.50	5.90	6.62	9.19	10.45	11.54	7.34	2.76	2.18	2.13	0.13	0.21	C92-C94,D45-47
1.55	1.83	2.67	2.62	4.72	5.94	7.55	8.55	10.14	10.95	2.46	2.02	2.09	0.12	0.19	C95
1.96	3.30	5.95	6.62	11.14	15.48	18.49	21.87	25.66	27.62	4.57	3.21	3.19	0.18	0.35	O&U
106.35	196.01	384.47	444.35	849.04	1 162.97	1 409.03	1 691.27	1 819.11	1 649.77	303.60	201.30	199.70	10.80	23.66	C00-96, D32-33, D42-43,D45-47
105.64	194.68	382.26	442.40	844.06	1 156.49	1 398.99	1 678.62	1 797.43	1 623.27	301.43	199.87	198.30	10.73	23.51	C00-96, D32-33, D42-43,D45-47 exc. C44

附表 1-9　2017 年全国农村肿瘤登记地区女性癌症发病主要指标

部位 Site		病例数 No. cases	构成 Freq. /%	年龄组								
				0~	1~4	5~9	10~14	15~19	20~24	25~29	30~34	35~39
唇	Lip	144	0.06	0.09	0.00	0.00	0.00	0.00	0.03	0.01	0.01	0.00
舌	Tongue	440	0.17	0.00	0.02	0.02	0.00	0.02	0.00	0.07	0.13	0.14
口	Mouth	762	0.29	0.09	0.02	0.05	0.02	0.11	0.05	0.13	0.13	0.19
唾液腺	Salivary glands	555	0.21	0.00	0.00	0.00	0.07	0.08	0.13	0.30	0.31	0.41
扁桃腺	Tonsil	82	0.03	0.00	0.00	0.00	0.00	0.00	0.03	0.00	0.01	0.02
其他口咽	Other oropharynx	83	0.03	0.00	0.00	0.00	0.00	0.00	0.01	0.01	0.04	0.02
鼻咽	Nasopharynx	2 364	0.91	0.09	0.00	0.03	0.11	0.21	0.26	0.56	1.20	1.62
下咽	Hypopharynx	86	0.03	0.09	0.00	0.02	0.00	0.00	0.00	0.02	0.01	0.05
咽,部位不明	Pharynx unspecified	136	0.05	0.00	0.00	0.00	0.02	0.00	0.03	0.01	0.00	0.02
食管	Esophagus	14 708	5.64	0.27	0.04	0.03	0.02	0.00	0.05	0.13	0.08	0.49
胃	Stomach	19 782	7.58	0.00	0.02	0.00	0.05	0.23	0.51	1.44	2.61	3.41
小肠	Small intestine	927	0.36	0.00	0.00	0.00	0.00	0.00	0.04	0.02	0.15	0.24
结肠	Colon	9 791	3.75	0.00	0.00	0.00	0.05	0.11	0.25	0.79	1.36	1.96
直肠	Rectum	11 732	4.50	0.09	0.02	0.00	0.07	0.02	0.13	0.72	1.19	1.86
肛门	Anus	339	0.13	0.00	0.00	0.00	0.00	0.00	0.01	0.01	0.01	0.12
肝脏	Liver	17 252	6.61	0.62	0.19	0.15	0.23	0.41	0.32	1.08	1.55	2.71
胆囊及其他	Gallbladder etc.	4 108	1.57	0.09	0.02	0.00	0.00	0.02	0.04	0.02	0.19	0.36
胰腺	Pancreas	5 642	2.16	0.09	0.02	0.05	0.04	0.08	0.13	0.14	0.28	0.66
鼻、鼻窦及其他	Nose,sinuses etc.	385	0.15	0.00	0.06	0.00	0.02	0.02	0.04	0.10	0.15	0.09
喉	Larynx	363	0.14	0.09	0.00	0.00	0.02	0.03	0.01	0.06	0.03	0.05
气管、支气管、肺	Trachea,bronchus & lung	43 751	16.77	0.00	0.06	0.00	0.11	0.15	0.51	1.49	3.15	5.33
其他胸腔器官	Other thoracic organs	725	0.28	0.00	0.04	0.05	0.04	0.13	0.08	0.13	0.17	0.27
骨	Bone	1 883	0.72	0.00	0.27	0.36	0.93	0.66	0.75	0.71	0.63	0.57
皮肤黑色素瘤	Melanoma of skin	467	0.18	0.00	0.04	0.03	0.02	0.02	0.08	0.13	0.15	0.22
皮肤其他	Other skin	2 502	0.96	0.18	0.08	0.13	0.11	0.16	0.24	0.25	0.32	0.49
间皮瘤	Mesothelioma	121	0.05	0.00	0.00	0.00	0.00	0.00	0.01	0.04	0.01	0.09
卡波氏肉瘤	Kaposi sarcoma	23	0.01	0.00	0.00	0.00	0.02	0.05	0.03	0.01	0.01	0.00
结缔组织、软组织	Connective & soft tissue	794	0.30	0.18	0.23	0.16	0.23	0.26	0.25	0.37	0.47	0.37
乳腺	Breast	37 749	14.47	0.00	0.00	0.00	0.21	0.44	2.26	6.48	15.24	26.27
外阴	Vulva	496	0.19	0.00	0.02	0.00	0.00	0.02	0.05	0.05	0.08	0.24
阴道	Vagina	262	0.10	0.09	0.02	0.00	0.00	0.02	0.00	0.00	0.07	0.10
子宫颈	Cervix uteri	19 182	7.35	0.00	0.00	0.00	0.00	0.13	0.63	3.11	7.92	13.77
子宫体	Corpus uteri	8 157	3.13	0.00	0.00	0.00	0.00	0.08	0.16	0.89	1.72	3.24
子宫,部位不明	Uterus unspecified	1 917	0.73	0.00	0.00	0.00	0.00	0.02	0.03	0.22	0.44	0.67
卵巢	Ovary	7 294	2.80	0.18	0.08	0.20	0.43	0.93	1.80	2.27	2.48	3.08
其他女性生殖器	Other female genital organs	556	0.21	0.00	0.02	0.00	0.02	0.08	0.09	0.19	0.16	0.31
胎盘	Placenta	107	0.04	0.00	0.00	0.02	0.02	0.02	0.14	0.32	0.35	0.10
阴茎	Penis	—	—	—	—	—	—	—	—	—	—	—
前列腺	Prostate	—	—	—	—	—	—	—	—	—	—	—
睾丸	Testis	—	—	—	—	—	—	—	—	—	—	—
其他男性生殖器	Other male genital organs	—	—	—	—	—	—	—	—	—	—	—
肾	Kidney	2 347	0.90	0.27	0.63	0.18	0.02	0.07	0.22	0.31	0.57	0.72
肾盂	Renal pelvis	306	0.12	0.00	0.02	0.02	0.02	0.00	0.03	0.00	0.07	0.01
输尿管	Ureter	375	0.14	0.09	0.00	0.00	0.00	0.00	0.00	0.00	0.03	0.01
膀胱	Bladder	2 220	0.85	0.18	0.00	0.02	0.02	0.02	0.11	0.28	0.16	0.35
其他泌尿器官	Other urinary organs	73	0.03	0.00	0.00	0.00	0.00	0.00	0.00	0.00	0.00	0.01
眼	Eye	190	0.07	1.07	0.48	0.08	0.02	0.00	0.00	0.02	0.01	0.06
脑、神经系统	Brain,nervous system	8 572	3.29	1.78	1.46	1.29	1.50	1.39	1.17	2.17	2.89	3.72
甲状腺	Thyroid	15 512	5.95	0.00	0.06	0.03	0.27	1.31	5.21	12.27	15.14	18.41
肾上腺	Adrenal gland	228	0.09	0.45	0.15	0.05	0.02	0.02	0.03	0.10	0.12	0.16
其他内分泌腺	Other endocrine	347	0.13	0.09	0.04	0.05	0.09	0.08	0.14	0.23	0.23	0.35
霍奇金淋巴瘤	Hodgkin lymphoma	258	0.10	0.00	0.00	0.00	0.05	0.11	0.13	0.13	0.29	0.15
非霍奇金淋巴瘤	Non-Hodgkin lymphoma	3 512	1.35	0.18	0.46	0.41	0.39	0.47	0.57	0.92	1.08	1.21
免疫增生性疾病	Immunoproliferative diseases	24	0.01	0.00	0.00	0.00	0.00	0.00	0.00	0.00	0.00	0.01
多发性骨髓瘤	Multiple myeloma	1 224	0.47	0.00	0.02	0.02	0.05	0.07	0.01	0.08	0.05	0.10
淋巴样白血病	Lymphoid leukemia	945	0.36	1.25	1.88	1.16	0.63	0.36	0.30	0.47	0.43	0.42
髓样白血病	Myeloid leukemia	2 461	0.94	0.80	0.59	0.60	0.73	0.75	0.87	1.08	1.09	1.37
白血病,未特指	Leukemia unspecified	2 083	0.80	2.14	1.42	1.11	0.64	0.75	0.67	0.78	0.97	0.85
其他或未指明部位	Other and unspecified	4 508	1.73	2.05	0.82	0.65	0.38	0.70	0.72	1.19	1.20	1.45
所有部位合计	All sites	260 852	100.00	12.58	9.32	6.94	7.67	10.61	19.36	42.33	67.13	98.94
所有部位除外 C44	All sites except C44	258 350	99.04	12.40	9.24	6.81	7.56	10.45	19.13	42.08	66.81	98.45

Appendix Table 1-9 Cancer incidence in rural registration areas of China, female in 2017

Age group										粗率 Crude rate/ $100\ 000^{-1}$	中标率 ASR China/ $100\ 000^{-1}$	世标率 ASR world/ $100\ 000^{-1}$	累积率 Cum. rate/%		ICD10
40~44	45~49	50~54	55~59	60~64	65~69	70~74	75~79	80~84	85+				0~64	0~74	
0. 02	0. 08	0. 15	0. 17	0. 19	0. 33	0. 67	0. 90	0. 98	1. 19	0. 13	0. 08	0. 08	0. 00	0. 01	C00
0. 23	0. 44	0. 55	0. 62	1. 18	0. 89	1. 62	1. 72	1. 26	1. 59	0. 40	0. 27	0. 26	0. 02	0. 03	C01-02
0. 24	0. 41	0. 76	0. 75	1. 88	2. 23	2. 83	4. 07	3. 73	3. 26	0. 70	0. 44	0. 44	0. 02	0. 05	C03-06
0. 44	0. 60	0. 92	0. 92	1. 07	1. 03	1. 27	1. 06	0. 98	1. 11	0. 51	0. 39	0. 36	0. 03	0. 04	C07-08
0. 12	0. 15	0. 06	0. 06	0. 16	0. 19	0. 35	0. 20	0. 06	0. 40	0. 08	0. 05	0. 05	0. 00	0. 01	C09
0. 03	0. 04	0. 10	0. 06	0. 22	0. 14	0. 40	0. 31	0. 29	0. 72	0. 08	0. 05	0. 05	0. 00	0. 01	C10
2. 63	3. 45	4. 49	2. 96	4. 75	5. 24	4. 25	3. 71	4. 02	4. 06	2. 17	1. 60	1. 49	0. 11	0. 16	C11
0. 06	0. 06	0. 12	0. 11	0. 17	0. 14	0. 35	0. 39	0. 17	0. 48	0. 08	0. 05	0. 05	0. 00	0. 01	C12-13
0. 03	0. 08	0. 11	0. 14	0. 38	0. 52	0. 55	0. 55	0. 34	1. 03	0. 12	0. 08	0. 08	0. 00	0. 01	C14
0. 77	2. 32	7. 25	11. 26	29. 98	53. 13	76. 59	97. 30	116. 52	108. 24	13. 50	7. 49	7. 48	0. 26	0. 91	C15
5. 83	9. 93	19. 58	19. 95	39. 11	62. 45	81. 16	106. 95	122. 95	121. 21	18. 15	10. 86	10. 62	0. 51	1. 23	C16
0. 28	0. 62	1. 18	1. 33	2. 33	2. 87	3. 70	3. 75	4. 02	3. 18	0. 85	0. 53	0. 52	0. 03	0. 06	C17
3. 52	6. 34	11. 94	11. 96	22. 73	29. 99	36. 16	45. 50	52. 12	40. 75	8. 99	5. 54	5. 42	0. 31	0. 64	C18
4. 20	7. 44	15. 03	14. 11	27. 61	36. 71	43. 42	54. 92	61. 48	50. 78	10. 77	6. 56	6. 46	0. 36	0. 76	C19-20
0. 15	0. 19	0. 44	0. 26	0. 62	0. 95	1. 01	2. 15	1. 89	2. 63	0. 31	0. 19	0. 18	0. 01	0. 02	C21
5. 68	10. 04	19. 27	20. 60	37. 78	53. 25	66. 09	81. 97	98. 67	97. 65	15. 83	9. 54	9. 44	0. 50	1. 10	C22
0. 66	1. 58	3. 94	4. 07	8. 80	12. 97	18. 60	22. 28	29. 68	26. 58	3. 77	2. 17	2. 15	0. 10	0. 26	C23-24
1. 25	2. 12	4. 49	5. 70	12. 54	18. 13	24. 73	32. 80	38. 34	34. 46	5. 18	3. 01	2. 98	0. 14	0. 35	C25
0. 25	0. 38	0. 63	0. 57	0. 68	0. 93	1. 39	1. 09	1. 21	1. 35	0. 35	0. 24	0. 23	0. 01	0. 03	C30-31
0. 10	0. 20	0. 29	0. 33	0. 96	0. 97	1. 71	2. 11	1. 95	1. 35	0. 33	0. 21	0. 20	0. 01	0. 02	C32
12. 79	24. 30	49. 04	51. 74	100. 57	137. 71	176. 99	210. 62	254. 17	234. 46	40. 15	23. 89	23. 69	1. 25	2. 82	C33-34
0. 40	0. 79	1. 36	0. 87	1. 56	2. 04	2. 17	2. 11	1. 49	1. 75	0. 67	0. 46	0. 45	0. 03	0. 05	C37-38
0. 94	1. 07	2. 38	2. 23	3. 74	4. 60	5. 52	5. 86	7. 00	7. 32	1. 73	1. 28	1. 25	0. 08	0. 13	C40-41
0. 18	0. 37	0. 60	0. 59	0. 88	1. 26	1. 42	2. 03	1. 44	2. 47	0. 43	0. 29	0. 28	0. 02	0. 03	C43
0. 78	1. 19	2. 09	2. 02	3. 82	5. 75	8. 62	13. 10	19. 11	31. 20	2. 30	1. 33	1. 32	0. 06	0. 13	C44
0. 03	0. 11	0. 16	0. 23	0. 39	0. 19	0. 46	0. 27	0. 46	0. 16	0. 11	0. 07	0. 07	0. 01	0. 01	C45
0. 01	0. 00	0. 02	0. 00	0. 06	0. 02	0. 09	0. 00	0. 17	0. 08	0. 02	0. 02	0. 02	0. 00	0. 00	C46
0. 75	1. 01	1. 10	1. 04	1. 44	1. 53	1. 59	1. 33	1. 26	1. 99	0. 73	0. 57	0. 55	0. 04	0. 05	C47;C49
50. 29	74. 60	85. 55	60. 50	71. 12	58. 78	45. 70	39. 79	36. 91	24. 11	34. 64	25. 55	23. 66	1. 96	2. 49	C50
0. 23	0. 37	0. 60	0. 63	0. 95	1. 38	1. 82	1. 92	2. 87	1. 91	0. 46	0. 29	0. 28	0. 02	0. 03	C51
0. 17	0. 30	0. 36	0. 41	0. 57	0. 72	0. 95	0. 86	0. 92	0. 24	0. 24	0. 16	0. 16	0. 01	0. 02	C52
23. 08	34. 70	45. 08	30. 60	33. 95	31. 51	29. 62	25. 53	24. 80	14. 88	17. 60	12. 87	11. 91	0. 96	1. 27	C53
7. 04	13. 27	24. 35	17. 27	17. 28	14. 56	11. 71	9. 11	6. 89	3. 74	7. 49	5. 22	5. 02	0. 43	0. 56	C54
1. 74	3. 21	4. 54	2. 76	3. 87	3. 92	3. 93	4. 46	3. 21	3. 26	1. 76	1. 21	1. 15	0. 09	0. 13	C55
6. 41	10. 72	16. 11	11. 76	14. 80	14. 73	14. 46	12. 67	9. 07	6. 13	6. 69	4. 88	4. 64	0. 36	0. 50	C56
0. 46	0. 80	1. 22	0. 89	1. 21	1. 01	0. 93	0. 78	1. 49	0. 48	0. 51	0. 37	0. 35	0. 03	0. 04	C57
0. 11	0. 10	0. 11	0. 03	0. 00	0. 00	0. 00	0. 04	0. 00	0. 00	0. 10	0. 11	0. 09	0. 01	0. 01	C58
—	—	—	—	—	—	—	—	—	—	—	—	—	—	—	C60
—	—	—	—	—	—	—	—	—	—	—	—	—	—	—	C61
—	—	—	—	—	—	—	—	—	—	—	—	—	—	—	C62
—	—	—	—	—	—	—	—	—	—	—	—	—	—	—	C63
1. 01	2. 22	4. 22	3. 54	5. 32	7. 03	7. 49	6. 37	5. 57	5. 41	2. 15	1. 45	1. 45	0. 09	0. 17	C64
0. 05	0. 18	0. 22	0. 29	0. 69	1. 07	1. 21	1. 95	1. 95	1. 11	0. 28	0. 17	0. 17	0. 01	0. 02	C65
0. 07	0. 11	0. 18	0. 54	0. 74	1. 20	2. 20	2. 27	2. 01	2. 31	0. 34	0. 20	0. 20	0. 01	0. 03	C66
0. 58	0. 71	1. 85	2. 20	4. 31	6. 33	9. 49	13. 56	16. 36	14. 72	2. 04	1. 19	1. 17	0. 05	0. 13	C67
0. 02	0. 02	0. 10	0. 12	0. 16	0. 21	0. 35	0. 35	0. 46	0. 24	0. 07	0. 04	0. 04	0. 00	0. 00	C68
0. 08	0. 07	0. 22	0. 11	0. 35	0. 62	0. 35	0. 47	0. 80	0. 96	0. 17	0. 13	0. 17	0. 01	0. 01	C69
5. 38	8. 30	13. 54	12. 56	18. 36	21. 96	21. 81	23. 30	22. 85	18. 70	7. 87	5. 63	5. 51	0. 37	0. 59	C70-72,D32-33,D42-43
21. 31	25. 65	33. 79	23. 25	20. 57	14. 17	10. 27	6. 49	5. 11	3. 98	14. 24	12. 04	10. 56	0. 89	1. 01	C73
0. 19	0. 23	0. 41	0. 21	0. 36	0. 39	0. 69	0. 47	0. 52	0. 40	0. 21	0. 16	0. 16	0. 01	0. 02	C74
0. 28	0. 42	0. 64	0. 48	0. 65	0. 54	0. 43	0. 27	0. 34	0. 80	0. 32	0. 26	0. 24	0. 02	0. 02	C75
0. 10	0. 18	0. 27	0. 29	0. 44	0. 60	0. 75	0. 86	0. 69	0. 64	0. 24	0. 19	0. 17	0. 01	0. 02	C81
1. 84	2. 68	4. 89	4. 34	7. 89	9. 86	11. 57	12. 04	12. 17	8. 04	3. 22	2. 23	2. 18	0. 14	0. 24	C82-C86;C96
0. 02	0. 01	0. 04	0. 05	0. 05	0. 08	0. 03	0. 16	0. 11	0. 00	0. 02	0. 01	0. 01	0. 00	0. 00	C88
0. 29	0. 67	1. 69	1. 93	3. 50	4. 66	5. 15	4. 61	3. 56	2. 39	1. 12	0. 70	0. 71	0. 04	0. 09	C90
0. 39	0. 59	1. 20	0. 83	1. 61	1. 51	2. 00	2. 11	1. 72	0. 88	0. 87	0. 76	0. 86	0. 05	0. 07	C91
1. 57	2. 22	3. 02	3. 12	4. 59	6. 33	6. 33	7. 00	6. 20	2. 79	2. 26	1. 74	1. 69	0. 11	0. 17	C92-C94,D45-47
1. 22	1. 41	2. 34	2. 22	3. 19	4. 72	5. 96	6. 25	7. 63	5. 41	1. 91	1. 48	1. 53	0. 09	0. 14	C95
2. 42	3. 89	6. 04	5. 13	8. 96	11. 10	12. 90	15. 95	18. 14	21. 73	4. 14	2. 81	2. 80	0. 17	0. 29	O&U
168. 75	262. 98	400. 66	340. 69	531. 10	655. 12	771. 84	898. 70	1 018. 11	926. 72	239. 38	159. 11	153. 05	9. 84	16. 97	C00-96, D32-33, D42-43,D45-47
167. 97	261. 79	398. 58	338. 67	527. 28	649. 37	763. 22	885. 60	998. 99	895. 52	237. 08	157. 78	151. 73	9. 78	16. 84	C00-96, D32-33, D42-43,D45-47 exc. C44

附表 1-10　2017 年全国肿瘤登记地区男女合计癌症死亡主要指标

部位 Site		死亡数 No. deaths	构成 Freq. /%	年龄组								
				0~	1~4	5~9	10~14	15~19	20~24	25~29	30~34	35~39
唇	Lip	346	0.04	0.00	0.00	0.00	0.00	0.00	0.00	0.00	0.00	0.01
舌	Tongue	2 067	0.27	0.00	0.01	0.00	0.00	0.01	0.01	0.02	0.07	0.10
口	Mouth	2 515	0.33	0.00	0.01	0.00	0.01	0.00	0.00	0.03	0.05	0.07
唾液腺	Salivary glands	800	0.10	0.00	0.00	0.00	0.01	0.01	0.02	0.02	0.01	0.07
扁桃腺	Tonsil	321	0.04	0.00	0.00	0.00	0.00	0.00	0.00	0.00	0.01	0.01
其他口咽	Other oropharynx	709	0.09	0.00	0.00	0.00	0.00	0.00	0.01	0.01	0.00	0.01
鼻咽	Nasopharynx	8 212	1.06	0.06	0.01	0.00	0.02	0.07	0.09	0.20	0.44	0.69
下咽	Hypopharynx	1 134	0.15	0.00	0.00	0.00	0.00	0.00	0.00	0.00	0.01	0.02
咽,部位不明	Pharynx unspecified	860	0.11	0.00	0.00	0.00	0.00	0.00	0.00	0.01	0.00	0.02
食管	Esophagus	66 371	8.59	0.24	0.03	0.00	0.01	0.01	0.02	0.04	0.09	0.23
胃	Stomach	91 166	11.79	0.77	0.02	0.01	0.01	0.08	0.26	0.62	1.27	1.86
小肠	Small intestine	3 115	0.40	0.02	0.00	0.00	0.00	0.00	0.01	0.02	0.03	0.11
结肠	Colon	27 904	3.61	0.24	0.01	0.00	0.02	0.05	0.15	0.26	0.59	0.72
直肠	Rectum	32 402	4.19	0.45	0.00	0.02	0.01	0.03	0.06	0.28	0.52	0.77
肛门	Anus	1 134	0.15	0.00	0.00	0.00	0.00	0.00	0.00	0.01	0.02	0.04
肝脏	Liver	108 691	14.06	1.63	0.24	0.08	0.15	0.22	0.42	1.31	3.08	5.68
胆囊及其他	Gallbladder etc.	13 178	1.70	0.13	0.01	0.00	0.00	0.01	0.02	0.06	0.09	0.13
胰腺	Pancreas	27 907	3.61	0.15	0.01	0.00	0.00	0.01	0.03	0.11	0.25	0.44
鼻、鼻窦及其他	Nose, sinuses etc.	980	0.13	0.02	0.02	0.01	0.01	0.02	0.02	0.02	0.05	0.06
喉	Larynx	4 712	0.61	0.02	0.02	0.01	0.00	0.03	0.01	0.02	0.03	0.06
气管、支气管、肺	Trachea, bronchus & lung	215 025	27.82	1.61	0.05	0.04	0.08	0.08	0.27	0.68	1.52	2.81
其他胸腔器官	Other thoracic organs	2 354	0.30	0.15	0.03	0.05	0.01	0.06	0.08	0.11	0.09	0.17
骨	Bone	5 795	0.75	0.06	0.02	0.11	0.28	0.43	0.28	0.23	0.27	0.23
皮肤黑色素瘤	Melanoma of skin	1 589	0.21	0.02	0.07	0.05	0.01	0.03	0.02	0.06	0.08	0.11
皮肤其他	Other skin	3 374	0.44	0.06	0.01	0.01	0.04	0.04	0.03	0.06	0.07	0.09
间皮瘤	Mesothelioma	517	0.07	0.00	0.00	0.00	0.00	0.00	0.00	0.01	0.03	0.03
卡波氏肉瘤	Kaposi sarcoma	1 157	0.15	0.02	0.02	0.01	0.02	0.03	0.02	0.04	0.03	0.04
结缔组织、软组织	Connective & soft tissue	1 688	0.22	0.28	0.12	0.10	0.07	0.10	0.08	0.10	0.11	0.11
乳腺	Breast	21 000	2.78	0.37	0.00	0.00	0.00	0.00	0.16	0.74	2.02	3.94
外阴	Vulva	384	0.05	0.00	0.00	0.00	0.00	0.00	0.02	0.01	0.02	0.04
阴道	Vagina	225	0.03	0.00	0.00	0.00	0.00	0.01	0.01	0.00	0.00	0.01
子宫颈	Cervix uteri	11 936	1.54	0.55	0.00	0.00	0.00	0.00	0.04	0.42	1.20	2.19
子宫体	Corpus uteri	3 453	0.45	0.00	0.00	0.00	0.00	0.01	0.05	0.08	0.13	0.32
子宫,部位不明	Uterus unspecified	1 793	0.23	0.09	0.01	0.00	0.00	0.00	0.01	0.04	0.13	0.18
卵巢	Ovary	7 751	1.00	0.09	0.02	0.01	0.08	0.06	0.14	0.27	0.49	0.73
其他女性生殖器	Other female genital organs	417	0.05	0.00	0.00	0.00	0.00	0.00	0.01	0.01	0.01	0.05
胎盘	Placenta	13	0.00	0.00	0.00	0.00	0.00	0.00	0.01	0.02	0.00	0.01
阴茎	Penis	531	0.07	0.00	0.00	0.00	0.00	0.02	0.00	0.02	0.02	0.04
前列腺	Prostate	10 688	1.38	0.00	0.00	0.00	0.00	0.03	0.03	0.01	0.04	0.03
睾丸	Testis	285	0.04	0.00	0.05	0.03	0.01	0.02	0.06	0.08	0.13	0.11
其他男性生殖器	Other male genital organs	107	0.01	0.00	0.01	0.00	0.00	0.01	0.01	0.01	0.01	0.01
肾	Kidney	6 049	0.78	0.19	0.13	0.09	0.01	0.03	0.03	0.07	0.13	0.15
肾盂	Renal pelvis	872	0.11	0.00	0.01	0.00	0.00	0.00	0.00	0.00	0.01	0.01
输尿管	Ureter	1 149	0.15	0.15	0.00	0.00	0.00	0.00	0.00	0.00	0.02	0.01
膀胱	Bladder	11 072	1.43	0.09	0.01	0.00	0.00	0.01	0.00	0.04	0.04	0.07
其他泌尿器官	Other urinary organs	228	0.03	0.00	0.01	0.00	0.00	0.00	0.00	0.00	0.00	0.01
眼	Eye	260	0.03	0.02	0.13	0.04	0.01	0.01	0.00	0.01	0.01	0.00
脑、神经系统	Brain, nervous system	17 255	2.23	0.90	1.03	1.00	0.86	0.66	0.49	0.91	1.13	1.39
甲状腺	Thyroid	2 551	0.33	0.06	0.00	0.00	0.01	0.01	0.02	0.08	0.09	0.16
肾上腺	Adrenal gland	647	0.08	0.11	0.10	0.06	0.01	0.01	0.00	0.02	0.03	0.02
其他内分泌腺	Other endocrine	440	0.06	0.02	0.02	0.01	0.03	0.04	0.03	0.03	0.05	0.04
霍奇金淋巴瘤	Hodgkin lymphoma	630	0.08	0.00	0.00	0.01	0.02	0.02	0.02	0.03	0.05	0.05
非霍奇金淋巴瘤	Non-Hodgkin lymphoma	10 999	1.42	0.06	0.14	0.13	0.18	0.20	0.20	0.30	0.45	0.50
免疫增生性疾病	Immunoproliferative diseases	83	0.01	0.02	0.00	0.00	0.00	0.00	0.00	0.00	0.00	0.00
多发性骨髓瘤	Multiple myeloma	4 239	0.55	0.02	0.05	0.02	0.04	0.05	0.03	0.02	0.05	0.09
淋巴样白血病	Lymphoid leukemia	3 551	0.46	0.92	0.45	0.42	0.38	0.51	0.32	0.38	0.32	0.29
髓样白血病	Myeloid leukemia	5 293	0.68	0.39	0.22	0.19	0.28	0.31	0.24	0.39	0.37	0.42
白血病,未特指	Leukemia unspecified	7 145	0.92	1.35	0.63	0.48	0.63	0.67	0.57	0.61	0.54	0.49
其他或未指明部位	Other and unspecified	15 423	2.00	0.73	0.38	0.21	0.25	0.31	0.26	0.38	0.52	0.56
所有部位合计	All sites	772 968	100.00	11.52	4.02	3.22	3.58	4.23	4.44	8.43	14.75	22.75
所有部位除外 C44	All sites except C44	769 594	99.56	11.45	4.01	3.21	3.54	4.19	4.41	8.37	14.68	22.66

Appendix Table 1-10 Cancer mortality in registration areas of China, both sexes in 2017

Age group										粗率 Crude rate/ 100 000^{-1}	中标率 ASR China/ 100 000^{-1}	世标率 ASR world/ 100 000^{-1}	累积率 Cum. rate/%		ICD10
40~44	45~49	50~54	55~59	60~64	65~69	70~74	75~79	80~84	85+				0~64	0~74	
0.01	0.03	0.03	0.07	0.16	0.24	0.31	0.51	0.73	1.40	0.08	0.04	0.04	0.00	0.00	C00
0.16	0.34	0.64	0.77	1.13	1.26	2.00	2.34	3.11	2.84	0.47	0.29	0.28	0.02	0.03	C01-02
0.11	0.24	0.58	0.66	1.42	1.83	2.42	3.57	4.62	5.07	0.58	0.33	0.33	0.02	0.04	C03-06
0.04	0.10	0.22	0.23	0.42	0.67	0.69	0.85	1.31	1.33	0.18	0.11	0.11	0.01	0.01	C07-08
0.01	0.05	0.11	0.14	0.19	0.26	0.22	0.38	0.45	0.31	0.07	0.04	0.04	0.00	0.01	C09
0.03	0.07	0.23	0.26	0.45	0.56	0.71	0.89	0.77	1.07	0.16	0.10	0.10	0.01	0.01	C10
1.40	2.01	3.35	3.16	4.39	5.74	6.24	6.54	6.20	6.31	1.88	1.24	1.20	0.08	0.14	C11
0.05	0.13	0.46	0.60	0.86	0.85	0.93	0.98	1.14	0.94	0.26	0.16	0.16	0.01	0.02	C12-13
0.02	0.10	0.26	0.23	0.49	0.59	0.83	1.25	1.47	1.62	0.20	0.11	0.11	0.01	0.01	C14
0.82	3.36	9.95	15.53	34.72	57.25	82.11	107.39	133.04	131.44	15.21	8.53	8.55	0.32	1.02	C15
3.69	7.11	15.34	21.18	43.82	70.05	104.68	148.33	184.12	181.90	20.89	11.95	11.81	0.48	1.35	C16
0.16	0.35	0.68	0.82	1.52	2.45	3.05	4.67	5.47	6.33	0.71	0.41	0.41	0.02	0.05	C17
1.29	2.34	4.57	6.22	11.90	17.87	26.91	42.45	67.45	81.07	6.40	3.57	3.54	0.14	0.36	C18
1.62	3.03	5.92	7.46	14.37	22.18	33.24	49.04	73.53	79.58	7.43	4.20	4.15	0.17	0.45	C19-20
0.09	0.11	0.25	0.21	0.51	0.76	1.15	1.75	2.16	3.14	0.26	0.15	0.15	0.01	0.02	C21
12.34	21.51	36.37	39.14	61.09	77.04	89.63	110.98	132.68	138.32	24.91	15.41	15.20	0.91	1.74	C22
0.42	0.96	2.13	3.14	6.25	9.75	13.66	21.77	29.29	31.57	3.02	1.68	1.68	0.07	0.18	C23-24
1.19	2.37	5.45	7.56	14.37	21.56	30.91	41.93	53.52	53.69	6.40	3.66	3.64	0.16	0.42	C25
0.10	0.15	0.31	0.31	0.59	0.59	0.68	1.02	1.37	1.75	0.22	0.14	0.14	0.01	0.01	C30-31
0.16	0.39	1.07	1.46	2.66	3.67	4.96	6.59	8.49	8.38	1.08	0.62	0.62	0.03	0.07	C32
7.31	16.10	39.91	56.09	114.51	175.69	243.25	331.55	405.32	396.28	49.28	28.14	28.08	1.20	3.29	C33-34
0.21	0.35	0.57	0.72	1.41	1.57	2.14	2.55	3.12	3.06	0.54	0.35	0.34	0.02	0.04	C37-38
0.43	0.65	1.25	1.39	2.76	4.17	5.87	7.59	8.58	9.08	1.33	0.86	0.85	0.04	0.09	C40-41
0.14	0.22	0.37	0.40	0.74	1.05	1.42	1.93	2.57	3.06	0.36	0.23	0.23	0.01	0.02	C43
0.14	0.29	0.47	0.48	0.88	1.56	2.53	4.43	8.92	19.52	0.77	0.41	0.42	0.01	0.03	C44
0.02	0.07	0.15	0.19	0.31	0.42	0.46	0.63	0.73	0.55	0.12	0.07	0.07	0.00	0.01	C45
0.06	0.09	0.22	0.25	0.44	0.78	1.23	1.91	2.35	2.64	0.27	0.16	0.16	0.01	0.02	C46
0.20	0.23	0.38	0.44	0.67	0.98	1.37	2.10	2.32	2.84	0.39	0.26	0.27	0.01	0.03	C47;C49
7.14	11.90	18.37	17.81	23.05	23.00	23.55	28.69	35.87	43.20	9.76	6.17	5.98	0.43	0.66	C50
0.05	0.06	0.15	0.21	0.23	0.65	0.57	1.01	1.35	2.22	0.18	0.10	0.10	0.00	0.01	C51
0.03	0.08	0.18	0.18	0.17	0.35	0.36	0.57	0.65	0.44	0.10	0.06	0.06	0.00	0.01	C52
3.87	7.37	11.81	9.05	11.54	13.49	15.43	18.06	18.82	18.25	5.55	3.56	3.42	0.24	0.38	C53
0.65	1.25	2.77	2.95	4.25	5.13	5.73	5.63	6.65	5.68	1.60	0.97	0.97	0.06	0.12	C54
0.44	0.73	1.36	1.23	1.83	2.41	2.86	3.49	3.95	4.44	0.83	0.50	0.49	0.03	0.06	C55
1.75	3.51	6.80	6.66	8.89	10.65	12.03	13.57	13.27	8.49	3.60	2.25	2.21	0.15	0.26	C56
0.06	0.15	0.24	0.30	0.40	0.64	0.61	0.92	1.14	1.38	0.19	0.11	0.11	0.01	0.01	C57
0.01	0.01	0.00	0.00	0.00	0.00	0.01	0.02	0.00	0.00	0.01	0.01	0.01	0.00	0.00	C58
0.08	0.17	0.23	0.20	0.42	0.62	1.19	1.27	2.81	3.33	0.24	0.15	0.14	0.01	0.02	C60
0.09	0.23	0.66	1.42	3.92	9.57	21.28	44.99	84.99	149.09	4.83	2.56	2.61	0.03	0.19	C61
0.09	0.07	0.08	0.12	0.14	0.27	0.27	0.74	0.92	1.36	0.13	0.10	0.09	0.00	0.01	C62
0.01	0.03	0.02	0.05	0.10	0.15	0.23	0.32	0.43	0.60	0.05	0.03	0.03	0.00	0.00	C63
0.29	0.66	1.22	1.82	2.97	4.53	5.36	8.02	11.68	13.56	1.39	0.81	0.81	0.04	0.09	C64
0.03	0.07	0.12	0.22	0.46	0.51	0.89	1.24	2.02	2.69	0.20	0.11	0.11	0.00	0.01	C65
0.03	0.05	0.09	0.26	0.36	0.73	1.15	2.30	3.45	3.34	0.26	0.14	0.14	0.00	0.01	C66
0.17	0.38	0.86	1.35	3.03	5.82	10.37	19.89	35.59	53.38	2.54	1.28	1.29	0.03	0.11	C67
0.01	0.02	0.03	0.03	0.08	0.10	0.24	0.35	0.79	0.74	0.05	0.03	0.03	0.00	0.00	C68
0.01	0.04	0.06	0.04	0.09	0.10	0.18	0.32	0.37	0.79	0.06	0.04	0.05	0.00	0.00	C69
2.07	3.19	5.00	5.12	8.48	11.12	13.67	17.16	20.20	17.75	3.95	2.72	2.70	0.16	0.28	C70-72,D32-33,D42-43
0.25	0.39	0.67	0.62	1.14	1.71	2.28	3.35	4.36	5.00	0.58	0.36	0.35	0.02	0.04	C73
0.04	0.07	0.16	0.24	0.28	0.41	0.64	0.81	0.88	0.79	0.15	0.10	0.10	0.01	0.01	C74
0.08	0.05	0.07	0.15	0.20	0.22	0.31	0.49	0.61	0.61	0.10	0.07	0.07	0.00	0.01	C75
0.08	0.07	0.14	0.13	0.33	0.34	0.61	0.89	0.86	1.07	0.14	0.09	0.09	0.00	0.01	C81
0.78	1.27	2.47	2.97	5.48	8.30	11.07	14.56	17.91	16.79	2.52	1.56	1.53	0.08	0.17	C82-C86;C96
0.00	0.01	0.01	0.01	0.05	0.06	0.07	0.16	0.16	0.15	0.02	0.01	0.01	0.00	0.00	C88
0.11	0.43	0.90	1.23	2.48	3.67	4.91	5.91	6.38	5.46	0.97	0.58	0.58	0.03	0.07	C90
0.39	0.47	0.84	0.92	1.39	2.01	2.44	3.30	4.10	3.49	0.81	0.63	0.65	0.04	0.06	C91
0.56	0.80	1.30	1.50	2.55	3.46	4.87	5.53	6.27	5.79	1.21	0.84	0.83	0.05	0.09	C92-C94,D45-47
0.79	1.07	1.60	1.69	3.11	4.18	5.63	7.67	9.01	8.60	1.64	1.19	1.20	0.07	0.11	C95
1.05	1.81	3.19	4.13	7.31	10.62	14.13	19.57	28.01	34.34	3.53	2.14	2.14	0.10	0.23	O&U
46.07	86.40	171.14	211.55	390.46	573.15	785.25	1 078.32	1 383.32	1 462.63	177.15	104.20	103.47	4.86	11.65	C00-96, D32-33, D42-43,D45-47
45.93	86.11	170.67	211.07	389.58	571.59	782.72	1 073.89	1 374.40	1 443.11	176.38	103.80	103.05	4.85	11.62	C00-96, D32-33, D42-43,D45-47 exc. C44

附表 1-11　2017 年全国肿瘤登记地区男性癌症死亡主要指标

部位 Site		死亡数 No. deaths	构成 Freq. /%	年龄组								
				0~	1~4	5~9	10~14	15~19	20~24	25~29	30~34	35~39
唇	Lip	237	0.05	0.00	0.00	0.00	0.00	0.01	0.00	0.00	0.01	0.01
舌	Tongue	1 436	0.29	0.00	0.00	0.00	0.00	0.01	0.02	0.04	0.11	0.14
口	Mouth	1 627	0.33	0.00	0.01	0.00	0.02	0.00	0.00	0.03	0.06	0.08
唾液腺	Salivary glands	536	0.11	0.00	0.00	0.00	0.00	0.01	0.02	0.01	0.01	0.08
扁桃腺	Tonsil	266	0.05	0.00	0.00	0.01	0.00	0.00	0.01	0.00	0.01	0.02
其他口咽	Other oropharynx	591	0.12	0.00	0.00	0.00	0.00	0.00	0.01	0.01	0.00	0.02
鼻咽	Nasopharynx	5 990	1.21	0.08	0.00	0.00	0.03	0.10	0.12	0.26	0.61	0.95
下咽	Hypopharynx	1 056	0.21	0.00	0.00	0.01	0.00	0.00	0.01	0.00	0.01	0.05
咽,部位不明	Pharynx unspecified	652	0.13	0.00	0.00	0.00	0.00	0.00	0.00	0.01	0.01	0.02
食管	Esophagus	48 719	9.86	0.41	0.03	0.00	0.03	0.02	0.04	0.05	0.14	0.33
胃	Stomach	63 514	12.85	1.01	0.02	0.02	0.01	0.11	0.28	0.50	1.26	1.91
小肠	Small intestine	1 853	0.37	0.00	0.00	0.00	0.01	0.00	0.01	0.03	0.02	0.09
结肠	Colon	15 662	3.17	0.32	0.01	0.00	0.03	0.03	0.18	0.24	0.62	0.77
直肠	Rectum	19 831	4.01	0.57	0.00	0.02	0.01	0.05	0.07	0.27	0.55	0.88
肛门	Anus	710	0.14	0.00	0.00	0.00	0.00	0.00	0.01	0.00	0.04	0.05
肝脏	Liver	79 885	16.16	2.23	0.28	0.10	0.19	0.23	0.62	2.02	5.05	9.59
胆囊及其他	Gallbladder etc.	6 149	1.24	0.04	0.01	0.00	0.00	0.01	0.03	0.07	0.12	0.15
胰腺	Pancreas	15 979	3.23	0.20	0.01	0.01	0.00	0.02	0.04	0.11	0.29	0.64
鼻、鼻窦及其他	Nose,sinuses etc.	601	0.12	0.04	0.03	0.00	0.01	0.03	0.01	0.02	0.07	0.07
喉	Larynx	3 947	0.80	0.04	0.02	0.02	0.01	0.04	0.01	0.02	0.04	0.08
气管、支气管、肺	Trachea,bronchus & lung	149 992	30.34	1.91	0.05	0.04	0.10	0.11	0.35	0.83	1.93	3.39
其他胸腔器官	Other thoracic organs	1 491	0.30	0.12	0.01	0.06	0.03	0.06	0.13	0.14	0.11	0.17
骨	Bone	3 422	0.69	0.04	0.00	0.15	0.26	0.56	0.31	0.29	0.33	0.27
皮肤黑色素瘤	Melanoma of skin	896	0.18	0.04	0.09	0.05	0.03	0.04	0.03	0.07	0.09	0.13
皮肤其他	Other skin	1 905	0.39	0.08	0.02	0.02	0.04	0.04	0.03	0.07	0.09	0.11
间皮瘤	Mesothelioma	308	0.06	0.00	0.00	0.00	0.00	0.00	0.00	0.01	0.03	0.02
卡波氏肉瘤	Kaposi sarcoma	727	0.15	0.00	0.02	0.02	0.02	0.04	0.03	0.04	0.03	0.05
结缔组织、软组织	Connective & soft tissue	1 023	0.21	0.24	0.15	0.14	0.09	0.12	0.11	0.12	0.11	0.12
乳腺	Breast	476	0.10	0.00	0.00	0.00	0.00	0.00	0.01	0.03	0.05	0.02
外阴	Vulva	—	—	—	—	—	—	—	—	—	—	—
阴道	Vagina	—	—	—	—	—	—	—	—	—	—	—
子宫颈	Cervix uteri	—	—	—	—	—	—	—	—	—	—	—
子宫体	Corpus uteri	—	—	—	—	—	—	—	—	—	—	—
子宫,部位不明	Uterus unspecified	—	—	—	—	—	—	—	—	—	—	—
卵巢	Ovary	—	—	—	—	—	—	—	—	—	—	—
其他女性生殖器	Other female genital organs	—	—	—	—	—	—	—	—	—	—	—
胎盘	Placenta	—	—	—	—	—	—	—	—	—	—	—
阴茎	Penis	531	0.11	0.00	0.00	0.00	0.00	0.02	0.00	0.02	0.02	0.04
前列腺	Prostate	10 688	2.16	0.00	0.00	0.00	0.00	0.03	0.03	0.01	0.04	0.03
睾丸	Testis	285	0.06	0.00	0.05	0.03	0.01	0.02	0.06	0.08	0.13	0.11
其他男性生殖器	Other male genital organs	107	0.02	0.00	0.01	0.00	0.00	0.01	0.01	0.01	0.01	0.01
肾	Kidney	3 998	0.81	0.24	0.13	0.13	0.01	0.05	0.02	0.08	0.14	0.19
肾盂	Renal pelvis	494	0.10	0.00	0.02	0.00	0.00	0.00	0.00	0.01	0.01	0.01
输尿管	Ureter	614	0.12	0.20	0.00	0.00	0.00	0.00	0.00	0.01	0.01	0.01
膀胱	Bladder	8 695	1.76	0.04	0.01	0.00	0.00	0.02	0.01	0.04	0.04	0.09
其他泌尿器官	Other urinary organs	145	0.03	0.00	0.00	0.01	0.00	0.00	0.01	0.01	0.00	0.01
眼	Eye	151	0.03	0.04	0.14	0.04	0.01	0.02	0.00	0.02	0.01	0.00
脑、神经系统	Brain,nervous system	9 656	1.95	1.01	1.15	1.16	0.91	0.71	0.59	1.11	1.35	1.62
甲状腺	Thyroid	979	0.20	0.04	0.00	0.00	0.01	0.00	0.01	0.06	0.05	0.12
肾上腺	Adrenal gland	386	0.08	0.08	0.10	0.07	0.01	0.02	0.01	0.02	0.04	0.04
其他内分泌腺	Other endocrine	248	0.05	0.00	0.01	0.02	0.05	0.07	0.04	0.02	0.06	0.06
霍奇金淋巴瘤	Hodgkin lymphoma	407	0.08	0.00	0.00	0.02	0.03	0.03	0.04	0.04	0.06	0.08
非霍奇金淋巴瘤	Non-Hodgkin lymphoma	6 725	1.36	0.04	0.18	0.18	0.25	0.29	0.26	0.34	0.59	0.61
免疫增生性疾病	Immunoproliferative diseases	59	0.01	0.04	0.00	0.00	0.00	0.00	0.00	0.00	0.00	0.00
多发性骨髓瘤	Multiple myeloma	2 499	0.51	0.04	0.07	0.03	0.05	0.06	0.04	0.03	0.06	0.11
淋巴样白血病	Lymphoid leukemia	2 081	0.42	0.93	0.59	0.47	0.49	0.66	0.37	0.39	0.42	0.34
髓样白血病	Myeloid leukemia	3 015	0.61	0.37	0.26	0.18	0.35	0.33	0.27	0.48	0.45	0.40
白血病,未特指	Leukemia unspecified	4 178	0.85	1.34	0.69	0.49	0.68	0.83	0.64	0.81	0.64	0.58
其他或未指明部位	Other and unspecified	8 908	1.80	0.65	0.43	0.25	0.35	0.38	0.26	0.42	0.61	0.61
所有部位合计	All sites	494 330	100.00	12.45	4.58	3.73	4.10	5.19	5.16	9.29	16.53	25.27
所有部位除外 C44	All sites except C44	492 425	99.61	12.37	4.56	3.72	4.05	5.15	5.12	9.22	16.44	25.16

Appendix Table 1-11 Cancer mortality in registration areas of China, male in 2017

Age group										粗率 Crude rate/ 100 000^{-1}	中标率 ASR China/ 100 000^{-1}	世标率 ASR world/ 100 000^{-1}	累积率 Cum. rate/%		ICD10
40~44	45~49	50~54	55~59	60~64	65~69	70~74	75~79	80~84	85+				0~64	0~74	
0.02	0.06	0.04	0.13	0.27	0.37	0.48	0.63	0.83	1.80	0.11	0.06	0.07	0.00	0.01	C00
0.24	0.50	1.03	1.26	1.61	2.01	2.46	2.94	3.80	3.98	0.65	0.41	0.41	0.02	0.05	C01-02
0.11	0.33	0.86	0.92	2.12	2.59	3.28	4.51	5.48	6.11	0.74	0.45	0.45	0.02	0.05	C03-06
0.03	0.13	0.24	0.36	0.65	0.95	0.98	1.27	1.88	1.91	0.24	0.15	0.15	0.01	0.02	C07-08
0.01	0.08	0.20	0.22	0.34	0.51	0.32	0.68	0.76	0.38	0.12	0.08	0.08	0.00	0.01	C09
0.07	0.12	0.39	0.48	0.82	1.07	1.11	1.40	1.26	1.53	0.27	0.17	0.17	0.01	0.02	C10
2.01	3.16	5.01	4.78	6.50	8.52	9.29	9.33	9.08	8.56	2.71	1.83	1.77	0.12	0.21	C11
0.08	0.26	0.86	1.14	1.67	1.61	1.67	1.88	2.25	1.74	0.48	0.30	0.30	0.02	0.04	C12-13
0.03	0.18	0.46	0.40	0.79	0.94	1.16	1.93	2.15	2.40	0.29	0.18	0.18	0.01	0.02	C14
1.38	5.80	17.26	26.78	56.79	89.83	121.85	156.00	182.33	185.67	22.03	13.13	13.22	0.54	1.60	C15
4.28	8.94	21.02	31.95	66.35	106.07	153.93	219.01	265.80	254.47	28.72	17.25	17.12	0.68	1.98	C16
0.20	0.40	0.92	0.97	1.90	3.10	3.95	5.37	6.57	8.61	0.84	0.51	0.51	0.02	0.06	C17
1.45	2.61	5.19	7.56	13.92	21.92	32.78	48.63	78.08	101.12	7.08	4.21	4.19	0.16	0.44	C18
1.76	3.44	7.20	9.40	19.09	29.71	42.83	63.02	94.27	105.43	8.97	5.35	5.32	0.21	0.58	C19-20
0.14	0.16	0.32	0.27	0.75	1.02	1.41	2.07	2.81	3.92	0.32	0.20	0.19	0.01	0.02	C21
21.13	36.20	59.56	63.03	94.45	112.40	123.94	150.07	172.62	184.20	36.12	23.43	23.07	1.46	2.65	C22
0.38	0.92	2.13	3.46	6.56	9.87	12.98	20.34	26.19	30.58	2.78	1.65	1.65	0.07	0.18	C23-24
1.54	3.08	6.82	9.79	17.95	25.42	36.08	46.83	59.42	63.51	7.23	4.37	4.37	0.20	0.51	C25
0.11	0.18	0.41	0.38	0.71	0.87	1.02	1.16	1.62	1.85	0.27	0.18	0.18	0.01	0.02	C30-31
0.27	0.65	1.86	2.55	4.81	6.43	8.43	11.11	14.70	15.26	1.78	1.07	1.08	0.05	0.13	C32
8.82	20.84	55.98	83.48	171.49	260.91	357.86	479.42	572.85	570.91	67.83	40.71	40.76	1.74	4.83	C33-34
0.30	0.46	0.73	0.91	1.85	2.09	2.93	3.03	4.36	3.92	0.67	0.45	0.44	0.02	0.05	C37-38
0.54	0.77	1.40	1.81	3.26	5.10	7.30	9.52	10.27	11.12	1.55	1.05	1.03	0.05	0.11	C40-41
0.15	0.26	0.40	0.52	0.78	1.27	1.56	2.35	3.27	3.54	0.41	0.27	0.26	0.01	0.03	C43
0.20	0.33	0.59	0.65	1.26	2.11	3.31	5.16	11.20	20.44	0.86	0.50	0.51	0.02	0.04	C44
0.02	0.08	0.19	0.21	0.35	0.53	0.53	0.91	0.92	0.65	0.14	0.09	0.09	0.00	0.01	C45
0.05	0.13	0.25	0.32	0.56	0.97	1.65	2.69	3.24	3.87	0.33	0.20	0.20	0.01	0.02	C46
0.27	0.23	0.50	0.57	0.79	1.27	1.82	2.62	2.64	4.03	0.46	0.32	0.33	0.02	0.03	C47;C49
0.08	0.15	0.28	0.18	0.48	0.62	0.95	1.21	1.75	2.40	0.22	0.14	0.13	0.01	0.01	C50
—	—	—	—	—	—	—	—	—	—	—	—	—	—	—	C51
—	—	—	—	—	—	—	—	—	—	—	—	—	—	—	C52
—	—	—	—	—	—	—	—	—	—	—	—	—	—	—	C53
—	—	—	—	—	—	—	—	—	—	—	—	—	—	—	C54
—	—	—	—	—	—	—	—	—	—	—	—	—	—	—	C55
—	—	—	—	—	—	—	—	—	—	—	—	—	—	—	C56
—	—	—	—	—	—	—	—	—	—	—	—	—	—	—	C57
—	—	—	—	—	—	—	—	—	—	—	—	—	—	—	C58
0.08	0.17	0.23	0.20	0.42	0.62	1.19	1.27	2.81	3.33	0.24	0.15	0.14	0.01	0.02	C60
0.09	0.23	0.66	1.42	3.92	9.57	21.28	44.99	84.99	149.09	4.83	2.56	2.61	0.03	0.19	C61
0.09	0.07	0.08	0.12	0.14	0.27	0.27	0.74	0.92	1.36	0.13	0.10	0.09	0.00	0.01	C62
0.01	0.03	0.02	0.05	0.10	0.15	0.23	0.32	0.43	0.60	0.05	0.03	0.03	0.00	0.00	C63
0.36	0.94	1.77	2.66	4.36	6.03	7.21	11.24	15.13	18.53	1.81	1.11	1.12	0.05	0.12	C64
0.05	0.08	0.16	0.29	0.59	0.64	0.99	1.27	2.25	3.38	0.22	0.13	0.13	0.01	0.01	C65
0.02	0.05	0.13	0.34	0.45	0.87	1.34	2.48	3.47	3.76	0.28	0.16	0.16	0.01	0.02	C66
0.24	0.59	1.36	2.21	5.06	9.37	17.21	33.05	60.41	101.12	3.93	2.15	2.19	0.05	0.18	C67
0.01	0.03	0.02	0.04	0.11	0.11	0.33	0.42	1.09	1.31	0.07	0.04	0.04	0.00	0.00	C68
0.01	0.04	0.07	0.04	0.15	0.09	0.24	0.44	0.43	0.98	0.07	0.05	0.06	0.00	0.00	C69
2.42	3.75	5.76	5.85	9.82	13.04	15.60	18.45	21.04	19.35	4.37	3.11	3.09	0.18	0.32	C70-72,D32-33,D42-43
0.16	0.28	0.48	0.49	0.90	1.39	1.76	2.81	3.70	4.91	0.44	0.28	0.27	0.01	0.03	C73
0.03	0.05	0.22	0.36	0.38	0.45	0.75	0.97	1.12	0.93	0.17	0.12	0.12	0.01	0.01	C74
0.06	0.05	0.09	0.16	0.23	0.20	0.42	0.72	0.66	0.76	0.11	0.08	0.08	0.00	0.01	C75
0.11	0.11	0.17	0.20	0.48	0.44	0.83	1.21	0.86	1.14	0.18	0.13	0.12	0.01	0.01	C81
0.95	1.57	3.08	3.74	7.03	10.65	13.99	17.92	21.64	22.84	3.04	1.97	1.94	0.10	0.22	C82-C86;C96
0.01	0.02	0.01	0.01	0.08	0.09	0.08	0.23	0.33	0.33	0.03	0.02	0.02	0.00	0.00	C88
0.15	0.45	1.04	1.47	3.09	4.26	5.76	6.94	8.69	8.01	1.13	0.70	0.70	0.03	0.08	C90
0.44	0.53	0.90	0.97	1.63	2.42	2.87	4.04	5.42	4.96	0.94	0.74	0.77	0.04	0.07	C91
0.67	0.84	1.41	1.67	2.77	4.11	5.98	6.54	8.22	7.80	1.36	0.97	0.95	0.05	0.10	C92-C94,D45-47
0.86	1.24	1.84	1.88	3.76	4.89	6.60	9.52	11.40	12.21	1.89	1.40	1.41	0.08	0.13	C95
1.19	2.09	3.88	4.88	9.02	13.26	17.40	23.17	32.80	40.72	4.03	2.56	2.57	0.12	0.28	O&U
53.70	103.66	215.51	283.56	533.33	783.00	1 060.17	1 443.84	1 830.20	2 011.36	223.54	137.23	136.84	6.33	15.54	C00-96, D32-33, D42-43,D45-47
53.50	103.33	214.92	282.91	532.07	780.88	1 056.86	1 438.68	1 819.00	1 990.92	222.68	136.73	136.33	6.31	15.50	C00-96, D32-33, D42-43,D45-47 exc. C44

附表 1-12　2017 年全国肿瘤登记地区女性癌症死亡主要指标

部位 Site		死亡数 No. deaths	构成 Freq. /%	年龄组								
				0~	1~4	5~9	10~14	15~19	20~24	25~29	30~34	35~39
唇	Lip	109	0.04	0.00	0.00	0.00	0.00	0.00	0.00	0.00	0.00	0.00
舌	Tongue	631	0.23	0.00	0.01	0.01	0.00	0.02	0.01	0.01	0.03	0.05
口	Mouth	888	0.32	0.00	0.01	0.00	0.01	0.01	0.00	0.03	0.04	0.07
唾液腺	Salivary glands	264	0.09	0.00	0.00	0.00	0.02	0.02	0.02	0.02	0.01	0.05
扁桃腺	Tonsil	55	0.02	0.00	0.00	0.00	0.01	0.00	0.00	0.00	0.01	0.00
其他口咽	Other oropharynx	118	0.04	0.00	0.00	0.00	0.00	0.00	0.01	0.01	0.01	0.00
鼻咽	Nasopharynx	2 222	0.80	0.05	0.01	0.00	0.01	0.04	0.06	0.13	0.26	0.43
下咽	Hypopharynx	78	0.03	0.00	0.00	0.00	0.00	0.00	0.00	0.00	0.01	0.00
咽,部位不明	Pharynx unspecified	208	0.07	0.00	0.00	0.00	0.01	0.01	0.00	0.00	0.00	0.02
食管	Esophagus	17 652	6.34	0.05	0.02	0.00	0.00	0.01	0.00	0.02	0.04	0.12
胃	Stomach	27 652	9.92	0.50	0.02	0.00	0.02	0.05	0.25	0.73	1.29	1.81
小肠	Small intestine	1 262	0.45	0.05	0.00	0.00	0.00	0.00	0.02	0.01	0.04	0.13
结肠	Colon	12 242	4.39	0.14	0.00	0.00	0.00	0.06	0.13	0.28	0.55	0.67
直肠	Rectum	12 571	4.51	0.32	0.00	0.02	0.02	0.01	0.04	0.28	0.48	0.65
肛门	Anus	424	0.15	0.00	0.00	0.00	0.00	0.01	0.00	0.01	0.00	0.02
肝脏	Liver	28 806	10.34	0.96	0.20	0.06	0.11	0.21	0.22	0.58	1.10	1.72
胆囊及其他	Gallbladder etc.	7 029	2.52	0.23	0.01	0.01	0.00	0.01	0.01	0.05	0.06	0.11
胰腺	Pancreas	11 928	4.28	0.09	0.00	0.00	0.01	0.00	0.01	0.11	0.21	0.25
鼻、鼻窦及其他	Nose, sinuses etc.	379	0.14	0.00	0.01	0.03	0.02	0.00	0.04	0.02	0.03	0.05
喉	Larynx	765	0.27	0.00	0.01	0.00	0.00	0.01	0.01	0.01	0.01	0.04
气管、支气管、肺	Trachea, bronchus & lung	65 033	23.34	1.28	0.05	0.04	0.06	0.04	0.18	0.52	1.12	2.23
其他胸腔器官	Other thoracic organs	863	0.31	0.18	0.05	0.04	0.00	0.05	0.03	0.08	0.08	0.17
骨	Bone	2 373	0.85	0.09	0.03	0.07	0.31	0.27	0.24	0.17	0.20	0.19
皮肤黑色素瘤	Melanoma of skin	693	0.25	0.00	0.04	0.04	0.00	0.01	0.01	0.05	0.08	0.08
皮肤其他	Other skin	1 469	0.53	0.05	0.00	0.01	0.03	0.04	0.02	0.05	0.06	0.07
间皮瘤	Mesothelioma	209	0.08	0.00	0.00	0.00	0.00	0.00	0.01	0.01	0.03	0.03
卡波氏肉瘤	Kaposi sarcoma	430	0.15	0.05	0.02	0.00	0.02	0.02	0.01	0.04	0.03	0.04
结缔组织、软组织	Connective & soft tissue	665	0.24	0.32	0.08	0.06	0.06	0.08	0.06	0.08	0.11	0.10
乳腺	Breast	21 000	7.54	0.37	0.00	0.00	0.00	0.00	0.16	0.74	2.02	3.94
外阴	Vulva	384	0.14	0.00	0.00	0.00	0.00	0.00	0.02	0.01	0.02	0.04
阴道	Vagina	225	0.08	0.00	0.00	0.00	0.00	0.01	0.01	0.00	0.00	0.01
子宫颈	Cervix uteri	11 936	4.28	0.55	0.00	0.00	0.00	0.00	0.04	0.42	1.20	2.19
子宫体	Corpus uteri	3 453	1.24	0.00	0.00	0.00	0.00	0.01	0.05	0.08	0.13	0.32
子宫,部位不明	Uterus unspecified	1 793	0.64	0.09	0.01	0.00	0.00	0.00	0.01	0.04	0.13	0.18
卵巢	Ovary	7 751	2.78	0.09	0.02	0.01	0.08	0.06	0.14	0.27	0.49	0.73
其他女性生殖器	Other female genital organs	417	0.15	0.00	0.00	0.00	0.00	0.00	0.01	0.01	0.01	0.05
胎盘	Placenta	13	0.00	0.00	0.00	0.00	0.00	0.00	0.01	0.02	0.00	0.01
阴茎	Penis	—	—	—	—	—	—	—	—	—	—	—
前列腺	Prostate	—	—	—	—	—	—	—	—	—	—	—
睾丸	Testis	—	—	—	—	—	—	—	—	—	—	—
其他男性生殖器	Other male genital organs	—	—	—	—	—	—	—	—	—	—	—
肾	Kidney	2 051	0.74	0.14	0.12	0.04	0.01	0.02	0.04	0.05	0.13	0.10
肾盂	Renal pelvis	378	0.14	0.00	0.00	0.00	0.00	0.00	0.00	0.00	0.01	0.01
输尿管	Ureter	535	0.19	0.09	0.00	0.00	0.00	0.00	0.00	0.00	0.03	0.01
膀胱	Bladder	2 377	0.85	0.14	0.00	0.01	0.00	0.00	0.00	0.04	0.03	0.04
其他泌尿器官	Other urinary organs	83	0.03	0.00	0.01	0.00	0.00	0.00	0.00	0.00	0.00	0.00
眼	Eye	109	0.04	0.00	0.12	0.04	0.01	0.00	0.00	0.01	0.01	0.01
脑、神经系统	Brain, nervous system	7 599	2.73	0.78	0.89	0.81	0.81	0.60	0.38	0.71	0.92	1.16
甲状腺	Thyroid	1 572	0.56	0.09	0.00	0.00	0.02	0.02	0.04	0.09	0.13	0.20
肾上腺	Adrenal gland	261	0.09	0.14	0.09	0.04	0.02	0.00	0.00	0.02	0.02	0.01
其他内分泌腺	Other endocrine	192	0.07	0.05	0.03	0.01	0.01	0.01	0.02	0.03	0.05	0.02
霍奇金淋巴瘤	Hodgkin lymphoma	223	0.08	0.00	0.00	0.00	0.01	0.00	0.01	0.02	0.04	0.02
非霍奇金淋巴瘤	Non-Hodgkin lymphoma	4 274	1.53	0.09	0.10	0.07	0.09	0.10	0.13	0.25	0.31	0.38
免疫增生性疾病	Immunoproliferative diseases	24	0.01	0.00	0.00	0.01	0.00	0.00	0.00	0.00	0.00	0.01
多发性骨髓瘤	Multiple myeloma	1 740	0.62	0.00	0.03	0.02	0.03	0.04	0.03	0.01	0.03	0.08
淋巴样白血病	Lymphoid leukemia	1 470	0.53	0.91	0.29	0.35	0.25	0.34	0.26	0.36	0.22	0.24
髓样白血病	Myeloid leukemia	2 278	0.82	0.41	0.18	0.19	0.21	0.28	0.22	0.29	0.29	0.44
白血病,未特指	Leukemia unspecified	2 967	1.06	1.37	0.55	0.47	0.58	0.50	0.49	0.41	0.43	0.40
其他或未指明部位	Other and unspecified	6 515	2.34	0.82	0.33	0.17	0.14	0.24	0.26	0.35	0.43	0.52
所有部位合计	All sites	278 638	100.00	10.46	3.37	2.65	2.98	3.18	3.70	7.55	12.96	20.21
所有部位除外 C44	All sites except C44	277 169	99.47	10.42	3.37	2.64	2.95	3.14	3.68	7.51	12.91	20.13

Appendix Table 1-12 Cancer mortality in registration areas of China, female in 2017

Age group										粗率 Crude rate/ $100\ 000^{-1}$	中标率 ASR China/ $100\ 000^{-1}$	世标率 ASR world/ $100\ 000^{-1}$	累积率 Cum. rate/%		ICD10
40~44	45~49	50~54	55~59	60~64	65~69	70~74	75~79	80~84	85+				0~64	0~74	
0.01	0.01	0.01	0.01	0.05	0.11	0.15	0.40	0.65	1.13	0.05	0.02	0.02	0.00	0.00	C00
0.07	0.17	0.24	0.27	0.65	0.52	1.55	1.79	2.54	2.08	0.29	0.17	0.16	0.01	0.02	C01-02
0.12	0.14	0.30	0.38	0.71	1.08	1.58	2.73	3.92	4.37	0.41	0.22	0.22	0.01	0.02	C03-06
0.05	0.07	0.20	0.10	0.19	0.39	0.42	0.48	0.84	0.95	0.12	0.08	0.07	0.00	0.01	C07-08
0.01	0.03	0.01	0.05	0.05	0.02	0.13	0.11	0.19	0.25	0.03	0.02	0.01	0.00	0.00	C09
0.00	0.02	0.06	0.03	0.09	0.06	0.32	0.44	0.38	0.76	0.05	0.03	0.03	0.00	0.00	C10
0.78	0.85	1.64	1.51	2.26	3.00	3.28	4.03	3.84	4.81	1.03	0.65	0.63	0.04	0.07	C11
0.02	0.01	0.04	0.05	0.05	0.09	0.22	0.17	0.24	0.40	0.04	0.02	0.02	0.00	0.00	C12-13
0.01	0.03	0.04	0.05	0.19	0.25	0.51	0.65	0.92	1.09	0.10	0.05	0.05	0.00	0.01	C14
0.25	0.90	2.41	4.08	12.48	24.95	43.68	63.53	92.70	95.21	8.20	4.10	4.06	0.10	0.44	C15
3.09	5.26	9.48	10.22	21.10	34.33	57.05	84.55	117.27	133.41	12.85	6.93	6.78	0.27	0.72	C16
0.12	0.31	0.44	0.66	1.13	1.80	2.18	4.03	4.57	4.81	0.59	0.32	0.32	0.01	0.03	C17
1.12	2.07	3.93	4.85	9.87	13.85	21.24	36.88	58.74	67.67	5.69	2.98	2.93	0.12	0.29	C18
1.48	2.61	4.59	5.49	9.62	14.72	23.98	36.43	56.55	62.32	5.84	3.12	3.07	0.13	0.32	C19-20
0.05	0.05	0.17	0.15	0.26	0.50	0.89	1.45	1.62	2.62	0.20	0.10	0.10	0.00	0.01	C21
3.40	6.65	12.47	14.82	27.45	41.98	56.45	75.71	100.00	107.66	13.39	7.47	7.41	0.35	0.84	C22
0.47	1.01	2.13	2.81	5.94	9.64	14.31	23.06	31.82	32.23	3.27	1.71	1.70	0.06	0.18	C23-24
0.84	1.65	4.03	5.29	10.77	17.74	25.91	37.51	48.69	47.13	5.54	2.96	2.94	0.12	0.33	C25
0.09	0.11	0.20	0.23	0.47	0.32	0.35	0.90	1.16	1.68	0.18	0.10	0.10	0.01	0.01	C30-31
0.05	0.12	0.25	0.35	0.50	0.92	1.61	2.52	3.41	3.79	0.36	0.19	0.19	0.01	0.02	C32
5.78	11.31	23.34	28.21	57.07	91.19	132.42	198.14	268.20	279.61	30.22	16.16	16.01	0.65	1.77	C33-34
0.12	0.23	0.40	0.53	0.97	1.04	1.38	2.12	2.11	2.48	0.40	0.25	0.25	0.01	0.03	C37-38
0.31	0.53	1.10	0.97	2.26	3.24	4.49	5.84	7.19	7.72	1.10	0.69	0.68	0.03	0.07	C40-41
0.13	0.18	0.35	0.29	0.70	0.84	1.28	1.55	2.00	2.73	0.32	0.19	0.19	0.01	0.02	C43
0.09	0.26	0.35	0.31	0.49	1.01	1.79	3.76	7.06	18.90	0.68	0.31	0.33	0.01	0.02	C44
0.02	0.05	0.10	0.16	0.26	0.31	0.39	0.38	0.57	0.47	0.10	0.06	0.06	0.00	0.01	C45
0.07	0.06	0.19	0.18	0.31	0.59	0.81	1.20	1.62	1.82	0.20	0.12	0.11	0.00	0.01	C46
0.12	0.24	0.27	0.31	0.56	0.69	0.94	1.62	2.05	2.04	0.31	0.20	0.20	0.01	0.02	C47;C49
7.14	11.90	18.37	17.81	23.05	23.00	23.55	28.69	35.87	43.20	9.76	6.17	5.98	0.43	0.66	C50
0.05	0.06	0.15	0.21	0.23	0.65	0.57	1.01	1.35	2.22	0.18	0.10	0.10	0.00	0.01	C51
0.03	0.08	0.18	0.18	0.17	0.35	0.36	0.57	0.65	0.44	0.10	0.06	0.06	0.00	0.01	C52
3.87	7.37	11.81	9.05	11.54	13.49	15.43	18.06	18.82	18.25	5.55	3.56	3.42	0.24	0.38	C53
0.65	1.25	2.77	2.95	4.25	5.13	5.73	5.63	6.65	5.68	1.60	0.97	0.97	0.06	0.12	C54
0.44	0.73	1.36	1.23	1.83	2.41	2.86	3.49	3.95	4.44	0.83	0.50	0.49	0.03	0.06	C55
1.75	3.51	6.80	6.66	8.89	10.65	12.03	13.57	13.27	8.49	3.60	2.25	2.21	0.15	0.26	C56
0.06	0.15	0.24	0.30	0.40	0.64	0.61	0.92	1.14	1.38	0.19	0.11	0.11	0.01	0.01	C57
0.01	0.01	0.00	0.00	0.00	0.00	0.01	0.02	0.00	0.00	0.01	0.01	0.01	0.00	0.00	C58
—	—	—	—	—	—	—	—	—	—	—	—	—	—	—	C60
—	—	—	—	—	—	—	—	—	—	—	—	—	—	—	C61
—	—	—	—	—	—	—	—	—	—	—	—	—	—	—	C62
—	—	—	—	—	—	—	—	—	—	—	—	—	—	—	C63
0.21	0.38	0.66	0.97	1.57	3.05	3.56	5.12	8.87	10.23	0.95	0.52	0.52	0.02	0.05	C64
0.01	0.05	0.09	0.15	0.33	0.39	0.80	1.22	1.84	2.22	0.18	0.09	0.09	0.00	0.01	C65
0.03	0.05	0.04	0.17	0.27	0.59	0.97	2.14	3.43	3.06	0.25	0.12	0.12	0.00	0.01	C66
0.09	0.16	0.35	0.47	0.98	2.29	3.76	8.02	15.27	21.49	1.10	0.51	0.51	0.01	0.04	C67
0.01	0.01	0.04	0.02	0.05	0.08	0.15	0.29	0.54	0.36	0.04	0.02	0.02	0.00	0.00	C68
0.01	0.04	0.06	0.03	0.04	0.11	0.12	0.21	0.32	0.66	0.05	0.03	0.04	0.00	0.00	C69
1.70	2.62	4.22	4.38	7.13	9.21	11.80	16.00	19.52	16.68	3.53	2.32	2.31	0.13	0.24	C70-72,D32-33,D42-43
0.33	0.51	0.86	0.75	1.38	2.02	2.79	3.84	4.89	5.06	0.73	0.43	0.42	0.02	0.05	C73
0.06	0.10	0.10	0.12	0.17	0.36	0.54	0.67	0.68	0.69	0.12	0.08	0.08	0.00	0.01	C74
0.10	0.05	0.05	0.14	0.17	0.25	0.20	0.29	0.57	0.51	0.09	0.06	0.06	0.00	0.01	C75
0.05	0.04	0.10	0.06	0.17	0.25	0.39	0.61	0.87	1.02	0.10	0.06	0.06	0.00	0.01	C81
0.61	0.97	1.85	2.19	3.93	5.96	8.24	11.53	14.87	12.75	1.99	1.16	1.14	0.05	0.13	C82-C86;C96
0.00	0.01	0.02	0.01	0.03	0.02	0.06	0.10	0.03	0.04	0.01	0.01	0.01	0.00	0.00	C88
0.07	0.41	0.75	0.98	1.87	3.08	4.08	4.98	4.49	3.75	0.81	0.47	0.47	0.02	0.06	C90
0.35	0.42	0.77	0.88	1.14	1.59	2.02	2.63	3.03	2.51	0.68	0.51	0.52	0.03	0.05	C91
0.44	0.77	1.19	1.33	2.34	2.81	3.79	4.62	4.68	4.44	1.06	0.71	0.71	0.04	0.07	C92-C94,D45-47
0.71	0.89	1.35	1.49	2.46	3.48	4.69	5.99	7.06	6.19	1.38	0.98	1.00	0.05	0.10	C95
0.91	1.53	2.48	3.37	5.58	8.01	10.97	16.32	24.09	30.08	3.03	1.73	1.73	0.08	0.18	O&U
38.30	68.94	125.41	138.27	246.44	365.06	519.43	748.55	1 017.58	1 096.00	129.48	72.77	71.77	3.38	7.80	C00-96, D32-33, D42-43,D45-47
38.22	68.68	125.06	137.96	245.95	364.05	517.64	744.79	1 010.52	1 077.10	128.79	72.45	71.45	3.37	7.78	C00-96, D32-33, D42-43,D45-47 exc. C44

附表 1-13 2017 年全国城市肿瘤登记地区男女合计癌症死亡主要指标

部位 Site		死亡数 No. deaths	构成 Freq./%	年龄组								
				0~	1~4	5~9	10~14	15~19	20~24	25~29	30~34	35~39
唇	Lip	144	0.04	0.00	0.00	0.00	0.00	0.00	0.00	0.00	0.00	0.00
舌	Tongue	1 132	0.29	0.00	0.00	0.00	0.00	0.01	0.02	0.02	0.05	0.07
口	Mouth	1 329	0.34	0.00	0.02	0.00	0.02	0.00	0.00	0.01	0.03	0.08
唾液腺	Salivary glands	462	0.12	0.00	0.00	0.00	0.01	0.03	0.01	0.01	0.01	0.08
扁桃腺	Tonsil	192	0.05	0.00	0.00	0.01	0.01	0.00	0.00	0.00	0.01	0.00
其他口咽	Other oropharynx	338	0.09	0.00	0.00	0.00	0.00	0.00	0.01	0.01	0.00	0.01
鼻咽	Nasopharynx	4 134	1.07	0.00	0.00	0.00	0.00	0.08	0.09	0.19	0.39	0.64
下咽	Hypopharynx	649	0.17	0.00	0.00	0.00	0.00	0.00	0.01	0.00	0.01	0.02
咽,部位不明	Pharynx unspecified	413	0.11	0.00	0.00	0.00	0.00	0.00	0.00	0.00	0.01	0.02
食管	Esophagus	25 601	6.63	0.00	0.02	0.00	0.03	0.01	0.02	0.02	0.07	0.19
胃	Stomach	39 707	10.28	0.00	0.01	0.00	0.01	0.06	0.21	0.56	1.13	1.83
小肠	Small intestine	1 868	0.48	0.00	0.00	0.00	0.00	0.00	0.01	0.02	0.02	0.12
结肠	Colon	18 105	4.69	0.00	0.01	0.00	0.03	0.04	0.16	0.25	0.71	0.76
直肠	Rectum	17 158	4.44	0.04	0.00	0.03	0.02	0.02	0.06	0.27	0.47	0.71
肛门	Anus	575	0.15	0.00	0.00	0.00	0.00	0.01	0.01	0.00	0.02	0.01
肝脏	Liver	50 549	13.09	0.44	0.25	0.06	0.14	0.17	0.32	0.97	2.62	4.73
胆囊及其他	Gallbladder etc.	7 386	1.91	0.09	0.01	0.01	0.00	0.01	0.02	0.08	0.08	0.11
胰腺	Pancreas	15 968	4.13	0.00	0.00	0.01	0.00	0.02	0.04	0.14	0.27	0.41
鼻、鼻窦及其他	Nose, sinuses etc.	504	0.13	0.00	0.00	0.02	0.03	0.01	0.04	0.02	0.03	0.04
喉	Larynx	2 531	0.66	0.04	0.00	0.01	0.01	0.02	0.02	0.01	0.00	0.05
气管、支气管、肺	Trachea, bronchus & lung	108 521	28.09	0.04	0.07	0.05	0.10	0.09	0.22	0.59	1.34	2.42
其他胸腔器官	Other thoracic organs	1 419	0.37	0.09	0.04	0.05	0.02	0.08	0.10	0.14	0.10	0.22
骨	Bone	2 634	0.68	0.04	0.02	0.10	0.27	0.39	0.26	0.19	0.31	0.20
皮肤黑色素瘤	Melanoma of skin	797	0.21	0.04	0.07	0.05	0.01	0.02	0.02	0.05	0.09	0.06
皮肤其他	Other skin	1 580	0.41	0.00	0.00	0.01	0.05	0.03	0.03	0.05	0.07	0.08
间皮瘤	Mesothelioma	352	0.09	0.00	0.00	0.00	0.00	0.00	0.01	0.02	0.02	0.04
卡波氏肉瘤	Kaposi sarcoma	727	0.19	0.00	0.01	0.02	0.00	0.01	0.02	0.03	0.03	0.04
结缔组织、软组织	Connective & soft tissue	1 023	0.26	0.27	0.15	0.12	0.10	0.11	0.08	0.12	0.17	0.15
乳腺	Breast	11 951	3.16	0.00	0.00	0.00	0.00	0.00	0.17	0.61	1.83	4.10
外阴	Vulva	199	0.05	0.00	0.00	0.00	0.00	0.00	0.00	0.02	0.01	0.03
阴道	Vagina	122	0.03	0.00	0.00	0.00	0.00	0.02	0.00	0.00	0.00	0.02
子宫颈	Cervix uteri	5 455	1.41	0.00	0.00	0.00	0.00	0.00	0.03	0.31	1.21	1.86
子宫体	Corpus uteri	1 831	0.47	0.00	0.00	0.00	0.00	0.00	0.06	0.09	0.14	0.29
子宫,部位不明	Uterus unspecified	787	0.20	0.00	0.02	0.00	0.00	0.00	0.02	0.06	0.09	0.16
卵巢	Ovary	4 531	1.17	0.00	0.02	0.02	0.04	0.10	0.17	0.23	0.45	0.91
其他女性生殖器	Other female genital organs	249	0.06	0.00	0.00	0.00	0.00	0.00	0.00	0.01	0.00	0.05
胎盘	Placenta	3	0.00	0.00	0.00	0.00	0.00	0.00	0.02	0.01	0.00	0.00
阴茎	Penis	230	0.06	0.00	0.00	0.00	0.00	0.00	0.00	0.02	0.04	0.05
前列腺	Prostate	6 642	1.72	0.00	0.00	0.00	0.00	0.04	0.06	0.02	0.06	0.05
睾丸	Testis	150	0.04	0.00	0.04	0.00	0.02	0.02	0.03	0.11	0.12	0.14
其他男性生殖器	Other male genital organs	73	0.02	0.00	0.02	0.00	0.00	0.00	0.01	0.00	0.00	0.01
肾	Kidney	3 772	0.98	0.31	0.06	0.10	0.02	0.03	0.03	0.06	0.12	0.13
肾盂	Renal pelvis	532	0.14	0.00	0.01	0.00	0.00	0.00	0.00	0.01	0.01	0.01
输尿管	Ureter	783	0.20	0.00	0.00	0.00	0.00	0.00	0.00	0.00	0.01	0.01
膀胱	Bladder	6 350	1.64	0.00	0.01	0.01	0.00	0.00	0.00	0.01	0.04	0.08
其他泌尿器官	Other urinary organs	161	0.04	0.00	0.01	0.00	0.00	0.00	0.01	0.00	0.00	0.01
眼	Eye	130	0.03	0.00	0.16	0.02	0.01	0.01	0.00	0.01	0.01	0.00
脑、神经系统	Brain, nervous system	8 292	2.15	0.93	1.09	0.96	0.89	0.65	0.43	0.86	1.01	1.30
甲状腺	Thyroid	1 471	0.38	0.00	0.00	0.00	0.02	0.00	0.01	0.05	0.08	0.16
肾上腺	Adrenal gland	363	0.09	0.04	0.05	0.07	0.02	0.00	0.01	0.02	0.04	0.01
其他内分泌腺	Other endocrine	251	0.06	0.00	0.02	0.01	0.06	0.05	0.03	0.03	0.05	0.02
霍奇金淋巴瘤	Hodgkin lymphoma	348	0.09	0.00	0.00	0.01	0.02	0.01	0.01	0.04	0.05	0.05
非霍奇金淋巴瘤	Non-Hodgkin lymphoma	6 015	1.56	0.04	0.11	0.16	0.17	0.27	0.18	0.27	0.53	0.49
免疫增生性疾病	Immunoproliferative diseases	49	0.01	0.04	0.00	0.00	0.00	0.00	0.00	0.00	0.00	0.00
多发性骨髓瘤	Multiple myeloma	2 480	0.64	0.00	0.04	0.02	0.04	0.02	0.03	0.01	0.01	0.09
淋巴样白血病	Lymphoid leukemia	1 873	0.48	1.02	0.46	0.54	0.40	0.56	0.34	0.33	0.33	0.30
髓样白血病	Myeloid leukemia	3 114	0.81	0.40	0.19	0.13	0.26	0.25	0.25	0.41	0.31	0.44
白血病,未特指	Leukemia unspecified	3 179	0.82	1.73	0.49	0.33	0.53	0.56	0.48	0.48	0.35	0.34
其他或未指明部位	Other and unspecified	8 822	2.28	0.36	0.47	0.17	0.22	0.32	0.23	0.41	0.51	0.59
所有部位合计	All sites	386 265	100.00	5.99	3.93	3.08	3.57	4.03	4.15	7.54	13.55	20.99
所有部位除外 C44	All sites except C44	384 685	99.59	5.99	3.93	3.08	3.52	4.00	4.12	7.49	13.48	20.90

Appendix Table 1-13 Cancer mortality in urban registration areas of China, both sexes in 2017

Age group										粗率 Crude rate/ 100 000^{-1}	中标率 ASR China/ 100 000^{-1}	世标率 ASR world/ 100 000^{-1}	累积率 Cum. rate/%		ICD10
40~44	45~49	50~54	55~59	60~64	65~69	70~74	75~79	80~84	85+				0~64	0~74	
0.02	0.03	0.02	0.06	0.13	0.18	0.18	0.38	0.65	1.31	0.07	0.03	0.03	0.00	0.00	C00
0.12	0.29	0.71	0.91	1.21	1.19	2.42	2.46	3.74	3.41	0.53	0.31	0.30	0.02	0.04	C01-02
0.12	0.26	0.57	0.73	1.46	1.97	2.27	3.78	4.90	5.36	0.62	0.34	0.34	0.02	0.04	C03-06
0.04	0.11	0.26	0.27	0.42	0.77	0.78	0.93	1.77	1.47	0.22	0.13	0.12	0.01	0.01	C07-08
0.01	0.06	0.15	0.17	0.21	0.29	0.29	0.46	0.48	0.40	0.09	0.05	0.05	0.00	0.01	C09
0.03	0.06	0.25	0.24	0.41	0.59	0.53	0.91	0.70	1.03	0.16	0.09	0.09	0.01	0.01	C10
1.39	1.99	3.31	3.32	4.15	6.03	6.24	6.89	6.19	6.19	1.94	1.23	1.20	0.08	0.14	C11
0.05	0.16	0.52	0.71	0.98	0.97	1.17	0.97	1.15	1.07	0.30	0.18	0.18	0.01	0.02	C12-13
0.05	0.08	0.26	0.27	0.48	0.48	0.74	1.09	1.58	1.35	0.19	0.11	0.11	0.01	0.01	C14
0.72	2.96	8.75	13.53	26.60	42.54	59.24	77.95	97.29	98.70	12.01	6.48	6.51	0.26	0.77	C15
3.50	5.98	13.09	19.18	35.84	56.82	87.06	127.74	162.93	164.41	18.62	10.17	10.03	0.41	1.13	C16
0.15	0.38	0.79	1.04	1.74	2.71	3.58	5.60	7.01	7.94	0.88	0.48	0.48	0.02	0.05	C17
1.41	2.55	5.34	7.98	14.51	22.01	33.91	55.50	88.34	110.32	8.49	4.46	4.42	0.17	0.45	C18
1.61	2.86	5.73	8.49	14.98	22.60	33.65	49.00	79.14	87.98	8.05	4.31	4.27	0.18	0.46	C19-20
0.09	0.11	0.23	0.22	0.41	0.68	1.22	1.87	2.19	3.57	0.27	0.14	0.14	0.01	0.01	C21
11.01	18.89	32.09	36.96	55.07	69.59	84.49	105.23	129.81	134.97	23.70	14.04	13.85	0.82	1.59	C22
0.44	0.98	2.24	3.34	6.29	11.05	14.44	24.58	33.48	36.79	3.46	1.83	1.82	0.07	0.20	C23-24
1.13	2.44	5.89	8.98	15.80	23.91	34.22	47.15	62.60	63.97	7.49	4.08	4.06	0.18	0.47	C25
0.09	0.14	0.25	0.35	0.63	0.53	0.65	1.17	1.55	2.06	0.24	0.14	0.14	0.01	0.01	C30-31
0.18	0.39	1.14	1.61	2.61	3.82	5.22	6.70	9.45	10.00	1.19	0.65	0.65	0.03	0.08	C32
6.78	14.22	37.75	55.96	110.72	170.50	238.80	334.64	423.67	418.39	50.89	27.64	27.58	1.15	3.20	C33-34
0.23	0.30	0.67	0.85	1.68	1.90	2.45	3.26	4.16	3.81	0.67	0.41	0.40	0.02	0.04	C37-38
0.35	0.57	1.11	1.24	2.31	3.52	4.90	7.33	8.44	9.09	1.24	0.78	0.76	0.04	0.08	C40-41
0.14	0.20	0.42	0.31	0.69	1.12	1.43	1.91	2.53	3.37	0.37	0.22	0.22	0.01	0.02	C43
0.09	0.28	0.43	0.57	0.76	1.41	2.11	4.07	7.79	18.02	0.74	0.37	0.37	0.01	0.03	C44
0.02	0.09	0.18	0.23	0.35	0.66	0.60	0.89	1.07	0.75	0.17	0.10	0.10	0.00	0.01	C45
0.07	0.13	0.23	0.30	0.49	0.93	1.44	2.42	3.29	3.77	0.34	0.19	0.18	0.01	0.02	C46
0.23	0.25	0.36	0.59	0.75	1.07	1.65	2.88	2.95	3.61	0.48	0.31	0.31	0.02	0.03	C47;C49
7.41	12.13	18.78	19.98	25.35	25.43	28.56	35.56	48.44	56.14	11.25	6.74	6.55	0.45	0.72	C50
0.04	0.02	0.14	0.16	0.25	0.73	0.53	1.12	1.43	2.48	0.19	0.09	0.09	0.00	0.01	C51
0.05	0.05	0.17	0.20	0.13	0.43	0.44	0.63	0.56	0.60	0.11	0.07	0.06	0.00	0.01	C52
3.87	7.20	11.30	8.73	9.98	10.62	12.88	16.19	15.38	16.92	5.13	3.23	3.09	0.22	0.34	C53
0.62	1.15	3.03	3.26	4.01	5.33	5.96	6.08	7.72	6.51	1.72	1.00	1.00	0.06	0.12	C54
0.43	0.62	1.03	1.06	1.60	2.25	2.31	3.10	3.17	4.16	0.74	0.43	0.43	0.03	0.05	C55
2.01	3.86	7.76	7.44	9.64	12.31	14.37	16.46	17.12	10.95	4.27	2.57	2.52	0.16	0.30	C56
0.04	0.18	0.25	0.30	0.44	0.75	0.82	1.04	1.48	2.08	0.23	0.13	0.13	0.01	0.01	C57
0.00	0.00	0.00	0.00	0.00	0.00	0.03	0.00	0.00	0.00	0.00	0.00	0.00	0.00	0.00	C58
0.09	0.16	0.19	0.21	0.42	0.46	0.93	1.15	2.38	2.13	0.21	0.13	0.12	0.01	0.01	C60
0.09	0.30	0.85	1.70	4.42	10.31	24.24	53.76	103.98	184.24	6.21	3.04	3.10	0.04	0.21	C61
0.12	0.10	0.05	0.11	0.18	0.27	0.28	0.72	1.00	1.36	0.14	0.10	0.09	0.01	0.01	C62
0.01	0.03	0.04	0.09	0.15	0.12	0.34	0.47	0.63	0.87	0.07	0.04	0.04	0.00	0.00	C63
0.35	0.71	1.48	2.10	3.55	5.42	6.59	10.01	15.73	17.78	1.77	0.97	0.98	0.04	0.10	C64
0.02	0.05	0.14	0.28	0.50	0.50	1.13	1.49	2.67	3.61	0.25	0.13	0.13	0.01	0.01	C65
0.03	0.06	0.11	0.30	0.46	0.93	1.44	3.20	4.90	4.72	0.37	0.18	0.18	0.00	0.02	C66
0.13	0.38	0.83	1.61	3.08	6.24	11.29	21.06	40.99	62.70	2.98	1.40	1.41	0.03	0.12	C67
0.01	0.03	0.01	0.04	0.11	0.15	0.33	0.56	1.15	0.87	0.08	0.04	0.04	0.00	0.00	C68
0.01	0.05	0.09	0.01	0.11	0.12	0.14	0.18	0.42	0.83	0.06	0.04	0.05	0.00	0.00	C69
1.81	2.89	4.63	4.80	7.58	10.60	13.52	17.21	21.07	18.53	3.89	2.58	2.57	0.14	0.26	C70-72,D32-33,D42-43
0.30	0.41	0.72	0.66	1.24	1.95	2.44	3.99	5.80	6.03	0.69	0.39	0.38	0.02	0.04	C73
0.06	0.09	0.17	0.30	0.30	0.45	0.83	0.76	0.90	1.11	0.17	0.11	0.11	0.01	0.01	C74
0.09	0.07	0.07	0.13	0.24	0.22	0.35	0.76	0.70	0.71	0.12	0.08	0.08	0.00	0.01	C75
0.08	0.06	0.17	0.16	0.27	0.41	0.71	0.89	1.01	1.47	0.16	0.10	0.10	0.00	0.01	C81
0.85	1.27	2.68	3.10	5.72	8.50	11.62	16.13	21.33	19.92	2.82	1.66	1.63	0.08	0.18	C82-C86;C96
0.00	0.02	0.02	0.01	0.07	0.06	0.11	0.22	0.11	0.12	0.02	0.01	0.01	0.00	0.00	C88
0.11	0.43	0.86	1.43	2.65	3.84	6.00	7.81	8.86	6.55	1.16	0.65	0.65	0.03	0.08	C90
0.43	0.48	0.88	0.99	1.26	2.12	2.38	3.70	4.95	4.05	0.88	0.66	0.68	0.04	0.06	C91
0.58	0.73	1.48	1.78	3.04	4.12	5.82	7.21	7.91	8.97	1.46	0.94	0.93	0.05	0.10	C92-C94,D45-47
0.60	0.95	1.31	1.55	2.57	3.78	5.25	7.61	8.72	8.69	1.49	1.02	1.04	0.05	0.10	C95
1.18	1.90	3.27	4.51	8.13	11.67	16.19	22.55	33.03	42.30	4.14	2.36	2.37	0.11	0.25	O&U
44.17	80.29	163.31	213.75	371.24	546.09	758.76	1 072.58	1 431.14	1 549.52	181.14	101.43	100.74	4.67	11.19	C00-96, D32-33, D42-43,D45-47
44.07	80.01	162.88	213.18	370.48	544.68	756.65	1 068.50	1 423.34	1 531.50	180.39	101.06	100.37	4.66	11.16	C00-96, D32-33, D42-43,D45-47 exc. C44

附表 1-14　2017 年全国城市肿瘤登记地区男性癌症死亡主要指标

部位 Site		死亡数 No. deaths	构成 Freq. /%	年龄组								
				0~	1~4	5~9	10~14	15~19	20~24	25~29	30~34	35~39
唇	Lip	91	0.04	0.00	0.00	0.00	0.00	0.00	0.00	0.00	0.00	0.00
舌	Tongue	774	0.32	0.00	0.00	0.00	0.00	0.02	0.04	0.04	0.07	0.08
口	Mouth	874	0.36	0.00	0.02	0.00	0.04	0.00	0.00	0.02	0.02	0.09
唾液腺	Salivary glands	305	0.12	0.00	0.00	0.00	0.00	0.02	0.00	0.00	0.00	0.09
扁桃腺	Tonsil	156	0.06	0.00	0.00	0.02	0.00	0.00	0.00	0.00	0.01	0.00
其他口咽	Other oropharynx	286	0.12	0.00	0.00	0.00	0.00	0.00	0.00	0.00	0.00	0.02
鼻咽	Nasopharynx	3 054	1.25	0.00	0.00	0.00	0.00	0.15	0.12	0.26	0.56	1.01
下咽	Hypopharynx	613	0.25	0.00	0.00	0.00	0.00	0.00	0.01	0.00	0.01	0.04
咽,部位不明	Pharynx unspecified	314	0.13	0.00	0.00	0.00	0.00	0.00	0.00	0.00	0.01	0.02
食管	Esophagus	19 504	7.96	0.00	0.02	0.00	0.06	0.02	0.04	0.01	0.11	0.26
胃	Stomach	27 563	11.25	0.00	0.00	0.00	0.00	0.07	0.23	0.45	1.03	1.80
小肠	Small intestine	1 109	0.45	0.00	0.00	0.00	0.00	0.00	0.01	0.02	0.02	0.06
结肠	Colon	10 167	4.15	0.00	0.02	0.00	0.06	0.02	0.20	0.21	0.77	0.80
直肠	Rectum	10 708	4.37	0.08	0.00	0.02	0.02	0.04	0.07	0.32	0.55	0.82
肛门	Anus	379	0.15	0.00	0.00	0.00	0.00	0.00	0.01	0.00	0.05	0.00
肝脏	Liver	37 123	15.15	0.51	0.24	0.09	0.20	0.17	0.47	1.57	4.32	8.01
胆囊及其他	Gallbladder etc.	3 478	1.42	0.08	0.02	0.00	0.00	0.00	0.03	0.09	0.11	0.12
胰腺	Pancreas	9 049	3.69	0.00	0.00	0.02	0.00	0.04	0.06	0.11	0.32	0.64
鼻、鼻窦及其他	Nose, sinuses etc.	316	0.13	0.00	0.00	0.00	0.02	0.02	0.03	0.02	0.05	0.05
喉	Larynx	2 156	0.88	0.08	0.00	0.02	0.02	0.04	0.01	0.01	0.00	0.09
气管、支气管、肺	Trachea, bronchus & lung	75 574	30.84	0.08	0.08	0.05	0.10	0.13	0.29	0.82	1.67	2.88
其他胸腔器官	Other thoracic organs	906	0.37	0.00	0.00	0.07	0.04	0.06	0.15	0.16	0.09	0.24
骨	Bone	1 575	0.64	0.00	0.00	0.16	0.22	0.50	0.34	0.27	0.33	0.26
皮肤黑色素瘤	Melanoma of skin	452	0.18	0.08	0.10	0.05	0.02	0.04	0.03	0.02	0.10	0.06
皮肤其他	Other skin	910	0.37	0.00	0.00	0.02	0.08	0.02	0.01	0.06	0.04	0.11
间皮瘤	Mesothelioma	217	0.09	0.00	0.00	0.00	0.00	0.00	0.00	0.02	0.02	0.04
卡波氏肉瘤	Kaposi sarcoma	455	0.19	0.00	0.00	0.03	0.00	0.00	0.03	0.04	0.05	0.05
结缔组织、软组织	Connective & soft tissue	630	0.26	0.08	0.18	0.17	0.12	0.11	0.12	0.15	0.19	0.15
乳腺	Breast	259	0.11	0.00	0.00	0.00	0.00	0.00	0.03	0.02	0.05	0.02
外阴	Vulva	—	—	—	—	—	—	—	—	—	—	—
阴道	Vagina	—	—	—	—	—	—	—	—	—	—	—
子宫颈	Cervix uteri	—	—	—	—	—	—	—	—	—	—	—
子宫体	Corpus uteri	—	—	—	—	—	—	—	—	—	—	—
子宫,部位不明	Uterus unspecified	—	—	—	—	—	—	—	—	—	—	—
卵巢	Ovary	—	—	—	—	—	—	—	—	—	—	—
其他女性生殖器	Other female genital organs	—	—	—	—	—	—	—	—	—	—	—
胎盘	Placenta	—	—	—	—	—	—	—	—	—	—	—
阴茎	Penis	230	0.09	0.00	0.00	0.00	0.00	0.00	0.00	0.02	0.04	0.05
前列腺	Prostate	6 642	2.71	0.00	0.00	0.00	0.00	0.04	0.06	0.02	0.06	0.05
睾丸	Testis	150	0.06	0.00	0.04	0.00	0.02	0.02	0.03	0.11	0.12	0.14
其他男性生殖器	Other male genital organs	73	0.03	0.00	0.02	0.00	0.00	0.00	0.01	0.00	0.00	0.01
肾	Kidney	2 546	1.04	0.34	0.04	0.16	0.02	0.04	0.03	0.06	0.10	0.16
肾盂	Renal pelvis	293	0.12	0.00	0.02	0.00	0.00	0.00	0.00	0.01	0.01	0.01
输尿管	Ureter	406	0.17	0.00	0.00	0.00	0.00	0.00	0.00	0.00	0.00	0.01
膀胱	Bladder	4 958	2.02	0.00	0.02	0.00	0.00	0.00	0.00	0.02	0.05	0.12
其他泌尿器官	Other urinary organs	98	0.04	0.00	0.00	0.00	0.00	0.00	0.01	0.00	0.00	0.01
眼	Eye	76	0.03	0.00	0.14	0.03	0.02	0.02	0.00	0.01	0.01	0.00
脑、神经系统	Brain, nervous system	4 587	1.87	1.10	1.19	1.16	0.84	0.63	0.50	0.98	1.22	1.48
甲状腺	Thyroid	590	0.24	0.00	0.00	0.00	0.02	0.00	0.01	0.02	0.06	0.09
肾上腺	Adrenal gland	219	0.09	0.00	0.04	0.09	0.02	0.00	0.01	0.02	0.06	0.01
其他内分泌腺	Other endocrine	143	0.06	0.00	0.02	0.02	0.10	0.09	0.04	0.02	0.07	0.04
霍奇金淋巴瘤	Hodgkin lymphoma	219	0.09	0.00	0.00	0.02	0.02	0.02	0.01	0.06	0.05	0.08
非霍奇金淋巴瘤	Non-Hodgkin lymphoma	3 647	1.49	0.00	0.10	0.24	0.22	0.39	0.25	0.30	0.73	0.67
免疫增生性疾病	Immunoproliferative diseases	33	0.01	0.08	0.00	0.00	0.00	0.00	0.00	0.00	0.00	0.00
多发性骨髓瘤	Multiple myeloma	1 437	0.59	0.00	0.06	0.02	0.04	0.04	0.04	0.01	0.02	0.11
淋巴样白血病	Lymphoid leukemia	1 096	0.45	0.84	0.65	0.61	0.56	0.75	0.41	0.37	0.40	0.34
髓样白血病	Myeloid leukemia	1 742	0.71	0.34	0.14	0.12	0.34	0.24	0.34	0.50	0.32	0.37
白血病,未特指	Leukemia unspecified	1 886	0.77	1.86	0.51	0.40	0.56	0.67	0.63	0.56	0.43	0.39
其他或未指明部位	Other and unspecified	4 996	2.04	0.42	0.49	0.21	0.30	0.39	0.23	0.46	0.51	0.61
所有部位合计	All sites	245 064	100.00	5.99	4.16	3.78	4.06	4.80	4.98	8.31	14.82	22.57
所有部位除外 C44	All sites except C44	244 154	99.63	5.99	4.16	3.76	3.98	4.78	4.96	8.25	14.78	22.47

Appendix Table 1-14 Cancer mortality in urban registration areas of China, male in 2017

Age group										粗率 Crude rate/ 100 000⁻¹	中标率 ASR China/ 100 000⁻¹	世标率 ASR world/ 100 000⁻¹	累积率 Cum. rate/%		ICD10
40~44	45~49	50~54	55~59	60~64	65~69	70~74	75~79	80~84	85+				0~64	0~74	
0.02	0.05	0.02	0.11	0.21	0.29	0.34	0.34	0.63	1.65	0.09	0.05	0.05	0.00	0.01	C00
0.16	0.44	1.16	1.47	1.72	2.06	2.91	2.93	4.51	4.75	0.72	0.44	0.44	0.03	0.05	C01-02
0.15	0.39	0.91	1.07	2.33	2.92	3.10	4.38	5.70	6.60	0.82	0.48	0.48	0.03	0.06	C03-06
0.02	0.14	0.27	0.42	0.65	1.17	1.09	1.32	2.69	2.04	0.29	0.17	0.17	0.01	0.02	C07-08
0.02	0.09	0.27	0.29	0.37	0.54	0.40	0.81	0.81	0.49	0.15	0.09	0.09	0.01	0.01	C09
0.06	0.10	0.45	0.44	0.73	1.17	0.74	1.49	1.25	1.65	0.27	0.16	0.16	0.01	0.02	C10
2.02	3.13	5.00	5.17	6.35	9.20	9.46	10.07	8.89	8.15	2.85	1.87	1.81	0.12	0.21	C11
0.08	0.31	1.00	1.35	1.93	1.83	2.20	1.96	2.25	2.23	0.57	0.34	0.35	0.02	0.04	C12-13
0.07	0.14	0.47	0.47	0.80	0.81	0.93	1.83	2.19	1.84	0.29	0.17	0.17	0.01	0.02	C14
1.32	5.18	15.65	24.49	46.18	69.59	93.71	116.97	136.66	140.00	18.23	10.46	10.55	0.47	1.28	C15
3.90	7.22	17.54	28.97	54.73	86.90	130.79	190.37	236.44	236.72	25.76	14.74	14.62	0.58	1.67	C16
0.22	0.42	1.16	1.30	2.27	3.39	4.77	6.16	8.14	10.48	1.04	0.60	0.60	0.03	0.07	C17
1.54	2.93	6.10	9.90	17.08	27.95	42.53	64.43	101.04	135.73	9.50	5.32	5.31	0.20	0.55	C18
1.76	3.24	6.97	11.13	20.89	31.94	44.86	64.56	103.42	114.97	10.01	5.66	5.65	0.23	0.61	C19-20
0.12	0.19	0.31	0.29	0.65	1.08	1.67	2.38	2.69	4.95	0.35	0.20	0.20	0.01	0.02	C21
19.04	32.40	53.24	60.87	86.85	103.06	118.64	141.83	168.77	179.29	34.69	21.57	21.26	1.34	2.45	C22
0.45	1.01	2.38	3.79	6.56	11.66	13.92	22.44	31.24	36.28	3.25	1.83	1.84	0.07	0.20	C23-24
1.48	3.23	7.43	12.00	20.04	28.17	40.05	51.98	67.29	74.99	8.46	4.88	4.89	0.23	0.57	C25
0.12	0.18	0.34	0.49	0.83	0.81	0.96	1.57	1.69	2.23	0.30	0.18	0.18	0.01	0.02	C30-31
0.32	0.66	2.03	2.88	4.83	6.91	9.33	11.31	16.84	18.34	2.01	1.15	1.17	0.05	0.14	C32
7.95	18.11	53.05	84.69	170.59	257.59	358.64	483.54	591.13	595.11	70.62	40.41	40.49	1.70	4.78	C33-34
0.34	0.45	0.85	1.15	2.33	2.60	3.29	4.00	5.57	5.24	0.85	0.53	0.53	0.03	0.06	C37-38
0.43	0.60	1.31	1.75	2.83	4.52	6.32	9.27	10.02	11.64	1.47	0.96	0.94	0.04	0.10	C40-41
0.15	0.25	0.41	0.44	0.71	1.33	1.67	2.51	3.07	4.56	0.42	0.26	0.26	0.01	0.03	C43
0.12	0.28	0.59	0.82	1.13	2.02	3.07	4.97	10.02	18.82	0.85	0.46	0.47	0.02	0.04	C44
0.04	0.12	0.28	0.32	0.39	0.87	0.59	1.23	1.50	0.97	0.20	0.12	0.12	0.01	0.01	C45
0.05	0.16	0.23	0.42	0.68	1.17	1.89	3.49	4.38	5.63	0.43	0.24	0.24	0.01	0.02	C46
0.33	0.27	0.48	0.82	0.92	1.33	2.26	3.70	3.63	5.24	0.59	0.40	0.40	0.02	0.04	C47;C49
0.09	0.12	0.29	0.14	0.49	0.67	1.09	1.15	2.25	3.10	0.24	0.14	0.14	0.01	0.02	C50
—	—	—	—	—	—	—	—	—	—	—	—	—	—	—	C51
—	—	—	—	—	—	—	—	—	—	—	—	—	—	—	C52
—	—	—	—	—	—	—	—	—	—	—	—	—	—	—	C53
—	—	—	—	—	—	—	—	—	—	—	—	—	—	—	C54
—	—	—	—	—	—	—	—	—	—	—	—	—	—	—	C55
—	—	—	—	—	—	—	—	—	—	—	—	—	—	—	C56
—	—	—	—	—	—	—	—	—	—	—	—	—	—	—	C57
—	—	—	—	—	—	—	—	—	—	—	—	—	—	—	C58
0.09	0.16	0.19	0.21	0.42	0.46	0.93	1.15	2.38	2.13	0.21	0.13	0.12	0.01	0.01	C60
0.09	0.30	0.85	1.70	4.42	10.31	24.24	53.76	103.98	184.24	6.21	3.04	3.10	0.04	0.21	C61
0.12	0.10	0.05	0.11	0.18	0.27	0.28	0.72	1.00	1.36	0.14	0.10	0.09	0.01	0.01	C62
0.01	0.03	0.04	0.09	0.15	0.12	0.34	0.47	0.63	0.87	0.07	0.04	0.04	0.00	0.00	C63
0.46	1.06	2.25	3.06	5.58	7.62	9.05	14.37	21.03	24.35	2.38	1.37	1.39	0.07	0.15	C64
0.04	0.07	0.17	0.39	0.65	0.67	1.21	1.32	2.94	4.37	0.27	0.15	0.15	0.01	0.02	C65
0.02	0.07	0.15	0.43	0.61	1.06	1.61	3.44	4.82	5.04	0.38	0.21	0.20	0.01	0.02	C66
0.21	0.60	1.33	2.65	5.22	10.22	18.76	35.19	68.80	116.03	4.63	2.36	2.40	0.05	0.20	C67
0.01	0.03	0.01	0.06	0.13	0.19	0.47	0.68	1.50	1.36	0.09	0.05	0.05	0.00	0.00	C68
0.01	0.03	0.08	0.03	0.18	0.12	0.19	0.26	0.50	1.16	0.07	0.05	0.06	0.00	0.00	C69
2.04	3.41	5.42	5.60	8.53	12.74	15.59	18.74	21.97	20.47	4.29	2.94	2.93	0.16	0.31	C70-72,D32-33,D42-43
0.20	0.30	0.59	0.53	1.10	1.56	1.98	3.66	4.69	6.50	0.55	0.32	0.32	0.01	0.03	C73
0.05	0.06	0.27	0.46	0.43	0.54	0.96	0.98	1.00	1.26	0.20	0.13	0.13	0.01	0.02	C74
0.02	0.07	0.07	0.16	0.28	0.17	0.40	1.15	0.75	1.16	0.13	0.10	0.09	0.01	0.01	C75
0.11	0.09	0.21	0.24	0.40	0.52	0.96	1.28	0.94	1.84	0.20	0.13	0.13	0.01	0.01	C81
0.96	1.56	3.35	4.05	7.29	10.95	14.79	19.47	25.60	27.75	3.41	2.11	2.07	0.10	0.23	C82-C86;C96
0.00	0.03	0.01	0.01	0.09	0.10	0.09	0.30	0.19	0.29	0.03	0.02	0.02	0.00	0.00	C88
0.15	0.47	0.94	1.75	3.30	4.52	6.51	9.31	11.77	9.70	1.34	0.78	0.78	0.03	0.09	C90
0.48	0.53	0.94	1.09	1.46	2.60	2.95	4.38	6.51	5.82	1.02	0.79	0.82	0.04	0.07	C91
0.74	0.73	1.66	1.99	3.23	4.96	7.25	8.20	10.14	11.74	1.63	1.07	1.06	0.05	0.11	C92-C94,D45-47
0.75	1.21	1.61	1.79	3.05	4.62	6.08	9.27	11.58	12.81	1.76	1.23	1.25	0.06	0.12	C95
1.34	2.10	3.92	5.40	10.32	14.58	19.31	26.61	38.12	48.80	4.67	2.80	2.82	0.13	0.30	O&U
50.29	94.85	204.30	289.24	513.12	752.49	1 035.20	1 427.64	1 875.56	2 122.75	229.00	133.80	133.59	6.10	15.04	C00-96, D32-33, D42-43,D45-47
50.17	94.57	203.71	288.42	511.99	750.47	1 032.13	1 422.67	1 865.54	2 103.93	228.15	133.33	133.12	6.08	14.99	C00-96, D32-33, D42-43,D45-47 exc. C44

附表 1-15　2017 年全国城市肿瘤登记地区女性癌症死亡主要指标

部位 Site		死亡数 No. deaths	构成 Freq. /%	年龄组								
				0~	1~4	5~9	10~14	15~19	20~24	25~29	30~34	35~39
唇	Lip	53	0.04	0.00	0.00	0.00	0.00	0.00	0.00	0.00	0.00	0.00
舌	Tongue	358	0.25	0.00	0.00	0.00	0.00	0.00	0.00	0.01	0.04	0.06
口	Mouth	455	0.32	0.00	0.02	0.00	0.00	0.00	0.00	0.00	0.04	0.06
唾液腺	Salivary glands	157	0.11	0.00	0.00	0.00	0.02	0.04	0.03	0.02	0.01	0.06
扁桃腺	Tonsil	36	0.03	0.00	0.00	0.00	0.02	0.00	0.00	0.00	0.01	0.00
其他口咽	Other oropharynx	52	0.04	0.00	0.00	0.00	0.00	0.00	0.02	0.01	0.00	0.00
鼻咽	Nasopharynx	1 080	0.76	0.00	0.00	0.00	0.00	0.00	0.06	0.12	0.22	0.28
下咽	Hypopharynx	36	0.03	0.00	0.00	0.00	0.00	0.00	0.00	0.00	0.01	0.00
咽,部位不明	Pharynx unspecified	99	0.07	0.00	0.00	0.00	0.00	0.00	0.00	0.00	0.00	0.01
食管	Esophagus	6 097	4.32	0.00	0.02	0.00	0.00	0.00	0.00	0.04	0.02	0.12
胃	Stomach	12 144	8.60	0.00	0.02	0.00	0.02	0.04	0.18	0.67	1.23	1.85
小肠	Small intestine	759	0.54	0.00	0.00	0.00	0.00	0.00	0.02	0.01	0.02	0.17
结肠	Colon	7 938	5.62	0.00	0.00	0.00	0.00	0.06	0.11	0.29	0.66	0.73
直肠	Rectum	6 450	4.57	0.00	0.00	0.04	0.02	0.00	0.05	0.21	0.39	0.60
肛门	Anus	196	0.14	0.00	0.00	0.00	0.00	0.02	0.00	0.00	0.00	0.01
肝脏	Liver	13 426	9.51	0.37	0.25	0.04	0.07	0.18	0.17	0.38	0.96	1.50
胆囊及其他	Gallbladder etc.	3 908	2.77	0.09	0.00	0.02	0.00	0.02	0.02	0.07	0.05	0.10
胰腺	Pancreas	6 919	4.90	0.00	0.00	0.00	0.00	0.00	0.03	0.16	0.22	0.20
鼻、鼻窦及其他	Nose, sinuses etc.	188	0.13	0.00	0.00	0.04	0.04	0.00	0.06	0.01	0.01	0.03
喉	Larynx	375	0.27	0.00	0.00	0.00	0.00	0.00	0.03	0.01	0.00	0.01
气管、支气管、肺	Trachea, bronchus & lung	32 947	23.33	0.00	0.07	0.06	0.09	0.04	0.15	0.37	1.02	1.96
其他胸腔器官	Other thoracic organs	513	0.36	0.19	0.09	0.02	0.00	0.10	0.06	0.11	0.11	0.21
骨	Bone	1 059	0.75	0.09	0.05	0.04	0.34	0.26	0.18	0.11	0.28	0.15
皮肤黑色素瘤	Melanoma of skin	345	0.24	0.00	0.05	0.06	0.00	0.00	0.02	0.07	0.08	0.07
皮肤其他	Other skin	670	0.47	0.00	0.00	0.00	0.02	0.04	0.05	0.04	0.09	0.06
间皮瘤	Mesothelioma	135	0.10	0.00	0.00	0.00	0.00	0.00	0.02	0.01	0.02	0.03
卡波氏肉瘤	Kaposi sarcoma	272	0.19	0.00	0.02	0.00	0.00	0.02	0.02	0.02	0.01	0.03
结缔组织、软组织	Connective & soft tissue	393	0.28	0.47	0.11	0.06	0.07	0.10	0.05	0.10	0.14	0.14
乳腺	Breast	11 951	8.46	0.00	0.00	0.00	0.00	0.00	0.17	0.61	1.83	4.10
外阴	Vulva	199	0.14	0.00	0.00	0.00	0.00	0.00	0.00	0.02	0.01	0.03
阴道	Vagina	122	0.09	0.00	0.00	0.00	0.00	0.02	0.00	0.00	0.00	0.02
子宫颈	Cervix uteri	5 455	3.86	0.00	0.00	0.00	0.00	0.00	0.03	0.31	1.21	1.86
子宫体	Corpus uteri	1 831	1.30	0.00	0.00	0.00	0.00	0.00	0.06	0.09	0.14	0.29
子宫,部位不明	Uterus unspecified	787	0.56	0.00	0.02	0.00	0.00	0.00	0.02	0.06	0.09	0.16
卵巢	Ovary	4 531	3.21	0.00	0.02	0.02	0.04	0.10	0.17	0.23	0.45	0.91
其他女性生殖器	Other female genital organs	249	0.18	0.00	0.00	0.00	0.00	0.00	0.00	0.01	0.00	0.05
胎盘	Placenta	3	0.00	0.00	0.00	0.00	0.00	0.00	0.02	0.01	0.00	0.00
阴茎	Penis	—	—	—	—	—	—	—	—	—	—	—
前列腺	Prostate	—	—	—	—	—	—	—	—	—	—	—
睾丸	Testis	—	—	—	—	—	—	—	—	—	—	—
其他男性生殖器	Other male genital organs	—	—	—	—	—	—	—	—	—	—	—
肾	Kidney	1 226	0.87	0.28	0.09	0.04	0.02	0.02	0.03	0.05	0.14	0.09
肾盂	Renal pelvis	239	0.17	0.00	0.00	0.00	0.00	0.00	0.00	0.00	0.01	0.00
输尿管	Ureter	377	0.27	0.00	0.00	0.00	0.00	0.00	0.00	0.00	0.02	0.00
膀胱	Bladder	1 392	0.99	0.00	0.00	0.02	0.00	0.00	0.00	0.00	0.04	0.05
其他泌尿器官	Other urinary organs	63	0.04	0.00	0.02	0.00	0.00	0.00	0.00	0.00	0.00	0.00
眼	Eye	54	0.04	0.00	0.18	0.00	0.00	0.00	0.00	0.01	0.00	0.00
脑、神经系统	Brain, nervous system	3 705	2.62	0.75	0.98	0.74	0.94	0.67	0.36	0.74	0.82	1.11
甲状腺	Thyroid	881	0.62	0.00	0.00	0.00	0.02	0.00	0.02	0.07	0.11	0.23
肾上腺	Adrenal gland	144	0.10	0.09	0.07	0.06	0.02	0.00	0.00	0.01	0.01	0.01
其他内分泌腺	Other endocrine	108	0.08	0.00	0.02	0.00	0.02	0.00	0.02	0.04	0.02	0.01
霍奇金淋巴瘤	Hodgkin lymphoma	129	0.09	0.00	0.00	0.00	0.02	0.00	0.02	0.02	0.06	0.02
非霍奇金淋巴瘤	Non-Hodgkin lymphoma	2 368	1.68	0.09	0.11	0.06	0.11	0.14	0.11	0.25	0.33	0.31
免疫增生性疾病	Immunoproliferative diseases	16	0.01	0.00	0.00	0.00	0.00	0.00	0.00	0.00	0.00	0.00
多发性骨髓瘤	Multiple myeloma	1 043	0.74	0.00	0.02	0.02	0.04	0.00	0.02	0.00	0.00	0.08
淋巴样白血病	Lymphoid leukemia	777	0.55	1.22	0.25	0.47	0.22	0.36	0.27	0.29	0.26	0.27
髓样白血病	Myeloid leukemia	1 372	0.97	0.47	0.25	0.14	0.18	0.26	0.17	0.32	0.30	0.51
白血病,未特指	Leukemia unspecified	1 293	0.92	1.59	0.48	0.25	0.49	0.45	0.32	0.40	0.28	0.29
其他或未指明部位	Other and unspecified	3 826	2.71	0.28	0.45	0.14	0.13	0.24	0.23	0.36	0.51	0.57
所有部位合计	All sites	141 201	100.00	5.99	3.68	2.31	3.01	3.20	3.29	6.78	12.32	19.43
所有部位除外 C44	All sites except C44	140 531	99.53	5.99	3.68	2.31	2.99	3.16	3.25	6.74	12.22	19.37

Appendix Table 1-15 Cancer mortality in urban registration areas of China, female in 2017

Age group										粗率 Crude rate/ $100\,000^{-1}$	中标率 ASR China/ $100\,000^{-1}$	世标率 ASR world/ $100\,000^{-1}$	累积率 Cum. rate/%		ICD10
40~44	45~49	50~54	55~59	60~64	65~69	70~74	75~79	80~84	85+				0~64	0~74	
0.01	0.00	0.02	0.01	0.06	0.08	0.03	0.41	0.66	1.07	0.05	0.02	0.02	0.00	0.00	C00
0.07	0.15	0.25	0.35	0.71	0.34	1.96	2.05	3.12	2.48	0.34	0.18	0.17	0.01	0.02	C01-02
0.09	0.14	0.22	0.38	0.60	1.05	1.49	3.25	4.24	4.50	0.43	0.21	0.21	0.01	0.02	C03-06
0.06	0.08	0.26	0.13	0.19	0.39	0.50	0.60	1.02	1.07	0.15	0.09	0.09	0.00	0.01	C07-08
0.00	0.03	0.02	0.06	0.06	0.04	0.18	0.15	0.20	0.34	0.03	0.02	0.02	0.00	0.00	C09
0.00	0.01	0.04	0.03	0.10	0.02	0.32	0.41	0.26	0.60	0.05	0.03	0.03	0.00	0.00	C10
0.77	0.85	1.57	1.45	1.98	2.94	3.21	4.10	3.99	4.84	1.02	0.61	0.59	0.04	0.07	C11
0.01	0.00	0.02	0.06	0.04	0.12	0.20	0.11	0.26	0.27	0.03	0.02	0.02	0.00	0.00	C12-13
0.02	0.03	0.04	0.06	0.16	0.16	0.55	0.45	1.07	1.01	0.09	0.05	0.05	0.00	0.01	C14
0.13	0.72	1.65	2.45	7.24	16.20	26.78	43.69	65.15	70.11	5.74	2.70	2.67	0.06	0.28	C15
3.10	4.73	8.52	9.28	17.16	27.53	45.87	72.76	102.92	114.36	11.43	5.93	5.77	0.23	0.60	C16
0.08	0.33	0.41	0.77	1.20	2.05	2.45	5.11	6.08	6.18	0.71	0.37	0.36	0.02	0.04	C17
1.29	2.18	4.56	6.04	11.96	16.24	25.78	47.65	77.98	92.74	7.47	3.66	3.61	0.14	0.35	C18
1.46	2.48	4.45	5.82	9.14	13.50	23.10	35.34	59.33	69.30	6.07	3.05	3.01	0.12	0.31	C19-20
0.06	0.04	0.14	0.14	0.16	0.28	0.79	1.42	1.79	2.62	0.18	0.09	0.09	0.00	0.01	C21
3.01	5.34	10.36	12.78	23.67	37.00	52.33	73.10	98.01	104.29	12.64	6.70	6.63	0.29	0.74	C22
0.43	0.95	2.09	2.88	6.02	10.46	14.92	26.46	35.31	37.14	3.68	1.82	1.80	0.06	0.19	C23-24
0.78	1.66	4.30	5.92	11.61	19.75	28.73	42.91	58.77	56.34	6.51	3.31	3.27	0.12	0.37	C25
0.06	0.10	0.16	0.20	0.43	0.26	0.35	0.82	1.43	1.95	0.18	0.10	0.10	0.01	0.01	C30-31
0.05	0.11	0.22	0.33	0.41	0.81	1.34	2.65	3.42	4.23	0.35	0.17	0.17	0.01	0.02	C32
5.62	10.32	22.02	26.92	51.56	85.70	125.91	203.92	286.98	296.08	31.01	15.68	15.48	0.60	1.66	C33-34
0.12	0.16	0.50	0.55	1.03	1.22	1.66	2.61	3.01	2.82	0.48	0.29	0.29	0.02	0.03	C37-38
0.27	0.53	0.92	0.72	1.79	2.55	3.56	5.63	7.15	7.32	1.00	0.60	0.59	0.03	0.06	C40-41
0.13	0.15	0.43	0.17	0.68	0.91	1.20	1.38	2.10	2.55	0.32	0.19	0.19	0.01	0.02	C43
0.07	0.27	0.26	0.32	0.40	0.81	1.20	3.28	5.98	17.46	0.63	0.27	0.28	0.01	0.02	C44
0.01	0.06	0.09	0.14	0.32	0.45	0.61	0.60	0.72	0.60	0.13	0.07	0.07	0.00	0.01	C45
0.09	0.10	0.22	0.19	0.29	0.71	1.02	1.49	2.40	2.48	0.26	0.14	0.13	0.01	0.01	C46
0.14	0.23	0.24	0.36	0.59	0.81	1.08	2.16	2.40	2.48	0.37	0.24	0.24	0.01	0.02	C47;C49
7.41	12.13	18.78	19.98	25.35	25.43	28.56	35.56	48.44	56.14	11.25	6.74	6.55	0.45	0.72	C50
0.04	0.02	0.14	0.16	0.25	0.73	0.53	1.12	1.43	2.48	0.19	0.09	0.09	0.00	0.01	C51
0.05	0.05	0.17	0.20	0.13	0.43	0.44	0.63	0.56	0.60	0.11	0.07	0.06	0.00	0.01	C52
3.87	7.20	11.30	8.73	9.98	10.62	12.88	16.19	15.38	16.92	5.13	3.23	3.09	0.22	0.34	C53
0.62	1.15	3.03	3.26	4.01	5.33	5.96	6.08	7.72	6.51	1.72	1.00	1.00	0.06	0.12	C54
0.43	0.62	1.03	1.06	1.60	2.25	2.31	3.10	3.17	4.16	0.74	0.43	0.43	0.03	0.05	C55
2.01	3.86	7.76	7.44	9.64	12.31	14.37	16.46	17.12	10.95	4.27	2.57	2.52	0.16	0.30	C56
0.04	0.18	0.25	0.30	0.44	0.75	0.82	1.04	1.48	2.08	0.23	0.13	0.13	0.01	0.01	C57
0.00	0.00	0.00	0.00	0.00	0.00	0.03	0.00	0.00	0.00	0.00	0.00	0.00	0.00	0.00	C58
—	—	—	—	—	—	—	—	—	—	—	—	—	—	—	C60
—	—	—	—	—	—	—	—	—	—	—	—	—	—	—	C61
—	—	—	—	—	—	—	—	—	—	—	—	—	—	—	C62
—	—	—	—	—	—	—	—	—	—	—	—	—	—	—	C63
0.23	0.37	0.70	1.13	1.56	3.28	4.26	6.19	11.40	13.23	1.15	0.59	0.59	0.02	0.06	C64
0.00	0.03	0.11	0.17	0.34	0.34	1.05	1.64	2.45	3.09	0.22	0.10	0.10	0.00	0.01	C65
0.04	0.05	0.07	0.17	0.31	0.81	1.28	2.99	4.96	4.50	0.35	0.16	0.16	0.00	0.01	C66
0.05	0.15	0.31	0.56	0.97	2.35	4.26	8.66	18.29	25.79	1.31	0.56	0.56	0.01	0.04	C67
0.01	0.02	0.01	0.03	0.09	0.12	0.20	0.45	0.87	0.54	0.06	0.03	0.03	0.00	0.00	C68
0.01	0.06	0.09	0.00	0.04	0.12	0.09	0.11	0.36	0.60	0.05	0.03	0.04	0.00	0.00	C69
1.58	2.37	3.83	4.00	6.63	8.52	11.56	15.86	20.34	17.19	3.49	2.23	2.22	0.12	0.22	C70-72,D32-33,D42-43
0.40	0.52	0.84	0.78	1.38	2.33	2.86	4.29	6.69	5.71	0.83	0.46	0.45	0.02	0.05	C73
0.08	0.13	0.06	0.14	0.16	0.36	0.70	0.56	0.82	1.01	0.14	0.08	0.09	0.00	0.01	C74
0.16	0.06	0.06	0.10	0.21	0.26	0.29	0.41	0.66	0.40	0.10	0.06	0.06	0.00	0.01	C75
0.05	0.03	0.14	0.07	0.15	0.30	0.47	0.56	1.07	1.21	0.12	0.07	0.07	0.00	0.01	C81
0.74	0.97	2.00	2.14	4.17	6.10	8.64	13.21	17.83	14.51	2.23	1.24	1.21	0.06	0.13	C82-C86;C96
0.00	0.00	0.02	0.01	0.04	0.02	0.12	0.15	0.05	0.00	0.02	0.01	0.01	0.00	0.00	C88
0.06	0.40	0.77	1.11	2.01	3.18	5.52	6.49	6.49	4.36	0.98	0.54	0.53	0.02	0.07	C90
0.37	0.43	0.82	0.88	1.07	1.64	1.84	3.10	3.68	2.82	0.73	0.53	0.55	0.03	0.05	C91
0.42	0.73	1.29	1.56	2.85	3.30	4.47	6.34	6.08	7.05	1.29	0.81	0.80	0.05	0.08	C92-C94,D45-47
0.44	0.70	1.01	1.30	2.10	2.96	4.47	6.16	6.39	5.84	1.22	0.82	0.84	0.04	0.08	C95
1.03	1.69	2.60	3.62	5.97	8.84	13.26	18.99	28.87	37.81	3.60	1.94	1.94	0.09	0.20	O&U
38.07	65.69	121.18	137.44	231.03	345.12	498.37	760.86	1 068.36	1 152.75	132.92	71.14	70.06	3.24	7.46	C00-96, D32-33, D42-43,D45-47
38.00	65.42	120.92	137.12	230.63	344.31	497.17	757.58	1 062.38	1 135.29	132.29	70.87	69.77	3.23	7.44	C00-96, D32-33, D42-43,D45-47 exc. C44

附表 1-16　2017 年全国农村肿瘤登记地区男女合计癌症死亡主要指标

部位 Site		死亡数 No. deaths	构成 Freq. /%	年龄组								
				0～	1～4	5～9	10～14	15～19	20～24	25～29	30～34	35～39
唇	Lip	202	0.05	0.00	0.00	0.00	0.00	0.01	0.00	0.00	0.01	0.01
舌	Tongue	935	0.24	0.00	0.01	0.01	0.00	0.02	0.01	0.02	0.08	0.12
口	Mouth	1 186	0.31	0.00	0.00	0.00	0.01	0.01	0.00	0.05	0.07	0.07
唾液腺	Salivary glands	338	0.09	0.00	0.00	0.00	0.01	0.00	0.03	0.02	0.01	0.06
扁桃腺	Tonsil	129	0.03	0.00	0.00	0.00	0.00	0.00	0.01	0.00	0.01	0.02
其他口咽	Other oropharynx	371	0.10	0.00	0.00	0.00	0.00	0.00	0.01	0.01	0.01	0.01
鼻咽	Nasopharynx	4 078	1.05	0.12	0.01	0.00	0.03	0.06	0.09	0.20	0.49	0.74
下咽	Hypopharynx	485	0.13	0.00	0.00	0.01	0.00	0.00	0.00	0.00	0.00	0.03
咽,部位不明	Pharynx unspecified	447	0.12	0.00	0.00	0.00	0.01	0.01	0.00	0.01	0.00	0.02
食管	Esophagus	40 770	10.54	0.46	0.03	0.00	0.00	0.02	0.02	0.05	0.12	0.27
胃	Stomach	51 459	13.31	1.50	0.03	0.02	0.02	0.10	0.31	0.67	1.43	1.89
小肠	Small intestine	1 247	0.32	0.04	0.00	0.00	0.01	0.00	0.01	0.02	0.04	0.10
结肠	Colon	9 799	2.53	0.46	0.00	0.00	0.01	0.05	0.15	0.27	0.44	0.67
直肠	Rectum	15 244	3.94	0.83	0.00	0.01	0.01	0.04	0.05	0.29	0.57	0.83
肛门	Anus	559	0.14	0.00	0.00	0.00	0.00	0.00	0.00	0.01	0.01	0.07
肝脏	Liver	58 142	15.04	2.75	0.24	0.10	0.17	0.25	0.51	1.62	3.59	6.67
胆囊及其他	Gallbladder etc.	5 792	1.50	0.17	0.01	0.00	0.00	0.01	0.01	0.04	0.10	0.16
胰腺	Pancreas	11 939	3.09	0.29	0.01	0.00	0.01	0.01	0.01	0.09	0.23	0.47
鼻、鼻窦及其他	Nose, sinuses etc.	476	0.12	0.04	0.04	0.01	0.00	0.02	0.01	0.02	0.07	0.08
喉	Larynx	2 181	0.56	0.00	0.03	0.01	0.00	0.03	0.01	0.02	0.05	0.07
气管、支气管、肺	Trachea, bronchus & lung	106 504	27.54	3.08	0.03	0.02	0.07	0.07	0.31	0.76	1.73	3.22
其他胸腔器官	Other thoracic organs	935	0.24	0.21	0.02	0.06	0.01	0.04	0.06	0.08	0.09	0.12
骨	Bone	3 161	0.82	0.08	0.01	0.12	0.29	0.45	0.29	0.27	0.22	0.25
皮肤黑色素瘤	Melanoma of skin	792	0.20	0.00	0.06	0.04	0.02	0.03	0.02	0.07	0.08	0.15
皮肤其他	Other skin	1 794	0.46	0.12	0.02	0.02	0.02	0.05	0.03	0.07	0.08	0.10
间皮瘤	Mesothelioma	165	0.04	0.00	0.00	0.00	0.00	0.00	0.00	0.01	0.04	0.02
卡波氏肉瘤	Kaposi sarcoma	430	0.11	0.04	0.03	0.01	0.03	0.05	0.02	0.04	0.03	0.04
结缔组织、软组织	Connective & soft tissue	665	0.17	0.29	0.09	0.09	0.06	0.10	0.08	0.08	0.05	0.07
乳腺	Breast	9 049	2.40	0.71	0.00	0.00	0.00	0.00	0.16	0.86	2.23	3.78
外阴	Vulva	185	0.05	0.00	0.00	0.00	0.00	0.00	0.04	0.00	0.03	0.05
阴道	Vagina	103	0.03	0.00	0.00	0.00	0.00	0.00	0.01	0.00	0.00	0.00
子宫颈	Cervix uteri	6 481	1.68	1.07	0.00	0.00	0.00	0.00	0.05	0.54	1.20	2.53
子宫体	Corpus uteri	1 622	0.42	0.00	0.00	0.00	0.00	0.02	0.04	0.08	0.11	0.35
子宫,部位不明	Uterus unspecified	1 006	0.26	0.18	0.00	0.00	0.00	0.00	0.01	0.01	0.17	0.20
卵巢	Ovary	3 220	0.83	0.18	0.02	0.00	0.11	0.03	0.12	0.30	0.53	0.54
其他女性生殖器	Other female genital organs	168	0.04	0.00	0.00	0.00	0.00	0.00	0.01	0.01	0.03	0.05
胎盘	Placenta	10	0.00	0.00	0.00	0.00	0.00	0.00	0.01	0.04	0.00	0.02
阴茎	Penis	301	0.08	0.00	0.00	0.00	0.00	0.03	0.00	0.02	0.01	0.04
前列腺	Prostate	4 046	1.05	0.00	0.00	0.00	0.00	0.03	0.01	0.00	0.01	0.01
睾丸	Testis	135	0.03	0.00	0.05	0.06	0.00	0.03	0.09	0.06	0.14	0.08
其他男性生殖器	Other male genital organs	34	0.01	0.00	0.00	0.00	0.00	0.01	0.00	0.01	0.01	0.00
肾	Kidney	2 277	0.59	0.08	0.18	0.08	0.00	0.04	0.03	0.08	0.15	0.17
肾盂	Renal pelvis	340	0.09	0.00	0.01	0.00	0.00	0.00	0.00	0.00	0.01	0.02
输尿管	Ureter	366	0.09	0.29	0.00	0.00	0.00	0.00	0.00	0.01	0.02	0.01
膀胱	Bladder	4 722	1.22	0.17	0.00	0.00	0.00	0.02	0.01	0.06	0.03	0.05
其他泌尿器官	Other urinary organs	67	0.02	0.00	0.00	0.01	0.00	0.00	0.00	0.01	0.00	0.01
眼	Eye	130	0.03	0.04	0.11	0.06	0.01	0.01	0.00	0.01	0.01	0.01
脑、神经系统	Brain, nervous system	8 963	2.32	0.87	0.97	1.03	0.84	0.66	0.54	0.96	1.26	1.49
甲状腺	Thyroid	1 080	0.28	0.12	0.00	0.00	0.01	0.02	0.03	0.10	0.10	0.15
肾上腺	Adrenal gland	284	0.07	0.17	0.13	0.05	0.01	0.02	0.00	0.02	0.03	0.04
其他内分泌腺	Other endocrine	189	0.05	0.04	0.02	0.02	0.01	0.03	0.03	0.02	0.06	0.06
霍奇金淋巴瘤	Hodgkin lymphoma	282	0.07	0.00	0.00	0.01	0.02	0.02	0.03	0.02	0.04	0.05
非霍奇金淋巴瘤	Non-Hodgkin lymphoma	4 984	1.29	0.08	0.17	0.11	0.18	0.14	0.21	0.32	0.37	0.50
免疫增生性疾病	Immunoproliferative diseases	34	0.01	0.00	0.00	0.01	0.00	0.00	0.00	0.00	0.00	0.01
多发性骨髓瘤	Multiple myeloma	1 759	0.45	0.04	0.06	0.03	0.04	0.07	0.04	0.03	0.08	0.09
淋巴样白血病	Lymphoid leukemia	1 678	0.43	0.83	0.44	0.31	0.36	0.47	0.30	0.41	0.31	0.28
髓样白血病	Myeloid leukemia	2 179	0.56	0.37	0.25	0.24	0.30	0.35	0.24	0.37	0.44	0.40
白血病,未特指	Leukemia unspecified	3 966	1.03	1.00	0.75	0.61	0.72	0.76	0.64	0.74	0.73	0.65
其他或未指明部位	Other and unspecified	6 601	1.71	1.08	0.30	0.24	0.27	0.30	0.29	0.36	0.54	0.54
所有部位合计	All sites	386 703	100.00	16.71	4.09	3.34	3.58	4.40	4.69	9.27	16.05	24.60
所有部位除外 C44	All sites except C44	384 909	99.54	16.58	4.07	3.33	3.56	4.35	4.67	9.20	15.97	24.50

Appendix Table 1-16 Cancer mortality in rural registration areas of China, both sexes in 2017

Age group										粗率 Crude rate/ 100 000^{-1}	中标率 ASR China/ 100 000^{-1}	世标率 ASR world/ 100 000^{-1}	累积率 Cum. rate/%		ICD10
40~44	45~49	50~54	55~59	60~64	65~69	70~74	75~79	80~84	85+				0~64	0~74	
0.01	0.04	0.03	0.07	0.19	0.30	0.44	0.65	0.82	1.50	0.09	0.05	0.05	0.00	0.01	C00
0.20	0.38	0.57	0.61	1.05	1.33	1.60	2.21	2.40	2.14	0.42	0.27	0.26	0.02	0.03	C01-02
0.11	0.21	0.59	0.58	1.37	1.69	2.56	3.37	4.32	4.71	0.53	0.32	0.32	0.02	0.04	C03-06
0.03	0.09	0.18	0.19	0.42	0.56	0.61	0.77	0.79	1.16	0.15	0.10	0.10	0.01	0.01	C07-08
0.01	0.04	0.07	0.10	0.17	0.24	0.16	0.30	0.41	0.19	0.06	0.04	0.04	0.00	0.00	C09
0.04	0.07	0.21	0.28	0.50	0.54	0.89	0.87	0.85	1.12	0.17	0.10	0.10	0.01	0.01	C10
1.40	2.03	3.40	3.00	4.63	5.46	6.23	6.19	6.21	6.46	1.83	1.24	1.20	0.08	0.14	C11
0.06	0.11	0.40	0.49	0.73	0.73	0.70	0.99	1.13	0.78	0.22	0.14	0.14	0.01	0.02	C12-13
0.00	0.12	0.25	0.19	0.51	0.70	0.91	1.42	1.36	1.94	0.20	0.12	0.12	0.01	0.01	C14
0.92	3.75	11.14	17.60	43.27	71.94	104.19	137.44	173.10	171.49	18.28	10.63	10.66	0.39	1.27	C15
3.87	8.19	17.55	23.25	52.21	83.26	121.69	169.34	207.87	203.28	23.07	13.75	13.63	0.55	1.57	C16
0.16	0.33	0.58	0.59	1.29	2.19	2.54	3.71	3.75	4.37	0.56	0.34	0.34	0.02	0.04	C17
1.17	2.13	3.81	4.40	9.16	13.73	20.16	29.14	44.04	45.29	4.39	2.64	2.60	0.11	0.28	C18
1.63	3.18	6.10	6.41	13.74	21.76	32.85	49.08	67.24	69.31	6.83	4.08	4.02	0.17	0.44	C19-20
0.09	0.10	0.27	0.20	0.61	0.84	1.07	1.62	2.11	2.62	0.25	0.15	0.15	0.01	0.02	C21
13.61	24.01	40.59	41.39	67.41	84.48	94.59	116.85	135.90	142.42	26.06	16.79	16.55	1.00	1.90	C22
0.41	0.95	2.02	2.93	6.21	8.46	12.91	18.90	24.59	25.19	2.60	1.53	1.52	0.06	0.17	C23-24
1.25	2.30	5.02	6.09	12.87	19.22	27.71	36.60	43.35	41.11	5.35	3.22	3.20	0.14	0.38	C25
0.11	0.15	0.36	0.27	0.55	0.65	0.71	0.87	1.17	1.36	0.21	0.14	0.14	0.01	0.02	C30-31
0.14	0.39	1.00	1.31	2.72	3.51	4.72	6.49	7.41	6.41	0.98	0.59	0.59	0.03	0.07	C32
7.82	17.89	42.04	56.22	118.49	180.88	247.54	328.39	384.75	369.24	47.74	28.59	28.54	1.25	3.39	C33-34
0.19	0.39	0.46	0.59	1.14	1.23	1.84	1.83	1.95	2.14	0.42	0.28	0.28	0.02	0.03	C37-38
0.50	0.73	1.39	1.56	3.24	4.81	6.81	7.85	8.73	9.08	1.42	0.95	0.94	0.05	0.10	C40-41
0.14	0.24	0.33	0.50	0.79	0.99	1.41	1.95	2.62	2.67	0.36	0.23	0.23	0.01	0.02	C43
0.19	0.31	0.52	0.39	1.00	1.71	2.95	4.79	10.18	21.36	0.80	0.45	0.46	0.01	0.04	C44
0.02	0.04	0.11	0.14	0.26	0.17	0.32	0.37	0.35	0.29	0.07	0.05	0.05	0.00	0.01	C45
0.04	0.05	0.21	0.19	0.38	0.63	1.02	1.38	1.29	1.26	0.19	0.13	0.13	0.01	0.01	C46
0.16	0.21	0.40	0.29	0.59	0.88	1.10	1.30	1.61	1.89	0.30	0.21	0.22	0.01	0.02	C47;C49
6.88	11.67	17.97	15.55	20.59	20.54	18.60	21.50	21.75	27.86	8.30	5.56	5.37	0.40	0.59	C50
0.07	0.09	0.16	0.26	0.21	0.58	0.61	0.90	1.26	1.91	0.17	0.10	0.10	0.00	0.01	C51
0.02	0.10	0.18	0.15	0.21	0.27	0.29	0.51	0.75	0.24	0.09	0.06	0.06	0.00	0.01	C52
3.87	7.53	12.31	9.38	13.22	16.40	17.96	20.01	22.67	19.82	5.95	3.90	3.76	0.25	0.43	C53
0.68	1.35	2.52	2.64	4.51	4.93	5.50	5.16	5.45	4.70	1.49	0.94	0.93	0.06	0.11	C54
0.44	0.84	1.69	1.40	2.08	2.58	3.41	3.91	4.82	4.78	0.92	0.57	0.56	0.03	0.06	C55
1.50	3.17	5.84	5.85	8.09	8.97	9.72	10.55	8.95	5.57	2.95	1.92	1.89	0.13	0.22	C56
0.08	0.12	0.23	0.30	0.35	0.54	0.40	0.78	0.75	0.56	0.15	0.10	0.09	0.01	0.01	C57
0.01	0.02	0.00	0.00	0.00	0.00	0.00	0.04	0.00	0.00	0.01	0.01	0.01	0.00	0.00	C58
0.07	0.19	0.26	0.18	0.43	0.78	1.43	1.39	3.29	4.85	0.26	0.17	0.17	0.01	0.02	C60
0.09	0.16	0.49	1.13	3.42	8.84	18.49	36.28	63.77	104.02	3.55	2.04	2.06	0.03	0.16	C61
0.07	0.04	0.11	0.12	0.09	0.27	0.26	0.76	0.84	1.37	0.12	0.10	0.09	0.00	0.01	C62
0.01	0.03	0.01	0.01	0.05	0.18	0.12	0.17	0.21	0.25	0.03	0.02	0.02	0.00	0.00	C63
0.23	0.62	0.97	1.53	2.36	3.64	4.17	5.98	7.16	8.40	1.02	0.64	0.64	0.03	0.07	C64
0.04	0.08	0.10	0.16	0.42	0.52	0.67	0.99	1.29	1.55	0.15	0.09	0.09	0.00	0.01	C65
0.02	0.03	0.07	0.21	0.26	0.52	0.87	1.38	1.83	1.65	0.16	0.10	0.10	0.00	0.01	C66
0.21	0.38	0.89	1.08	2.98	5.40	9.48	18.70	29.54	41.99	2.12	1.15	1.15	0.03	0.10	C67
0.00	0.01	0.05	0.02	0.04	0.04	0.15	0.14	0.38	0.58	0.03	0.02	0.02	0.00	0.00	C68
0.01	0.03	0.04	0.06	0.08	0.08	0.22	0.47	0.32	0.73	0.06	0.04	0.05	0.00	0.00	C69
2.31	3.47	5.36	5.45	9.43	11.64	13.81	17.12	19.23	16.79	4.02	2.85	2.83	0.17	0.30	C70-72,D32-33,D42-43
0.19	0.38	0.62	0.59	1.03	1.47	2.13	2.70	2.74	3.74	0.48	0.31	0.31	0.02	0.03	C73
0.02	0.05	0.16	0.17	0.26	0.36	0.46	0.87	0.85	0.39	0.13	0.09	0.09	0.00	0.01	C74
0.06	0.03	0.07	0.17	0.16	0.23	0.28	0.22	0.50	0.49	0.08	0.06	0.06	0.00	0.01	C75
0.08	0.08	0.11	0.10	0.38	0.28	0.51	0.89	0.69	0.58	0.13	0.09	0.08	0.00	0.01	C81
0.72	1.28	2.27	2.83	5.23	8.10	10.53	12.96	14.09	12.96	2.23	1.45	1.43	0.07	0.16	C82-C86;C96
0.01	0.01	0.01	0.00	0.04	0.05	0.03	0.10	0.22	0.19	0.02	0.01	0.01	0.00	0.00	C88
0.12	0.42	0.94	1.02	2.30	3.49	3.85	3.97	3.59	4.13	0.79	0.50	0.51	0.03	0.06	C90
0.36	0.47	0.79	0.86	1.52	1.90	2.50	2.90	3.15	2.82	0.75	0.59	0.61	0.03	0.06	C91
0.53	0.88	1.13	1.21	2.04	2.80	3.95	3.81	4.44	1.89	0.98	0.73	0.72	0.04	0.08	C92-C94,D45-47
0.97	1.17	1.89	1.83	3.68	4.58	6.00	7.73	9.33	8.49	1.78	1.35	1.35	0.08	0.13	C95
0.93	1.73	3.11	3.74	6.44	9.57	12.14	16.53	22.38	24.61	2.96	1.90	1.90	0.09	0.20	O&U
47.88	92.23	178.86	209.27	410.69	600.17	810.85	1 084.17	1 329.74	1 356.35	173.34	106.86	106.05	5.06	12.11	C00-96, D32-33, D42-43,D45-47
47.69	91.93	178.35	208.88	409.68	598.46	807.90	1 079.39	1 319.56	1 334.99	172.53	106.41	105.59	5.04	12.08	C00-96, D32-33, D42-43,D45-47 exc. C44

附表 1-17　2017 年全国农村肿瘤登记地区男性癌症死亡主要指标

部位 Site		死亡数 No. deaths	构成 Freq. /%	年龄组								
				0～	1～4	5～9	10～14	15～19	20～24	25～29	30～34	35～39
唇	Lip	146	0. 06	0. 00	0. 00	0. 00	0. 00	0. 01	0. 00	0. 00	0. 01	0. 02
舌	Tongue	662	0. 27	0. 00	0. 00	0. 00	0. 00	0. 00	0. 00	0. 03	0. 14	0. 19
口	Mouth	753	0. 30	0. 00	0. 00	0. 00	0. 00	0. 00	0. 00	0. 03	0. 09	0. 06
唾液腺	Salivary glands	231	0. 09	0. 00	0. 00	0. 00	0. 00	0. 00	0. 04	0. 01	0. 01	0. 07
扁桃腺	Tonsil	110	0. 04	0. 00	0. 00	0. 00	0. 00	0. 00	0. 01	0. 00	0. 00	0. 05
其他口咽	Other oropharynx	305	0. 12	0. 00	0. 00	0. 00	0. 00	0. 00	0. 01	0. 02	0. 00	0. 02
鼻咽	Nasopharynx	2 936	1. 18	0. 16	0. 00	0. 00	0. 05	0. 06	0. 13	0. 26	0. 67	0. 89
下咽	Hypopharynx	443	0. 18	0. 00	0. 00	0. 01	0. 00	0. 00	0. 00	0. 00	0. 00	0. 06
咽,部位不明	Pharynx unspecified	338	0. 14	0. 00	0. 00	0. 00	0. 00	0. 00	0. 00	0. 02	0. 00	0. 01
食管	Esophagus	29 215	11. 72	0. 78	0. 04	0. 00	0. 00	0. 01	0. 04	0. 09	0. 18	0. 41
胃	Stomach	35 951	14. 42	1. 95	0. 04	0. 03	0. 02	0. 15	0. 31	0. 55	1. 49	2. 01
小肠	Small intestine	744	0. 30	0. 00	0. 00	0. 00	0. 02	0. 00	0. 00	0. 03	0. 01	0. 12
结肠	Colon	5 495	2. 20	0. 63	0. 00	0. 00	0. 02	0. 04	0. 15	0. 27	0. 47	0. 73
直肠	Rectum	9 123	3. 66	1. 02	0. 00	0. 01	0. 00	0. 06	0. 08	0. 23	0. 55	0. 95
肛门	Anus	331	0. 13	0. 00	0. 00	0. 00	0. 00	0. 00	0. 00	0. 00	0. 03	0. 11
肝脏	Liver	42 762	17. 16	3. 83	0. 32	0. 11	0. 18	0. 28	0. 75	2. 43	5. 83	11. 19
胆囊及其他	Gallbladder etc.	2 671	1. 07	0. 00	0. 00	0. 00	0. 00	0. 01	0. 03	0. 05	0. 13	0. 19
胰腺	Pancreas	6 930	2. 78	0. 39	0. 02	0. 00	0. 00	0. 01	0. 03	0. 11	0. 27	0. 64
鼻、鼻窦及其他	Nose, sinuses etc.	285	0. 11	0. 08	0. 05	0. 00	0. 00	0. 04	0. 00	0. 02	0. 10	0. 10
喉	Larynx	1 791	0. 72	0. 00	0. 04	0. 01	0. 00	0. 04	0. 01	0. 02	0. 08	0. 07
气管、支气管、肺	Trachea, bronchus & lung	74 418	29. 85	3. 60	0. 02	0. 03	0. 09	0. 10	0. 40	0. 84	2. 21	3. 89
其他胸腔器官	Other thoracic organs	585	0. 23	0. 23	0. 02	0. 06	0. 02	0. 06	0. 11	0. 11	0. 13	0. 11
骨	Bone	1 847	0. 74	0. 08	0. 00	0. 14	0. 29	0. 61	0. 29	0. 31	0. 33	0. 28
皮肤黑色素瘤	Melanoma of skin	444	0. 18	0. 00	0. 07	0. 04	0. 03	0. 04	0. 03	0. 10	0. 08	0. 20
皮肤其他	Other skin	995	0. 40	0. 16	0. 04	0. 01	0. 02	0. 06	0. 05	0. 08	0. 14	0. 12
间皮瘤	Mesothelioma	91	0. 04	0. 00	0. 00	0. 00	0. 00	0. 00	0. 00	0. 00	0. 04	0. 01
卡波氏肉瘤	Kaposi sarcoma	272	0. 11	0. 00	0. 04	0. 01	0. 03	0. 07	0. 03	0. 03	0. 01	0. 05
结缔组织、软组织	Connective & soft tissue	393	0. 16	0. 39	0. 13	0. 11	0. 06	0. 13	0. 10	0. 10	0. 03	0. 10
乳腺	Breast	217	0. 09	0. 00	0. 00	0. 00	0. 00	0. 00	0. 00	0. 03	0. 05	0. 01
外阴	Vulva	—	—	—	—	—	—	—	—	—	—	—
阴道	Vagina	—	—	—	—	—	—	—	—	—	—	—
子宫颈	Cervix uteri	—	—	—	—	—	—	—	—	—	—	—
子宫体	Corpus uteri	—	—	—	—	—	—	—	—	—	—	—
子宫,部位不明	Uterus unspecified	—	—	—	—	—	—	—	—	—	—	—
卵巢	Ovary	—	—	—	—	—	—	—	—	—	—	—
其他女性生殖器	Other female genital organs	—	—	—	—	—	—	—	—	—	—	—
胎盘	Placenta	—	—	—	—	—	—	—	—	—	—	—
阴茎	Penis	301	0. 12	0. 00	0. 00	0. 00	0. 00	0. 03	0. 00	0. 02	0. 01	0. 04
前列腺	Prostate	4 046	1. 62	0. 00	0. 00	0. 00	0. 00	0. 03	0. 01	0. 00	0. 01	0. 01
睾丸	Testis	135	0. 05	0. 00	0. 05	0. 06	0. 00	0. 03	0. 09	0. 06	0. 14	0. 08
其他男性生殖器	Other male genital organs	34	0. 01	0. 00	0. 00	0. 00	0. 00	0. 01	0. 00	0. 01	0. 01	0. 00
肾	Kidney	1 452	0. 58	0. 16	0. 21	0. 11	0. 00	0. 06	0. 01	0. 09	0. 18	0. 22
肾盂	Renal pelvis	201	0. 08	0. 00	0. 02	0. 00	0. 00	0. 00	0. 00	0. 00	0. 01	0. 01
输尿管	Ureter	208	0. 08	0. 39	0. 00	0. 00	0. 00	0. 00	0. 00	0. 01	0. 01	0. 00
膀胱	Bladder	3 737	1. 50	0. 08	0. 00	0. 00	0. 00	0. 03	0. 01	0. 05	0. 04	0. 06
其他泌尿器官	Other urinary organs	47	0. 02	0. 00	0. 00	0. 01	0. 00	0. 00	0. 00	0. 01	0. 00	0. 01
眼	Eye	75	0. 03	0. 08	0. 14	0. 04	0. 00	0. 01	0. 00	0. 02	0. 00	0. 00
脑、神经系统	Brain, nervous system	5 069	2. 03	0. 94	1. 11	1. 16	0. 97	0. 77	0. 68	1. 23	1. 49	1. 76
甲状腺	Thyroid	389	0. 16	0. 08	0. 00	0. 00	0. 00	0. 00	0. 01	0. 09	0. 04	0. 14
肾上腺	Adrenal gland	167	0. 07	0. 16	0. 16	0. 06	0. 00	0. 03	0. 00	0. 02	0. 03	0. 06
其他内分泌腺	Other endocrine	105	0. 04	0. 00	0. 00	0. 01	0. 02	0. 04	0. 04	0. 02	0. 04	0. 08
霍奇金淋巴瘤	Hodgkin lymphoma	188	0. 08	0. 00	0. 00	0. 01	0. 03	0. 04	0. 06	0. 02	0. 06	0. 07
非霍奇金淋巴瘤	Non-Hodgkin lymphoma	3 078	1. 23	0. 08	0. 25	0. 13	0. 28	0. 20	0. 28	0. 38	0. 45	0. 54
免疫增生性疾病	Immunoproliferative diseases	26	0. 01	0. 00	0. 00	0. 00	0. 00	0. 00	0. 00	0. 00	0. 00	0. 00
多发性骨髓瘤	Multiple myeloma	1 062	0. 43	0. 08	0. 07	0. 04	0. 06	0. 07	0. 04	0. 05	0. 10	0. 11
淋巴样白血病	Lymphoid leukemia	985	0. 40	1. 02	0. 54	0. 36	0. 44	0. 60	0. 34	0. 41	0. 44	0. 34
髓样白血病	Myeloid leukemia	1 273	0. 51	0. 39	0. 36	0. 23	0. 35	0. 39	0. 21	0. 47	0. 59	0. 43
白血病,未特指	Leukemia unspecified	2 292	0. 92	0. 86	0. 86	0. 57	0. 78	0. 96	0. 65	1. 04	0. 87	0. 78
其他或未指明部位	Other and unspecified	3 912	1. 57	0. 86	0. 38	0. 29	0. 38	0. 36	0. 29	0. 38	0. 72	0. 61
所有部位合计	All sites	249 266	100. 00	18. 45	4. 95	3. 70	4. 12	5. 49	5. 31	10. 19	18. 33	28. 02
所有部位除外 C44	All sites except C44	248 271	99. 60	18. 29	4. 91	3. 69	4. 11	5. 44	5. 26	10. 11	18. 18	27. 90

Appendix Table 1-17 Cancer mortality in rural registration areas of China, male in 2017

Age group										粗率 Crude rate/ 100 000⁻¹	中标率 ASR China/ 100 000⁻¹	世标率 ASR world/ 100 000⁻¹	累积率 Cum. rate/%		ICD10
40~44	45~49	50~54	55~59	60~64	65~69	70~74	75~79	80~84	85+				0~64	0~74	
0.02	0.07	0.06	0.15	0.34	0.45	0.61	0.93	1.05	1.99	0.13	0.08	0.08	0.00	0.01	C00
0.32	0.56	0.90	1.03	1.49	1.96	2.04	2.95	3.01	2.99	0.58	0.39	0.38	0.02	0.04	C01-02
0.08	0.29	0.81	0.77	1.90	2.27	3.44	4.64	5.24	5.47	0.66	0.42	0.42	0.02	0.05	C03-06
0.03	0.13	0.21	0.31	0.64	0.74	0.88	1.22	0.98	1.74	0.20	0.13	0.13	0.01	0.02	C07-08
0.00	0.06	0.14	0.16	0.31	0.47	0.23	0.55	0.70	0.25	0.10	0.06	0.06	0.00	0.01	C09
0.08	0.13	0.33	0.52	0.90	0.98	1.46	1.31	1.26	1.37	0.27	0.17	0.17	0.01	0.02	C10
1.99	3.18	5.02	4.39	6.65	7.84	9.13	8.60	9.30	9.08	2.57	1.79	1.74	0.12	0.20	C11
0.09	0.22	0.72	0.93	1.39	1.39	1.17	1.81	2.24	1.12	0.39	0.25	0.25	0.02	0.03	C12-13
0.00	0.22	0.45	0.32	0.78	1.06	1.37	2.02	2.10	3.11	0.30	0.19	0.19	0.01	0.02	C14
1.45	6.39	18.84	29.14	67.73	109.67	148.32	194.70	233.35	244.25	25.60	15.84	15.95	0.62	1.91	C15
4.64	10.56	24.44	35.01	78.34	124.87	175.71	247.42	298.59	277.22	31.50	19.75	19.63	0.79	2.29	C16
0.17	0.38	0.69	0.62	1.52	2.82	3.18	4.59	4.83	6.22	0.65	0.42	0.41	0.02	0.05	C17
1.37	2.30	4.30	5.17	10.65	16.01	23.60	32.96	52.45	56.74	4.82	3.06	3.02	0.13	0.33	C18
1.75	3.63	7.42	7.62	17.23	27.51	40.92	61.49	84.05	93.20	7.99	5.03	4.98	0.20	0.54	C19-20
0.15	0.14	0.32	0.25	0.86	0.96	1.17	1.77	2.94	2.61	0.29	0.19	0.18	0.01	0.02	C21
23.07	39.80	65.77	65.25	102.29	121.56	128.92	158.25	176.92	190.50	37.47	25.28	24.86	1.59	2.84	C22
0.32	0.84	1.88	3.12	6.56	8.11	12.10	18.25	20.56	23.27	2.34	1.46	1.46	0.07	0.17	C23-24
1.59	2.94	6.22	7.52	15.79	22.71	32.35	41.72	50.63	48.78	6.07	3.86	3.84	0.18	0.45	C25
0.11	0.19	0.49	0.28	0.58	0.92	1.08	0.76	1.54	1.37	0.25	0.17	0.17	0.01	0.02	C30-31
0.23	0.64	1.70	2.22	4.78	5.96	7.58	10.91	12.31	11.32	1.57	0.99	1.00	0.05	0.12	C32
9.62	23.41	58.86	82.25	172.41	264.17	357.13	475.33	552.43	539.89	65.21	40.96	40.97	1.77	4.88	C33-34
0.26	0.47	0.62	0.66	1.35	1.59	2.60	2.06	3.01	2.24	0.51	0.36	0.35	0.02	0.04	C37-38
0.64	0.93	1.50	1.88	3.71	5.68	8.23	9.78	10.56	10.45	1.62	1.13	1.11	0.05	0.12	C40-41
0.14	0.28	0.39	0.59	0.84	1.20	1.46	2.19	3.50	2.24	0.39	0.27	0.26	0.01	0.03	C43
0.27	0.37	0.59	0.49	1.39	2.21	3.53	5.35	12.52	22.52	0.87	0.54	0.55	0.02	0.05	C44
0.01	0.04	0.11	0.10	0.32	0.18	0.47	0.59	0.28	0.25	0.08	0.05	0.05	0.00	0.01	C45
0.04	0.10	0.26	0.22	0.43	0.78	1.43	1.90	1.96	1.62	0.24	0.16	0.16	0.01	0.02	C46
0.22	0.19	0.51	0.32	0.66	1.20	1.40	1.56	1.54	2.49	0.34	0.25	0.26	0.01	0.03	C47;C49
0.08	0.18	0.27	0.22	0.48	0.57	0.82	1.26	1.19	1.49	0.19	0.13	0.12	0.01	0.01	C50
—	—	—	—	—	—	—	—	—	—	—	—	—	—	—	C51
—	—	—	—	—	—	—	—	—	—	—	—	—	—	—	C52
—	—	—	—	—	—	—	—	—	—	—	—	—	—	—	C53
—	—	—	—	—	—	—	—	—	—	—	—	—	—	—	C54
—	—	—	—	—	—	—	—	—	—	—	—	—	—	—	C55
—	—	—	—	—	—	—	—	—	—	—	—	—	—	—	C56
—	—	—	—	—	—	—	—	—	—	—	—	—	—	—	C57
—	—	—	—	—	—	—	—	—	—	—	—	—	—	—	C58
0.07	0.19	0.26	0.18	0.43	0.78	1.43	1.39	3.29	4.85	0.26	0.17	0.17	0.01	0.02	C60
0.09	0.16	0.49	1.13	3.42	8.84	18.49	36.28	63.77	104.02	3.55	2.04	2.06	0.03	0.16	C61
0.07	0.04	0.11	0.12	0.09	0.27	0.26	0.76	0.84	1.37	0.12	0.10	0.09	0.00	0.01	C62
0.01	0.03	0.01	0.01	0.05	0.18	0.12	0.17	0.21	0.25	0.03	0.02	0.02	0.00	0.00	C63
0.27	0.83	1.29	2.25	3.11	4.47	5.48	8.13	8.53	11.07	1.27	0.83	0.84	0.04	0.09	C64
0.07	0.09	0.14	0.19	0.52	0.61	0.79	1.22	1.47	2.12	0.18	0.11	0.11	0.01	0.01	C65
0.02	0.03	0.12	0.25	0.28	0.67	1.08	1.52	1.96	2.12	0.18	0.11	0.12	0.00	0.01	C66
0.27	0.57	1.39	1.77	4.90	8.54	15.75	30.93	51.05	82.00	3.27	1.93	1.95	0.05	0.17	C67
0.00	0.03	0.02	0.03	0.08	0.04	0.20	0.17	0.63	1.24	0.04	0.03	0.03	0.00	0.00	C68
0.00	0.05	0.05	0.06	0.12	0.06	0.29	0.63	0.35	0.75	0.07	0.05	0.06	0.00	0.00	C69
2.78	4.08	6.09	6.11	11.14	13.34	15.60	18.16	20.00	17.92	4.44	3.27	3.24	0.20	0.34	C70-72,D32-33,D42-43
0.12	0.26	0.37	0.46	0.69	1.23	1.55	1.98	2.59	2.86	0.34	0.23	0.22	0.01	0.02	C73
0.01	0.04	0.18	0.25	0.34	0.37	0.55	0.97	1.26	0.50	0.15	0.10	0.11	0.01	0.01	C74
0.09	0.03	0.11	0.16	0.17	0.22	0.44	0.29	0.56	0.25	0.09	0.07	0.07	0.00	0.01	C75
0.12	0.12	0.14	0.16	0.55	0.37	0.70	1.14	0.77	0.25	0.16	0.12	0.11	0.01	0.01	C81
0.94	1.58	2.83	3.41	6.76	10.35	13.24	16.39	17.20	16.55	2.70	1.82	1.80	0.09	0.21	C82-C86;C96
0.01	0.01	0.00	0.00	0.06	0.08	0.06	0.17	0.49	0.37	0.02	0.01	0.01	0.00	0.00	C88
0.15	0.42	1.14	1.19	2.87	4.00	5.05	4.59	5.24	5.85	0.93	0.61	0.62	0.03	0.08	C90
0.39	0.52	0.87	0.84	1.81	2.25	2.80	3.71	4.20	3.86	0.86	0.70	0.72	0.04	0.07	C91
0.61	0.95	1.18	1.34	2.30	3.29	4.78	4.89	6.08	2.74	1.12	0.86	0.83	0.05	0.09	C92-C94,D45-47
0.97	1.28	2.08	1.97	4.49	5.15	7.09	9.78	11.19	11.45	2.01	1.56	1.56	0.09	0.15	C95
1.06	2.09	3.84	4.36	7.68	11.97	15.60	19.76	26.85	30.36	3.43	2.31	2.30	0.11	0.25	O&U
56.86	112.00	226.52	277.73	554.17	812.92	1 083.66	1 459.90	1 779.53	1 868.51	218.42	140.43	139.81	6.55	16.03	C00-96, D32-33, D42-43,D45-47
56.59	111.62	225.93	277.24	552.78	810.71	1 080.13	1 454.55	1 767.01	1 845.99	217.55	139.89	139.26	6.53	15.99	C00-96, D32-33, D42-43,D45-47 exc. C44

附表 1-18　2017 年全国农村肿瘤登记地区女性癌症死亡主要指标

	部位 Site	死亡数 No. deaths	构成 Freq. /%	年龄组								
				0~	1~4	5~9	10~14	15~19	20~24	25~29	30~34	35~39
唇	Lip	56	0.04	0.00	0.00	0.00	0.00	0.00	0.00	0.00	0.00	0.00
舌	Tongue	273	0.20	0.00	0.02	0.02	0.00	0.03	0.01	0.00	0.03	0.05
口	Mouth	433	0.32	0.00	0.00	0.00	0.02	0.02	0.00	0.06	0.04	0.07
唾液腺	Salivary glands	107	0.08	0.00	0.00	0.00	0.02	0.00	0.01	0.02	0.01	0.04
扁桃腺	Tonsil	19	0.01	0.00	0.00	0.00	0.00	0.00	0.00	0.00	0.01	0.00
其他口咽	Other oropharynx	66	0.05	0.00	0.00	0.00	0.00	0.00	0.00	0.00	0.01	0.00
鼻咽	Nasopharynx	1 142	0.83	0.09	0.02	0.00	0.02	0.07	0.05	0.13	0.31	0.59
下咽	Hypopharynx	42	0.03	0.00	0.00	0.00	0.00	0.00	0.00	0.00	0.00	0.00
咽,部位不明	Pharynx unspecified	109	0.08	0.00	0.00	0.00	0.02	0.02	0.00	0.00	0.00	0.02
食管	Esophagus	11 555	8.41	0.09	0.02	0.00	0.00	0.02	0.00	0.01	0.05	0.12
胃	Stomach	15 508	11.28	0.98	0.02	0.00	0.02	0.05	0.30	0.79	1.36	1.76
小肠	Small intestine	503	0.37	0.09	0.00	0.00	0.00	0.00	0.03	0.00	0.07	0.09
结肠	Colon	4 304	3.13	0.27	0.00	0.00	0.00	0.07	0.14	0.26	0.41	0.61
直肠	Rectum	6 121	4.45	0.62	0.00	0.00	0.02	0.02	0.03	0.36	0.59	0.71
肛门	Anus	228	0.17	0.00	0.00	0.00	0.00	0.00	0.00	0.02	0.00	0.02
肝脏	Liver	15 380	11.19	1.52	0.15	0.08	0.14	0.23	0.26	0.78	1.27	1.96
胆囊及其他	Gallbladder etc.	3 121	2.27	0.36	0.02	0.00	0.00	0.00	0.00	0.04	0.08	0.12
胰腺	Pancreas	5 009	3.64	0.18	0.00	0.00	0.02	0.00	0.00	0.06	0.19	0.30
鼻、鼻窦及其他	Nose, sinuses etc.	191	0.14	0.00	0.02	0.02	0.00	0.00	0.01	0.02	0.04	0.06
喉	Larynx	390	0.28	0.00	0.02	0.00	0.00	0.02	0.00	0.01	0.03	0.07
气管、支气管、肺	Trachea, bronchus & lung	32 086	23.35	2.50	0.04	0.02	0.04	0.03	0.21	0.67	1.23	2.52
其他胸腔器官	Other thoracic organs	350	0.25	0.18	0.02	0.07	0.00	0.02	0.00	0.05	0.05	0.12
骨	Bone	1 314	0.96	0.09	0.02	0.10	0.29	0.28	0.29	0.23	0.11	0.22
皮肤黑色素瘤	Melanoma of skin	348	0.25	0.00	0.04	0.03	0.00	0.02	0.01	0.04	0.08	0.10
皮肤其他	Other skin	799	0.58	0.09	0.00	0.02	0.04	0.03	0.00	0.06	0.01	0.09
间皮瘤	Mesothelioma	74	0.05	0.00	0.00	0.00	0.00	0.00	0.00	0.01	0.04	0.02
卡波氏肉瘤	Kaposi sarcoma	158	0.11	0.09	0.02	0.00	0.04	0.02	0.01	0.05	0.04	0.04
结缔组织、软组织	Connective & soft tissue	272	0.20	0.18	0.04	0.07	0.05	0.07	0.07	0.06	0.08	0.05
乳腺	Breast	9 049	6.58	0.71	0.00	0.00	0.00	0.00	0.16	0.86	2.23	3.78
外阴	Vulva	185	0.13	0.00	0.00	0.00	0.00	0.00	0.04	0.00	0.03	0.05
阴道	Vagina	103	0.07	0.00	0.00	0.00	0.00	0.00	0.01	0.00	0.00	0.00
子宫颈	Cervix uteri	6 481	4.72	1.07	0.00	0.00	0.00	0.00	0.05	0.54	1.20	2.53
子宫体	Corpus uteri	1 622	1.18	0.00	0.00	0.00	0.00	0.02	0.04	0.08	0.11	0.35
子宫,部位不明	Uterus unspecified	1 006	0.73	0.18	0.00	0.00	0.00	0.00	0.01	0.01	0.17	0.20
卵巢	Ovary	3 220	2.34	0.18	0.02	0.00	0.11	0.03	0.12	0.30	0.53	0.54
其他女性生殖器	Other female genital organs	168	0.12	0.00	0.00	0.00	0.00	0.00	0.01	0.01	0.03	0.05
胎盘	Placenta	10	0.01	0.00	0.00	0.00	0.00	0.00	0.01	0.04	0.00	0.02
阴茎	Penis	—	—	—	—	—	—	—	—	—	—	—
前列腺	Prostate	—	—	—	—	—	—	—	—	—	—	—
睾丸	Testis	—	—	—	—	—	—	—	—	—	—	—
其他男性生殖器	Other male genital organs	—	—	—	—	—	—	—	—	—	—	—
肾	Kidney	825	0.60	0.00	0.15	0.05	0.00	0.02	0.05	0.06	0.12	0.11
肾盂	Renal pelvis	139	0.10	0.00	0.00	0.00	0.00	0.00	0.00	0.00	0.01	0.02
输尿管	Ureter	158	0.11	0.18	0.00	0.00	0.00	0.00	0.00	0.00	0.03	0.01
膀胱	Bladder	985	0.72	0.27	0.00	0.00	0.00	0.00	0.00	0.07	0.03	0.04
其他泌尿器官	Other urinary organs	20	0.01	0.00	0.00	0.00	0.00	0.00	0.00	0.00	0.00	0.00
眼	Eye	55	0.04	0.00	0.06	0.08	0.02	0.00	0.00	0.00	0.01	0.01
脑、神经系统	Brain, nervous system	3 894	2.83	0.80	0.82	0.88	0.70	0.54	0.39	0.68	1.03	1.21
甲状腺	Thyroid	691	0.50	0.18	0.00	0.00	0.02	0.03	0.05	0.11	0.16	0.16
肾上腺	Adrenal gland	117	0.09	0.18	0.10	0.03	0.02	0.00	0.00	0.02	0.03	0.01
其他内分泌腺	Other endocrine	84	0.06	0.09	0.04	0.02	0.00	0.02	0.03	0.02	0.08	0.04
霍奇金淋巴瘤	Hodgkin lymphoma	94	0.07	0.00	0.00	0.00	0.00	0.00	0.00	0.02	0.01	0.02
非霍奇金淋巴瘤	Non-Hodgkin lymphoma	1 906	1.39	0.09	0.08	0.08	0.07	0.07	0.14	0.26	0.29	0.46
免疫增生性疾病	Immunoproliferative diseases	8	0.01	0.00	0.00	0.02	0.00	0.00	0.00	0.00	0.00	0.01
多发性骨髓瘤	Multiple myeloma	697	0.51	0.00	0.04	0.02	0.02	0.07	0.04	0.01	0.07	0.07
淋巴样白血病	Lymphoid leukemia	693	0.50	0.62	0.33	0.26	0.27	0.33	0.25	0.42	0.17	0.21
髓样白血病	Myeloid leukemia	906	0.66	0.36	0.13	0.24	0.23	0.29	0.26	0.26	0.29	0.36
白血病,未特指	Leukemia unspecified	1 674	1.22	1.16	0.63	0.65	0.64	0.54	0.63	0.42	0.59	0.51
其他或未指明部位	Other and unspecified	2 689	1.96	1.34	0.21	0.20	0.14	0.23	0.29	0.35	0.35	0.46
所有部位合计	All sites	137 437	100.00	14.72	3.09	2.93	2.95	3.16	4.05	8.31	13.69	21.05
所有部位除外 C44	All sites except C44	136 638	99.42	14.63	3.09	2.92	2.91	3.13	4.05	8.25	13.68	20.96

Appendix Table 1-18 Cancer mortality in rural registration areas of China, female in 2017

Age group										粗率 Crude rate/ 100 000^{-1}	中标率 ASR China/ 100 000^{-1}	世标率 ASR world/ 100 000^{-1}	累积率 Cum. rate/%		ICD10
40~44	45~49	50~54	55~59	60~64	65~69	70~74	75~79	80~84	85+				0~64	0~74	
0.00	0.01	0.00	0.00	0.05	0.14	0.26	0.39	0.63	1.19	0.05	0.02	0.03	0.00	0.00	C00
0.08	0.20	0.23	0.18	0.60	0.70	1.16	1.52	1.89	1.59	0.25	0.15	0.15	0.01	0.02	C01-02
0.14	0.14	0.37	0.39	0.82	1.11	1.68	2.19	3.56	4.22	0.40	0.23	0.23	0.01	0.02	C03-06
0.03	0.06	0.15	0.08	0.19	0.39	0.35	0.35	0.63	0.80	0.10	0.06	0.06	0.00	0.01	C07-08
0.01	0.02	0.00	0.05	0.03	0.00	0.09	0.08	0.17	0.16	0.02	0.01	0.01	0.00	0.00	C09
0.00	0.02	0.09	0.03	0.08	0.10	0.32	0.47	0.52	0.96	0.06	0.03	0.03	0.00	0.00	C10
0.78	0.85	1.72	1.58	2.56	3.05	3.36	3.95	3.67	4.78	1.05	0.69	0.67	0.04	0.08	C11
0.02	0.01	0.06	0.05	0.05	0.06	0.23	0.23	0.23	0.56	0.04	0.02	0.02	0.00	0.00	C12-13
0.00	0.02	0.05	0.05	0.22	0.33	0.46	0.86	0.75	1.19	0.10	0.06	0.06	0.00	0.01	C14
0.36	1.06	3.17	5.78	18.10	33.84	60.42	84.32	123.64	124.95	10.60	5.57	5.53	0.14	0.61	C15
3.07	5.77	10.42	11.20	25.32	41.25	68.12	96.91	133.40	155.99	14.23	7.96	7.83	0.30	0.85	C16
0.15	0.28	0.47	0.56	1.06	1.55	1.91	2.89	2.87	3.18	0.46	0.27	0.27	0.01	0.03	C17
0.95	1.96	3.31	3.62	7.62	11.43	16.75	25.60	37.14	37.96	3.95	2.25	2.21	0.10	0.24	C18
1.51	2.72	4.74	5.16	10.14	15.96	24.85	37.57	53.44	54.04	5.62	3.19	3.12	0.13	0.33	C19-20
0.03	0.06	0.21	0.15	0.36	0.72	0.98	1.49	1.44	2.63	0.21	0.12	0.12	0.00	0.01	C21
3.77	7.90	14.56	16.95	31.51	47.04	60.54	78.46	102.23	111.66	14.11	8.27	8.21	0.40	0.94	C22
0.50	1.06	2.17	2.73	5.85	8.81	13.71	19.51	27.90	26.42	2.86	1.59	1.58	0.06	0.18	C23-24
0.90	1.64	3.77	4.63	9.88	15.69	23.11	31.86	37.37	36.21	4.60	2.60	2.58	0.11	0.30	C25
0.11	0.12	0.23	0.26	0.52	0.37	0.35	0.98	0.86	1.35	0.18	0.11	0.11	0.01	0.01	C30-31
0.06	0.13	0.27	0.38	0.60	1.03	1.88	2.38	3.39	3.26	0.36	0.20	0.20	0.01	0.02	C32
5.94	12.26	24.65	29.56	62.98	96.77	138.87	192.09	247.11	260.09	29.44	16.62	16.53	0.70	1.88	C33-34
0.12	0.30	0.31	0.51	0.92	0.87	1.10	1.60	1.09	2.07	0.32	0.21	0.21	0.01	0.02	C37-38
0.35	0.53	1.28	1.22	2.76	3.94	5.41	6.06	7.23	8.20	1.21	0.77	0.77	0.04	0.09	C40-41
0.14	0.21	0.26	0.41	0.73	0.76	1.36	1.72	1.89	2.94	0.32	0.20	0.19	0.01	0.02	C43
0.10	0.24	0.44	0.30	0.60	1.22	2.37	4.26	8.27	20.61	0.73	0.36	0.37	0.01	0.03	C44
0.02	0.04	0.11	0.18	0.19	0.16	0.17	0.16	0.40	0.32	0.07	0.04	0.04	0.00	0.00	C45
0.05	0.01	0.15	0.17	0.33	0.47	0.61	0.90	0.75	1.03	0.14	0.09	0.09	0.00	0.01	C46
0.10	0.24	0.29	0.26	0.52	0.56	0.81	1.06	1.66	1.51	0.25	0.17	0.17	0.01	0.02	C47;C49
6.88	11.67	17.97	15.55	20.59	20.54	18.60	21.50	21.75	27.86	8.30	5.56	5.37	0.40	0.59	C50
0.07	0.09	0.16	0.26	0.21	0.58	0.61	0.90	1.26	1.91	0.17	0.10	0.10	0.00	0.01	C51
0.02	0.10	0.18	0.15	0.21	0.27	0.29	0.51	0.75	0.24	0.09	0.06	0.06	0.00	0.01	C52
3.87	7.53	12.31	9.38	13.22	16.40	17.96	20.01	22.67	19.82	5.95	3.90	3.76	0.25	0.43	C53
0.68	1.35	2.52	2.64	4.51	4.93	5.50	5.16	5.45	4.70	1.49	0.94	0.93	0.06	0.11	C54
0.44	0.84	1.69	1.40	2.08	2.58	3.41	3.91	4.82	4.78	0.92	0.57	0.56	0.03	0.06	C55
1.50	3.17	5.84	5.85	8.09	8.97	9.72	10.55	8.95	5.57	2.95	1.92	1.89	0.13	0.22	C56
0.08	0.12	0.23	0.30	0.35	0.54	0.40	0.78	0.75	0.56	0.15	0.10	0.09	0.01	0.01	C57
0.01	0.02	0.00	0.00	0.00	0.00	0.00	0.04	0.00	0.00	0.01	0.01	0.01	0.00	0.00	C58
—	—	—	—	—	—	—	—	—	—	—	—	—	—	—	C60
—	—	—	—	—	—	—	—	—	—	—	—	—	—	—	C61
—	—	—	—	—	—	—	—	—	—	—	—	—	—	—	C62
—	—	—	—	—	—	—	—	—	—	—	—	—	—	—	C63
0.19	0.40	0.63	0.80	1.58	2.80	2.86	3.99	6.03	6.69	0.76	0.45	0.45	0.02	0.05	C64
0.01	0.07	0.06	0.12	0.32	0.43	0.55	0.78	1.15	1.19	0.13	0.07	0.07	0.00	0.01	C65
0.02	0.04	0.01	0.17	0.24	0.37	0.67	1.25	1.72	1.35	0.14	0.08	0.08	0.00	0.01	C66
0.14	0.18	0.38	0.38	0.99	2.23	3.27	7.35	11.88	16.39	0.90	0.46	0.46	0.01	0.04	C67
0.00	0.00	0.07	0.02	0.00	0.04	0.09	0.12	0.17	0.16	0.02	0.01	0.01	0.00	0.00	C68
0.01	0.02	0.04	0.06	0.03	0.10	0.14	0.31	0.29	0.72	0.05	0.03	0.04	0.00	0.00	C69
1.82	2.85	4.60	4.78	7.67	9.92	12.03	16.14	18.60	16.08	3.57	2.42	2.40	0.14	0.25	C70-72,D32-33,D42-43
0.27	0.50	0.87	0.72	1.39	1.71	2.72	3.36	2.87	4.30	0.63	0.40	0.39	0.02	0.04	C73
0.03	0.07	0.14	0.09	0.19	0.35	0.38	0.78	0.52	0.32	0.11	0.07	0.08	0.00	0.01	C74
0.03	0.04	0.04	0.18	0.14	0.23	0.12	0.16	0.46	0.64	0.08	0.06	0.06	0.00	0.01	C75
0.05	0.05	0.07	0.05	0.21	0.19	0.32	0.66	0.63	0.80	0.09	0.05	0.05	0.00	0.00	C81
0.49	0.97	1.69	2.23	3.66	5.82	7.84	9.77	11.54	10.66	1.75	1.08	1.06	0.05	0.12	C82-C86;C96
0.00	0.01	0.01	0.00	0.02	0.02	0.00	0.04	0.00	0.08	0.01	0.01	0.01	0.00	0.00	C88
0.09	0.42	0.72	0.84	1.72	2.97	2.66	3.40	2.24	3.02	0.64	0.39	0.40	0.02	0.05	C90
0.32	0.41	0.71	0.87	1.21	1.55	2.20	2.15	2.30	2.15	0.64	0.49	0.50	0.03	0.05	C91
0.45	0.80	1.09	1.09	1.78	2.31	3.12	2.81	3.10	1.35	0.83	0.61	0.60	0.04	0.06	C92-C94,D45-47
0.96	1.06	1.69	1.69	2.86	4.00	4.92	5.82	7.81	6.61	1.54	1.13	1.15	0.06	0.11	C95
0.79	1.37	2.37	3.11	5.17	7.16	8.71	13.53	18.71	20.93	2.47	1.50	1.51	0.08	0.16	O&U
38.53	72.07	129.59	139.12	262.99	385.34	540.30	735.65	960.53	1 028.75	126.12	74.34	73.44	3.52	8.15	C00-96, D32-33, D42-43,D45-47
38.43	71.83	129.15	138.82	262.39	384.12	537.92	731.39	952.27	1 008.13	125.39	73.99	73.07	3.51	8.12	C00-96, D32-33, D42-43,D45-47 exc. C44

附录 2　2017 年全国东中西部肿瘤登记地区癌症发病和死亡结果

Appendix 2　Cancer incidence and mortality in Eastern, Central and Western registration areas of China, 2017

附表 2-1　2017 年全国东部肿瘤登记地区癌症发病主要指标

Appendix Table 2-1　Cancer incidence in Eastern registration areas of China, 2017

部位 Site		男性 Male						女性 Female						ICD10
		病例数 No. cases	构成 Freq. /%	粗率 Crude rate/ 100 000^{-1}	世标率 ASR world/ 100 000^{-1}	累积率 Cum. rate/%		病例数 No. cases	构成 Freq. /%	粗率 Crude rate/ 100 000^{-1}	世标率 ASR world/ 100 000^{-1}	累积率 Cum. rate/%		
						0~64	0~74					0~64	0~74	
唇	Lip	204	0.06	0.21	0.11	0.00	0.01	169	0.06	0.17	0.08	0.00	0.01	C00
舌	Tongue	1 092	0.31	1.10	0.67	0.05	0.08	675	0.22	0.69	0.38	0.02	0.04	C01-02
口	Mouth	1 385	0.39	1.39	0.82	0.05	0.10	864	0.28	0.88	0.47	0.02	0.05	C03-06
唾液腺	Salivary glands	760	0.21	0.76	0.50	0.03	0.05	577	0.19	0.59	0.40	0.03	0.04	C07-08
扁桃腺	Tonsil	248	0.07	0.25	0.15	0.01	0.02	94	0.03	0.10	0.06	0.00	0.01	C09
其他口咽	Other oropharynx	416	0.12	0.42	0.25	0.02	0.03	85	0.03	0.09	0.05	0.00	0.01	C10
鼻咽	Nasopharynx	4 908	1.38	4.93	3.27	0.25	0.35	1 968	0.65	2.00	1.31	0.10	0.14	C11
下咽	Hypopharynx	1 167	0.33	1.17	0.70	0.05	0.09	76	0.02	0.08	0.04	0.00	0.00	C12-13
咽,部位不明	Pharynx unspecified	300	0.08	0.30	0.18	0.01	0.02	83	0.03	0.08	0.04	0.00	0.00	C14
食管	Esophagus	27 629	7.75	27.77	15.52	0.76	1.96	10 468	3.44	10.64	5.01	0.16	0.60	C15
胃	Stomach	43 357	12.17	43.57	24.52	1.20	3.04	18 706	6.14	19.01	9.85	0.49	1.14	C16
小肠	Small intestine	1 584	0.44	1.59	0.93	0.05	0.11	1 162	0.38	1.18	0.62	0.03	0.07	C17
结肠	Colon	20 400	5.73	20.50	11.66	0.60	1.39	16 163	5.31	16.43	8.48	0.45	0.98	C18
直肠	Rectum	19 143	5.37	19.24	11.03	0.62	1.35	12 041	3.95	12.24	6.44	0.36	0.75	C19-20
肛门	Anus	341	0.10	0.34	0.20	0.01	0.02	265	0.09	0.27	0.14	0.01	0.01	C21
肝脏	Liver	38 634	10.84	38.82	23.32	1.58	2.71	13 857	4.55	14.08	7.25	0.37	0.83	C22
胆囊及其他	Gallbladder etc.	4 764	1.34	4.79	2.65	0.12	0.31	4 880	1.60	4.96	2.40	0.10	0.27	C23-24
胰腺	Pancreas	9 980	2.80	10.03	5.59	0.27	0.66	7 653	2.51	7.78	3.80	0.16	0.44	C25
鼻、鼻窦及其他	Nose, sinuses etc.	598	0.17	0.60	0.38	0.02	0.04	315	0.10	0.32	0.19	0.01	0.02	C30-31
喉	Larynx	3 609	1.01	3.63	2.10	0.13	0.27	277	0.09	0.28	0.15	0.01	0.02	C32
气管、支气管、肺	Trachea, bronchus & lung	87 382	24.53	87.81	49.25	2.39	6.12	50 381	16.54	51.20	26.80	1.47	3.17	C33-34
其他胸腔器官	Other thoracic organs	1 324	0.37	1.33	0.89	0.06	0.10	802	0.26	0.82	0.51	0.03	0.05	C37-38
骨	Bone	1 836	0.52	1.85	1.31	0.07	0.13	1 464	0.48	1.49	0.99	0.06	0.10	C40-41
皮肤黑色素瘤	Melanoma of skin	596	0.17	0.60	0.36	0.02	0.04	579	0.19	0.59	0.34	0.02	0.04	C43
皮肤其他	Other skin	3 077	0.86	3.09	1.77	0.08	0.19	3 120	1.02	3.17	1.57	0.07	0.16	C44
间皮瘤	Mesothelioma	220	0.06	0.22	0.13	0.01	0.02	173	0.06	0.18	0.10	0.01	0.01	C45
卡波氏肉瘤	Kaposi sarcoma	30	0.01	0.03	0.02	0.00	0.00	23	0.01	0.02	0.02	0.00	0.00	C46
结缔组织、软组织	Connective & soft tissue	1 157	0.32	1.16	0.82	0.05	0.08	982	0.32	1.00	0.71	0.05	0.07	C47;C49
乳腺	Breast	551	0.15	0.55	0.34	0.02	0.04	51 902	17.04	52.74	33.30	2.70	3.60	C50
外阴	Vulva	—	—	—	—	—	—	524	0.17	0.53	0.29	0.02	0.03	C51
阴道	Vagina	—	—	—	—	—	—	280	0.09	0.28	0.17	0.01	0.02	C52
子宫颈	Cervix uteri	—	—	—	—	—	—	15 191	4.99	15.44	9.92	0.83	1.04	C53
子宫体	Corpus uteri	—	—	—	—	—	—	9 907	3.25	10.07	6.22	0.53	0.71	C54
子宫,部位不明	Uterus unspecified	—	—	—	—	—	—	1 564	0.51	1.59	0.94	0.07	0.10	C55
卵巢	Ovary	—	—	—	—	—	—	8 311	2.73	8.45	5.41	0.41	0.59	C56
其他女性生殖器	Other female genital organs	—	—	—	—	—	—	687	0.23	0.70	0.43	0.03	0.05	C57
胎盘	Placenta	—	—	—	—	—	—	86	0.03	0.09	0.08	0.01	0.01	C58
阴茎	Penis	803	0.23	0.81	0.47	0.03	0.05	—	—	—	—	—	—	C60
前列腺	Prostate	15 628	4.39	15.71	8.09	0.18	0.91	—	—	—	—	—	—	C61
睾丸	Testis	533	0.15	0.54	0.47	0.03	0.04	—	—	—	—	—	—	C62
其他男性生殖器	Other male genital organs	246	0.07	0.25	0.15	0.01	0.02	—	—	—	—	—	—	C63
肾	Kidney	7 260	2.04	7.30	4.50	0.31	0.53	3 731	1.23	3.79	2.27	0.15	0.26	C64
肾盂	Renal pelvis	757	0.21	0.76	0.43	0.02	0.05	526	0.17	0.53	0.26	0.01	0.03	C65
输尿管	Ureter	811	0.23	0.82	0.46	0.02	0.06	658	0.22	0.67	0.31	0.01	0.04	C66
膀胱	Bladder	11 484	3.22	11.54	6.32	0.28	0.71	3 071	1.01	3.12	1.54	0.07	0.17	C67
其他泌尿器官	Other urinary organs	190	0.05	0.19	0.10	0.00	0.01	103	0.03	0.10	0.05	0.00	0.01	C68
眼	Eye	164	0.05	0.16	0.17	0.01	0.01	153	0.05	0.16	0.16	0.01	0.01	C69
脑、神经系统	Brain, nervous system	7 835	2.20	7.87	5.54	0.36	0.56	9 858	3.24	10.02	6.46	0.43	0.68	C70-72, D32-33, D42-43
甲状腺	Thyroid	9 967	2.80	10.02	7.52	0.61	0.70	31 026	10.19	31.53	22.76	1.91	2.15	C73
肾上腺	Adrenal gland	302	0.08	0.30	0.23	0.01	0.02	219	0.07	0.22	0.18	0.01	0.02	C74
其他内分泌腺	Other endocrine	380	0.11	0.38	0.30	0.02	0.03	373	0.12	0.38	0.27	0.02	0.03	C75
霍奇金淋巴瘤	Hodgkin lymphoma	396	0.11	0.40	0.32	0.02	0.03	278	0.09	0.28	0.22	0.01	0.02	C81
非霍奇金淋巴瘤	Non-Hodgkin lymphoma	6 461	1.81	6.49	4.14	0.24	0.45	4 865	1.60	4.94	2.96	0.18	0.33	C82-C86;C96
免疫增生性疾病	Immunoproliferative diseases	102	0.03	0.10	0.06	0.00	0.01	51	0.02	0.05	0.03	0.00	0.00	C88
多发性骨髓瘤	Multiple myeloma	2 176	0.61	2.19	1.26	0.07	0.16	1 618	0.53	1.64	0.90	0.05	0.11	C90
淋巴样白血病	Lymphoid leukemia	1 750	0.49	1.76	1.77	0.09	0.13	1 242	0.41	1.26	1.28	0.07	0.09	C91
髓样白血病	Myeloid leukemia	4 833	1.36	4.86	3.34	0.20	0.34	3 737	1.23	3.80	2.54	0.16	0.26	C92-C94, D45-47
白血病,未特指	Leukemia unspecified	1 825	0.51	1.83	1.36	0.07	0.12	1 334	0.44	1.36	0.96	0.05	0.09	C95
其他或未指明部位	Other and unspecified	5 699	1.60	5.73	3.47	0.18	0.37	5 333	1.75	5.42	3.12	0.18	0.32	O&U
所有部位合计	All sites	356 294	100.00	358.05	209.88	11.29	24.64	304 530	100.00	309.47	181.20	11.97	19.80	C00-96, D32-33, D42-43, D45-47
所有部位除外 C44	All sites except C44	353 217	99.14	354.96	208.11	11.21	24.45	301 410	98.98	306.30	179.63	11.90	19.64	C00-96, D32-33, D42-43, D45-47 exc. C44

附表 2-2 2017 年全国东部城市肿瘤登记地区癌症发病主要指标

Appendix Table 2-2 Cancer incidence in Eastern urban registration areas of China, 2017

部位 Site		男性 Male						女性 Female						ICD10
		病例数 No. cases	构成 Freq. /%	粗率 Crude rate/ $100\,000^{-1}$	世标率 ASR world/ $100\,000^{-1}$	累积率 Cum. rate/% 0~64	累积率 Cum. rate/% 0~74	病例数 No. cases	构成 Freq. /%	粗率 Crude rate/ $100\,000^{-1}$	世标率 ASR world/ $100\,000^{-1}$	累积率 Cum. rate/% 0~64	累积率 Cum. rate/% 0~74	
唇	Lip	109	0. 05	0. 20	0. 11	0. 00	0. 01	101	0. 05	0. 18	0. 08	0. 00	0. 01	C00
舌	Tongue	743	0. 36	1. 34	0. 80	0. 06	0. 09	478	0. 26	0. 86	0. 47	0. 03	0. 06	C01-02
口	Mouth	859	0. 41	1. 55	0. 88	0. 06	0. 10	526	0. 28	0. 94	0. 49	0. 02	0. 06	C03-06
唾液腺	Salivary glands	476	0. 23	0. 86	0. 56	0. 04	0. 06	348	0. 19	0. 62	0. 42	0. 03	0. 04	C07-08
扁桃腺	Tonsil	162	0. 08	0. 29	0. 18	0. 01	0. 02	61	0. 03	0. 11	0. 07	0. 01	0. 01	C09
其他口咽	Other oropharynx	290	0. 14	0. 52	0. 31	0. 02	0. 04	57	0. 03	0. 10	0. 06	0. 00	0. 01	C10
鼻咽	Nasopharynx	3 015	1. 45	5. 44	3. 58	0. 28	0. 38	1 201	0. 64	2. 15	1. 40	0. 11	0. 15	C11
下咽	Hypopharynx	728	0. 35	1. 31	0. 76	0. 05	0. 09	39	0. 02	0. 07	0. 04	0. 00	0. 00	C12-13
咽,部位不明	Pharynx unspecified	175	0. 08	0. 32	0. 18	0. 01	0. 02	47	0. 03	0. 08	0. 04	0. 00	0. 00	C14
食管	Esophagus	11 985	5. 75	21. 62	11. 83	0. 62	1. 49	3 842	2. 05	6. 89	3. 12	0. 09	0. 37	C15
胃	Stomach	22 478	10. 79	40. 55	22. 21	1. 09	2. 76	10 131	5. 42	18. 16	9. 26	0. 48	1. 06	C16
小肠	Small intestine	997	0. 48	1. 80	1. 01	0. 06	0. 12	739	0. 40	1. 32	0. 68	0. 04	0. 08	C17
结肠	Colon	14 134	6. 79	25. 50	14. 03	0. 70	1. 67	11 276	6. 03	20. 21	10. 15	0. 52	1. 17	C18
直肠	Rectum	11 916	5. 72	21. 49	12. 02	0. 68	1. 47	7 249	3. 88	12. 99	6. 70	0. 38	0. 78	C19-20
肛门	Anus	192	0. 09	0. 35	0. 20	0. 01	0. 02	161	0. 09	0. 29	0. 14	0. 01	0. 02	C21
肝脏	Liver	21 061	10. 11	37. 99	22. 31	1. 52	2. 59	7 532	4. 03	13. 50	6. 71	0. 33	0. 76	C22
胆囊及其他	Gallbladder etc.	2 919	1. 40	5. 27	2. 83	0. 13	0. 33	2 994	1. 60	5. 37	2. 52	0. 11	0. 28	C23-24
胰腺	Pancreas	6 004	2. 88	10. 83	5. 85	0. 29	0. 69	4 731	2. 53	8. 48	4. 01	0. 17	0. 46	C25
鼻、鼻窦及其他	Nose, sinuses etc.	346	0. 17	0. 62	0. 39	0. 03	0. 04	181	0. 10	0. 32	0. 20	0. 01	0. 02	C30-31
喉	Larynx	2 297	1. 10	4. 14	2. 34	0. 15	0. 30	173	0. 09	0. 31	0. 16	0. 01	0. 02	C32
气管、支气管、肺	Trachea, bronchus & lung	49 954	23. 99	90. 11	49. 19	2. 43	6. 10	30 212	16. 16	54. 16	27. 89	1. 57	3. 26	C33-34
其他胸腔器官	Other thoracic organs	881	0. 42	1. 59	1. 05	0. 07	0. 11	523	0. 28	0. 94	0. 58	0. 04	0. 06	C37-38
骨	Bone	955	0. 46	1. 72	1. 20	0. 07	0. 12	773	0. 41	1. 39	0. 89	0. 05	0. 09	C40-41
皮肤黑色素瘤	Melanoma of skin	362	0. 17	0. 65	0. 37	0. 02	0. 04	373	0. 20	0. 67	0. 38	0. 02	0. 04	C43
皮肤其他	Other skin	2 000	0. 96	3. 61	2. 02	0. 10	0. 22	1 935	1. 03	3. 47	1. 72	0. 08	0. 18	C44
间皮瘤	Mesothelioma	146	0. 07	0. 26	0. 15	0. 01	0. 02	102	0. 05	0. 18	0. 11	0. 01	0. 01	C45
卡波氏肉瘤	Kaposi sarcoma	22	0. 01	0. 04	0. 03	0. 00	0. 00	13	0. 01	0. 02	0. 02	0. 00	0. 00	C46
结缔组织、软组织	Connective & soft tissue	739	0. 35	1. 33	0. 93	0. 06	0. 09	632	0. 34	1. 13	0. 81	0. 05	0. 08	C47;C49
乳腺	Breast	345	0. 17	0. 62	0. 37	0. 02	0. 04	33 672	18. 01	60. 36	37. 45	3. 02	4. 08	C50
外阴	Vulva	—	—	—	—	—	—	340	0. 18	0. 61	0. 32	0. 02	0. 04	C51
阴道	Vagina	—	—	—	—	—	—	179	0. 10	0. 32	0. 18	0. 01	0. 02	C52
子宫颈	Cervix uteri	—	—	—	—	—	—	8 495	4. 54	15. 23	9. 79	0. 83	1. 02	C53
子宫体	Corpus uteri	—	—	—	—	—	—	6 182	3. 31	11. 08	6. 78	0. 57	0. 77	C54
子宫,部位不明	Uterus unspecified	—	—	—	—	—	—	876	0. 47	1. 57	0. 92	0. 07	0. 10	C55
卵巢	Ovary	—	—	—	—	—	—	5 132	2. 74	9. 20	5. 85	0. 44	0. 63	C56
其他女性生殖器	Other female genital organs	—	—	—	—	—	—	419	0. 22	0. 75	0. 45	0. 03	0. 05	C57
胎盘	Placenta	—	—	—	—	—	—	53	0. 03	0. 10	0. 08	0. 01	0. 01	C58
阴茎	Penis	434	0. 21	0. 78	0. 44	0. 02	0. 05	—	—	—	—	—	—	C60
前列腺	Prostate	10 693	5. 13	19. 29	9. 64	0. 21	1. 11	—	—	—	—	—	—	C61
睾丸	Testis	368	0. 18	0. 66	0. 58	0. 04	0. 05	—	—	—	—	—	—	C62
其他男性生殖器	Other male genital organs	177	0. 08	0. 32	0. 19	0. 01	0. 02	—	—	—	—	—	—	C63
肾	Kidney	5 105	2. 45	9. 21	5. 54	0. 38	0. 65	2 520	1. 35	4. 52	2. 63	0. 17	0. 30	C64
肾盂	Renal pelvis	501	0. 24	0. 90	0. 49	0. 02	0. 06	368	0. 20	0. 66	0. 31	0. 01	0. 04	C65
输尿管	Ureter	544	0. 26	0. 98	0. 52	0. 02	0. 06	463	0. 25	0. 83	0. 37	0. 01	0. 04	C66
膀胱	Bladder	7 331	3. 52	13. 22	7. 01	0. 31	0. 79	2 024	1. 08	3. 63	1. 72	0. 07	0. 20	C67
其他泌尿器官	Other urinary organs	139	0. 07	0. 25	0. 13	0. 00	0. 01	72	0. 04	0. 13	0. 06	0. 00	0. 01	C68
眼	Eye	90	0. 04	0. 16	0. 17	0. 01	0. 01	81	0. 04	0. 15	0. 14	0. 01	0. 01	C69
脑、神经系统	Brain, nervous system	4 613	2. 21	8. 32	5. 81	0. 37	0. 59	6 017	3. 22	10. 79	6. 83	0. 46	0. 72	C70-72, D32-33, D42-43
甲状腺	Thyroid	7 165	3. 44	12. 92	9. 66	0. 78	0. 89	21 584	11. 54	38. 69	27. 80	2. 33	2. 62	C73
肾上腺	Adrenal gland	174	0. 08	0. 31	0. 23	0. 01	0. 02	129	0. 07	0. 23	0. 17	0. 01	0. 02	C74
其他内分泌腺	Other endocrine	231	0. 11	0. 42	0. 33	0. 02	0. 03	230	0. 12	0. 41	0. 29	0. 02	0. 03	C75
霍奇金淋巴瘤	Hodgkin lymphoma	250	0. 12	0. 45	0. 38	0. 02	0. 03	165	0. 09	0. 30	0. 25	0. 02	0. 02	C81
非霍奇金淋巴瘤	Non-Hodgkin lymphoma	3 994	1. 92	7. 20	4. 52	0. 26	0. 50	3 120	1. 67	5. 59	3. 26	0. 20	0. 37	C82-C86;C96
免疫增生性疾病	Immunoproliferative diseases	69	0. 03	0. 12	0. 07	0. 00	0. 01	36	0. 02	0. 06	0. 04	0. 00	0. 00	C88
多发性骨髓瘤	Multiple myeloma	1 363	0. 65	2. 46	1. 36	0. 07	0. 17	972	0. 52	1. 74	0. 91	0. 05	0. 12	C90
淋巴样白血病	Lymphoid leukemia	1 029	0. 49	1. 86	1. 92	0. 10	0. 14	762	0. 41	1. 37	1. 37	0. 07	0. 10	C91
髓样白血病	Myeloid leukemia	2 996	1. 44	5. 40	3. 61	0. 21	0. 36	2 350	1. 26	4. 21	2. 75	0. 17	0. 28	C92-C94, D45-47
白血病,未特指	Leukemia unspecified	930	0. 45	1. 68	1. 17	0. 06	0. 11	652	0. 35	1. 17	0. 81	0. 05	0. 07	C95
其他或未指明部位	Other and unspecified	3780	1. 81	6. 82	3. 99	0. 20	0. 43	3 680	1. 97	6. 60	3. 68	0. 21	0. 37	O&U
所有部位合计	All sites	208 266	100. 00	375. 67	215. 45	11. 74	25. 14	187 003	100. 00	335. 21	194. 32	13. 02	21. 10	C00-96, D32-33, D42-43, D45-47
所有部位除外 C44	All sites except C44	206 266	99. 04	372. 07	213. 43	11. 65	24. 92	185 068	98. 97	331. 74	192. 60	12. 94	20. 93	C00-96, D32-33, D42-43, D45-47 exc. C44

附表 2-3 2017 年全国东部农村肿瘤登记地区癌症发病主要指标

Appendix Table 2-3 Cancer incidence in Eastern rural registration areas of China, 2017

部位 Site		男性 Male						女性 Female						ICD10
		病例数 No. cases	构成 Freq. /%	粗率 Crude rate/ 100 000⁻¹	世标率 ASR world/ 100 000⁻¹	累积率 Cum. rate/% 0~64	累积率 Cum. rate/% 0~74	病例数 No. cases	构成 Freq. /%	粗率 Crude rate/ 100 000⁻¹	世标率 ASR world/ 100 000⁻¹	累积率 Cum. rate/% 0~64	累积率 Cum. rate/% 0~74	
唇	Lip	95	0.06	0.22	0.12	0.01	0.01	68	0.06	0.16	0.08	0.00	0.01	C00
舌	Tongue	349	0.24	0.79	0.50	0.04	0.06	197	0.17	0.46	0.26	0.02	0.03	C01-02
口	Mouth	526	0.36	1.19	0.74	0.04	0.09	338	0.29	0.79	0.44	0.02	0.05	C03-06
唾液腺	Salivary glands	284	0.19	0.64	0.43	0.03	0.05	229	0.19	0.54	0.36	0.03	0.04	C07-08
扁桃腺	Tonsil	86	0.06	0.20	0.12	0.01	0.01	33	0.03	0.08	0.05	0.00	0.01	C09
其他口咽	Other oropharynx	126	0.09	0.29	0.18	0.01	0.02	28	0.02	0.07	0.04	0.00	0.00	C10
鼻咽	Nasopharynx	1 893	1.28	4.30	2.88	0.22	0.31	767	0.65	1.80	1.20	0.09	0.12	C11
下咽	Hypopharynx	439	0.30	1.00	0.62	0.04	0.08	37	0.03	0.09	0.05	0.00	0.00	C12-13
咽,部位不明	Pharynx unspecified	125	0.08	0.28	0.17	0.01	0.02	36	0.03	0.08	0.05	0.00	0.01	C14
食管	Esophagus	15 644	10.57	35.50	20.48	0.94	2.58	6 626	5.64	15.55	7.59	0.25	0.91	C15
胃	Stomach	20 879	14.10	47.38	27.57	1.35	3.41	8 575	7.30	20.12	10.67	0.51	1.25	C16
小肠	Small intestine	587	0.40	1.33	0.81	0.05	0.10	423	0.36	0.99	0.55	0.03	0.06	C17
结肠	Colon	6 266	4.23	14.22	8.47	0.45	1.02	4 887	4.16	11.47	6.20	0.34	0.72	C18
直肠	Rectum	7 227	4.88	16.40	9.71	0.53	1.18	4 792	4.08	11.24	6.08	0.34	0.71	C19-20
肛门	Anus	149	0.10	0.34	0.20	0.01	0.02	104	0.09	0.24	0.12	0.01	0.01	C21
肝脏	Liver	17 573	11.87	39.87	24.65	1.65	2.86	6 325	5.38	14.84	7.96	0.42	0.92	C22
胆囊及其他	Gallbladder etc.	1 845	1.25	4.19	2.41	0.11	0.29	1 886	1.60	4.43	2.22	0.09	0.26	C23-24
胰腺	Pancreas	3 976	2.69	9.02	5.21	0.24	0.62	2 922	2.49	6.86	3.50	0.15	0.41	C25
鼻、鼻窦及其他	Nose, sinuses etc.	252	0.17	0.57	0.37	0.02	0.04	134	0.11	0.31	0.19	0.01	0.02	C30-31
喉	Larynx	1 312	0.89	2.98	1.77	0.11	0.23	104	0.09	0.24	0.13	0.01	0.02	C32
气管、支气管、肺	Trachea, bronchus & lung	37 428	25.28	84.93	49.29	2.33	6.15	20 169	17.16	47.32	25.35	1.34	3.04	C33-34
其他胸腔器官	Other thoracic organs	443	0.30	1.01	0.69	0.04	0.08	279	0.24	0.65	0.40	0.03	0.05	C37-38
骨	Bone	881	0.60	2.00	1.44	0.08	0.14	691	0.59	1.62	1.11	0.06	0.11	C40-41
皮肤黑色素瘤	Melanoma of skin	234	0.16	0.53	0.33	0.02	0.03	206	0.18	0.48	0.28	0.02	0.03	C43
皮肤其他	Other skin	1 077	0.73	2.44	1.45	0.07	0.15	1 185	1.01	2.78	1.38	0.06	0.13	C44
间皮瘤	Mesothelioma	74	0.05	0.17	0.10	0.01	0.01	71	0.06	0.17	0.10	0.01	0.01	C45
卡波氏肉瘤	Kaposi sarcoma	8	0.01	0.02	0.01	0.00	0.00	10	0.01	0.02	0.02	0.00	0.00	C46
结缔组织、软组织	Connective & soft tissue	418	0.28	0.95	0.68	0.04	0.07	350	0.30	0.82	0.59	0.04	0.06	C47;C49
乳腺	Breast	206	0.14	0.47	0.29	0.02	0.03	18 230	15.51	42.78	27.72	2.28	2.96	C50
外阴	Vulva	—	—	—	—	—	—	184	0.16	0.43	0.24	0.01	0.03	C51
阴道	Vagina	—	—	—	—	—	—	101	0.09	0.24	0.15	0.01	0.02	C52
子宫颈	Cervix uteri	—	—	—	—	—	—	6 696	5.70	15.71	10.12	0.82	1.07	C53
子宫体	Corpus uteri	—	—	—	—	—	—	3 725	3.17	8.74	5.48	0.47	0.62	C54
子宫,部位不明	Uterus unspecified	—	—	—	—	—	—	688	0.59	1.61	0.97	0.07	0.11	C55
卵巢	Ovary	—	—	—	—	—	—	3 179	2.70	7.46	4.84	0.37	0.52	C56
其他女性生殖器	Other female genital organs	—	—	—	—	—	—	268	0.23	0.63	0.42	0.03	0.04	C57
胎盘	Placenta	—	—	—	—	—	—	33	0.03	0.08	0.07	0.01	0.01	C58
阴茎	Penis	369	0.25	0.84	0.50	0.03	0.06	—	—	—	—	—	—	C60
前列腺	Prostate	4 935	3.33	11.20	6.01	0.13	0.66	—	—	—	—	—	—	C61
睾丸	Testis	165	0.11	0.37	0.33	0.02	0.03	—	—	—	—	—	—	C62
其他男性生殖器	Other male genital organs	69	0.05	0.16	0.10	0.00	0.01	—	—	—	—	—	—	C63
肾	Kidney	2 155	1.46	4.89	3.13	0.21	0.36	1 211	1.03	2.84	1.78	0.12	0.21	C64
肾盂	Renal pelvis	256	0.17	0.58	0.34	0.02	0.04	158	0.13	0.37	0.20	0.01	0.02	C65
输尿管	Ureter	267	0.18	0.61	0.36	0.02	0.05	195	0.17	0.46	0.23	0.01	0.03	C66
膀胱	Bladder	4 153	2.81	9.42	5.40	0.24	0.61	1 047	0.89	2.46	1.28	0.06	0.15	C67
其他泌尿器官	Other urinary organs	51	0.03	0.12	0.06	0.00	0.01	31	0.03	0.07	0.04	0.00	0.00	C68
眼	Eye	74	0.05	0.17	0.17	0.01	0.01	72	0.06	0.17	0.18	0.01	0.01	C69
脑、神经系统	Brain, nervous system	3 222	2.18	7.31	5.20	0.34	0.53	3 841	3.27	9.01	5.96	0.40	0.62	C70-72, D32-33, D42-43
甲状腺	Thyroid	2 802	1.89	6.36	4.76	0.38	0.45	9 442	8.03	22.15	16.05	1.35	1.52	C73
肾上腺	Adrenal gland	128	0.09	0.29	0.22	0.01	0.02	90	0.08	0.21	0.18	0.01	0.02	C74
其他内分泌腺	Other endocrine	149	0.10	0.34	0.26	0.02	0.03	143	0.12	0.34	0.24	0.02	0.02	C75
霍奇金淋巴瘤	Hodgkin lymphoma	146	0.10	0.33	0.24	0.02	0.02	113	0.10	0.27	0.18	0.01	0.02	C81
非霍奇金淋巴瘤	Non-Hodgkin lymphoma	2 467	1.67	5.60	3.64	0.21	0.40	1 745	1.48	4.09	2.54	0.15	0.28	C82-C86;C96
免疫增生性疾病	Immunoproliferative diseases	33	0.02	0.07	0.04	0.00	0.01	15	0.01	0.04	0.02	0.00	0.00	C88
多发性骨髓瘤	Multiple myeloma	813	0.55	1.84	1.12	0.06	0.14	646	0.55	1.52	0.87	0.05	0.11	C90
淋巴样白血病	Lymphoid leukemia	721	0.49	1.64	1.60	0.09	0.12	480	0.41	1.13	1.15	0.07	0.08	C91
髓样白血病	Myeloid leukemia	1 837	1.24	4.17	3.00	0.18	0.30	1 387	1.18	3.25	2.25	0.14	0.23	C92-C94, D45-47
白血病,未特指	Leukemia unspecified	895	0.60	2.03	1.59	0.09	0.15	682	0.58	1.60	1.17	0.07	0.11	C95
其他或未指明部位	Other and unspecified	1 919	1.30	4.35	2.77	0.15	0.30	1 653	1.41	3.88	2.36	0.14	0.24	O&U
所有部位合计	All sites	148 028	100.00	335.89	202.57	10.71	24.00	117 527	100.00	275.77	163.66	10.57	18.06	C00-96, D32-33, D42-43, D45-47
所有部位除外 C44	All sites except C44	146 951	99.27	333.44	201.12	10.64	23.85	116 342	98.99	272.99	162.28	10.51	17.93	C00-96, D32-33, D42-43, D45-47 exc. C44

附表 2-4　2017 年全国中部肿瘤登记地区癌症发病主要指标

Appendix Table 2-4　Cancer incidence in Central registration areas of China, 2017

部位 Site		男性 Male						女性 Female						ICD10
		病例数 No. cases	构成 Freq. /%	粗率 Crude rate/ $100\,000^{-1}$	世标率 ASR world/ $100\,000^{-1}$	累积率 Cum. rate/% 0~64	累积率 Cum. rate/% 0~74	病例数 No. cases	构成 Freq. /%	粗率 Crude rate/ $100\,000^{-1}$	世标率 ASR world/ $100\,000^{-1}$	累积率 Cum. rate/% 0~64	累积率 Cum. rate/% 0~74	
唇	Lip	95	0.06	0.16	0.12	0.01	0.01	68	0.05	0.12	0.08	0.00	0.01	C00
舌	Tongue	662	0.40	1.13	0.81	0.06	0.09	240	0.18	0.43	0.28	0.02	0.03	C01-02
口	Mouth	784	0.47	1.33	0.96	0.06	0.11	355	0.26	0.63	0.41	0.02	0.05	C03-06
唾液腺	Salivary glands	366	0.22	0.62	0.47	0.03	0.05	321	0.24	0.57	0.41	0.03	0.05	C07-08
扁桃腺	Tonsil	122	0.07	0.21	0.15	0.01	0.02	52	0.04	0.09	0.07	0.01	0.01	C09
其他口咽	Other oropharynx	249	0.15	0.42	0.31	0.02	0.04	48	0.04	0.09	0.06	0.00	0.01	C10
鼻咽	Nasopharynx	2 462	1.47	4.19	3.06	0.23	0.34	1 037	0.77	1.84	1.30	0.10	0.14	C11
下咽	Hypopharynx	388	0.23	0.66	0.47	0.03	0.06	34	0.03	0.06	0.04	0.00	0.00	C12-13
咽,部位不明	Pharynx unspecified	187	0.11	0.32	0.22	0.01	0.03	52	0.04	0.09	0.06	0.00	0.01	C14
食管	Esophagus	14 574	8.72	24.78	17.16	0.77	2.20	6 416	4.78	11.40	6.89	0.25	0.84	C15
胃	Stomach	23 107	13.83	39.28	27.28	1.34	3.44	10 051	7.49	17.86	11.23	0.55	1.30	C16
小肠	Small intestine	655	0.39	1.11	0.78	0.05	0.10	526	0.39	0.93	0.62	0.04	0.08	C17
结肠	Colon	6 921	4.14	11.77	8.17	0.44	0.96	5 503	4.10	9.78	6.27	0.35	0.75	C18
直肠	Rectum	8 054	4.82	13.69	9.59	0.53	1.18	5 515	4.11	9.80	6.32	0.36	0.75	C19-20
肛门	Anus	225	0.13	0.38	0.27	0.01	0.03	158	0.12	0.28	0.17	0.01	0.02	C21
肝脏	Liver	22 942	13.73	39.00	27.56	1.76	3.20	9 045	6.74	16.08	10.19	0.51	1.18	C22
胆囊及其他	Gallbladder etc.	1 653	0.99	2.81	1.94	0.09	0.24	2 162	1.61	3.84	2.37	0.11	0.28	C23-24
胰腺	Pancreas	3 486	2.09	5.93	4.08	0.21	0.49	2 567	1.91	4.56	2.85	0.14	0.33	C25
鼻、鼻窦及其他	Nose, sinuses etc.	286	0.17	0.49	0.36	0.02	0.04	197	0.15	0.35	0.24	0.02	0.03	C30-31
喉	Larynx	1 819	1.09	3.09	2.17	0.13	0.27	206	0.15	0.37	0.24	0.01	0.03	C32
气管、支气管、肺	Trachea, bronchus & lung	44 807	26.82	76.18	52.50	2.52	6.51	19 622	14.62	34.88	21.88	1.12	2.57	C33-34
其他胸腔器官	Other thoracic organs	545	0.33	0.93	0.70	0.04	0.08	405	0.30	0.72	0.52	0.03	0.06	C37-38
骨	Bone	1 223	0.73	2.08	1.68	0.10	0.17	914	0.68	1.62	1.22	0.07	0.12	C40-41
皮肤黑色素瘤	Melanoma of skin	286	0.17	0.49	0.36	0.02	0.04	231	0.17	0.41	0.29	0.02	0.03	C43
皮肤其他	Other skin	1 230	0.74	2.09	1.45	0.06	0.16	1 138	0.85	2.02	1.25	0.05	0.12	C44
间皮瘤	Mesothelioma	57	0.03	0.10	0.07	0.01	0.01	55	0.04	0.10	0.07	0.01	0.01	C45
卡波氏肉瘤	Kaposi sarcoma	11	0.01	0.02	0.02	0.00	0.00	9	0.01	0.02	0.02	0.00	0.00	C46
结缔组织、软组织	Connective & soft tissue	496	0.30	0.84	0.69	0.05	0.07	430	0.32	0.76	0.59	0.04	0.06	C47;C49
乳腺	Breast	324	0.19	0.55	0.39	0.03	0.04	21 613	16.10	38.42	26.97	2.21	2.87	C50
外阴	Vulva	—	—	—	—	—	—	240	0.18	0.43	0.27	0.02	0.03	C51
阴道	Vagina	—	—	—	—	—	—	127	0.09	0.23	0.16	0.01	0.02	C52
子宫颈	Cervix uteri	—	—	—	—	—	—	11 180	8.33	19.87	13.86	1.12	1.49	C53
子宫体	Corpus uteri	—	—	—	—	—	—	4 260	3.17	7.57	5.31	0.44	0.59	C54
子宫,部位不明	Uterus unspecified	—	—	—	—	—	—	927	0.69	1.65	1.13	0.09	0.13	C55
卵巢	Ovary	—	—	—	—	—	—	3 993	2.97	7.10	5.12	0.39	0.56	C56
其他女性生殖器	Other female genital organs	—	—	—	—	—	—	274	0.20	0.49	0.33	0.03	0.04	C57
胎盘	Placenta	—	—	—	—	—	—	62	0.05	0.11	0.09	0.01	0.01	C58
阴茎	Penis	392	0.23	0.67	0.47	0.03	0.06	—	—	—	—	—	—	C60
前列腺	Prostate	4 411	2.64	7.50	4.84	0.10	0.52	—	—	—	—	—	—	C61
睾丸	Testis	213	0.13	0.36	0.32	0.02	0.03	—	—	—	—	—	—	C62
其他男性生殖器	Other male genital organs	73	0.04	0.12	0.09	0.01	0.01	—	—	—	—	—	—	C63
肾	Kidney	2 218	1.33	3.77	2.73	0.17	0.32	1 314	0.98	2.34	1.64	0.10	0.19	C64
肾盂	Renal pelvis	229	0.14	0.39	0.28	0.01	0.04	179	0.13	0.32	0.20	0.01	0.02	C65
输尿管	Ureter	251	0.15	0.43	0.29	0.01	0.03	231	0.17	0.41	0.25	0.01	0.03	C66
膀胱	Bladder	4 309	2.58	7.33	4.99	0.23	0.57	1 130	0.84	2.01	1.22	0.05	0.14	C67
其他泌尿器官	Other urinary organs	63	0.04	0.11	0.07	0.00	0.01	40	0.03	0.07	0.04	0.00	0.01	C68
眼	Eye	106	0.06	0.18	0.18	0.01	0.01	89	0.07	0.16	0.15	0.01	0.01	C69
脑、神经系统	Brain, nervous system	3 812	2.28	6.48	5.08	0.32	0.53	3 958	2.95	7.04	5.13	0.34	0.55	C70-72, D32-33, D42-43
甲状腺	Thyroid	2 715	1.62	4.62	3.53	0.28	0.34	9 012	6.71	16.02	11.98	1.01	1.15	C73
肾上腺	Adrenal gland	162	0.10	0.28	0.21	0.01	0.02	144	0.11	0.26	0.19	0.01	0.02	C74
其他内分泌腺	Other endocrine	149	0.09	0.25	0.22	0.01	0.02	148	0.11	0.26	0.21	0.02	0.02	C75
霍奇金淋巴瘤	Hodgkin lymphoma	211	0.13	0.36	0.30	0.02	0.03	146	0.11	0.26	0.20	0.01	0.02	C81
非霍奇金淋巴瘤	Non-Hodgkin lymphoma	2 472	1.48	4.20	3.15	0.19	0.35	1 841	1.37	3.27	2.33	0.15	0.25	C82-C86;C96
免疫增生性疾病	Immunoproliferative diseases	24	0.01	0.04	0.03	0.00	0.00	11	0.01	0.02	0.01	0.00	0.00	C88
多发性骨髓瘤	Multiple myeloma	851	0.51	1.45	1.05	0.06	0.13	633	0.47	1.13	0.75	0.04	0.09	C90
淋巴样白血病	Lymphoid leukemia	613	0.37	1.04	1.05	0.06	0.08	492	0.37	0.87	0.85	0.05	0.07	C91
髓样白血病	Myeloid leukemia	1331	0.80	2.26	1.80	0.11	0.18	1 098	0.82	1.95	1.53	0.09	0.15	C92-C94,D45-47
白血病,未特指	Leukemia unspecified	1 497	0.90	2.55	2.25	0.13	0.20	1 098	0.82	1.95	1.64	0.10	0.15	C95
其他或未指明部位	Other and unspecified	2 974	1.78	5.06	3.70	0.20	0.41	2 630	1.96	4.67	3.27	0.19	0.34	O&U
所有部位合计	All sites	167 092	100.00	284.08	200.37	10.61	23.85	134 227	100.00	238.58	160.78	10.38	17.82	C00-96, D32-33, D42-43, D45-47
所有部位除外 C44	All sites except C44	165 862	99.26	281.99	198.92	10.54	23.69	133 089	99.15	236.56	159.52	10.32	17.69	C00-96, D32-33, D42-43, D45-47 exc. C44

附表 2-5 2017 年全国中部城市肿瘤登记地区癌症发病主要指标

Appendix Table 2-5 Cancer incidence in Central urban registration areas of China, 2017

部位 Site		男性 Male						女性 Female						ICD10
		病例数 No. cases	构成 Freq. /%	粗率 Crude rate/ 100 000^{-1}	世标率 ASR world/ 100 000^{-1}	累积率 Cum. rate/% 0~64	累积率 Cum. rate/% 0~74	病例数 No. cases	构成 Freq. /%	粗率 Crude rate/ 100 000^{-1}	世标率 ASR world/ 100 000^{-1}	累积率 Cum. rate/% 0~64	累积率 Cum. rate/% 0~74	
唇	Lip	35	0.05	0.16	0.11	0.01	0.01	28	0.05	0.13	0.08	0.00	0.01	C00
舌	Tongue	332	0.51	1.53	1.03	0.08	0.11	135	0.24	0.63	0.38	0.02	0.04	C01-02
口	Mouth	366	0.56	1.68	1.11	0.08	0.12	161	0.29	0.75	0.45	0.02	0.05	C03-06
唾液腺	Salivary glands	148	0.23	0.68	0.48	0.03	0.05	113	0.20	0.53	0.36	0.02	0.04	C07-08
扁桃腺	Tonsil	59	0.09	0.27	0.18	0.01	0.02	30	0.05	0.14	0.10	0.01	0.01	C09
其他口咽	Other oropharynx	93	0.14	0.43	0.28	0.02	0.03	22	0.04	0.10	0.07	0.00	0.01	C10
鼻咽	Nasopharynx	861	1.31	3.96	2.71	0.20	0.32	328	0.59	1.54	1.04	0.07	0.11	C11
下咽	Hypopharynx	202	0.31	0.93	0.62	0.05	0.08	11	0.02	0.05	0.03	0.00	0.00	C12-13
咽,部位不明	Pharynx unspecified	73	0.11	0.34	0.22	0.01	0.03	15	0.03	0.07	0.05	0.00	0.00	C14
食管	Esophagus	4 619	7.03	21.23	13.54	0.66	1.72	1 672	3.03	7.83	4.30	0.14	0.51	C15
胃	Stomach	7 168	10.91	32.94	20.95	1.03	2.59	3 193	5.78	14.95	8.77	0.44	1.00	C16
小肠	Small intestine	297	0.45	1.36	0.88	0.05	0.11	238	0.43	1.11	0.68	0.04	0.08	C17
结肠	Colon	3 641	5.54	16.73	10.61	0.53	1.25	2 779	5.03	13.01	7.65	0.41	0.90	C18
直肠	Rectum	3 434	5.23	15.78	10.13	0.57	1.23	2 249	4.07	10.53	6.30	0.35	0.75	C19-20
肛门	Anus	67	0.10	0.31	0.20	0.01	0.03	50	0.09	0.23	0.13	0.01	0.01	C21
肝脏	Liver	7 654	11.65	35.17	23.04	1.48	2.68	2 982	5.40	13.96	8.14	0.40	0.93	C22
胆囊及其他	Gallbladder etc.	782	1.19	3.59	2.26	0.10	0.27	944	1.71	4.42	2.50	0.11	0.29	C23-24
胰腺	Pancreas	1 596	2.43	7.33	4.62	0.23	0.55	1 228	2.22	5.75	3.29	0.15	0.37	C25
鼻、鼻窦及其他	Nose, sinuses etc.	107	0.16	0.49	0.34	0.02	0.04	79	0.14	0.37	0.25	0.02	0.03	C30-31
喉	Larynx	837	1.27	3.85	2.49	0.15	0.31	76	0.14	0.36	0.21	0.01	0.02	C32
气管、支气管、肺	Trachea, bronchus & lung	17 981	27.37	82.63	52.39	2.54	6.52	7 948	14.38	37.21	21.61	1.11	2.53	C33-34
其他胸腔器官	Other thoracic organs	229	0.35	1.05	0.73	0.05	0.09	163	0.29	0.76	0.53	0.03	0.06	C37-38
骨	Bone	401	0.61	1.84	1.36	0.08	0.14	294	0.53	1.38	0.94	0.05	0.09	C40-41
皮肤黑色素瘤	Melanoma of skin	118	0.18	0.54	0.35	0.02	0.04	98	0.18	0.46	0.30	0.02	0.03	C43
皮肤其他	Other skin	518	0.79	2.38	1.52	0.06	0.16	445	0.81	2.08	1.18	0.05	0.11	C44
间皮瘤	Mesothelioma	31	0.05	0.14	0.10	0.01	0.01	31	0.06	0.15	0.09	0.01	0.01	C45
卡波氏肉瘤	Kaposi sarcoma	5	0.01	0.02	0.01	0.00	0.00	3	0.01	0.01	0.02	0.00	0.00	C46
结缔组织、软组织	Connective & soft tissue	240	0.37	1.10	0.81	0.05	0.08	204	0.37	0.96	0.68	0.04	0.06	C47;C49
乳腺	Breast	143	0.22	0.66	0.44	0.03	0.05	10 111	18.29	47.34	31.29	2.53	3.42	C50
外阴	Vulva	—	—	—	—	—	—	78	0.14	0.37	0.22	0.01	0.02	C51
阴道	Vagina	—	—	—	—	—	—	51	0.09	0.24	0.15	0.01	0.02	C52
子宫颈	Cervix uteri	—	—	—	—	—	—	3 968	7.18	18.58	12.27	1.01	1.31	C53
子宫体	Corpus uteri	—	—	—	—	—	—	1 663	3.01	7.79	5.16	0.42	0.59	C54
子宫,部位不明	Uterus unspecified	—	—	—	—	—	—	264	0.48	1.24	0.81	0.06	0.10	C55
卵巢	Ovary	—	—	—	—	—	—	1 709	3.09	8.00	5.40	0.40	0.59	C56
其他女性生殖器	Other female genital organs	—	—	—	—	—	—	121	0.22	0.57	0.36	0.03	0.04	C57
胎盘	Placenta	—	—	—	—	—	—	16	0.03	0.07	0.06	0.00	0.00	C58
阴茎	Penis	158	0.24	0.73	0.46	0.03	0.05	—	—	—	—	—	—	C60
前列腺	Prostate	2 426	3.69	11.15	6.47	0.12	0.69	—	—	—	—	—	—	C61
睾丸	Testis	93	0.14	0.43	0.38	0.02	0.03	—	—	—	—	—	—	C62
其他男性生殖器	Other male genital organs	40	0.06	0.18	0.12	0.01	0.01	—	—	—	—	—	—	C63
肾	Kidney	1 154	1.76	5.30	3.52	0.22	0.42	642	1.16	3.01	1.98	0.13	0.23	C64
肾盂	Renal pelvis	118	0.18	0.54	0.35	0.02	0.05	98	0.18	0.46	0.26	0.01	0.03	C65
输尿管	Ureter	126	0.19	0.58	0.36	0.02	0.04	138	0.25	0.65	0.35	0.01	0.04	C66
膀胱	Bladder	2 086	3.18	9.59	5.96	0.27	0.68	515	0.93	2.41	1.34	0.05	0.15	C67
其他泌尿器官	Other urinary organs	23	0.04	0.11	0.07	0.00	0.01	18	0.03	0.08	0.05	0.00	0.01	C68
眼	Eye	39	0.06	0.18	0.16	0.01	0.01	30	0.05	0.14	0.12	0.01	0.01	C69
脑、神经系统	Brain, nervous system	1 275	1.94	5.86	4.29	0.26	0.45	1 444	2.61	6.76	4.67	0.31	0.49	C70-72, D32-33, D42-43
甲状腺	Thyroid	1 700	2.59	7.81	5.70	0.46	0.53	5 310	9.61	24.86	17.99	1.52	1.71	C73
肾上腺	Adrenal gland	64	0.10	0.29	0.20	0.01	0.02	49	0.09	0.23	0.17	0.01	0.02	C74
其他内分泌腺	Other endocrine	46	0.07	0.21	0.19	0.01	0.02	34	0.06	0.16	0.13	0.01	0.01	C75
霍奇金淋巴瘤	Hodgkin lymphoma	84	0.13	0.39	0.31	0.02	0.03	50	0.09	0.23	0.19	0.01	0.02	C81
非霍奇金淋巴瘤	Non-Hodgkin lymphoma	1 077	1.64	4.95	3.45	0.20	0.39	848	1.53	3.97	2.61	0.16	0.29	C82-C86;C96
免疫增生性疾病	Immunoproliferative diseases	15	0.02	0.07	0.06	0.00	0.01	6	0.01	0.03	0.02	0.00	0.00	C88
多发性骨髓瘤	Multiple myeloma	403	0.61	1.85	1.23	0.07	0.15	303	0.55	1.42	0.87	0.04	0.11	C90
淋巴样白血病	Lymphoid leukemia	291	0.44	1.34	1.28	0.07	0.10	248	0.45	1.16	1.13	0.06	0.10	C91
髓样白血病	Myeloid leukemia	631	0.96	2.90	2.07	0.11	0.23	532	0.96	2.49	1.81	0.11	0.19	C92-C94, D45-47
白血病,未特指	Leukemia unspecified	428	0.65	1.97	1.62	0.09	0.14	290	0.52	1.36	1.07	0.06	0.10	C95
其他或未指明部位	Other and unspecified	1 376	2.09	6.32	4.18	0.22	0.45	1 212	2.19	5.67	3.63	0.21	0.38	O&U
所有部位合计	All sites	65 690	100.00	301.87	195.94	10.42	23.14	55 267	100.00	258.77	164.24	10.73	18.06	C00-96, D32-33, D42-43, D45-47
所有部位除外 C44	All sites except C44	65 172	99.21	299.49	194.43	10.36	22.98	54 822	99.19	256.69	163.05	10.68	17.94	C00-96, D32-33, D42-43, D45-47 exc. C44

附表 2-6　2017 年全国中部农村肿瘤登记地区癌症发病主要指标

Appendix Table 2-6　Cancer incidence in Central rural registration areas of China, 2017

部位 Site		男性 Male						女性 Female						ICD10
		病例数 No. cases	构成 Freq. /%	粗率 Crude rate/ $100\,000^{-1}$	世标率 ASR world/ $100\,000^{-1}$	累积率 Cum. rate/% 0~64	累积率 Cum. rate/% 0~74	病例数 No. cases	构成 Freq. /%	粗率 Crude rate/ $100\,000^{-1}$	世标率 ASR world/ $100\,000^{-1}$	累积率 Cum. rate/% 0~64	累积率 Cum. rate/% 0~74	
唇	Lip	60	0.06	0.16	0.13	0.01	0.01	40	0.05	0.11	0.07	0.00	0.01	C00
舌	Tongue	330	0.33	0.89	0.67	0.05	0.07	105	0.13	0.30	0.21	0.01	0.03	C01-02
口	Mouth	418	0.41	1.13	0.85	0.05	0.10	194	0.25	0.56	0.39	0.02	0.05	C03-06
唾液腺	Salivary glands	218	0.21	0.59	0.46	0.03	0.05	208	0.26	0.60	0.44	0.03	0.05	C07-08
扁桃腺	Tonsil	63	0.06	0.17	0.13	0.01	0.01	22	0.03	0.06	0.05	0.00	0.01	C09
其他口咽	Other oropharynx	156	0.15	0.42	0.32	0.02	0.04	26	0.03	0.07	0.05	0.00	0.01	C10
鼻咽	Nasopharynx	1 601	1.58	4.32	3.27	0.26	0.36	709	0.90	2.03	1.48	0.11	0.16	C11
下咽	Hypopharynx	186	0.18	0.50	0.38	0.02	0.05	23	0.03	0.07	0.05	0.00	0.01	C12-13
咽,部位不明	Pharynx unspecified	114	0.11	0.31	0.22	0.01	0.03	37	0.05	0.11	0.07	0.00	0.01	C14
食管	Esophagus	9 955	9.82	26.86	19.58	0.83	2.52	4 744	6.01	13.59	8.66	0.32	1.07	C15
胃	Stomach	15 939	15.72	43.01	31.47	1.54	3.99	6 858	8.69	19.65	12.91	0.63	1.51	C16
小肠	Small intestine	358	0.35	0.97	0.71	0.04	0.09	288	0.36	0.83	0.57	0.03	0.07	C17
结肠	Colon	3 280	3.23	8.85	6.52	0.38	0.77	2 724	3.45	7.80	5.32	0.31	0.64	C18
直肠	Rectum	4 620	4.56	12.47	9.21	0.50	1.14	3 266	4.14	9.36	6.32	0.36	0.75	C19-20
肛门	Anus	158	0.16	0.43	0.31	0.02	0.04	108	0.14	0.31	0.20	0.01	0.02	C21
肝脏	Liver	15 288	15.08	41.25	30.54	1.94	3.54	6 063	7.68	17.37	11.58	0.59	1.35	C22
胆囊及其他	Gallbladder etc.	871	0.86	2.35	1.72	0.08	0.22	1 218	1.54	3.49	2.28	0.10	0.28	C23-24
胰腺	Pancreas	1 890	1.86	5.10	3.70	0.19	0.45	1 339	1.70	3.84	2.55	0.13	0.31	C25
鼻、鼻窦及其他	Nose, sinuses etc.	179	0.18	0.48	0.37	0.02	0.04	118	0.15	0.34	0.24	0.01	0.03	C30-31
喉	Larynx	982	0.97	2.65	1.95	0.11	0.25	130	0.16	0.37	0.26	0.01	0.03	C32
气管、支气管、肺	Trachea, bronchus & lung	26 826	26.46	72.39	52.54	2.50	6.49	11 674	14.78	33.45	22.06	1.13	2.60	C33-34
其他胸腔器官	Other thoracic organs	316	0.31	0.85	0.67	0.04	0.07	242	0.31	0.69	0.52	0.04	0.06	C37-38
骨	Bone	822	0.81	2.22	1.87	0.11	0.19	620	0.79	1.78	1.39	0.09	0.14	C40-41
皮肤黑色素瘤	Melanoma of skin	168	0.17	0.45	0.36	0.02	0.04	133	0.17	0.38	0.28	0.02	0.03	C43
皮肤其他	Other skin	712	0.70	1.92	1.41	0.07	0.15	693	0.88	1.99	1.29	0.06	0.13	C44
间皮瘤	Mesothelioma	26	0.03	0.07	0.05	0.00	0.01	24	0.03	0.07	0.05	0.00	0.01	C45
卡波氏肉瘤	Kaposi sarcoma	6	0.01	0.02	0.02	0.00	0.00	6	0.01	0.02	0.02	0.00	0.00	C46
结缔组织、软组织	Connective & soft tissue	256	0.25	0.69	0.60	0.04	0.06	226	0.29	0.65	0.53	0.04	0.05	C47;C49
乳腺	Breast	181	0.18	0.49	0.37	0.02	0.04	11 502	14.57	32.95	24.02	1.99	2.49	C50
外阴	Vulva	—	—	—	—	—	—	162	0.21	0.46	0.31	0.02	0.04	C51
阴道	Vagina	—	—	—	—	—	—	76	0.10	0.22	0.16	0.01	0.02	C52
子宫颈	Cervix uteri	—	—	—	—	—	—	7 212	9.13	20.66	14.91	1.20	1.61	C53
子宫体	Corpus uteri	—	—	—	—	—	—	2 597	3.29	7.44	5.40	0.46	0.59	C54
子宫,部位不明	Uterus unspecified	—	—	—	—	—	—	663	0.84	1.90	1.35	0.11	0.14	C55
卵巢	Ovary	—	—	—	—	—	—	2 284	2.89	6.54	4.92	0.38	0.54	C56
其他女性生殖器	Other female genital organs	—	—	—	—	—	—	153	0.19	0.44	0.31	0.02	0.03	C57
胎盘	Placenta	—	—	—	—	—	—	46	0.06	0.13	0.11	0.01	0.01	C58
阴茎	Penis	234	0.23	0.63	0.47	0.03	0.06	—	—	—	—	—	—	C60
前列腺	Prostate	1 985	1.96	5.36	3.71	0.08	0.40	—	—	—	—	—	—	C61
睾丸	Testis	120	0.12	0.32	0.28	0.02	0.02	—	—	—	—	—	—	C62
其他男性生殖器	Other male genital organs	33	0.03	0.09	0.07	0.00	0.01	—	—	—	—	—	—	C63
肾	Kidney	1 064	1.05	2.87	2.20	0.13	0.26	672	0.85	1.93	1.41	0.09	0.16	C64
肾盂	Renal pelvis	111	0.11	0.30	0.23	0.01	0.03	81	0.10	0.23	0.16	0.01	0.02	C65
输尿管	Ureter	125	0.12	0.34	0.24	0.01	0.03	93	0.12	0.27	0.18	0.01	0.02	C66
膀胱	Bladder	2 223	2.19	6.00	4.32	0.20	0.49	615	0.78	1.76	1.14	0.05	0.13	C67
其他泌尿器官	Other urinary organs	40	0.04	0.11	0.08	0.00	0.01	22	0.03	0.06	0.04	0.00	0.00	C68
眼	Eye	67	0.07	0.18	0.19	0.01	0.02	59	0.07	0.17	0.17	0.01	0.01	C69
脑、神经系统	Brain, nervous system	2 537	2.50	6.85	5.56	0.35	0.58	2 514	3.18	7.20	5.43	0.37	0.59	C70-72, D32-33, D42-43
甲状腺	Thyroid	1 015	1.00	2.74	2.16	0.17	0.21	3 702	4.69	10.61	8.09	0.68	0.79	C73
肾上腺	Adrenal gland	98	0.10	0.26	0.21	0.02	0.02	95	0.12	0.27	0.20	0.01	0.02	C74
其他内分泌腺	Other endocrine	103	0.10	0.28	0.24	0.02	0.02	114	0.14	0.33	0.27	0.02	0.03	C75
霍奇金淋巴瘤	Hodgkin lymphoma	127	0.13	0.34	0.29	0.02	0.03	96	0.12	0.28	0.21	0.01	0.02	C81
非霍奇金淋巴瘤	Non-Hodgkin lymphoma	1 395	1.38	3.76	2.95	0.18	0.33	993	1.26	2.84	2.13	0.14	0.23	C82-C86;C96
免疫增生性疾病	Immunoproliferative diseases	9	0.01	0.02	0.02	0.00	0.00	5	0.01	0.01	0.01	0.00	0.00	C88
多发性骨髓瘤	Multiple myeloma	448	0.44	1.21	0.93	0.05	0.11	330	0.42	0.95	0.67	0.04	0.08	C90
淋巴样白血病	Lymphoid leukemia	322	0.32	0.87	0.91	0.05	0.07	244	0.31	0.70	0.69	0.04	0.06	C91
髓样白血病	Myeloid leukemia	700	0.69	1.89	1.60	0.10	0.15	566	0.72	1.62	1.34	0.09	0.13	C92-C94, D45-47
白血病,未特指	Leukemia unspecified	1 069	1.05	2.88	2.62	0.16	0.24	808	1.02	2.31	2.00	0.12	0.19	C95
其他或未指明部位	Other and unspecified	1 598	1.58	4.31	3.35	0.19	0.37	1 418	1.80	4.06	3.02	0.18	0.31	O&U
所有部位合计	All sites	101 402	100.00	273.63	203.01	10.73	24.30	78 960	100.00	226.22	158.48	10.14	17.66	C00-96, D32-33, D42-43, D45-47
所有部位除外 C44	All sites except C44	100 690	99.30	271.71	201.60	10.66	24.15	78 267	99.12	224.24	157.19	10.09	17.53	C00-96, D32-33, D42-43, D45-47 exc. C44

附表 2-7　2017 年全国西部肿瘤登记地区癌症发病主要指标

Appendix Table 2-7　Cancer incidence in Western registration areas of China, 2017

部位 Site		男性 Male 病例数 No. cases	构成 Freq. /%	粗率 Crude rate/ 100 000⁻¹	世标率 ASR world/ 100 000⁻¹	累积率 Cum. rate/% 0~64	累积率 Cum. rate/% 0~74	女性 Female 病例数 No. cases	构成 Freq. /%	粗率 Crude rate/ 100 000⁻¹	世标率 ASR world/ 100 000⁻¹	累积率 Cum. rate/% 0~64	累积率 Cum. rate/% 0~74	ICD10
唇	Lip	128	0.07	0.20	0.13	0.01	0.01	90	0.07	0.15	0.10	0.00	0.01	C00
舌	Tongue	555	0.29	0.88	0.58	0.04	0.07	273	0.21	0.45	0.30	0.02	0.03	C01-02
口	Mouth	826	0.44	1.32	0.86	0.05	0.10	441	0.34	0.73	0.47	0.03	0.05	C03-06
唾液腺	Salivary glands	349	0.19	0.56	0.39	0.03	0.04	226	0.17	0.37	0.26	0.02	0.03	C07-08
扁桃腺	Tonsil	145	0.08	0.23	0.16	0.01	0.02	57	0.04	0.09	0.06	0.00	0.01	C09
其他口咽	Other oropharynx	326	0.17	0.52	0.34	0.02	0.04	54	0.04	0.09	0.06	0.00	0.01	C10
鼻咽	Nasopharynx	3 815	2.03	6.07	4.24	0.33	0.46	1 648	1.26	2.72	1.88	0.14	0.20	C11
下咽	Hypopharynx	435	0.23	0.69	0.47	0.03	0.06	39	0.03	0.06	0.05	0.00	0.01	C12-13
咽,部位不明	Pharynx unspecified	335	0.18	0.53	0.36	0.02	0.04	100	0.08	0.17	0.11	0.01	0.01	C14
食管	Esophagus	19 382	10.30	30.86	20.12	1.01	2.61	5 432	4.15	8.97	5.28	0.20	0.65	C15
胃	Stomach	19 760	10.50	31.46	20.47	1.10	2.54	8 219	6.27	13.58	8.30	0.42	0.95	C16
小肠	Small intestine	686	0.36	1.09	0.73	0.04	0.09	502	0.38	0.83	0.53	0.03	0.06	C17
结肠	Colon	7 235	3.84	11.52	7.50	0.40	0.87	5 391	4.12	8.91	5.52	0.30	0.64	C18
直肠	Rectum	11 306	6.01	18.00	11.68	0.60	1.40	7 126	5.44	11.77	7.28	0.40	0.86	C19-20
肛门	Anus	349	0.19	0.56	0.36	0.02	0.04	220	0.17	0.36	0.22	0.01	0.02	C21
肝脏	Liver	29 191	15.51	46.48	31.32	2.14	3.58	9 229	7.05	15.25	9.45	0.51	1.09	C22
胆囊及其他	Gallbladder etc.	1 789	0.95	2.85	1.83	0.09	0.21	2 194	1.68	3.62	2.18	0.11	0.26	C23-24
胰腺	Pancreas	4 266	2.27	6.79	4.39	0.23	0.51	2 917	2.23	4.82	2.89	0.14	0.34	C25
鼻、鼻窦及其他	Nose, sinuses etc.	386	0.21	0.61	0.42	0.03	0.05	247	0.19	0.41	0.27	0.02	0.03	C30-31
喉	Larynx	1 862	0.99	2.96	1.96	0.12	0.24	243	0.19	0.40	0.25	0.01	0.03	C32
气管、支气管、肺	Trachea, bronchus & lung	49 770	26.44	79.24	51.49	2.76	6.31	22 728	17.35	37.54	22.94	1.21	2.69	C33-34
其他胸腔器官	Other thoracic organs	642	0.34	1.02	0.72	0.05	0.08	427	0.33	0.71	0.49	0.03	0.05	C37-38
骨	Bone	1 460	0.78	2.32	1.70	0.10	0.18	1 070	0.82	1.77	1.29	0.08	0.13	C40-41
皮肤黑色素瘤	Melanoma of skin	284	0.15	0.45	0.31	0.02	0.04	249	0.19	0.41	0.27	0.02	0.03	C43
皮肤其他	Other skin	1 405	0.75	2.24	1.48	0.07	0.16	1 310	1.00	2.16	1.32	0.06	0.14	C44
间皮瘤	Mesothelioma	68	0.04	0.11	0.07	0.00	0.01	56	0.04	0.09	0.06	0.00	0.01	C45
卡波氏肉瘤	Kaposi sarcoma	25	0.01	0.04	0.03	0.00	0.00	9	0.01	0.01	0.01	0.00	0.00	C46
结缔组织、软组织	Connective & soft tissue	482	0.26	0.77	0.58	0.04	0.06	461	0.35	0.76	0.59	0.04	0.06	C47;C49
乳腺	Breast	341	0.18	0.54	0.36	0.02	0.04	17 960	13.71	29.67	20.27	1.69	2.13	C50
外阴	Vulva	—	—	—	—	—	—	292	0.22	0.48	0.31	0.02	0.03	C51
阴道	Vagina	—	—	—	—	—	—	183	0.14	0.30	0.19	0.01	0.02	C52
子宫颈	Cervix uteri	—	—	—	—	—	—	10 369	7.92	17.13	11.72	0.96	1.25	C53
子宫体	Corpus uteri	—	—	—	—	—	—	4 000	3.05	6.61	4.50	0.38	0.50	C54
子宫,部位不明	Uterus unspecified	—	—	—	—	—	—	988	0.75	1.63	1.10	0.08	0.12	C55
卵巢	Ovary	—	—	—	—	—	—	4 175	3.19	6.90	4.84	0.37	0.52	C56
其他女性生殖器	Other female genital organs	—	—	—	—	—	—	293	0.22	0.48	0.33	0.03	0.04	C57
胎盘	Placenta	—	—	—	—	—	—	54	0.04	0.09	0.08	0.01	0.01	C58
阴茎	Penis	503	0.27	0.80	0.53	0.03	0.06	—	—	—	—	—	—	C60
前列腺	Prostate	5 538	2.94	8.82	5.23	0.10	0.53	—	—	—	—	—	—	C61
睾丸	Testis	278	0.15	0.44	0.36	0.02	0.03	—	—	—	—	—	—	C62
其他男性生殖器	Other male genital organs	72	0.04	0.11	0.08	0.00	0.01	—	—	—	—	—	—	C63
肾	Kidney	1 768	0.94	2.81	1.93	0.12	0.22	1 125	0.86	1.86	1.25	0.08	0.14	C64
肾盂	Renal pelvis	235	0.12	0.37	0.25	0.01	0.03	183	0.14	0.30	0.18	0.01	0.02	C65
输尿管	Ureter	251	0.13	0.40	0.24	0.01	0.03	234	0.18	0.39	0.22	0.01	0.03	C66
膀胱	Bladder	4 692	2.49	7.47	4.71	0.20	0.52	1 235	0.94	2.04	1.20	0.05	0.13	C67
其他泌尿器官	Other urinary organs	60	0.03	0.10	0.06	0.00	0.01	40	0.03	0.07	0.04	0.00	0.01	C68
眼	Eye	111	0.06	0.18	0.16	0.01	0.01	104	0.08	0.17	0.14	0.01	0.01	C69
脑、神经系统	Brain, nervous system	4 143	2.20	6.60	5.01	0.32	0.51	4 363	3.33	7.21	5.13	0.33	0.55	C70-72, D32-33, D42-43
甲状腺	Thyroid	1 890	1.00	3.01	2.27	0.18	0.21	6 083	4.64	10.05	7.51	0.62	0.70	C73
肾上腺	Adrenal gland	111	0.06	0.18	0.13	0.01	0.01	95	0.07	0.16	0.13	0.01	0.01	C74
其他内分泌腺	Other endocrine	208	0.11	0.33	0.25	0.02	0.03	191	0.15	0.32	0.24	0.02	0.02	C75
霍奇金淋巴瘤	Hodgkin lymphoma	226	0.12	0.36	0.28	0.02	0.03	108	0.08	0.18	0.14	0.01	0.01	C81
非霍奇金淋巴瘤	Non-Hodgkin lymphoma	2 509	1.33	3.99	2.89	0.18	0.31	1 718	1.31	2.84	1.94	0.12	0.22	C82-C86;C96
免疫增生性疾病	Immunoproliferative diseases	44	0.02	0.07	0.06	0.00	0.00	29	0.02	0.05	0.04	0.00	0.00	C88
多发性骨髓瘤	Multiple myeloma	796	0.42	1.27	0.84	0.05	0.10	614	0.47	1.01	0.65	0.04	0.09	C90
淋巴样白血病	Lymphoid leukemia	679	0.36	1.08	1.06	0.06	0.08	464	0.35	0.77	0.75	0.04	0.06	C91
髓样白血病	Myeloid leukemia	1 416	0.75	2.25	1.76	0.11	0.17	1 111	0.85	1.84	1.42	0.09	0.14	C92-C94, D45-47
白血病,未特指	Leukemia unspecified	1 523	0.81	2.42	2.03	0.12	0.19	1 117	0.85	1.85	1.50	0.09	0.14	C95
其他或未指明部位	Other and unspecified	3 576	1.90	5.69	4.06	0.23	0.44	2 896	2.21	4.78	3.33	0.20	0.35	O&U
所有部位合计	All sites	188 232	100.00	299.70	199.25	11.18	23.37	130 982	100.00	216.37	141.56	9.07	15.66	C00-96, D32-33, D42-43, D45-47
所有部位除外 C44	All sites except C44	186 827	99.25	297.46	197.77	11.11	23.21	129 672	99.00	214.20	140.24	9.01	15.52	C00-96, D32-33, D42-43, D45-47 exc. C44

附表 2-8 2017 年全国西部城市肿瘤登记地区癌症发病主要指标

Appendix Table 2-8 Cancer incidence in Western urban registration areas of China, 2017

部位 Site		男性 Male						女性 Female						ICD10
		病例数 No. cases	构成 Freq./%	粗率 Crude rate/ $100\,000^{-1}$	世标率 ASR world/ $100\,000^{-1}$	累积率 Cum. rate/% 0~64	0~74	病例数 No. cases	构成 Freq./%	粗率 Crude rate/ $100\,000^{-1}$	世标率 ASR world/ $100\,000^{-1}$	累积率 Cum. rate/% 0~64	0~74	
唇	Lip	64	0.07	0.21	0.14	0.01	0.01	54	0.08	0.19	0.12	0.01	0.01	C00
舌	Tongue	242	0.27	0.81	0.55	0.03	0.07	135	0.20	0.46	0.30	0.02	0.04	C01-02
口	Mouth	395	0.43	1.32	0.88	0.05	0.10	211	0.32	0.73	0.46	0.02	0.05	C03-06
唾液腺	Salivary glands	188	0.21	0.63	0.45	0.03	0.05	108	0.16	0.37	0.27	0.02	0.03	C07-08
扁桃腺	Tonsil	78	0.09	0.26	0.17	0.01	0.02	30	0.05	0.10	0.07	0.01	0.01	C09
其他口咽	Other oropharynx	159	0.17	0.53	0.36	0.02	0.04	25	0.04	0.09	0.06	0.00	0.01	C10
鼻咽	Nasopharynx	1 775	1.95	5.95	4.16	0.33	0.45	760	1.14	2.61	1.80	0.14	0.20	C11
下咽	Hypopharynx	237	0.26	0.79	0.54	0.04	0.07	13	0.02	0.04	0.03	0.00	0.00	C12-13
咽,部位不明	Pharynx unspecified	148	0.16	0.50	0.34	0.02	0.04	37	0.06	0.13	0.08	0.01	0.01	C14
食管	Esophagus	7 478	8.20	25.08	16.76	0.84	2.17	2 094	3.14	7.20	4.31	0.16	0.52	C15
胃	Stomach	9 261	10.16	31.06	20.63	1.12	2.55	3 870	5.81	13.30	8.31	0.44	0.95	C16
小肠	Small intestine	367	0.40	1.23	0.83	0.05	0.10	286	0.43	0.98	0.62	0.04	0.07	C17
结肠	Colon	4 276	4.69	14.34	9.44	0.48	1.11	3 211	4.82	11.04	6.82	0.35	0.78	C18
直肠	Rectum	5 552	6.09	18.62	12.32	0.62	1.50	3 452	5.18	11.87	7.37	0.39	0.86	C19-20
肛门	Anus	164	0.18	0.55	0.36	0.02	0.04	93	0.14	0.32	0.20	0.01	0.02	C21
肝脏	Liver	13 295	14.58	44.59	30.29	2.02	3.49	4 365	6.55	15.01	9.35	0.49	1.06	C22
胆囊及其他	Gallbladder etc.	931	1.02	3.12	2.04	0.10	0.23	1 190	1.79	4.09	2.46	0.11	0.28	C23-24
胰腺	Pancreas	2 189	2.40	7.34	4.81	0.25	0.55	1 536	2.31	5.28	3.19	0.15	0.37	C25
鼻、鼻窦及其他	Nose, sinuses etc.	178	0.20	0.60	0.41	0.03	0.05	114	0.17	0.39	0.25	0.02	0.03	C30-31
喉	Larynx	1 044	1.14	3.50	2.35	0.13	0.29	114	0.17	0.39	0.25	0.01	0.03	C32
气管、支气管、肺	Trachea, bronchus & lung	23 989	26.31	80.46	53.34	2.75	6.59	10 820	16.24	37.20	22.92	1.18	2.67	C33-34
其他胸腔器官	Other thoracic organs	341	0.37	1.14	0.82	0.05	0.10	223	0.33	0.77	0.54	0.04	0.06	C37-38
骨	Bone	671	0.74	2.25	1.63	0.09	0.17	498	0.75	1.71	1.23	0.07	0.13	C40-41
皮肤黑色素瘤	Melanoma of skin	149	0.16	0.50	0.35	0.02	0.04	121	0.18	0.42	0.26	0.01	0.03	C43
皮肤其他	Other skin	725	0.80	2.43	1.64	0.08	0.18	686	1.03	2.36	1.42	0.07	0.14	C44
间皮瘤	Mesothelioma	39	0.04	0.13	0.09	0.01	0.01	30	0.05	0.10	0.07	0.00	0.01	C45
卡波氏肉瘤	Kaposi sarcoma	11	0.01	0.04	0.03	0.00	0.00	2	0.00	0.01	0.00	0.00	0.00	C46
结缔组织、软组织	Connective & soft tissue	267	0.29	0.90	0.65	0.04	0.06	243	0.36	0.84	0.66	0.04	0.06	C47;C49
乳腺	Breast	189	0.21	0.63	0.43	0.03	0.05	9 943	14.93	34.18	23.15	1.89	2.47	C50
外阴	Vulva	—	—	—	—	—	—	142	0.21	0.49	0.32	0.02	0.04	C51
阴道	Vagina	—	—	—	—	—	—	98	0.15	0.34	0.22	0.01	0.03	C52
子宫颈	Cervix uteri	—	—	—	—	—	—	5 095	7.65	17.52	11.97	0.98	1.27	C53
子宫体	Corpus uteri	—	—	—	—	—	—	2 165	3.25	7.44	5.08	0.43	0.57	C54
子宫,部位不明	Uterus unspecified	—	—	—	—	—	—	422	0.63	1.45	0.98	0.07	0.10	C55
卵巢	Ovary	—	—	—	—	—	—	2 344	3.52	8.06	5.64	0.43	0.61	C56
其他女性生殖器	Other female genital organs	—	—	—	—	—	—	158	0.24	0.54	0.38	0.03	0.04	C57
胎盘	Placenta	—	—	—	—	—	—	26	0.04	0.09	0.08	0.01	0.01	C58
阴茎	Penis	245	0.27	0.82	0.55	0.03	0.07	—	—	—	—	—	—	C60
前列腺	Prostate	3 424	3.75	11.48	6.95	0.14	0.69	—	—	—	—	—	—	C61
睾丸	Testis	141	0.15	0.47	0.38	0.03	0.03	—	—	—	—	—	—	C62
其他男性生殖器	Other male genital organs	45	0.05	0.15	0.10	0.00	0.01	—	—	—	—	—	—	C63
肾	Kidney	1 090	1.20	3.66	2.50	0.16	0.28	661	0.99	2.27	1.52	0.10	0.17	C64
肾盂	Renal pelvis	132	0.14	0.44	0.30	0.02	0.04	116	0.17	0.40	0.24	0.01	0.03	C65
输尿管	Ureter	161	0.18	0.54	0.33	0.02	0.03	147	0.22	0.51	0.29	0.01	0.03	C66
膀胱	Bladder	2 513	2.76	8.43	5.42	0.22	0.60	677	1.02	2.33	1.37	0.05	0.15	C67
其他泌尿器官	Other urinary organs	29	0.03	0.10	0.06	0.00	0.01	20	0.03	0.07	0.04	0.00	0.01	C68
眼	Eye	55	0.06	0.18	0.17	0.01	0.02	45	0.07	0.15	0.14	0.01	0.01	C69
脑、神经系统	Brain, nervous system	1 931	2.12	6.48	4.90	0.32	0.50	2 146	3.22	7.38	5.27	0.34	0.55	C70-72, D32-33, D42-43
甲状腺	Thyroid	1 182	1.30	3.96	2.93	0.23	0.28	3 715	5.58	12.77	9.34	0.78	0.88	C73
肾上腺	Adrenal gland	59	0.06	0.20	0.14	0.01	0.01	52	0.08	0.18	0.15	0.01	0.01	C74
其他内分泌腺	Other endocrine	98	0.11	0.33	0.25	0.02	0.03	101	0.15	0.35	0.25	0.02	0.02	C75
霍奇金淋巴瘤	Hodgkin lymphoma	118	0.13	0.40	0.31	0.02	0.03	59	0.09	0.20	0.18	0.01	0.02	C81
非霍奇金淋巴瘤	Non-Hodgkin lymphoma	1 356	1.49	4.55	3.28	0.20	0.34	944	1.42	3.25	2.22	0.13	0.25	C82-C86;C96
免疫增生性疾病	Immunoproliferative diseases	31	0.03	0.10	0.09	0.01	0.01	25	0.04	0.09	0.07	0.00	0.01	C88
多发性骨髓瘤	Multiple myeloma	445	0.49	1.49	1.01	0.05	0.12	366	0.55	1.26	0.81	0.04	0.11	C90
淋巴样白血病	Lymphoid leukemia	374	0.41	1.25	1.20	0.06	0.10	243	0.36	0.84	0.82	0.05	0.06	C91
髓样白血病	Myeloid leukemia	805	0.88	2.70	2.09	0.13	0.20	603	0.91	2.07	1.60	0.10	0.16	C92-C94, D45-47
白血病,未特指	Leukemia unspecified	675	0.74	2.26	1.87	0.10	0.18	524	0.79	1.80	1.50	0.08	0.14	C95
其他或未指明部位	Other and unspecified	1 883	2.06	6.32	4.58	0.25	0.50	1 459	2.19	5.02	3.50	0.20	0.37	O&U
所有部位合计	All sites	91 194	100.00	305.86	206.23	11.29	24.19	66 617	100.00	229.02	150.54	9.60	16.57	C00-96, D32-33, D42-43, D45-47
所有部位除外 C44	All sites except C44	90 469	99.20	303.43	204.59	11.22	24.02	65 931	98.97	226.66	149.12	9.53	16.43	C00-96, D32-33, D42-43, D45-47 exc. C44

附表 2-9　2017 年全国西部农村肿瘤登记地区癌症发病主要指标
Appendix Table 2-9　Cancer incidence in Western rural registration areas of China, 2017

部位 Site		男性 Male						女性 Female						ICD10
		病例数 No. cases	构成 Freq. /%	粗率 Crude rate/ 100 000⁻¹	世标率 ASR world/ 100 000⁻¹	累积率 Cum. rate/% 0~64	累积率 Cum. rate/% 0~74	病例数 No. cases	构成 Freq. /%	粗率 Crude rate/ 100 000⁻¹	世标率 ASR world/ 100 000⁻¹	累积率 Cum. rate/% 0~64	累积率 Cum. rate/% 0~74	
唇	Lip	64	0.07	0.19	0.13	0.01	0.01	36	0.06	0.11	0.07	0.00	0.01	C00
舌	Tongue	313	0.32	0.95	0.61	0.04	0.07	138	0.21	0.44	0.30	0.02	0.03	C01-02
口	Mouth	431	0.44	1.31	0.85	0.05	0.10	230	0.36	0.73	0.48	0.03	0.05	C03-06
唾液腺	Salivary glands	161	0.17	0.49	0.34	0.02	0.04	118	0.18	0.38	0.26	0.02	0.03	C07-08
扁桃腺	Tonsil	67	0.07	0.20	0.14	0.01	0.02	27	0.04	0.09	0.06	0.00	0.01	C09
其他口咽	Other oropharynx	167	0.17	0.51	0.33	0.02	0.04	29	0.05	0.09	0.06	0.00	0.01	C10
鼻咽	Nasopharynx	2 040	2.10	6.18	4.32	0.34	0.46	888	1.38	2.82	1.96	0.15	0.21	C11
下咽	Hypopharynx	198	0.20	0.60	0.41	0.03	0.05	26	0.04	0.08	0.06	0.00	0.01	C12-13
咽,部位不明	Pharynx unspecified	187	0.19	0.57	0.37	0.02	0.04	63	0.10	0.20	0.13	0.01	0.02	C14
食管	Esophagus	11 904	12.27	36.08	23.01	1.16	2.98	3 338	5.19	10.61	6.14	0.23	0.76	C15
胃	Stomach	10 499	10.82	31.82	20.35	1.08	2.53	4 349	6.76	13.83	8.28	0.41	0.94	C16
小肠	Small intestine	319	0.33	0.97	0.64	0.04	0.08	216	0.34	0.69	0.44	0.03	0.06	C17
结肠	Colon	2 959	3.05	8.97	5.83	0.33	0.68	2 180	3.39	6.93	4.35	0.25	0.51	C18
直肠	Rectum	5 754	5.93	17.44	11.15	0.58	1.33	3 674	5.71	11.68	7.22	0.40	0.85	C19-20
肛门	Anus	185	0.19	0.56	0.36	0.02	0.05	127	0.20	0.40	0.25	0.01	0.03	C21
肝脏	Liver	15 896	16.38	48.18	32.30	2.24	3.67	4 864	7.56	15.47	9.56	0.54	1.12	C22
胆囊及其他	Gallbladder etc.	858	0.88	2.60	1.66	0.09	0.20	1 004	1.56	3.19	1.93	0.10	0.24	C23-24
胰腺	Pancreas	2 077	2.14	6.30	4.04	0.22	0.47	1 381	2.15	4.39	2.63	0.13	0.32	C25
鼻、鼻窦及其他	Nose, sinuses etc.	208	0.21	0.63	0.43	0.03	0.05	133	0.21	0.42	0.29	0.02	0.03	C30-31
喉	Larynx	818	0.84	2.48	1.62	0.10	0.20	129	0.20	0.41	0.26	0.01	0.03	C32
气管、支气管、肺	Trachea, bronchus & lung	25 781	26.57	78.14	50.02	2.77	6.08	11 908	18.50	37.87	22.98	1.23	2.72	C33-34
其他胸腔器官	Other thoracic organs	301	0.31	0.91	0.65	0.04	0.07	204	0.32	0.65	0.43	0.03	0.05	C37-38
骨	Bone	789	0.81	2.39	1.76	0.10	0.19	572	0.89	1.82	1.35	0.08	0.14	C40-41
皮肤黑色素瘤	Melanoma of skin	135	0.14	0.41	0.28	0.02	0.03	128	0.20	0.41	0.28	0.02	0.03	C43
皮肤其他	Other skin	680	0.70	2.06	1.34	0.07	0.14	624	0.97	1.98	1.23	0.06	0.13	C44
间皮瘤	Mesothelioma	29	0.03	0.09	0.06	0.00	0.01	26	0.04	0.08	0.06	0.00	0.01	C45
卡波氏肉瘤	Kaposi sarcoma	14	0.01	0.04	0.03	0.00	0.00	7	0.01	0.02	0.02	0.00	0.00	C46
结缔组织、软组织	Connective & soft tissue	215	0.22	0.65	0.50	0.03	0.05	218	0.34	0.69	0.53	0.04	0.05	C47;C49
乳腺	Breast	152	0.16	0.46	0.30	0.02	0.03	8 017	12.46	25.49	17.67	1.51	1.81	C50
外阴	Vulva	—	—	—	—	—	—	150	0.23	0.48	0.31	0.02	0.03	C51
阴道	Vagina	—	—	—	—	—	—	85	0.13	0.27	0.17	0.01	0.02	C52
子宫颈	Cervix uteri	—	—	—	—	—	—	5 274	8.19	16.77	11.49	0.94	1.23	C53
子宫体	Corpus uteri	—	—	—	—	—	—	1 835	2.85	5.83	3.97	0.33	0.44	C54
子宫,部位不明	Uterus unspecified	—	—	—	—	—	—	566	0.88	1.80	1.21	0.09	0.14	C55
卵巢	Ovary	—	—	—	—	—	—	1 831	2.84	5.82	4.10	0.32	0.44	C56
其他女性生殖器	Other female genital organs	—	—	—	—	—	—	135	0.21	0.43	0.29	0.02	0.03	C57
胎盘	Placenta	—	—	—	—	—	—	28	0.04	0.09	0.09	0.01	0.01	C58
阴茎	Penis	258	0.27	0.78	0.52	0.03	0.06	—	—	—	—	—	—	C60
前列腺	Prostate	2 114	2.18	6.41	3.73	0.07	0.39	—	—	—	—	—	—	C61
睾丸	Testis	137	0.14	0.42	0.35	0.02	0.03	—	—	—	—	—	—	C62
其他男性生殖器	Other male genital organs	27	0.03	0.08	0.06	0.00	0.01	—	—	—	—	—	—	C63
肾	Kidney	678	0.70	2.06	1.44	0.09	0.16	464	0.72	1.48	1.00	0.06	0.11	C64
肾盂	Renal pelvis	103	0.11	0.31	0.20	0.01	0.02	67	0.10	0.21	0.13	0.01	0.01	C65
输尿管	Ureter	90	0.09	0.27	0.17	0.01	0.02	87	0.14	0.28	0.16	0.01	0.02	C66
膀胱	Bladder	2 179	2.25	6.60	4.09	0.18	0.45	558	0.87	1.77	1.04	0.05	0.12	C67
其他泌尿器官	Other urinary organs	31	0.03	0.09	0.06	0.00	0.01	20	0.03	0.06	0.04	0.00	0.01	C68
眼	Eye	56	0.06	0.17	0.16	0.01	0.01	59	0.09	0.19	0.15	0.01	0.02	C69
脑、神经系统	Brain, nervous system	2 212	2.28	6.70	5.11	0.33	0.51	2 217	3.44	7.05	5.02	0.33	0.54	C70-72, D32-33, D42-43
甲状腺	Thyroid	708	0.73	2.15	1.64	0.13	0.16	2 368	3.68	7.53	5.75	0.47	0.53	C73
肾上腺	Adrenal gland	52	0.05	0.16	0.11	0.01	0.01	43	0.07	0.14	0.11	0.01	0.01	C74
其他内分泌腺	Other endocrine	110	0.11	0.33	0.25	0.02	0.03	90	0.14	0.29	0.23	0.02	0.02	C75
霍奇金淋巴瘤	Hodgkin lymphoma	108	0.11	0.33	0.27	0.02	0.03	49	0.08	0.16	0.11	0.01	0.01	C81
非霍奇金淋巴瘤	Non-Hodgkin lymphoma	1 153	1.19	3.49	2.54	0.16	0.27	774	1.20	2.46	1.69	0.11	0.19	C82-C86;C96
免疫增生性疾病	Immunoproliferative diseases	13	0.01	0.04	0.03	0.00	0.00	4	0.01	0.01	0.01	0.00	0.00	C88
多发性骨髓瘤	Multiple myeloma	351	0.36	1.06	0.70	0.04	0.09	248	0.39	0.79	0.51	0.03	0.07	C90
淋巴样白血病	Lymphoid leukemia	305	0.31	0.92	0.95	0.05	0.07	221	0.34	0.70	0.69	0.04	0.06	C91
髓样白血病	Myeloid leukemia	611	0.63	1.85	1.48	0.09	0.14	508	0.79	1.62	1.27	0.08	0.13	C92-C94, D45-47
白血病,未特指	Leukemia unspecified	848	0.87	2.57	2.17	0.13	0.19	593	0.92	1.89	1.50	0.09	0.14	C95
其他或未指明部位	Other and unspecified	1 693	1.74	5.13	3.62	0.21	0.39	1 437	2.23	4.57	3.19	0.20	0.34	O&U
所有部位合计	All sites	97 038	100.00	294.13	193.46	11.10	22.70	64 365	100.00	204.67	133.49	8.59	14.84	C00-96, D32-33, D42-43, D45-47
所有部位除外 C44	All sites except C44	96 358	99.30	292.07	192.12	11.04	22.57	63 741	99.03	202.68	132.25	8.53	14.71	C00-96, D32-33, D42-43, D45-47 exc. C44

附表 2-10　2017 年全国东部肿瘤登记地区癌症死亡主要指标

Appendix Table 2-10　Cancer mortality in Eastern registration areas of China, 2017

部位 Site		男性 Male						女性 Female						ICD10
		死亡数 No. deaths	构成 Freq. /%	粗率 Crude rate/ 100 000⁻¹	世标率 ASR world/ 100 000⁻¹	累积率 Cum. rate/% 0~64	累积率 Cum. rate/% 0~74	死亡数 No. deaths	构成 Freq. /%	粗率 Crude rate/ 100 000⁻¹	世标率 ASR world/ 100 000⁻¹	累积率 Cum. rate/% 0~64	累积率 Cum. rate/% 0~74	
唇	Lip	113	0. 05	0. 11	0. 06	0. 00	0. 01	49	0. 03	0. 05	0. 02	0. 00	0. 00	C00
舌	Tongue	705	0. 29	0. 71	0. 41	0. 02	0. 05	329	0. 23	0. 33	0. 16	0. 01	0. 02	C01-02
口	Mouth	708	0. 29	0. 71	0. 39	0. 02	0. 05	484	0. 34	0. 49	0. 23	0. 01	0. 02	C03-06
唾液腺	Salivary glands	302	0. 13	0. 30	0. 17	0. 01	0. 02	132	0. 09	0. 13	0. 07	0. 00	0. 01	C07-08
扁桃腺	Tonsil	125	0. 05	0. 13	0. 07	0. 00	0. 01	26	0. 02	0. 03	0. 01	0. 00	0. 00	C09
其他口咽	Other oropharynx	248	0. 10	0. 25	0. 14	0. 01	0. 02	53	0. 04	0. 05	0. 03	0. 00	0. 00	C10
鼻咽	Nasopharynx	2 852	1. 18	2. 87	1. 76	0. 12	0. 21	956	0. 68	0. 97	0. 55	0. 03	0. 06	C11
下咽	Hypopharynx	617	0. 26	0. 62	0. 36	0. 03	0. 04	45	0. 03	0. 05	0. 02	0. 00	0. 00	C12-13
咽,部位不明	Pharynx unspecified	255	0. 11	0. 26	0. 14	0. 01	0. 02	72	0. 05	0. 07	0. 03	0. 00	0. 00	C14
食管	Esophagus	22 819	9. 48	22. 93	12. 42	0. 51	1. 48	8 720	6. 17	8. 86	3. 83	0. 09	0. 41	C15
胃	Stomach	31 465	13. 07	31. 62	16. 98	0. 64	1. 94	13 579	9. 61	13. 80	6. 52	0. 25	0. 69	C16
小肠	Small intestine	1 025	0. 43	1. 03	0. 57	0. 02	0. 06	696	0. 49	0. 71	0. 34	0. 02	0. 04	C17
结肠	Colon	9 147	3. 80	9. 19	4. 89	0. 19	0. 51	7 314	5. 17	7. 43	3. 37	0. 13	0. 33	C18
直肠	Rectum	9 479	3. 94	9. 53	5. 08	0. 20	0. 54	6 065	4. 29	6. 16	2. 84	0. 12	0. 28	C19-20
肛门	Anus	182	0. 08	0. 18	0. 10	0. 00	0. 01	161	0. 11	0. 16	0. 07	0. 00	0. 01	C21
肝脏	Liver	34 611	14. 37	34. 78	20. 50	1. 31	2. 37	12 659	8. 96	12. 86	6. 36	0. 29	0. 72	C22
胆囊及其他	Gallbladder etc.	3 617	1. 50	3. 63	1. 95	0. 08	0. 22	3 855	2. 73	3. 92	1. 79	0. 07	0. 19	C23-24
胰腺	Pancreas	9 205	3. 82	9. 25	5. 07	0. 23	0. 59	7 180	5. 08	7. 30	3. 44	0. 13	0. 39	C25
鼻、鼻窦及其他	Nose, sinuses etc.	299	0. 12	0. 30	0. 18	0. 01	0. 02	157	0. 11	0. 16	0. 08	0. 01	0. 01	C30-31
喉	Larynx	1 874	0. 78	1. 88	1. 03	0. 05	0. 12	377	0. 27	0. 38	0. 18	0. 01	0. 02	C32
气管、支气管、肺	Trachea, bronchus & lung	71 952	29. 88	72. 31	39. 22	1. 58	4. 65	33 485	23. 69	34. 03	16. 03	0. 63	1. 75	C33-34
其他胸腔器官	Other thoracic organs	728	0. 30	0. 73	0. 44	0. 02	0. 05	420	0. 30	0. 43	0. 24	0. 01	0. 02	C37-38
骨	Bone	1 485	0. 62	1. 49	0. 93	0. 04	0. 10	1 151	0. 81	1. 17	0. 67	0. 03	0. 07	C40-41
皮肤黑色素瘤	Melanoma of skin	453	0. 19	0. 46	0. 28	0. 01	0. 03	400	0. 28	0. 41	0. 23	0. 01	0. 02	C43
皮肤其他	Other skin	860	0. 36	0. 86	0. 44	0. 01	0. 03	697	0. 49	0. 71	0. 28	0. 01	0. 02	C44
间皮瘤	Mesothelioma	204	0. 08	0. 21	0. 12	0. 01	0. 01	139	0. 10	0. 14	0. 08	0. 00	0. 01	C45
卡波氏肉瘤	Kaposi sarcoma	571	0. 24	0. 57	0. 32	0. 01	0. 03	335	0. 24	0. 34	0. 17	0. 01	0. 02	C46
结缔组织、软组织	Connective & soft tissue	545	0. 23	0. 55	0. 37	0. 02	0. 03	368	0. 26	0. 37	0. 23	0. 01	0. 02	C47;C49
乳腺	Breast	157	0. 07	0. 16	0. 09	0. 00	0. 01	11 290	7. 99	11. 47	6. 41	0. 44	0. 71	C50
外阴	Vulva	—	—	—	—	—	—	192	0. 14	0. 20	0. 09	0. 00	0. 01	C51
阴道	Vagina	—	—	—	—	—	—	101	0. 07	0. 10	0. 05	0. 00	0. 01	C52
子宫颈	Cervix uteri	—	—	—	—	—	—	4 636	3. 28	4. 71	2. 71	0. 19	0. 30	C53
子宫体	Corpus uteri	—	—	—	—	—	—	1 644	1. 16	1. 67	0. 91	0. 06	0. 11	C54
子宫,部位不明	Uterus unspecified	—	—	—	—	—	—	831	0. 59	0. 84	0. 45	0. 03	0. 05	C55
卵巢	Ovary	—	—	—	—	—	—	4 208	2. 98	4. 28	2. 42	0. 16	0. 29	C56
其他女性生殖器	Other female genital organs	—	—	—	—	—	—	218	0. 15	0. 22	0. 11	0. 01	0. 01	C57
胎盘	Placenta	—	—	—	—	—	—	4	0. 00	0. 00	0. 00	0. 00	0. 00	C58
阴茎	Penis	253	0. 11	0. 25	0. 14	0. 01	0. 01	—	—	—	—	—	—	C60
前列腺	Prostate	6 155	2. 56	6. 19	2. 94	0. 03	0. 21	—	—	—	—	—	—	C61
睾丸	Testis	133	0. 06	0. 13	0. 09	0. 00	0. 01	—	—	—	—	—	—	C62
其他男性生殖器	Other male genital organs	67	0. 03	0. 07	0. 04	0. 00	0. 00	—	—	—	—	—	—	C63
肾	Kidney	2 385	0. 99	2. 40	1. 35	0. 06	0. 14	1 231	0. 87	1. 25	0. 61	0. 03	0. 06	C64
肾盂	Renal pelvis	271	0. 11	0. 27	0. 15	0. 01	0. 02	201	0. 14	0. 20	0. 09	0. 00	0. 01	C65
输尿管	Ureter	394	0. 16	0. 40	0. 21	0. 01	0. 02	351	0. 25	0. 36	0. 15	0. 00	0. 01	C66
膀胱	Bladder	4 836	2. 01	4. 86	2. 37	0. 05	0. 19	1 302	0. 92	1. 32	0. 52	0. 01	0. 04	C67
其他泌尿器官	Other urinary organs	97	0. 04	0. 10	0. 05	0. 00	0. 00	54	0. 04	0. 05	0. 02	0. 00	0. 00	C68
眼	Eye	71	0. 03	0. 07	0. 06	0. 00	0. 00	41	0. 03	0. 04	0. 03	0. 00	0. 00	C69
脑、神经系统	Brain, nervous system	4 402	1. 83	4. 42	2. 92	0. 17	0. 31	3 684	2. 61	3. 74	2. 23	0. 13	0. 23	C70-72, D32-33, D42-43
甲状腺	Thyroid	512	0. 21	0. 51	0. 28	0. 01	0. 03	799	0. 57	0. 81	0. 41	0. 02	0. 05	C73
肾上腺	Adrenal gland	198	0. 08	0. 20	0. 14	0. 01	0. 01	123	0. 09	0. 12	0. 08	0. 00	0. 01	C74
其他内分泌腺	Other endocrine	122	0. 05	0. 12	0. 08	0. 00	0. 01	85	0. 06	0. 09	0. 05	0. 00	0. 01	C75
霍奇金淋巴瘤	Hodgkin lymphoma	196	0. 08	0. 20	0. 12	0. 01	0. 01	127	0. 09	0. 13	0. 07	0. 00	0. 01	C81
非霍奇金淋巴瘤	Non-Hodgkin lymphoma	3 694	1. 53	3. 71	2. 16	0. 10	0. 24	2 464	1. 74	2. 50	1. 27	0. 06	0. 14	C82-C86;C96
免疫增生性疾病	Immunoproliferative diseases	33	0. 01	0. 03	0. 02	0. 00	0. 00	14	0. 01	0. 01	0. 01	0. 00	0. 00	C88
多发性骨髓瘤	Multiple myeloma	1 409	0. 59	1. 42	0. 78	0. 03	0. 10	1 015	0. 72	1. 03	0. 53	0. 02	0. 07	C90
淋巴样白血病	Lymphoid leukemia	1 046	0. 43	1. 05	0. 82	0. 04	0. 07	763	0. 54	0. 78	0. 55	0. 03	0. 05	C91
髓样白血病	Myeloid leukemia	1 783	0. 74	1. 79	1. 13	0. 06	0. 12	1 342	0. 95	1. 36	0. 84	0. 05	0. 09	C92-C94,D45-47
白血病,未特指	Leukemia unspecified	1 882	0. 78	1. 89	1. 28	0. 07	0. 12	1 355	0. 96	1. 38	0. 87	0. 05	0. 09	C95
其他或未指明部位	Other and unspecified	4 266	1. 77	4. 29	2. 44	0. 11	0. 26	3 379	2. 39	3. 43	1. 71	0. 08	0. 17	O&U
所有部位合计	All sites	240 808	100. 00	242. 00	134. 04	5. 96	15. 12	141 358	100. 00	143. 65	71. 08	3. 26	7. 64	C00-96, D32-33, D42-43, D45-47
所有部位除外 C44	All sites except C44	239 948	99. 64	241. 13	133. 60	5. 95	15. 08	140 661	99. 51	142. 94	70. 80	3. 25	7. 62	C00-96, D32-33, D42-43, D45-47 exc. C44

附表 2-11　2017 年全国东部城市肿瘤登记地区癌症死亡主要指标

Appendix Table 2-11　Cancer mortality in Eastern urban registration areas of China, 2017

部位 Site		男性 Male						女性 Female						ICD10
		死亡数 No. deaths	构成 Freq. /%	粗率 Crude rate/ 100 000^{-1}	世标率 ASR world/ 100 000^{-1}	累积率 Cum. rate/% 0~64	累积率 Cum. rate/% 0~74	死亡数 No. deaths	构成 Freq. /%	粗率 Crude rate/ 100 000^{-1}	世标率 ASR world/ 100 000^{-1}	累积率 Cum. rate/% 0~64	累积率 Cum. rate/% 0~74	
唇	Lip	30	0.02	0.05	0.03	0.00	0.00	22	0.03	0.04	0.01	0.00	0.00	C00
舌	Tongue	405	0.30	0.73	0.40	0.03	0.05	207	0.26	0.37	0.17	0.01	0.02	C01-02
口	Mouth	422	0.31	0.76	0.41	0.02	0.05	280	0.35	0.50	0.22	0.01	0.02	C03-06
唾液腺	Salivary glands	187	0.14	0.34	0.18	0.01	0.02	87	0.11	0.16	0.08	0.00	0.01	C07-08
扁桃腺	Tonsil	81	0.06	0.15	0.08	0.00	0.01	22	0.03	0.04	0.02	0.00	0.00	C09
其他口咽	Other oropharynx	140	0.10	0.25	0.14	0.01	0.02	28	0.03	0.05	0.03	0.00	0.00	C10
鼻咽	Nasopharynx	1 724	1.28	3.11	1.88	0.13	0.22	541	0.67	0.97	0.54	0.03	0.06	C11
下咽	Hypopharynx	382	0.28	0.69	0.39	0.03	0.05	21	0.03	0.04	0.02	0.00	0.00	C12-13
咽,部位不明	Pharynx unspecified	149	0.11	0.27	0.14	0.01	0.02	42	0.05	0.08	0.03	0.00	0.00	C14
食管	Esophagus	10 062	7.47	18.15	9.62	0.44	1.16	3 261	4.03	5.85	2.40	0.05	0.24	C15
胃	Stomach	15 774	11.71	28.45	14.73	0.56	1.66	6 919	8.56	12.40	5.70	0.23	0.58	C16
小肠	Small intestine	631	0.47	1.14	0.61	0.03	0.07	449	0.56	0.80	0.37	0.01	0.04	C17
结肠	Colon	6 378	4.74	11.50	5.86	0.22	0.60	5 154	6.38	9.24	4.00	0.16	0.38	C18
直肠	Rectum	5 841	4.34	10.54	5.41	0.22	0.58	3 557	4.40	6.38	2.84	0.12	0.28	C19-20
肛门	Anus	110	0.08	0.20	0.11	0.00	0.01	92	0.11	0.16	0.07	0.00	0.01	C21
肝脏	Liver	18 673	13.86	33.68	19.30	1.23	2.24	6 872	8.50	12.32	5.85	0.26	0.65	C22
胆囊及其他	Gallbladder etc.	2 205	1.64	3.98	2.06	0.08	0.23	2 338	2.89	4.19	1.85	0.07	0.19	C23-24
胰腺	Pancreas	5 622	4.17	10.14	5.39	0.25	0.63	4 417	5.46	7.92	3.61	0.13	0.41	C25
鼻、鼻窦及其他	Nose, sinuses etc.	187	0.14	0.34	0.19	0.01	0.02	86	0.11	0.15	0.08	0.00	0.01	C30-31
喉	Larynx	1 115	0.83	2.01	1.06	0.05	0.12	228	0.28	0.41	0.18	0.01	0.02	C32
气管、支气管、肺	Trachea, bronchus & lung	40 579	30.13	73.20	38.32	1.54	4.50	19 067	23.59	34.18	15.40	0.59	1.64	C33-34
其他胸腔器官	Other thoracic organs	495	0.37	0.89	0.52	0.03	0.06	286	0.35	0.51	0.28	0.01	0.03	C37-38
骨	Bone	740	0.55	1.33	0.80	0.04	0.08	551	0.68	0.99	0.54	0.03	0.05	C40-41
皮肤黑色素瘤	Melanoma of skin	261	0.19	0.47	0.28	0.01	0.03	211	0.26	0.38	0.21	0.01	0.02	C43
皮肤其他	Other skin	515	0.38	0.93	0.45	0.01	0.04	359	0.44	0.64	0.24	0.01	0.01	C44
间皮瘤	Mesothelioma	145	0.11	0.26	0.14	0.01	0.02	99	0.12	0.18	0.09	0.00	0.01	C45
卡波氏肉瘤	Kaposi sarcoma	380	0.28	0.69	0.35	0.01	0.04	222	0.27	0.40	0.18	0.01	0.02	C46
结缔组织、软组织	Connective & soft tissue	370	0.27	0.67	0.43	0.02	0.04	237	0.29	0.42	0.26	0.01	0.02	C47;C49
乳腺	Breast	97	0.07	0.17	0.09	0.00	0.01	7 116	8.80	12.76	6.87	0.46	0.76	C50
外阴	Vulva	—	—	—	—	—	—	111	0.14	0.20	0.08	0.00	0.01	C51
阴道	Vagina	—	—	—	—	—	—	66	0.08	0.12	0.06	0.00	0.01	C52
子宫颈	Cervix uteri	—	—	—	—	—	—	2 477	3.06	4.44	2.56	0.19	0.28	C53
子宫体	Corpus uteri	—	—	—	—	—	—	1 039	1.29	1.86	0.99	0.06	0.12	C54
子宫,部位不明	Uterus unspecified	—	—	—	—	—	—	432	0.53	0.77	0.42	0.03	0.05	C55
卵巢	Ovary	—	—	—	—	—	—	2 619	3.24	4.69	2.60	0.16	0.31	C56
其他女性生殖器	Other female genital organs	—	—	—	—	—	—	142	0.18	0.25	0.12	0.01	0.01	C57
胎盘	Placenta	—	—	—	—	—	—	1	0.00	0.00	0.00	0.00	0.00	C58
阴茎	Penis	128	0.10	0.23	0.12	0.01	0.01	—	—	—	—	—	—	C60
前列腺	Prostate	4 017	2.98	7.25	3.23	0.04	0.22	—	—	—	—	—	—	C61
睾丸	Testis	86	0.06	0.16	0.10	0.01	0.01	—	—	—	—	—	—	C62
其他男性生殖器	Other male genital organs	49	0.04	0.09	0.05	0.00	0.01	—	—	—	—	—	—	C63
肾	Kidney	1 658	1.23	2.99	1.61	0.08	0.17	799	0.99	1.43	0.66	0.03	0.07	C64
肾盂	Renal pelvis	184	0.14	0.33	0.17	0.01	0.02	140	0.17	0.25	0.10	0.00	0.01	C65
输尿管	Ureter	275	0.20	0.50	0.25	0.01	0.03	260	0.32	0.47	0.18	0.00	0.02	C66
膀胱	Bladder	3 013	2.24	5.43	2.50	0.05	0.20	852	1.05	1.53	0.56	0.01	0.04	C67
其他泌尿器官	Other urinary organs	72	0.05	0.13	0.06	0.00	0.01	46	0.06	0.08	0.03	0.00	0.00	C68
眼	Eye	41	0.03	0.07	0.05	0.00	0.00	23	0.03	0.04	0.03	0.00	0.00	C69
脑、神经系统	Brain, nervous system	2 363	1.75	4.26	2.76	0.15	0.29	1 981	2.45	3.55	2.07	0.12	0.21	C70-72, D32-33, D42-43
甲状腺	Thyroid	350	0.26	0.63	0.33	0.01	0.04	514	0.64	0.92	0.45	0.02	0.05	C73
肾上腺	Adrenal gland	112	0.08	0.20	0.13	0.01	0.01	72	0.09	0.13	0.09	0.00	0.01	C74
其他内分泌腺	Other endocrine	72	0.05	0.13	0.09	0.01	0.01	49	0.06	0.09	0.05	0.00	0.01	C75
霍奇金淋巴瘤	Hodgkin lymphoma	117	0.09	0.21	0.12	0.01	0.01	82	0.10	0.15	0.08	0.00	0.01	C81
非霍奇金淋巴瘤	Non-Hodgkin lymphoma	2 171	1.61	3.92	2.21	0.10	0.25	1 466	1.81	2.63	1.30	0.06	0.14	C82-C86;C96
免疫增生性疾病	Immunoproliferative diseases	20	0.01	0.04	0.02	0.00	0.00	9	0.01	0.02	0.01	0.00	0.00	C88
多发性骨髓瘤	Multiple myeloma	866	0.64	1.56	0.82	0.03	0.10	633	0.78	1.13	0.56	0.02	0.07	C90
淋巴样白血病	Lymphoid leukemia	557	0.41	1.00	0.78	0.04	0.06	413	0.51	0.74	0.54	0.03	0.05	C91
髓样白血病	Myeloid leukemia	1 115	0.83	2.01	1.22	0.06	0.13	873	1.08	1.56	0.91	0.05	0.09	C92-C94, D45-47
白血病,未特指	Leukemia unspecified	988	0.73	1.78	1.16	0.06	0.11	685	0.85	1.23	0.74	0.04	0.07	C95
其他或未指明部位	Other and unspecified	2 734	2.03	4.93	2.68	0.12	0.29	2 287	2.83	4.10	1.97	0.09	0.20	O&U
所有部位合计	All sites	134 688	100.00	242.95	129.84	5.78	14.51	80 842	100.00	144.91	69.31	3.17	7.32	C00-96, D32-33, D42-43, D45-47
所有部位除外 C44	All sites except C44	134 173	99.62	242.02	129.39	5.76	14.47	80 483	99.56	144.27	69.07	3.16	7.31	C00-96, D32-33, D42-43, D45-47 exc. C44

附表 2-12　2017 年全国东部农村肿瘤登记地区癌症死亡主要指标
Appendix Table 2-12　Cancer mortality in Eastern rural registration areas of China, 2017

部位 Site		男性 Male						女性 Female						ICD10
		死亡数 No. deaths	构成 Freq. /%	粗率 Crude rate/ 100 000^{-1}	世标率 ASR world/ 100 000^{-1}	累积率 Cum. rate/% 0~64	累积率 Cum. rate/% 0~74	死亡数 No. deaths	构成 Freq. /%	粗率 Crude rate/ 100 000^{-1}	世标率 ASR world/ 100 000^{-1}	累积率 Cum. rate/% 0~64	累积率 Cum. rate/% 0~74	
唇	Lip	83	0.08	0.19	0.11	0.00	0.01	27	0.04	0.06	0.03	0.00	0.00	C00
舌	Tongue	300	0.28	0.68	0.41	0.02	0.05	122	0.20	0.29	0.14	0.01	0.02	C01-02
口	Mouth	286	0.27	0.65	0.38	0.02	0.04	204	0.34	0.48	0.23	0.01	0.02	C03-06
唾液腺	Salivary glands	115	0.11	0.26	0.16	0.01	0.02	45	0.07	0.11	0.06	0.00	0.01	C07-08
扁桃腺	Tonsil	44	0.04	0.10	0.06	0.00	0.01	4	0.01	0.01	0.00	0.00	0.00	C09
其他口咽	Other oropharynx	108	0.10	0.25	0.14	0.01	0.02	25	0.04	0.06	0.03	0.00	0.00	C10
鼻咽	Nasopharynx	1 128	1.06	2.56	1.60	0.10	0.19	415	0.69	0.97	0.58	0.04	0.07	C11
下咽	Hypopharynx	235	0.22	0.53	0.31	0.02	0.04	24	0.04	0.06	0.03	0.00	0.00	C12-13
咽,部位不明	Pharynx unspecified	106	0.10	0.24	0.14	0.01	0.01	30	0.05	0.07	0.03	0.00	0.00	C14
食管	Esophagus	12 757	12.02	28.95	16.23	0.62	1.91	5 459	9.02	12.81	5.82	0.14	0.62	C15
胃	Stomach	15 691	14.79	35.60	19.96	0.76	2.30	6 660	11.01	15.63	7.65	0.28	0.83	C16
小肠	Small intestine	394	0.37	0.89	0.51	0.02	0.06	247	0.41	0.58	0.30	0.02	0.03	C17
结肠	Colon	2 769	2.61	6.28	3.57	0.14	0.38	2 160	3.57	5.07	2.49	0.10	0.25	C18
直肠	Rectum	3 638	3.43	8.25	4.62	0.18	0.49	2 508	4.14	5.88	2.84	0.11	0.29	C19-20
肛门	Anus	72	0.07	0.16	0.09	0.00	0.01	69	0.11	0.16	0.08	0.00	0.01	C21
肝脏	Liver	15 938	15.02	36.16	22.07	1.42	2.55	5 787	9.56	13.58	7.03	0.34	0.80	C22
胆囊及其他	Gallbladder etc.	1 412	1.33	3.20	1.80	0.08	0.20	1 517	2.51	3.56	1.71	0.06	0.18	C23-24
胰腺	Pancreas	3 583	3.38	8.13	4.63	0.20	0.54	2 763	4.57	6.48	3.20	0.12	0.37	C25
鼻、鼻窦及其他	Nose, sinuses etc.	112	0.11	0.25	0.16	0.01	0.02	71	0.12	0.17	0.09	0.01	0.01	C30-31
喉	Larynx	759	0.72	1.72	0.99	0.05	0.11	149	0.25	0.35	0.17	0.00	0.02	C32
气管、支气管、肺	Trachea, bronchus & lung	31 373	29.56	71.19	40.35	1.63	4.84	14 418	23.83	33.83	16.86	0.70	1.90	C33-34
其他胸腔器官	Other thoracic organs	233	0.22	0.53	0.34	0.02	0.04	134	0.22	0.31	0.18	0.01	0.02	C37-38
骨	Bone	745	0.70	1.69	1.10	0.05	0.12	600	0.99	1.41	0.84	0.04	0.09	C40-41
皮肤黑色素瘤	Melanoma of skin	192	0.18	0.44	0.28	0.01	0.03	189	0.31	0.44	0.25	0.01	0.03	C43
皮肤其他	Other skin	345	0.33	0.78	0.44	0.01	0.03	338	0.56	0.79	0.33	0.01	0.02	C44
间皮瘤	Mesothelioma	59	0.06	0.13	0.08	0.01	0.01	40	0.07	0.09	0.05	0.00	0.01	C45
卡波氏肉瘤	Kaposi sarcoma	191	0.18	0.43	0.26	0.01	0.03	113	0.19	0.27	0.15	0.01	0.02	C46
结缔组织、软组织	Connective & soft tissue	175	0.16	0.40	0.30	0.01	0.03	131	0.22	0.31	0.19	0.01	0.02	C47;C49
乳腺	Breast	60	0.06	0.14	0.08	0.00	0.01	4 174	6.90	9.79	5.76	0.41	0.64	C50
外阴	Vulva	—	—	—	—	—	—	81	0.13	0.19	0.10	0.01	0.01	C51
阴道	Vagina	—	—	—	—	—	—	35	0.06	0.08	0.04	0.00	0.01	C52
子宫颈	Cervix uteri	—	—	—	—	—	—	2 159	3.57	5.07	2.92	0.20	0.32	C53
子宫体	Corpus uteri	—	—	—	—	—	—	605	1.00	1.42	0.80	0.05	0.10	C54
子宫,部位不明	Uterus unspecified	—	—	—	—	—	—	399	0.66	0.94	0.50	0.03	0.05	C55
卵巢	Ovary	—	—	—	—	—	—	1 589	2.63	3.73	2.17	0.15	0.26	C56
其他女性生殖器	Other female genital organs	—	—	—	—	—	—	76	0.13	0.18	0.10	0.01	0.01	C57
胎盘	Placenta	—	—	—	—	—	—	3	0.00	0.01	0.01	0.00	0.00	C58
阴茎	Penis	125	0.12	0.28	0.16	0.00	0.02	—	—	—	—	—	—	C60
前列腺	Prostate	2 138	2.01	4.85	2.50	0.03	0.19	—	—	—	—	—	—	C61
睾丸	Testis	47	0.04	0.11	0.07	0.00	0.01	—	—	—	—	—	—	C62
其他男性生殖器	Other male genital organs	18	0.02	0.04	0.02	0.00	0.00	—	—	—	—	—	—	C63
肾	Kidney	727	0.69	1.65	0.99	0.05	0.11	432	0.71	1.01	0.54	0.03	0.06	C64
肾盂	Renal pelvis	87	0.08	0.20	0.11	0.00	0.01	61	0.10	0.14	0.07	0.00	0.01	C65
输尿管	Ureter	119	0.11	0.27	0.17	0.01	0.02	91	0.15	0.21	0.11	0.00	0.01	C66
膀胱	Bladder	1 823	1.72	4.14	2.18	0.04	0.18	450	0.74	1.06	0.45	0.01	0.04	C67
其他泌尿器官	Other urinary organs	25	0.02	0.06	0.03	0.00	0.00	8	0.01	0.02	0.01	0.00	0.00	C68
眼	Eye	30	0.03	0.07	0.06	0.00	0.00	18	0.03	0.04	0.03	0.00	0.00	C69
脑、神经系统	Brain, nervous system	2 039	1.92	4.63	3.14	0.19	0.34	1 703	2.81	4.00	2.45	0.14	0.25	C70-72, D32-33, D42-43
甲状腺	Thyroid	162	0.15	0.37	0.22	0.01	0.02	285	0.47	0.67	0.36	0.02	0.04	C73
肾上腺	Adrenal gland	86	0.08	0.20	0.15	0.01	0.01	51	0.08	0.12	0.08	0.00	0.01	C74
其他内分泌腺	Other endocrine	50	0.05	0.11	0.07	0.00	0.01	36	0.06	0.08	0.05	0.00	0.00	C75
霍奇金淋巴瘤	Hodgkin lymphoma	79	0.07	0.18	0.11	0.01	0.01	45	0.07	0.11	0.05	0.00	0.00	C81
非霍奇金淋巴瘤	Non-Hodgkin lymphoma	1 523	1.44	3.46	2.10	0.10	0.24	998	1.65	2.34	1.23	0.06	0.14	C82-C86;C96
免疫增生性疾病	Immunoproliferative diseases	13	0.01	0.03	0.02	0.00	0.00	5	0.01	0.01	0.01	0.00	0.00	C88
多发性骨髓瘤	Multiple myeloma	543	0.51	1.23	0.72	0.03	0.09	382	0.63	0.90	0.49	0.02	0.06	C90
淋巴样白血病	Lymphoid leukemia	489	0.46	1.11	0.87	0.05	0.08	350	0.58	0.82	0.58	0.03	0.05	C91
髓样白血病	Myeloid leukemia	668	0.63	1.52	1.01	0.05	0.11	469	0.78	1.10	0.74	0.04	0.08	C92-C94, D45-47
白血病,未特指	Leukemia unspecified	894	0.84	2.03	1.43	0.07	0.14	670	1.11	1.57	1.05	0.06	0.10	C95
其他或未指明部位	Other and unspecified	1 532	1.44	3.48	2.10	0.10	0.23	1 092	1.80	2.56	1.36	0.07	0.14	O&U
所有部位合计	All sites	106 120	100.00	240.80	139.38	6.21	15.90	60 516	100.00	142.00	73.42	3.39	8.06	C00-96, D32-33, D42-43, D45-47
所有部位除外 C44	All sites except C44	105 775	99.67	240.01	138.95	6.20	15.87	60 178	99.44	141.20	73.09	3.38	8.04	C00-96, D32-33, D42-43, D45-47 exc. C44

附表 2-13　2017 年全国中部肿瘤登记地区癌症死亡主要指标
Appendix Table 2-13　Cancer mortality in Central registration areas of China, 2017

部位 Site		男性 Male						女性 Female						ICD10
		死亡数 No. deaths	构成 Freq. /%	粗率 Crude rate/ 100 000⁻¹	世标率 ASR world/ 100 000⁻¹	累积率 Cum. rate/%		死亡数 No. deaths	构成 Freq. /%	粗率 Crude rate/ 100 000⁻¹	世标率 ASR world/ 100 000⁻¹	累积率 Cum. rate/%		
						0~64	0~74					0~64	0~74	
唇	Lip	61	0.05	0.10	0.07	0.00	0.01	33	0.05	0.06	0.03	0.00	0.00	C00
舌	Tongue	345	0.29	0.59	0.41	0.03	0.05	138	0.20	0.25	0.15	0.01	0.02	C01-02
口	Mouth	435	0.36	0.74	0.51	0.03	0.06	179	0.26	0.32	0.19	0.01	0.02	C03-06
唾液腺	Salivary glands	130	0.11	0.22	0.15	0.01	0.02	70	0.10	0.12	0.08	0.00	0.01	C07-08
扁桃腺	Tonsil	63	0.05	0.11	0.07	0.00	0.01	11	0.02	0.02	0.01	0.00	0.00	C09
其他口咽	Other oropharynx	154	0.13	0.26	0.19	0.01	0.02	28	0.04	0.05	0.03	0.00	0.00	C10
鼻咽	Nasopharynx	1 281	1.07	2.18	1.55	0.10	0.18	527	0.78	0.94	0.61	0.04	0.07	C11
下咽	Hypopharynx	208	0.17	0.35	0.25	0.02	0.03	16	0.02	0.03	0.02	0.00	0.00	C12-13
咽,部位不明	Pharynx unspecified	141	0.12	0.24	0.16	0.01	0.02	47	0.07	0.08	0.05	0.00	0.01	C14
食管	Esophagus	11 165	9.32	18.98	12.86	0.48	1.55	4 720	6.95	8.39	4.76	0.13	0.53	C15
胃	Stomach	17 257	14.41	29.34	19.82	0.79	2.34	7 712	11.35	13.71	8.16	0.33	0.90	C16
小肠	Small intestine	446	0.37	0.76	0.52	0.02	0.06	294	0.43	0.52	0.32	0.01	0.04	C17
结肠	Colon	3 321	2.77	5.65	3.80	0.16	0.41	2 644	3.89	4.70	2.80	0.12	0.30	C18
直肠	Rectum	4 411	3.68	7.50	5.04	0.21	0.56	2 881	4.24	5.12	3.06	0.13	0.34	C19-20
肛门	Anus	168	0.14	0.29	0.20	0.01	0.02	98	0.14	0.17	0.11	0.00	0.01	C21
肝脏	Liver	20 327	16.97	34.56	24.25	1.47	2.78	7 972	11.73	14.17	8.75	0.41	0.99	C22
胆囊及其他	Gallbladder etc.	1 320	1.10	2.24	1.52	0.07	0.18	1 624	2.39	2.89	1.69	0.06	0.19	C23-24
胰腺	Pancreas	3 123	2.61	5.31	3.65	0.17	0.44	2 270	3.34	4.03	2.44	0.10	0.28	C25
鼻、鼻窦及其他	Nose, sinuses etc.	122	0.10	0.21	0.15	0.01	0.02	97	0.14	0.17	0.11	0.01	0.01	C30-31
喉	Larynx	1 003	0.84	1.71	1.18	0.06	0.14	202	0.30	0.36	0.22	0.01	0.02	C32
气管、支气管、肺	Trachea, bronchus & lung	37 234	31.09	63.30	42.92	1.78	5.11	14 568	21.44	25.89	15.43	0.63	1.71	C33-34
其他胸腔器官	Other thoracic organs	344	0.29	0.58	0.42	0.02	0.05	207	0.30	0.37	0.25	0.01	0.03	C37-38
骨	Bone	848	0.71	1.44	1.05	0.05	0.12	527	0.78	0.94	0.63	0.03	0.07	C40-41
皮肤黑色素瘤	Melanoma of skin	297	0.25	0.50	0.35	0.02	0.03	192	0.28	0.34	0.22	0.01	0.02	C43
皮肤其他	Other skin	467	0.39	0.79	0.53	0.02	0.05	389	0.57	0.69	0.38	0.01	0.03	C44
间皮瘤	Mesothelioma	58	0.05	0.10	0.07	0.00	0.01	40	0.06	0.07	0.05	0.00	0.01	C45
卡波氏肉瘤	Kaposi sarcoma	97	0.08	0.16	0.12	0.01	0.01	71	0.10	0.13	0.08	0.00	0.01	C46
结缔组织、软组织	Connective & soft tissue	232	0.19	0.39	0.31	0.02	0.03	153	0.23	0.27	0.19	0.01	0.02	C47;C49
乳腺	Breast	114	0.10	0.19	0.13	0.01	0.02	5 114	7.53	9.09	6.14	0.45	0.69	C50
外阴	Vulva	—	—	—	—	—	—	89	0.13	0.16	0.10	0.00	0.01	C51
阴道	Vagina	—	—	—	—	—	—	47	0.07	0.08	0.06	0.00	0.01	C52
子宫颈	Cervix uteri	—	—	—	—	—	—	3 652	5.37	6.49	4.30	0.29	0.49	C53
子宫体	Corpus uteri	—	—	—	—	—	—	885	1.30	1.57	1.04	0.06	0.12	C54
子宫,部位不明	Uterus unspecified	—	—	—	—	—	—	410	0.60	0.73	0.47	0.03	0.05	C55
卵巢	Ovary	—	—	—	—	—	—	1 816	2.67	3.23	2.17	0.15	0.26	C56
其他女性生殖器	Other female genital organs	—	—	—	—	—	—	100	0.15	0.18	0.11	0.01	0.01	C57
胎盘	Placenta	—	—	—	—	—	—	7	0.01	0.01	0.01	0.00	0.00	C58
阴茎	Penis	142	0.12	0.24	0.16	0.01	0.02	—	—	—	—	—	—	C60
前列腺	Prostate	2 031	1.70	3.45	2.16	0.03	0.15	—	—	—	—	—	—	C61
睾丸	Testis	69	0.06	0.12	0.09	0.00	0.01	—	—	—	—	—	—	C62
其他男性生殖器	Other male genital organs	25	0.02	0.04	0.03	0.00	0.00	—	—	—	—	—	—	C63
肾	Kidney	851	0.71	1.45	1.01	0.05	0.12	424	0.62	0.75	0.48	0.02	0.05	C64
肾盂	Renal pelvis	109	0.09	0.19	0.13	0.01	0.01	93	0.14	0.17	0.10	0.00	0.01	C65
输尿管	Ureter	108	0.09	0.18	0.12	0.00	0.01	97	0.14	0.17	0.09	0.00	0.01	C66
膀胱	Bladder	1 829	1.53	3.11	2.00	0.05	0.18	530	0.78	0.94	0.50	0.01	0.04	C67
其他泌尿器官	Other urinary organs	22	0.02	0.04	0.03	0.00	0.00	16	0.02	0.03	0.02	0.00	0.00	C68
眼	Eye	30	0.03	0.05	0.04	0.00	0.00	37	0.05	0.07	0.06	0.00	0.00	C69
脑、神经系统	Brain, nervous system	2 411	2.01	4.10	3.13	0.18	0.33	1 877	2.76	3.34	2.39	0.14	0.25	C70-72, D32-33, D42-43
甲状腺	Thyroid	250	0.21	0.43	0.30	0.01	0.03	434	0.64	0.77	0.49	0.03	0.05	C73
肾上腺	Adrenal gland	109	0.09	0.19	0.14	0.01	0.02	80	0.12	0.14	0.10	0.01	0.01	C74
其他内分泌腺	Other endocrine	70	0.06	0.12	0.09	0.00	0.01	35	0.05	0.06	0.05	0.00	0.00	C75
霍奇金淋巴瘤	Hodgkin lymphoma	99	0.08	0.17	0.12	0.01	0.01	46	0.07	0.08	0.05	0.00	0.01	C81
非霍奇金淋巴瘤	Non-Hodgkin lymphoma	1 499	1.25	2.55	1.81	0.09	0.21	967	1.42	1.72	1.12	0.06	0.12	C82-C86;C96
免疫增生性疾病	Immunoproliferative diseases	13	0.01	0.02	0.02	0.00	0.00	5	0.01	0.01	0.01	0.00	0.00	C88
多发性骨髓瘤	Multiple myeloma	621	0.52	1.06	0.75	0.04	0.09	404	0.59	0.72	0.47	0.02	0.06	C90
淋巴样白血病	Lymphoid leukemia	494	0.41	0.84	0.72	0.04	0.07	345	0.51	0.61	0.50	0.03	0.05	C91
髓样白血病	Myeloid leukemia	565	0.47	0.96	0.75	0.04	0.08	451	0.66	0.80	0.58	0.03	0.06	C92-C94, D45-47
白血病,未特指	Leukemia unspecified	1 152	0.96	1.96	1.58	0.09	0.15	777	1.14	1.38	1.09	0.06	0.10	C95
其他或未指明部位	Other and unspecified	2 102	1.75	3.57	2.54	0.12	0.28	1 497	2.20	2.66	1.69	0.08	0.17	O&U
所有部位合计	All sites	119 773	100.00	203.63	140.00	6.36	16.10	67 945	100.00	120.77	75.01	3.57	8.30	C00-96, D32-33, D42-43, D45-47
所有部位除外 C44	All sites except C44	119 306	99.61	202.84	139.47	6.34	16.05	67 556	99.43	120.08	74.62	3.56	8.27	C00-96, D32-33, D42-43, D45-47 exc. C44

附表 2-14 2017 年全国中部城市肿瘤登记地区癌症死亡主要指标

Appendix Table 2-14 Cancer mortality in Central urban registration areas of China, 2017

部位 Site		男性 Male						女性 Female						ICD10
		死亡数 No. deaths	构成 Freq. /%	粗率 Crude rate/ 100 000^{-1}	世标率 ASR world/ 100 000^{-1}	累积率 Cum. rate/%		死亡数 No. deaths	构成 Freq. /%	粗率 Crude rate/ 100 000^{-1}	世标率 ASR world/ 100 000^{-1}	累积率 Cum. rate/%		
						0~64	0~74					0~64	0~74	
唇	Lip	31	0.07	0.14	0.09	0.01	0.01	15	0.06	0.07	0.03	0.00	0.00	C00
舌	Tongue	192	0.41	0.88	0.58	0.04	0.07	82	0.31	0.38	0.21	0.01	0.02	C01-02
口	Mouth	201	0.43	0.92	0.60	0.04	0.07	78	0.29	0.37	0.19	0.01	0.02	C03-06
唾液腺	Salivary glands	65	0.14	0.30	0.18	0.01	0.02	34	0.13	0.16	0.10	0.01	0.01	C07-08
扁桃腺	Tonsil	29	0.06	0.13	0.09	0.01	0.01	3	0.01	0.01	0.01	0.00	0.00	C09
其他口咽	Other oropharynx	50	0.11	0.23	0.15	0.01	0.02	7	0.03	0.03	0.02	0.00	0.00	C10
鼻咽	Nasopharynx	451	0.97	2.07	1.37	0.08	0.16	193	0.72	0.90	0.54	0.03	0.06	C11
下咽	Hypopharynx	108	0.23	0.50	0.33	0.02	0.04	5	0.02	0.02	0.02	0.00	0.00	C12-13
咽,部位不明	Pharynx unspecified	58	0.12	0.27	0.17	0.01	0.02	15	0.06	0.07	0.03	0.00	0.00	C14
食管	Esophagus	3 609	7.73	16.58	10.31	0.44	1.23	1 204	4.52	5.64	2.87	0.06	0.30	C15
胃	Stomach	5 298	11.34	24.35	14.98	0.61	1.72	2 442	9.16	11.43	6.29	0.25	0.67	C16
小肠	Small intestine	239	0.51	1.10	0.69	0.03	0.08	157	0.59	0.74	0.41	0.02	0.04	C17
结肠	Colon	1 805	3.86	8.29	5.04	0.19	0.53	1 356	5.09	6.35	3.40	0.13	0.35	C18
直肠	Rectum	1 935	4.14	8.89	5.42	0.22	0.60	1 141	4.28	5.34	2.89	0.12	0.30	C19-20
肛门	Anus	80	0.17	0.37	0.23	0.01	0.03	34	0.13	0.16	0.08	0.00	0.01	C21
肝脏	Liver	7 177	15.37	32.98	21.34	1.29	2.43	2 752	10.32	12.89	7.24	0.31	0.80	C22
胆囊及其他	Gallbladder etc.	628	1.34	2.89	1.78	0.08	0.20	752	2.82	3.52	1.87	0.06	0.21	C23-24
胰腺	Pancreas	1 487	3.18	6.83	4.29	0.20	0.50	1 126	4.22	5.27	2.89	0.11	0.32	C25
鼻、鼻窦及其他	Nose, sinuses etc.	48	0.10	0.22	0.15	0.01	0.01	38	0.14	0.18	0.11	0.01	0.01	C30-31
喉	Larynx	442	0.95	2.03	1.28	0.06	0.15	64	0.24	0.30	0.15	0.01	0.01	C32
气管、支气管、肺	Trachea, bronchus & lung	15 171	32.48	69.72	43.12	1.78	5.13	5 987	22.45	28.03	15.12	0.59	1.60	C33-34
其他胸腔器官	Other thoracic organs	160	0.34	0.74	0.49	0.03	0.06	90	0.34	0.42	0.26	0.01	0.03	C37-38
骨	Bone	324	0.69	1.49	1.04	0.05	0.11	186	0.70	0.87	0.54	0.03	0.05	C40-41
皮肤黑色素瘤	Melanoma of skin	106	0.23	0.49	0.31	0.01	0.03	80	0.30	0.37	0.22	0.01	0.02	C43
皮肤其他	Other skin	157	0.34	0.72	0.44	0.01	0.04	125	0.47	0.59	0.30	0.01	0.03	C44
间皮瘤	Mesothelioma	44	0.09	0.20	0.13	0.01	0.02	24	0.09	0.11	0.07	0.00	0.01	C45
卡波氏肉瘤	Kaposi sarcoma	42	0.09	0.19	0.12	0.01	0.01	34	0.13	0.16	0.09	0.00	0.01	C46
结缔组织、软组织	Connective & soft tissue	121	0.26	0.56	0.39	0.02	0.04	85	0.32	0.40	0.27	0.01	0.02	C47;C49
乳腺	Breast	40	0.09	0.18	0.12	0.01	0.01	2 321	8.70	10.87	6.81	0.47	0.77	C50
外阴	Vulva	—	—	—	—	—	—	28	0.11	0.13	0.07	0.00	0.01	C51
阴道	Vagina	—	—	—	—	—	—	15	0.06	0.07	0.05	0.00	0.01	C52
子宫颈	Cervix uteri	—	—	—	—	—	—	1 292	4.85	6.05	3.72	0.26	0.40	C53
子宫体	Corpus uteri	—	—	—	—	—	—	326	1.22	1.53	0.92	0.05	0.11	C54
子宫,部位不明	Uterus unspecified	—	—	—	—	—	—	134	0.50	0.63	0.38	0.02	0.04	C55
卵巢	Ovary	—	—	—	—	—	—	867	3.25	4.06	2.53	0.17	0.30	C56
其他女性生殖器	Other female genital organs	—	—	—	—	—	—	54	0.20	0.25	0.14	0.01	0.01	C57
胎盘	Placenta	—	—	—	—	—	—	1	0.00	0.00	0.01	0.00	0.00	C58
阴茎	Penis	39	0.08	0.18	0.11	0.01	0.01	—	—	—	—	—	—	C60
前列腺	Prostate	1 079	2.31	4.96	2.68	0.03	0.17	—	—	—	—	—	—	C61
睾丸	Testis	29	0.06	0.13	0.09	0.00	0.01	—	—	—	—	—	—	C62
其他男性生殖器	Other male genital organs	13	0.03	0.06	0.04	0.00	0.00	—	—	—	—	—	—	C63
肾	Kidney	429	0.92	1.97	1.25	0.06	0.14	201	0.75	0.94	0.54	0.02	0.06	C64
肾盂	Renal pelvis	55	0.12	0.25	0.16	0.01	0.02	47	0.18	0.22	0.12	0.00	0.01	C65
输尿管	Ureter	57	0.12	0.26	0.15	0.00	0.01	67	0.25	0.31	0.15	0.00	0.01	C66
膀胱	Bladder	872	1.87	4.01	2.30	0.06	0.20	240	0.90	1.12	0.53	0.01	0.04	C67
其他泌尿器官	Other urinary organs	10	0.02	0.05	0.03	0.00	0.00	8	0.03	0.04	0.02	0.00	0.00	C68
眼	Eye	11	0.02	0.05	0.04	0.00	0.00	18	0.07	0.08	0.06	0.00	0.01	C69
脑、神经系统	Brain, nervous system	910	1.95	4.18	2.97	0.17	0.32	720	2.70	3.37	2.31	0.13	0.22	C70-72, D32-33, D42-43
甲状腺	Thyroid	109	0.23	0.50	0.32	0.02	0.03	172	0.65	0.81	0.46	0.02	0.05	C73
肾上腺	Adrenal gland	62	0.13	0.28	0.20	0.01	0.02	38	0.14	0.18	0.11	0.00	0.01	C74
其他内分泌腺	Other endocrine	38	0.08	0.17	0.12	0.01	0.01	19	0.07	0.09	0.07	0.00	0.01	C75
霍奇金淋巴瘤	Hodgkin lymphoma	35	0.07	0.16	0.10	0.00	0.01	16	0.06	0.07	0.04	0.00	0.00	C81
非霍奇金淋巴瘤	Non-Hodgkin lymphoma	668	1.43	3.07	1.98	0.09	0.22	440	1.65	2.06	1.24	0.06	0.14	C82-C86;C96
免疫增生性疾病	Immunoproliferative diseases	8	0.02	0.04	0.03	0.00	0.00	5	0.02	0.02	0.01	0.00	0.00	C88
多发性骨髓瘤	Multiple myeloma	317	0.68	1.46	0.92	0.05	0.10	198	0.74	0.93	0.54	0.02	0.07	C90
淋巴样白血病	Lymphoid leukemia	239	0.51	1.10	0.89	0.05	0.08	186	0.70	0.87	0.66	0.04	0.06	C91
髓样白血病	Myeloid leukemia	251	0.54	1.15	0.79	0.04	0.09	213	0.80	1.00	0.64	0.03	0.07	C92-C94, D45-47
白血病,未特指	Leukemia unspecified	371	0.79	1.70	1.28	0.06	0.12	216	0.81	1.01	0.73	0.04	0.07	C95
其他或未指明部位	Other and unspecified	1 007	2.16	4.63	2.99	0.14	0.33	715	2.68	3.35	1.94	0.09	0.20	O&U
所有部位合计	All sites	46 707	100.00	214.64	134.66	6.07	15.26	26 666	100.00	124.86	71.02	3.28	7.61	C00-96, D32-33, D42-43, D45-47
所有部位除外 C44	All sites except C44	46 550	99.66	213.92	134.22	6.06	15.22	26 541	99.53	124.27	70.72	3.27	7.59	C00-96, D32-33, D42-43, D45-47 exc. C44

附表 2-15　2017 年全国中部农村肿瘤登记地区癌症死亡主要指标

Appendix Table 2-15　Cancer mortality in Central rural registration areas of China, 2017

部位 Site		男性 Male						女性 Female						ICD10
		死亡数 No. deaths	构成 Freq. /%	粗率 Crude rate/ 100 000^{-1}	世标率 ASR world/ 100 000^{-1}	累积率 Cum. rate/% 0~64	累积率 Cum. rate/% 0~74	死亡数 No. deaths	构成 Freq. /%	粗率 Crude rate/ 100 000^{-1}	世标率 ASR world/ 100 000^{-1}	累积率 Cum. rate/% 0~64	累积率 Cum. rate/% 0~74	
唇	Lip	30	0.04	0.08	0.06	0.00	0.01	18	0.04	0.05	0.03	0.00	0.00	C00
舌	Tongue	153	0.21	0.41	0.30	0.02	0.03	56	0.14	0.16	0.11	0.01	0.01	C01-02
口	Mouth	234	0.32	0.63	0.46	0.02	0.06	101	0.24	0.29	0.19	0.01	0.02	C03-06
唾液腺	Salivary glands	65	0.09	0.18	0.13	0.01	0.02	36	0.09	0.10	0.07	0.00	0.01	C07-08
扁桃腺	Tonsil	34	0.05	0.09	0.07	0.00	0.01	8	0.02	0.02	0.02	0.00	0.00	C09
其他口咽	Other oropharynx	104	0.14	0.28	0.21	0.01	0.03	21	0.05	0.06	0.04	0.00	0.00	C10
鼻咽	Nasopharynx	830	1.14	2.24	1.67	0.12	0.19	334	0.81	0.96	0.65	0.04	0.07	C11
下咽	Hypopharynx	100	0.14	0.27	0.20	0.01	0.02	11	0.03	0.03	0.02	0.00	0.00	C12-13
咽,部位不明	Pharynx unspecified	83	0.11	0.22	0.16	0.01	0.02	32	0.08	0.09	0.06	0.00	0.01	C14
食管	Esophagus	7 556	10.34	20.39	14.60	0.51	1.76	3 516	8.52	10.07	6.07	0.17	0.69	C15
胃	Stomach	11 959	16.37	32.27	23.05	0.91	2.75	5 270	12.77	15.10	9.45	0.38	1.04	C16
小肠	Small intestine	207	0.28	0.56	0.41	0.02	0.05	137	0.33	0.39	0.26	0.01	0.03	C17
结肠	Colon	1 516	2.07	4.09	2.93	0.13	0.33	1 288	3.12	3.69	2.37	0.11	0.27	C18
直肠	Rectum	2 476	3.39	6.68	4.77	0.21	0.54	1 740	4.22	4.99	3.17	0.14	0.36	C19-20
肛门	Anus	88	0.12	0.24	0.18	0.01	0.02	64	0.16	0.18	0.12	0.01	0.01	C21
肝脏	Liver	13 150	18.00	35.48	26.17	1.59	3.00	5 220	12.65	14.96	9.77	0.47	1.12	C22
胆囊及其他	Gallbladder etc.	692	0.95	1.87	1.35	0.06	0.16	872	2.11	2.50	1.57	0.06	0.18	C23-24
胰腺	Pancreas	1 636	2.24	4.41	3.21	0.15	0.39	1 144	2.77	3.28	2.13	0.10	0.26	C25
鼻、鼻窦及其他	Nose, sinuses etc.	74	0.10	0.20	0.15	0.01	0.02	59	0.14	0.17	0.12	0.01	0.01	C30-31
喉	Larynx	561	0.77	1.51	1.11	0.05	0.13	138	0.33	0.40	0.26	0.01	0.03	C32
气管、支气管、肺	Trachea, bronchus & lung	22 063	30.20	59.54	42.75	1.79	5.10	8 581	20.79	24.58	15.62	0.66	1.79	C33-34
其他胸腔器官	Other thoracic organs	184	0.25	0.50	0.38	0.02	0.04	117	0.28	0.34	0.24	0.02	0.03	C37-38
骨	Bone	524	0.72	1.41	1.07	0.05	0.12	341	0.83	0.98	0.69	0.03	0.08	C40-41
皮肤黑色素瘤	Melanoma of skin	191	0.26	0.52	0.38	0.02	0.04	112	0.27	0.32	0.21	0.01	0.02	C43
皮肤其他	Other skin	310	0.42	0.84	0.60	0.02	0.06	264	0.64	0.76	0.44	0.01	0.03	C44
间皮瘤	Mesothelioma	14	0.02	0.04	0.03	0.00	0.00	16	0.04	0.05	0.03	0.00	0.00	C45
卡波氏肉瘤	Kaposi sarcoma	55	0.08	0.15	0.11	0.01	0.01	37	0.09	0.11	0.08	0.00	0.01	C46
结缔组织、软组织	Connective & soft tissue	111	0.15	0.30	0.25	0.01	0.03	68	0.16	0.19	0.15	0.01	0.02	C47;C49
乳腺	Breast	74	0.10	0.20	0.14	0.01	0.02	2 793	6.77	8.00	5.69	0.43	0.64	C50
外阴	Vulva	—	—	—	—	—	—	61	0.15	0.17	0.11	0.00	0.01	C51
阴道	Vagina	—	—	—	—	—	—	32	0.08	0.09	0.06	0.00	0.01	C52
子宫颈	Cervix uteri	—	—	—	—	—	—	2 360	5.72	6.76	4.69	0.31	0.55	C53
子宫体	Corpus uteri	—	—	—	—	—	—	559	1.35	1.60	1.12	0.07	0.14	C54
子宫,部位不明	Uterus unspecified	—	—	—	—	—	—	276	0.67	0.79	0.53	0.03	0.06	C55
卵巢	Ovary	—	—	—	—	—	—	949	2.30	2.72	1.92	0.14	0.23	C56
其他女性生殖器	Other female genital organs	—	—	—	—	—	—	46	0.11	0.13	0.09	0.01	0.01	C57
胎盘	Placenta	—	—	—	—	—	—	6	0.01	0.02	0.01	0.00	0.00	C58
阴茎	Penis	103	0.14	0.28	0.20	0.01	0.02	—	—	—	—	—	—	C60
前列腺	Prostate	952	1.30	2.57	1.76	0.02	0.15	—	—	—	—	—	—	C61
睾丸	Testis	40	0.05	0.11	0.09	0.00	0.01	—	—	—	—	—	—	C62
其他男性生殖器	Other male genital organs	12	0.02	0.03	0.03	0.00	0.00	—	—	—	—	—	—	C63
肾	Kidney	422	0.58	1.14	0.85	0.04	0.10	223	0.54	0.64	0.43	0.02	0.05	C64
肾盂	Renal pelvis	54	0.07	0.15	0.11	0.01	0.01	46	0.11	0.13	0.09	0.01	0.01	C65
输尿管	Ureter	51	0.07	0.14	0.10	0.00	0.01	30	0.07	0.09	0.05	0.00	0.00	C66
膀胱	Bladder	957	1.31	2.58	1.78	0.05	0.16	290	0.70	0.83	0.48	0.01	0.04	C67
其他泌尿器官	Other urinary organs	12	0.02	0.03	0.02	0.00	0.00	8	0.02	0.02	0.01	0.00	0.00	C68
眼	Eye	19	0.03	0.05	0.04	0.00	0.00	19	0.05	0.05	0.05	0.00	0.00	C69
脑、神经系统	Brain, nervous system	1 501	2.05	4.05	3.22	0.19	0.34	1 157	2.80	3.31	2.44	0.14	0.26	C70-72, D32-33, D42-43
甲状腺	Thyroid	141	0.19	0.38	0.28	0.01	0.03	262	0.63	0.75	0.52	0.03	0.06	C73
肾上腺	Adrenal gland	47	0.06	0.13	0.11	0.01	0.01	42	0.10	0.12	0.10	0.01	0.01	C74
其他内分泌腺	Other endocrine	32	0.04	0.09	0.07	0.00	0.01	16	0.04	0.05	0.04	0.00	0.00	C75
霍奇金淋巴瘤	Hodgkin lymphoma	64	0.09	0.17	0.13	0.01	0.02	30	0.07	0.09	0.06	0.00	0.01	C81
非霍奇金淋巴瘤	Non-Hodgkin lymphoma	831	1.14	2.24	1.68	0.09	0.20	527	1.28	1.51	1.04	0.05	0.12	C82-C86;C96
免疫增生性疾病	Immunoproliferative diseases	5	0.01	0.01	0.01	0.00	0.00	0	0.00	0.00	0.00	0.00	0.00	C88
多发性骨髓瘤	Multiple myeloma	304	0.42	0.82	0.63	0.03	0.08	206	0.50	0.59	0.42	0.02	0.06	C90
淋巴样白血病	Lymphoid leukemia	255	0.35	0.69	0.61	0.03	0.06	159	0.39	0.46	0.40	0.03	0.04	C91
髓样白血病	Myeloid leukemia	314	0.43	0.85	0.72	0.04	0.07	238	0.58	0.68	0.54	0.03	0.06	C92-C94, D45-47
白血病,未特指	Leukemia unspecified	781	1.07	2.11	1.76	0.10	0.17	561	1.36	1.61	1.31	0.07	0.12	C95
其他或未指明部位	Other and unspecified	1 095	1.50	2.95	2.24	0.10	0.25	782	1.89	2.24	1.51	0.07	0.16	O&U
所有部位合计	All sites	73 066	100.00	197.16	143.32	6.54	16.65	41 279	100.00	118.27	77.65	3.77	8.76	C00-96, D32-33, D42-43, D45-47
所有部位除外 C44	All sites except C44	72 756	99.58	196.33	142.72	6.52	16.59	41 015	99.36	117.51	77.20	3.76	8.73	C00-96, D32-33, D42-43, D45-47 exc. C44

附表 2-16　2017 年全国西部肿瘤登记地区癌症死亡主要指标

Appendix Table 2-16　Cancer mortality in Western registration areas of China, 2017

部位 Site		男性 Male						女性 Female						ICD10
		死亡数 No. deaths	构成 Freq. /%	粗率 Crude rate/ 100 000^{-1}	世标率 ASR world/ 100 000^{-1}	累积率 Cum. rate/% 0~64	累积率 Cum. rate/% 0~74	死亡数 No. deaths	构成 Freq. /%	粗率 Crude rate/ 100 000^{-1}	世标率 ASR world/ 100 000^{-1}	累积率 Cum. rate/% 0~64	累积率 Cum. rate/% 0~74	
唇	Lip	63	0.05	0.10	0.07	0.00	0.01	27	0.04	0.04	0.02	0.00	0.00	C00
舌	Tongue	386	0.29	0.61	0.40	0.02	0.05	164	0.24	0.27	0.17	0.01	0.02	C01-02
口	Mouth	484	0.36	0.77	0.50	0.02	0.06	225	0.32	0.37	0.22	0.01	0.02	C03-06
唾液腺	Salivary glands	104	0.08	0.17	0.11	0.01	0.01	62	0.09	0.10	0.07	0.00	0.01	C07-08
扁桃腺	Tonsil	78	0.06	0.12	0.08	0.01	0.01	18	0.03	0.03	0.02	0.00	0.00	C09
其他口咽	Other oropharynx	189	0.14	0.30	0.20	0.01	0.02	37	0.05	0.06	0.03	0.00	0.00	C10
鼻咽	Nasopharynx	1 857	1.39	2.96	2.00	0.13	0.23	739	1.07	1.22	0.81	0.06	0.09	C11
下咽	Hypopharynx	231	0.17	0.37	0.25	0.02	0.03	17	0.02	0.03	0.02	0.00	0.00	C12-13
咽,部位不明	Pharynx unspecified	256	0.19	0.41	0.26	0.01	0.03	89	0.13	0.15	0.09	0.00	0.01	C14
食管	Esophagus	14 735	11.02	23.46	15.04	0.66	1.86	4 212	6.07	6.96	3.90	0.11	0.44	C15
胃	Stomach	14 792	11.06	23.55	15.05	0.67	1.77	6 361	9.17	10.51	6.10	0.24	0.64	C16
小肠	Small intestine	382	0.29	0.61	0.40	0.02	0.05	272	0.39	0.45	0.27	0.01	0.03	C17
结肠	Colon	3 194	2.39	5.09	3.22	0.13	0.34	2 284	3.29	3.77	2.18	0.09	0.23	C18
直肠	Rectum	5 941	4.44	9.46	5.98	0.24	0.66	3 625	5.23	5.99	3.49	0.15	0.37	C19-20
肛门	Anus	360	0.27	0.57	0.36	0.02	0.04	165	0.24	0.27	0.15	0.01	0.02	C21
肝脏	Liver	24 947	18.65	39.72	26.64	1.73	3.01	8 175	11.79	13.50	8.23	0.40	0.93	C22
胆囊及其他	Gallbladder etc.	1 212	0.91	1.93	1.22	0.06	0.13	1 550	2.24	2.56	1.50	0.06	0.17	C23-24
胰腺	Pancreas	3 651	2.73	5.81	3.73	0.18	0.43	2 478	3.57	4.09	2.42	0.11	0.28	C25
鼻、鼻窦及其他	Nose, sinuses etc.	180	0.13	0.29	0.21	0.01	0.02	125	0.18	0.21	0.13	0.01	0.01	C30-31
喉	Larynx	1 070	0.80	1.70	1.10	0.06	0.13	186	0.27	0.31	0.17	0.01	0.02	C32
气管、支气管、肺	Trachea, bronchus & lung	40 806	30.51	64.97	41.78	2.00	4.95	16 980	24.49	28.05	16.54	0.71	1.86	C33-34
其他胸腔器官	Other thoracic organs	419	0.31	0.67	0.46	0.03	0.05	236	0.34	0.39	0.26	0.02	0.03	C37-38
骨	Bone	1 089	0.81	1.73	1.19	0.06	0.13	695	1.00	1.15	0.75	0.04	0.08	C40-41
皮肤黑色素瘤	Melanoma of skin	146	0.11	0.23	0.16	0.01	0.02	101	0.15	0.17	0.10	0.01	0.01	C43
皮肤其他	Other skin	578	0.43	0.92	0.60	0.03	0.06	383	0.55	0.63	0.36	0.01	0.03	C44
间皮瘤	Mesothelioma	46	0.03	0.07	0.05	0.00	0.01	30	0.04	0.05	0.03	0.00	0.00	C45
卡波氏肉瘤	Kaposi sarcoma	59	0.04	0.09	0.07	0.00	0.01	24	0.03	0.04	0.03	0.00	0.00	C46
结缔组织、软组织	Connective & soft tissue	246	0.18	0.39	0.27	0.02	0.03	144	0.21	0.24	0.17	0.01	0.02	C47;C49
乳腺	Breast	205	0.15	0.33	0.21	0.01	0.02	4 596	6.63	7.59	5.00	0.38	0.54	C50
外阴	Vulva	—	—	—	—	—	—	103	0.15	0.17	0.11	0.01	0.01	C51
阴道	Vagina	—	—	—	—	—	—	77	0.11	0.13	0.08	0.00	0.01	C52
子宫颈	Cervix uteri	—	—	—	—	—	—	3 648	5.26	6.03	3.96	0.27	0.45	C53
子宫体	Corpus uteri	—	—	—	—	—	—	924	1.33	1.53	1.00	0.07	0.12	C54
子宫,部位不明	Uterus unspecified	—	—	—	—	—	—	552	0.80	0.91	0.59	0.04	0.07	C55
卵巢	Ovary	—	—	—	—	—	—	1 727	2.49	2.85	1.87	0.13	0.21	C56
其他女性生殖器	Other female genital organs	—	—	—	—	—	—	99	0.14	0.16	0.10	0.01	0.01	C57
胎盘	Placenta	—	—	—	—	—	—	2	0.00	0.00	0.00	0.00	0.00	C58
阴茎	Penis	136	0.10	0.22	0.14	0.01	0.02	—	—	—	—	—	—	C60
前列腺	Prostate	2 502	1.87	3.98	2.36	0.04	0.18	—	—	—	—	—	—	C61
睾丸	Testis	83	0.06	0.13	0.10	0.01	0.01	—	—	—	—	—	—	C62
其他男性生殖器	Other male genital organs	15	0.01	0.02	0.02	0.00	0.00	—	—	—	—	—	—	C63
肾	Kidney	762	0.57	1.21	0.80	0.04	0.08	396	0.57	0.65	0.39	0.02	0.04	C64
肾盂	Renal pelvis	114	0.09	0.18	0.12	0.01	0.01	84	0.12	0.14	0.08	0.00	0.01	C65
输尿管	Ureter	112	0.08	0.18	0.11	0.00	0.01	87	0.13	0.14	0.08	0.00	0.01	C66
膀胱	Bladder	2 030	1.52	3.23	1.96	0.05	0.17	545	0.79	0.90	0.49	0.01	0.04	C67
其他泌尿器官	Other urinary organs	26	0.02	0.04	0.02	0.00	0.00	13	0.02	0.02	0.02	0.00	0.00	C68
眼	Eye	50	0.04	0.08	0.07	0.00	0.01	31	0.04	0.05	0.04	0.00	0.00	C69
脑、神经系统	Brain, nervous system	2 843	2.13	4.53	3.35	0.20	0.34	2 038	2.94	3.37	2.37	0.13	0.24	C70-72, D32-33, D42-43
甲状腺	Thyroid	217	0.16	0.35	0.22	0.01	0.02	339	0.49	0.56	0.36	0.02	0.04	C73
肾上腺	Adrenal gland	79	0.06	0.13	0.08	0.01	0.01	58	0.08	0.10	0.06	0.00	0.01	C74
其他内分泌腺	Other endocrine	56	0.04	0.09	0.07	0.00	0.01	72	0.10	0.12	0.08	0.01	0.01	C75
霍奇金淋巴瘤	Hodgkin lymphoma	112	0.08	0.18	0.13	0.01	0.01	50	0.07	0.08	0.05	0.00	0.01	C81
非霍奇金淋巴瘤	Non-Hodgkin lymphoma	1 532	1.15	2.44	1.67	0.09	0.19	843	1.22	1.39	0.89	0.04	0.10	C82-C86;C96
免疫增生性疾病	Immunoproliferative diseases	13	0.01	0.02	0.01	0.00	0.00	5	0.01	0.01	0.01	0.00	0.00	C88
多发性骨髓瘤	Multiple myeloma	469	0.35	0.75	0.50	0.03	0.06	321	0.46	0.53	0.34	0.02	0.04	C90
淋巴样白血病	Lymphoid leukemia	541	0.40	0.86	0.74	0.04	0.06	362	0.52	0.60	0.49	0.03	0.05	C91
髓样白血病	Myeloid leukemia	667	0.50	1.06	0.80	0.05	0.08	485	0.70	0.80	0.58	0.03	0.06	C92-C94, D45-47
白血病,未特指	Leukemia unspecified	1 144	0.86	1.82	1.45	0.08	0.14	835	1.20	1.38	1.10	0.06	0.10	C95
其他或未指明部位	Other and unspecified	2 540	1.90	4.04	2.78	0.15	0.30	1 639	2.36	2.71	1.76	0.09	0.19	O&U
所有部位合计	All sites	133 749	100.00	212.95	139.08	6.97	15.87	69 335	100.00	114.53	70.14	3.44	7.69	C00-96, D32-33, D42-43, D45-47
所有部位除外 C44	All sites except C44	133 171	99.57	212.03	138.48	6.95	15.81	68 952	99.45	113.90	69.78	3.43	7.67	C00-96, D32-33, D42-43, D45-47 exc. C44

附表 2-17 2017 年全国西部城市肿瘤登记地区癌症死亡主要指标

Appendix Table 2-17 Cancer mortality in Western urban registration areas of China,2017

部位 Site		男性 Male						女性 Female						ICD10
		死亡数 No. deaths	构成 Freq. /%	粗率 Crude rate/ 100 000^{-1}	世标率 ASR world/ 100 000^{-1}	累积率 Cum. rate/%		死亡数 No. deaths	构成 Freq. /%	粗率 Crude rate/ 100 000^{-1}	世标率 ASR world/ 100 000^{-1}	累积率 Cum. rate/%		
						0~64	0~74					0~64	0~74	
唇	Lip	30	0.05	0.10	0.07	0.00	0.01	16	0.05	0.06	0.03	0.00	0.00	C00
舌	Tongue	177	0.28	0.59	0.40	0.02	0.05	69	0.20	0.24	0.15	0.01	0.02	C01-02
口	Mouth	251	0.39	0.84	0.56	0.03	0.06	97	0.29	0.33	0.19	0.01	0.02	C03-06
唾液腺	Salivary glands	53	0.08	0.18	0.12	0.01	0.01	36	0.11	0.12	0.08	0.00	0.01	C07-08
扁桃腺	Tonsil	46	0.07	0.15	0.11	0.01	0.01	11	0.03	0.04	0.03	0.00	0.00	C09
其他口咽	Other oropharynx	96	0.15	0.32	0.21	0.01	0.02	17	0.05	0.06	0.03	0.00	0.00	C10
鼻咽	Nasopharynx	879	1.38	2.95	2.00	0.13	0.23	346	1.03	1.19	0.77	0.05	0.09	C11
下咽	Hypopharynx	123	0.19	0.41	0.29	0.02	0.04	10	0.03	0.03	0.02	0.00	0.00	C12-13
咽,部位不明	Pharynx unspecified	107	0.17	0.36	0.23	0.01	0.02	42	0.12	0.14	0.08	0.00	0.01	C14
食管	Esophagus	5 833	9.16	19.56	12.87	0.56	1.60	1 632	4.84	5.61	3.20	0.09	0.34	C15
胃	Stomach	6 491	10.19	21.77	14.09	0.61	1.67	2 783	8.26	9.57	5.61	0.22	0.59	C16
小肠	Small intestine	239	0.38	0.80	0.53	0.03	0.06	153	0.45	0.53	0.31	0.01	0.03	C17
结肠	Colon	1 984	3.12	6.65	4.27	0.16	0.45	1 428	4.24	4.91	2.83	0.11	0.28	C18
直肠	Rectum	2 932	4.61	9.83	6.31	0.25	0.70	1 752	5.20	6.02	3.50	0.14	0.36	C19-20
肛门	Anus	189	0.30	0.63	0.41	0.01	0.04	70	0.21	0.24	0.14	0.00	0.01	C21
肝脏	Liver	11 273	17.71	37.81	25.43	1.61	2.90	3 802	11.28	13.07	7.96	0.36	0.89	C22
胆囊及其他	Gallbladder etc.	645	1.01	2.16	1.38	0.06	0.14	818	2.43	2.81	1.64	0.06	0.18	C23-24
胰腺	Pancreas	1 940	3.05	6.51	4.22	0.21	0.48	1 376	4.08	4.73	2.79	0.12	0.31	C25
鼻、鼻窦及其他	Nose,sinuses etc.	81	0.13	0.27	0.18	0.01	0.02	64	0.19	0.22	0.14	0.01	0.01	C30-31
喉	Larynx	599	0.94	2.01	1.32	0.07	0.16	83	0.25	0.29	0.16	0.01	0.01	C32
气管、支气管、肺	Trachea,bronchus & lung	19 824	31.14	66.49	43.47	2.02	5.18	7 893	23.43	27.13	16.05	0.66	1.77	C33-34
其他胸腔器官	Other thoracic organs	251	0.39	0.84	0.58	0.03	0.07	137	0.41	0.47	0.31	0.02	0.03	C37-38
骨	Bone	511	0.80	1.71	1.18	0.06	0.13	322	0.96	1.11	0.73	0.03	0.08	C40-41
皮肤黑色素瘤	Melanoma of skin	85	0.13	0.29	0.20	0.01	0.02	54	0.16	0.19	0.12	0.01	0.01	C43
皮肤其他	Other skin	238	0.37	0.80	0.53	0.02	0.05	186	0.55	0.64	0.36	0.01	0.02	C44
间皮瘤	Mesothelioma	28	0.04	0.09	0.06	0.00	0.01	12	0.04	0.04	0.03	0.00	0.00	C45
卡波氏肉瘤	Kaposi sarcoma	33	0.05	0.11	0.08	0.00	0.01	16	0.05	0.06	0.05	0.00	0.00	C46
结缔组织、软组织	Connective & soft tissue	139	0.22	0.47	0.32	0.02	0.03	71	0.21	0.24	0.17	0.01	0.02	C47;C49
乳腺	Breast	122	0.19	0.41	0.28	0.01	0.03	2 514	7.46	8.64	5.60	0.41	0.61	C50
外阴	Vulva	—	—	—	—	—	—	60	0.18	0.21	0.13	0.01	0.02	C51
阴道	Vagina	—	—	—	—	—	—	41	0.12	0.14	0.09	0.00	0.01	C52
子宫颈	Cervix uteri	—	—	—	—	—	—	1 686	5.00	5.80	3.80	0.26	0.43	C53
子宫体	Corpus uteri	—	—	—	—	—	—	466	1.38	1.60	1.06	0.07	0.13	C54
子宫,部位不明	Uterus unspecified	—	—	—	—	—	—	221	0.66	0.76	0.48	0.03	0.05	C55
卵巢	Ovary	—	—	—	—	—	—	1 045	3.10	3.59	2.34	0.16	0.27	C56
其他女性生殖器	Other female genital organs	—	—	—	—	—	—	53	0.16	0.18	0.12	0.01	0.02	C57
胎盘	Placenta	—	—	—	—	—	—	1	0.00	0.00	0.00	0.00	0.00	C58
阴茎	Penis	63	0.10	0.21	0.14	0.01	0.02	—	—	—	—	—	—	C60
前列腺	Prostate	1 546	2.43	5.19	3.11	0.05	0.22	—	—	—	—	—	—	C61
睾丸	Testis	35	0.05	0.12	0.09	0.01	0.01	—	—	—	—	—	—	C62
其他男性生殖器	Other male genital organs	11	0.02	0.04	0.02	0.00	0.00	—	—	—	—	—	—	C63
肾	Kidney	459	0.72	1.54	0.98	0.05	0.10	226	0.67	0.78	0.46	0.02	0.05	C64
肾盂	Renal pelvis	54	0.08	0.18	0.12	0.01	0.01	52	0.15	0.18	0.10	0.00	0.01	C65
输尿管	Ureter	74	0.12	0.25	0.15	0.00	0.01	50	0.15	0.17	0.10	0.00	0.01	C66
膀胱	Bladder	1 073	1.69	3.60	2.21	0.05	0.19	300	0.89	1.03	0.56	0.01	0.05	C67
其他泌尿器官	Other urinary organs	16	0.03	0.05	0.03	0.00	0.00	9	0.03	0.03	0.02	0.00	0.00	C68
眼	Eye	24	0.04	0.08	0.07	0.00	0.01	13	0.04	0.04	0.05	0.00	0.00	C69
脑、神经系统	Brain,nervous system	1 314	2.06	4.41	3.26	0.19	0.34	1 004	2.98	3.45	2.47	0.13	0.25	C70-72,D32-33,D42-43
甲状腺	Thyroid	131	0.21	0.44	0.27	0.01	0.02	195	0.58	0.67	0.42	0.02	0.04	C73
肾上腺	Adrenal gland	45	0.07	0.15	0.10	0.01	0.01	34	0.10	0.12	0.08	0.00	0.01	C74
其他内分泌腺	Other endocrine	33	0.05	0.11	0.08	0.00	0.01	40	0.12	0.14	0.09	0.01	0.01	C75
霍奇金淋巴瘤	Hodgkin lymphoma	67	0.11	0.22	0.16	0.01	0.02	31	0.09	0.11	0.07	0.00	0.01	C81
非霍奇金淋巴瘤	Non-Hodgkin lymphoma	808	1.27	2.71	1.85	0.10	0.20	462	1.37	1.59	1.01	0.05	0.11	C82-C86;C96
免疫增生性疾病	Immunoproliferative diseases	5	0.01	0.02	0.01	0.00	0.00	2	0.01	0.01	0.01	0.00	0.00	C88
多发性骨髓瘤	Multiple myeloma	254	0.40	0.85	0.57	0.03	0.07	212	0.63	0.73	0.45	0.02	0.06	C90
淋巴样白血病	Lymphoid leukemia	300	0.47	1.01	0.86	0.04	0.07	178	0.53	0.61	0.49	0.03	0.05	C91
髓样白血病	Myeloid leukemia	376	0.59	1.26	0.92	0.05	0.10	286	0.85	0.98	0.70	0.04	0.08	C92-C94,D45-47
白血病,未特指	Leukemia unspecified	527	0.83	1.77	1.40	0.07	0.13	392	1.16	1.35	1.11	0.06	0.10	C95
其他或未指明部位	Other and unspecified	1 255	1.97	4.21	2.92	0.15	0.31	824	2.45	2.83	1.83	0.09	0.20	O&U
所有部位合计	All sites	63 669	100.00	213.54	141.03	6.84	16.07	33 693	100.00	115.83	71.10	3.40	7.68	C00-96, D32-33, D42-43, D45-47
所有部位除外 C44	All sites except C44	63 431	99.63	212.74	140.50	6.82	16.01	33 507	99.45	115.19	70.74	3.38	7.65	C00-96, D32-33, D42-43, D45-47 exc. C44

附表 2-18　2017 年全国西部农村肿瘤登记地区癌症死亡主要指标

Appendix Table 2-18　Cancer mortality in Western rural registration areas of China, 2017

部位 Site		男性 Male						女性 Female						ICD10
		死亡数 No. deaths	构成 Freq. /%	粗率 Crude rate/ 100 000⁻¹	世标率 ASR world/ 100 000⁻¹	累积率 Cum. rate/% 0~64	累积率 Cum. rate/% 0~74	死亡数 No. deaths	构成 Freq. /%	粗率 Crude rate/ 100 000⁻¹	世标率 ASR world/ 100 000⁻¹	累积率 Cum. rate/% 0~64	累积率 Cum. rate/% 0~74	
唇	Lip	33	0.05	0.10	0.06	0.00	0.01	11	0.03	0.03	0.02	0.00	0.00	C00
舌	Tongue	209	0.30	0.63	0.41	0.03	0.05	95	0.27	0.30	0.19	0.01	0.02	C01-02
口	Mouth	233	0.33	0.71	0.44	0.02	0.05	128	0.36	0.41	0.25	0.01	0.03	C03-06
唾液腺	Salivary glands	51	0.07	0.15	0.10	0.00	0.01	26	0.07	0.08	0.06	0.00	0.01	C07-08
扁桃腺	Tonsil	32	0.05	0.10	0.06	0.00	0.01	7	0.02	0.02	0.01	0.00	0.00	C09
其他口咽	Other oropharynx	93	0.13	0.28	0.18	0.01	0.02	20	0.06	0.06	0.04	0.00	0.00	C10
鼻咽	Nasopharynx	978	1.40	2.96	1.99	0.14	0.23	393	1.10	1.25	0.84	0.06	0.09	C11
下咽	Hypopharynx	108	0.15	0.33	0.22	0.01	0.03	7	0.02	0.02	0.01	0.00	0.00	C12-13
咽,部位不明	Pharynx unspecified	149	0.21	0.45	0.29	0.01	0.03	47	0.13	0.15	0.09	0.00	0.01	C14
食管	Esophagus	8 902	12.70	26.98	16.92	0.74	2.08	2 580	7.24	8.20	4.52	0.12	0.53	C15
胃	Stomach	8 301	11.85	25.16	15.90	0.72	1.86	3 578	10.04	11.38	6.55	0.26	0.69	C16
小肠	Small intestine	143	0.20	0.43	0.28	0.01	0.03	119	0.33	0.38	0.24	0.01	0.03	C17
结肠	Colon	1 210	1.73	3.67	2.31	0.10	0.25	856	2.40	2.72	1.60	0.07	0.18	C18
直肠	Rectum	3 009	4.29	9.12	5.70	0.22	0.62	1 873	5.26	5.96	3.49	0.15	0.38	C19-20
肛门	Anus	171	0.24	0.52	0.33	0.02	0.04	95	0.27	0.30	0.17	0.01	0.02	C21
肝脏	Liver	13 674	19.51	41.45	27.77	1.85	3.12	4 373	12.27	13.91	8.49	0.43	0.97	C22
胆囊及其他	Gallbladder etc.	567	0.81	1.72	1.09	0.05	0.12	732	2.05	2.33	1.37	0.06	0.16	C23-24
胰腺	Pancreas	1 711	2.44	5.19	3.30	0.17	0.38	1 102	3.09	3.50	2.08	0.10	0.25	C25
鼻、鼻窦及其他	Nose, sinuses etc.	99	0.14	0.30	0.23	0.01	0.03	61	0.17	0.19	0.13	0.01	0.01	C30-31
喉	Larynx	471	0.67	1.43	0.90	0.05	0.10	103	0.29	0.33	0.18	0.01	0.02	C32
气管、支气管、肺	Trachea, bronchus & lung	20 982	29.94	63.60	40.38	1.99	4.77	9 087	25.50	28.89	17.00	0.76	1.94	C33-34
其他胸腔器官	Other thoracic organs	168	0.24	0.51	0.35	0.02	0.04	99	0.28	0.31	0.21	0.01	0.02	C37-38
骨	Bone	578	0.82	1.75	1.19	0.06	0.13	373	1.05	1.19	0.77	0.04	0.09	C40-41
皮肤黑色素瘤	Melanoma of skin	61	0.09	0.18	0.12	0.01	0.01	47	0.13	0.15	0.09	0.01	0.01	C43
皮肤其他	Other skin	340	0.49	1.03	0.67	0.03	0.06	197	0.55	0.63	0.35	0.01	0.03	C44
间皮瘤	Mesothelioma	18	0.03	0.05	0.03	0.00	0.00	18	0.05	0.06	0.04	0.00	0.00	C45
卡波氏肉瘤	Kaposi sarcoma	26	0.04	0.08	0.06	0.00	0.01	8	0.02	0.03	0.02	0.00	0.00	C46
结缔组织、软组织	Connective & soft tissue	107	0.15	0.32	0.23	0.01	0.02	73	0.20	0.23	0.17	0.01	0.02	C47;C49
乳腺	Breast	83	0.12	0.25	0.16	0.01	0.02	2 082	5.84	6.62	4.46	0.35	0.48	C50
外阴	Vulva	—	—	—	—	—	—	43	0.12	0.14	0.08	0.00	0.01	C51
阴道	Vagina	—	—	—	—	—	—	36	0.10	0.11	0.07	0.00	0.01	C52
子宫颈	Cervix uteri	—	—	—	—	—	—	1 962	5.50	6.24	4.11	0.28	0.46	C53
子宫体	Corpus uteri	—	—	—	—	—	—	458	1.29	1.46	0.95	0.07	0.11	C54
子宫,部位不明	Uterus unspecified	—	—	—	—	—	—	331	0.93	1.05	0.69	0.04	0.08	C55
卵巢	Ovary	—	—	—	—	—	—	682	1.91	2.17	1.45	0.11	0.16	C56
其他女性生殖器	Other female genital organs	—	—	—	—	—	—	46	0.13	0.15	0.09	0.01	0.01	C57
胎盘	Placenta	—	—	—	—	—	—	1	0.00	0.00	0.00	0.00	0.00	C58
阴茎	Penis	73	0.10	0.22	0.14	0.01	0.02	—	—	—	—	—	—	C60
前列腺	Prostate	956	1.36	2.90	1.69	0.03	0.15	—	—	—	—	—	—	C61
睾丸	Testis	48	0.07	0.15	0.11	0.01	0.01	—	—	—	—	—	—	C62
其他男性生殖器	Other male genital organs	4	0.01	0.01	0.01	0.00	0.00	—	—	—	—	—	—	C63
肾	Kidney	303	0.43	0.92	0.64	0.04	0.07	170	0.48	0.54	0.33	0.02	0.04	C64
肾盂	Renal pelvis	60	0.09	0.18	0.11	0.01	0.01	32	0.09	0.10	0.06	0.00	0.01	C65
输尿管	Ureter	38	0.05	0.12	0.07	0.00	0.01	37	0.10	0.12	0.07	0.00	0.01	C66
膀胱	Bladder	957	1.37	2.90	1.75	0.05	0.16	245	0.69	0.78	0.43	0.01	0.04	C67
其他泌尿器官	Other urinary organs	10	0.01	0.03	0.02	0.00	0.00	4	0.01	0.01	0.01	0.00	0.00	C68
眼	Eye	26	0.04	0.08	0.07	0.00	0.01	18	0.05	0.06	0.04	0.00	0.00	C69
脑、神经系统	Brain, nervous system	1 529	2.18	4.63	3.43	0.21	0.35	1 034	2.90	3.29	2.29	0.13	0.24	C70-72, D32-33, D42-43
甲状腺	Thyroid	86	0.12	0.26	0.17	0.01	0.02	144	0.40	0.46	0.30	0.02	0.03	C73
肾上腺	Adrenal gland	34	0.05	0.10	0.07	0.00	0.01	24	0.07	0.08	0.05	0.00	0.00	C74
其他内分泌腺	Other endocrine	23	0.03	0.07	0.05	0.00	0.01	32	0.09	0.10	0.08	0.01	0.01	C75
霍奇金淋巴瘤	Hodgkin lymphoma	45	0.06	0.14	0.10	0.01	0.01	19	0.05	0.06	0.03	0.00	0.00	C81
非霍奇金淋巴瘤	Non-Hodgkin lymphoma	724	1.03	2.19	1.50	0.08	0.18	381	1.07	1.21	0.79	0.04	0.10	C82-C86;C96
免疫增生性疾病	Immunoproliferative diseases	8	0.01	0.02	0.01	0.00	0.00	3	0.01	0.01	0.01	0.00	0.00	C88
多发性骨髓瘤	Multiple myeloma	215	0.31	0.65	0.45	0.02	0.05	109	0.31	0.35	0.23	0.01	0.03	C90
淋巴样白血病	Lymphoid leukemia	241	0.34	0.73	0.64	0.04	0.06	184	0.52	0.59	0.49	0.03	0.05	C91
髓样白血病	Myeloid leukemia	291	0.42	0.88	0.70	0.04	0.07	199	0.56	0.63	0.47	0.03	0.05	C92-C94, D45-47
白血病,未特指	Leukemia unspecified	617	0.88	1.87	1.51	0.09	0.14	443	1.24	1.41	1.09	0.07	0.11	C95
其他或未指明部位	Other and unspecified	1 285	1.83	3.89	2.65	0.14	0.28	815	2.29	2.59	1.71	0.09	0.18	O&U
所有部位合计	All sites	70 080	100.00	212.42	137.58	7.10	15.73	35 642	100.00	113.33	69.36	3.48	7.71	C00-96, D32-33, D42-43, D45-47
所有部位除外 C44	All sites except C44	69 740	99.51	211.39	136.91	7.07	15.67	35 445	99.45	112.71	69.01	3.47	7.68	C00-96, D32-33, D42-43, D45-47 exc. C44

鸣　谢

《中国肿瘤登记年报》编委会对各肿瘤登记处的相关工作人员在本年报出版过程中给予的大力协助，尤其在整理、补充、审核登记资料，以及建档、建库等方面所做出的贡献表示感谢。衷心感谢编写组成员在年报撰写工作付出的辛苦努力。

Acknowledgement

The editorial committee of *China Cancer Registry Annual Report* would like to express their gratitude to all staff of cancer registries who have made a great contribution for the report, especially on data reduction, supplements, auditing and cancer registration database management. Sincere thanks go to all members of the contributors for their great efforts.

肿瘤登记处名单 List of Cancer Registries and Registrars

省(自治区、直辖市) Province (autonomous region, municipality)	肿瘤登记处 Cancer registry	登记处所在单位 Affiliation	主要工作人员 Staff
北京市	北京市	北京大学肿瘤医院暨北京市肿瘤防治研究所	季加孚 王　宁 杨　雷 刘　硕 李慧超 张　希 李晴雨 程杨杨
天津市	天津市	天津市疾病预防控制中心	江国虹 王德征 沈成凤 王　冲 孙　坤 张　爽 张　辉 宋桂德
河北省	河北省	河北医科大学第四医院	单保恩 贺宇彤 李道娟 刘言玉 梁　迪 温登瑰 靳　晶 师　金 瞿　峰
	石家庄市	石家庄市疾病预防控制中心	马新颜 梁震宇 高　从 范志磊 张幸岩 曹朴芳 赵　炜
	石家庄市郊区	石家庄市疾病预防控制中心	高　从 梁震宇 马新颜 田密格 任军辉 张玉峰 张玉伟 邓莉莉
	赞皇县	赞皇县疾病预防控制中心	王树革 李　丽 郝月红 吕晓红
	迁西县	迁西县疾病预防控制中心	盛振海 赵金鸽 陈晓东 王伟光 赵　珊 赵　丹
	迁安市	迁安市疾病预防控制中心	刘　芳 王翠玲 邵舰伟 谌华卿
	秦皇岛市	秦皇岛市第四医院	熊润红 赵　月 杨　晋 窦雅琳
	邯郸市邯山区	邯郸市邯山区疾病预防控制中心	张瑞欣 李金娥 王晓燕 白银燕
	大名县	大名县疾病预防控制中心	任永彪 刘肖单 孙成旭 孙建冰 杨永华 张　赛 李欣欣
	涉县	涉县肿瘤防治所	李永伟 温登瑰 杨保证 张书宾 贾瑞强 张　喻
	磁县	磁县肿瘤防治研究所	宋国慧 陈　超 孟凡书 龚妍玮 冀鸿新 张　金 路晓雪 高志光
	武安市	武安市疾病预防控制中心	杨　慧 魏延其 郭秀杰 崔亚宁
	邢台市	邢台市人民医院	刘登湘 王军辉 贾丹丹 张亚琛 刘淑娴 韩　蕾 孟亚飞 王艳霞
	邢台县	邢台县疾病预防控制中心	董　玲 贾丹丹 刘淑娴 王德旗 赵书云

省(自治区、直辖市) Province (autonomous region, municipality)	肿瘤登记处 Cancer registry	登记处所在单位 Affiliation	主要工作人员 Staff
	临城县	临城县人民医院	和丽娜　王　童
	内丘县	内丘县疾病预防控制中心	龙　云　石胜民　智　玉　房晓芳
	任县	河北省任县医院	赵雅芳　吉国强　孟　飞
	保定市	保定市疾病预防控制中心	张　雁　赵凤芹　侯　烨　和丽娜　张卫君　曹　帅　孙　明　张　利
	望都县	望都县疾病预防控制中心	梁鹏涛　田红梅　谷朝华
	安国市	安国市疾病预防控制中心	刘树生　李　辉　魏泽永
	张家口市宣化区	张家口市宣化区疾病预防控制中心	左存锐　李少英　支　雯
	张北县	张北县疾病预防控制中心	刘　会　刘东雍
	承德市双桥区	承德市双桥区疾病预防控制中心	管丽娟　李广鲲　王明慧　平　萍　彭媛媛
	丰宁满族自治县	丰宁满族自治县医院	梁树军　颜学文　付杨健娇
	沧州市	沧州市疾病预防控制中心	杨希晨　鲁文慧　安连芹　高哲敏　李文娟　仝建玲　付素红　杨秀敏
	海兴县	海兴县疾病预防控制中心	韩明明　张　策
	盐山县	盐山县疾病预防控制中心	巩吉良　陈清彦　边梅芳　侯美娟
	衡水市冀州区	衡水市冀州区疾病预防控制中心	魏　丹　郭志超　贾向勇　酒梅洁　王英林
	辛集市	辛集市疾病预防控制中心	郝士卿　万真真　耿　兵
山西省	山西省	山西省肿瘤医院	张永贞　郭雪蓉　马朝辉　曹　凌　王昕琛　崔王飞
	太原市杏花岭区	太原市杏花岭区疾病预防控制中心	荆国旗　倪　芳　薛秀丽　赵　虹　李芝玲
	阳泉市	阳泉市肿瘤防治研究所	高秋生　吕利成　冯俊青　蒋书琼
	平定县	平定县疾病预防控制中心	贾源瑶　李春霞
	盂县	盂县疾病预防控制中心	李俊才　郭长青　韩瑞贞
	平顺县	平顺县疾病预防控制中心	贾艳芳　王丽娟
	沁源县	沁源县疾病预防控制中心	关鹏飞
	阳城县	阳城县肿瘤医院	王新正　元芳梅　李　阳
	晋中市榆次区	晋中市榆次区疾病预防控制中心	郑永萍　郭秀峰　董小平　智　伟　李巧凤　闫梦娇　郭　磊
	昔阳县	昔阳县疾病预防控制中心	王晓霞
	寿阳县	寿阳县疾病预防控制中心	张慧玲　郝佐文　霍志强　杨晓静　胡旭强　王俊红
	稷山县	稷山县疾病预防控制中心	谭万霞　赵夏娟

续表

省(自治区、直辖市) Province (autonomous region, municipality)	肿瘤登记处 Cancer registry	登记处所在单位 Affiliation	主要工作人员 Staff
	绛县	绛县疾病预防控制中心	李姣霞　高丽莉
	垣曲县	垣曲县疾病预防控制中心	张红霞　武茹燕
	芮城县	芮城县疾病预防控制中心	范夏莉　王康宁
	洪洞县	洪洞县疾病预防控制中心	侯晓艳　焦燕燕
	临县	临县疾病预防控制中心	刘秀娥　高旭亮
	孝义市	孝义市疾病预防控制中心	冀德恩　张学慧　黄　丽　张剑荣
内蒙古自治区	内蒙古自治区	内蒙古自治区综合疾病预防控制中心	席云峰　乔丽颖
	呼和浩特市	呼和浩特市疾病预防控制中心	汪洋杰　李　娜　董连英
	呼伦贝尔市	呼伦贝尔市疾病预防控制中心	王　勇　蔡静明
	通辽市	通辽市疾病预防控制中心	李智慧
	赤峰市	赤峰市疾病预防控制中心	张竞丹　谢景学　王化彬　迟艳玲
	锡林郭勒盟	锡林郭勒盟疾病预防控制中心	彭爱云　格日勒　王树丽
	巴彦淖尔市	巴彦淖尔市疾病预防控制中心	张　琳　韩爱英　邓海凤
	武川县	武川县疾病预防控制中心	郭建平　赵晓钢
	土默特右旗	土默特右旗疾病预防控制中心	贾卫军　王　峰　田晓丽　邬燕慧　刘茂林
	赤峰市红山区	赤峰市红山区疾病预防控制中心	何　丽
	赤峰市元宝山区	赤峰市元宝山区疾病预防控制中心	韩小玉　孟晓东
	赤峰市松山区	赤峰市松山区疾病预防控制中心	王梦元　许建斌　夏丽红
	巴林左旗	巴林左旗疾病预防控制中心	凌海杰　宫　明
	赤峰市敖汉旗	敖汉旗疾病预防控制中心	耿文飞　崔海华
	通辽市科尔沁区	通辽市科尔沁区疾病预防控制中心	周婷婷　高　晶
	科尔沁左翼中旗	科尔沁左翼中旗疾病预防控制中心	李伟杰　刘艳玲
	开鲁县	开鲁县疾病预防控制中心	吴艳伟　丁秀鸿　曹　亮
	库伦旗	库伦旗疾病预防控制中心	于鑫刚　王朝民
	奈曼旗	奈曼旗疾病预防控制中心	李丽媛　倪志华　张永红
	扎鲁特旗	扎鲁特旗疾病预防控制中心	王晓琪　婷　婷
	呼伦贝尔市海拉尔区	呼伦贝尔市海拉尔区疾病预防控制中心	孔程程　孙溯苑

省(自治区、直辖市) Province (autonomous region, municipality)	肿瘤登记处 Cancer registry	登记处所在单位 Affiliation	主要工作人员 Staff
	呼伦贝尔市扎赉诺尔区	呼伦贝尔市扎赉诺尔区疾病预防控制中心	刘杰峰　过　亮
	阿荣旗	阿荣旗疾病预防控制中心	郭天骅　高　智　林鸿鸣　张银华
	莫力达瓦达斡尔族自治旗	莫力达瓦达斡尔族自治旗疾病预防控制中心	赵占峰
	鄂温克族自治旗	鄂温克族自治旗疾病预防控制中心	张艺杰　田伟伟
	陈巴尔虎旗	陈巴尔虎旗疾病预防控制中心	永　梅
	满洲里市	满洲里市疾病预防控制中心	刘　伟　张欣越　张美燕
	牙克石市	牙克石市疾病预防控制中心	苏　燕　李覆男　夏　宇
	扎兰屯市	扎兰屯市疾病预防控制中心	李　静　陈　丽
	额尔古纳市	额尔古纳市疾病预防控制中心	张　欢
	根河市	根河市疾病预防控制中心	谷寒峰
	巴彦淖尔市临河区	巴彦淖尔市临河区疾病预防控制中心	马　萍　安　静　刘美丽　丁建平
	锡林浩特市	锡林浩特市疾病预防控制中心	刘福生　闫永峰　李智鹏　樊翠玲
辽宁省	辽宁省	辽宁省疾病预防控制中心	穆慧娟
	沈阳市	沈阳市疾病预防控制中心	白　杉　刘　岩　许秀莹　刘新雨
	康平县	康平县疾病预防控制中心	彭红伟　白宇南
	法库县	法库县疾病预防控制中心	马云丽　张宝桐　曹海洋　白鹤楠
	大连市	大连市疾病预防控制中心	王晓锋　梅　丹　林　红　张新慧
	庄河市	庄河市疾病预防控制中心	王丽娜　姜金宏
	鞍山市	鞍山市疾病预防控制中心	徐绍和　王丽娟　邹青春　尹　晔　张微微　王肖琳　林立强　李绯璇　刘美玲　陈康境　张　颖　洪圣茹
	本溪市	本溪市疾病预防控制中心	安晓霞　李海娜
	丹东市	丹东市疾病预防控制中心	孙继绪　邹晓琳　盛禹萌
	东港市	东港市疾病预防控制中心	张武武　程笛珈
	营口市	营口市疾病预防控制中心	白明宇　刘　洋　陈丽莉　李　颖
	阜新市	阜新市疾病预防控制中心	代晓泽　刘　辉　徐　飒
	彰武县	彰武县疾病预防控制中心	王静艳　王　楠
	辽阳县	辽阳县疾病预防控制中心	何秀玲　李迎秋　李修竹
	盘锦市大洼区	盘锦市大洼区疾病预防控制中心	吕建峰　陆　阳

续表

省(自治区、直辖市) Province (autonomous region, municipality)	肿瘤登记处 Cancer registry	登记处所在单位 Affiliation	主要工作人员 Staff
	建平县	建平县疾病预防控制中心	杨晓光　马佳杰　熊丽杰　吕广艳
吉林省	吉林省	吉林省疾病预防控制中心慢病所	朱颖俐　侯筑林　贾湑媛
	德惠市	德惠市疾病预防控制中心	程志芳　凌命新　邢　健
	吉林市	吉林市疾病预防控制中心	张　迪　孙殿伟　刘　晔　王丽宇　王　刚
	吉林市昌邑区	吉林市昌邑区疾病预防控制中心	闫　双　何　冰　徐　翠　靳程程
	吉林市龙潭区	吉林市龙潭区疾病预防控制中心	代肖瑶
	吉林市船营区	吉林市船营区疾病预防控制中心	刘亚卓
	吉林市丰满区	吉林市丰满区疾病预防控制中心	周兴超　周　岩
	永吉县	永吉县疾病预防控制中心	王晓妍　何晓峰
	蛟河市	蛟河市疾病预防控制中心	张黎黎
	桦甸市	桦甸市疾病预防控制中心	王晓丽　李忠诚　于彩霞
	磐石市	磐石市疾病预防控制中心	冀　鹏　步　颖
	通化市	通化市疾病预防控制中心	何　柳　张　琳　魏　霞　王晓雪
	柳河县	柳河县疾病预防控制中心	季洪伟
	梅河口市	梅河口市疾病预防控制中心	王　彬　刘　宏　潘培丰　李红云
	大安市	大安市疾病预防控制中心	王　越　王　威　李晓秋　刘艳萍
	延吉市	延吉市疾病预防控制中心	方学哲　孙铭徽　谢　瑶
	图们市	图们市疾病预防控制中心	宋立军　王嘉玉　郑玉凤
	敦化市	敦化市疾病预防控制中心	李秀英　朱晓梅　马桂君
	珲春市	珲春市疾病预防控制中心	任爱芳　李美子
	龙井市	龙井市疾病预防控制中心	罗艳丽　金秀颖
	和龙市	和龙市疾病预防控制中心	张春英　马晓宇　徐桐欣
	汪清县	汪清县疾病预防控制中心	李美娜　刘　宇
	安图县	安图县疾病预防控制中心	朴顺姬　段丽雪　方立强
黑龙江省	黑龙江省	黑龙江省癌症中心	宋冰冰　孙惠昕　张茂祥　王婉莹　贾海晗
	哈尔滨市道里区	哈尔滨市道里区疾病预防控制中心	王　欣　康　娟　杨媛媛　那　倩　张希羽
	哈尔滨市南岗区	哈尔滨市南岗区疾病预防控制中心	王　驰　于　波　单晓丽　王威娜
	哈尔滨市香坊区	哈尔滨市香坊区疾病预防控制中心	曲　洋　高艳丽

省(自治区、直辖市) Province (autonomous region, municipality)	肿瘤登记处 Cancer registry	登记处所在单位 Affiliation	主要工作人员 Staff
	尚志市	尚志市疾病预防控制中心	姜　欣
	五常市	五常市疾病预防控制中心	周　锐　田伟成
	勃利县	勃利县疾病预防控制中心	石旭蕾　胡　月
	牡丹江市东安区	牡丹江市东安区疾病预防控制中心	常　蓉
	牡丹江市阳明区	牡丹江市阳明区疾病预防控制中心	姚　琳
	牡丹江市爱民区	牡丹江市爱民区疾病预防控制中心	郝庆华
	牡丹江市西安区	牡丹江市西安区疾病预防控制中心	邱　红　严海莹　付　饶
	海林市	海林市疾病预防控制中心	佘　斌　龙　江　牛春英
上海市	上海市	上海市疾病预防控制中心	付　晨　施　燕　吴春晓　顾　凯　庞　怡　王春芳　鲍萍萍　龚杨明　施　亮　窦剑明　向咏梅　吴梦吟
江苏省	江苏省	江苏市疾病预防控制中心(江苏省公共卫生研究院)	武　鸣　韩仁强　周金意　罗鹏飞　俞　浩　缪伟刚
	无锡市	无锡市疾病预防控制中心	王　璐　钱　云　杨志杰　董昀球　陈　海　刘　佳　申　倩　刘雅琦
	无锡市	无锡市锡山区疾病预防控制中心	徐红艳　顾　月　邹丽艳　薛文涛　姚吕航　夏　焱　华　芬　浦佳林　张　丹　徐　芳
	无锡市	无锡市惠山区疾病预防控制中心	陈顺平　曹　军　蒋金彪　茹　炯　李心意　赵　悦
	无锡市	无锡市滨湖区疾病预防控制中心	徐汉顺　刘俊华　杜　明　许丽佳　肖静燕　叶文斌　许　敏　王　菁　顾　飞　朱　漪　陶燕君
	无锡市	无锡市梁溪区疾病预防控制中心	沈晓文　陈　鑫　王　琳　包海明　徐凌云
	无锡市	无锡市新吴区疾病预防控制中心	陆绍琦　胡　磊　李　纯　吴晓慧　颜锁芳　张　芳　殷锡琴　钱　郁　钱嘉红　华　怡　朱明玉
	无锡市	无锡市经开区疾病预防控制中心	王礼华　高敏国　陈善辉　邹志红　王　景　周梦迪　姚成帅　陈汉哲　段春晓
	江阴市	江阴市疾病预防控制中心	章　剑　朱爱萍　李　莹　刘　娟　王敏洁　汤海波　张燕茹
	宜兴市	宜兴市疾病预防控制中心	胡　静　任露露　闵艺璇
	徐州市	徐州市疾病预防控制中心	娄培安　常桂秋　张　盼　董宗美　陈培培　张　宁　乔　程　李　婷

省(自治区、直辖市) Province (autonomous region, municipality)	肿瘤登记处 Cancer registry	登记处所在单位 Affiliation	主要工作人员 Staff
	徐州市	徐州市鼓楼区疾病预防控制中心	刘娅娴　祁艳秋
	徐州市	徐州市云龙区疾病预防控制中心	李玉波　宋兆芬　渠漫漫　刘　云
	徐州市	徐州市贾汪区疾病预防控制中心	宗　华　张　迪　李金宇
	徐州市	徐州市泉山区疾病预防控制中心	吴海宏　李　念　王艳梅　张　培　赵梦晨
	徐州市	徐州市铜山区疾病预防控制中心	唐士涛　侯书莹
	徐州市	丰县疾病预防控制中心	王友林　韩红芳　李爽爽
	徐州市	沛县疾病预防控制中心	独梅芝　陈　峰　徐　丽　梁艳静　赵欲辉　倪　萌　魏文静
	徐州市	睢宁县疾病预防控制中心	仲崇义　张申亮　赵梦洁　姚建英
	徐州市	新沂市疾病预防控制中心	王　志　张　奇
	徐州市	邳州市疾病预防控制中心	温之花　刘　杰　李军政
	常州市	常州市疾病预防控制中心	徐文超　骆文书　李贵英　周孟孟
	常州市新北区	常州市新北区疾病预防控制中心	张　友　郑蜀贞　何　怡
	常州市天宁区	常州市天宁区疾病预防控制中心	陈燕芬　施鸿飞
	常州市武进区	常州市武进区疾病预防控制中心	强德仁　宗　菁　石素逸　杨佳成　孔晓玲　闫于飘
	常州市钟楼区	常州市钟楼区疾病预防控制中心	崔艳丽　吴振霞　陈志华　戴安迪
	常州市金坛区	常州市金坛区疾病预防控制中心	周　鑫　程　鑫
	溧阳市	溧阳市疾病预防控制中心	刘建平　狄　静　曹　磊　石一辰　朱阿仙
	苏州市	苏州市疾病预防控制中心	陆　艳　王临池　黄春妍　华钰洁
	苏州市	苏州高新区疾病预防控制中心	王从菊　归国平　季　文　顾　晴
	苏州市	苏州市吴中区疾病预防控制中心	顾建芬　周　游　刘景超　马菊萍
	苏州市	苏州市相城区疾病预防控制中心	古娜利　吴向青　张　群　任玮叶
	苏州市	苏州市姑苏区疾病预防控制中心	张　秋　孔芳芳　吴新凡　徐　燚　陈　丽

省(自治区、直辖市) Province (autonomous region, municipality)	肿瘤登记处 Cancer registry	登记处所在单位 Affiliation	主要工作人员 Staff
	苏州市	苏州市吴江区疾病预防控制中心	沈建新 沈红梅 张荣艳 姚小燕 彭晓楚 杨 梅 沈 霞 俞哲宇
	苏州市	苏州市工业园区疾病预防控制中心	周 慧 周靓玥 翟 静 景 阳
	常熟市	常熟市疾病预防控制中心	陈冰霞 盛红艳 吴 叶 薛雨星 陈丽枫 顾亦斌 叶映丹
	张家港市	张家港市疾病预防控制中心	杜国明 邱 晶 秦敏晔 赵丽霞 王夏冬 王洵之 朱晓炜
	昆山市	昆山市疾病预防控制中心	张 婷 秦 威 金亦徐 陆吕霖 周 杰 仝 岚 邱和泉 贺方荣 朱琴花
	太仓市	太仓市疾病预防控制中心	张建安 高玲琳 颜小銮 陆鸿滋
	南通市	南通市疾病预防控制中心	徐 红 王 秦 韩颖颖 潘少聪 梁潇静
	南通市	南通市崇川区疾病预防控制中心	刘海峰 郑会燕
	南通市	南通市通州区疾病预防控制中心	赵 培 刘 玉
	海安市	海安市疾病预防控制中心	王小健 童海燕 孙 静
	如东县	如东县疾病预防控制中心	张爱红 纪桂勤 张红星 孙艳丽 吴双玲 季佳慧 周晓云
	启东市	启东肝癌防治研究所	朱 健 陈永胜 王 军 张永辉 丁璐璐 陈建国
	如皋市	如皋市疾病预防控制中心	吕家爱 王书兰 徐周洲 吴 坚
	南通市海门区	南通市海门区疾病预防控制中心	杨艳蕾 唐锦高 倪倬健 邱 敏 施 华
	连云港市	连云港市疾病预防控制中心	董建梅 张春道 李伟伟 马昭君 秦绪成 柴丽丽
	连云港市	连云港市海州区疾病预防控制中心	李炎炎 李佳雨 邓鑫鑫
	连云港市	连云港市连云区疾病预防控制中心	付艳云 刘 敏 张 琦 李绪磊 惠康琴
	连云港市	连云港市经济技术开发区疾病预防控制中心	李存禄 宋家胜
	连云港市	连云港市赣榆区疾病预防控制中心	张晓峰 金 凤 顾绍生
	东海县	东海县疾病预防控制中心	吴同浩 仲 进 王 勇 马 进 吉园园 陈 晓
	灌云县	灌云县疾病预防控制中心	马士化 宋 靖 严春华

省(自治区、直辖市) Province (autonomous region, municipality)	肿瘤登记处 Cancer registry	登记处所在单位 Affiliation	主要工作人员 Staff
	灌南县	灌南县疾病预防控制中心	张源生　陈学琴　丁梦秋　孟忆宁
	淮安市	淮安市疾病预防控制中心	沈　欢　潘恩春　孙中明　张　芹　文进博　缪丹丹　王　璐　唐　勇
	淮安市淮安区	淮安市淮安区疾病预防控制中心	宋　光　王　昕　苏　明　颜庆洋　朱丽萍　开海涛　马建玲　顾忠祥
	淮安市淮阴区	淮安市淮阴区疾病预防控制中心	罗国良　袁　瑛　刘　丹　徐　静　滕笑雨　高晓清　李　敏
	淮安市清江浦区	淮安市清江浦区疾病预防控制中心	曹慷慷　万福萍
	涟水县	涟水县疾病预防控制中心	叶建玲　孙维新　浦继尹
	淮安市洪泽区	淮安市洪泽区疾病预防控制中心	李　栋　陈思红　张举巧　袁翠莲　王庶安　曹巧力
	盱眙县	盱眙县疾病预防控制中心	王　裕　姜其家　袁守国
	金湖县	金湖县疾病预防控制中心	陈茂勇　何士林　吴　婷　雷茵子
	盐城市	盐城市疾病预防控制中心	刘付东　吴玲玲　梁　季　郑春早　祁朝霞
	盐城市亭湖区	盐城市亭湖区疾病预防控制中心	严莉丽　开志琴　王　静
	盐城市盐都区	盐城市盐都区疾病预防控制中心	何　飞　王建康　黄海涌
	响水县	响水县疾病预防控制中心	潘永富　陈玥华　王　超　徐红云　刘宇春
	滨海县	滨海县疾病预防控制中心	蔡　伟　赵　鹏　李　明　陈希冀　王　瑞　胡　裕　樊明静
	阜宁县	阜宁县疾病预防控制中心	梁从凯　杨尚波　支　杰
	射阳县	射阳县疾病预防控制中心	戴曙光　戴春云　王颖莹　陈星宇　戴　利
	建湖县	建湖县疾病预防控制中心	王　剑　肖　丽　孔文娟
	东台市	东台市疾病预防控制中心	郑小祥　赵建华　丁海健　史春兰
	盐城市大丰区	盐城市大丰区疾病预防控制中心	顾晓平　顾　昕　盛　凤　王银存　智恒奎
	扬州市	扬州市疾病预防控制中心	解　晔　李秋梅　杨文彬　时巧梅　赵　培　蒋　萌　胡乃元
	宝应县	宝应县疾病预防控制中心	梁永春　朱立文　任　涛　王元霞　潘艳玉
	镇江市	镇江市疾病预防控制中心	姜方平　徐　璐　王宏宇　古孝勇　何佳佳
	丹阳市	丹阳市疾病预防控制中心	应洪琰　周　超　陈丽黎　胡佳慧　王佳烨
	扬中市	扬中市肿瘤防治研究所	朱进华　华召来　周　琴　施爱武　冯　祥　宋统球
	泰州市	泰州市疾病预防控制中心	赵小兰　卢海燕　张德坤　杨玉雪　张慧琴　周　永　浦　栋

省(自治区、直辖市) Province (autonomous region, municipality)	肿瘤登记处 Cancer registry	登记处所在单位 Affiliation	主要工作人员 Staff
	泰兴市	泰兴市疾病预防控制中心	黄素勤 范 敏 徐 兴 封军莉 丁华萍 刘静琦 蒋 慧
	宿迁市	宿迁市疾病预防控制中心	卢道山 于 蕾 邱玉保 高 歌
	宿迁市宿城区	宿迁市宿城区疾病预防控制中心	漆苏洋 陈 英 张恋恋 朱 敏 于蒙蒙
	宿迁市宿豫区	宿迁市宿豫区疾病预防控制中心	朱 雷 郭鑫雨 陶 欣 孙绪远 王松梅 胡彩红
	泗阳县	泗阳县疾病预防控制中心	韩 奎 李红霞 符地宝 陈淑婷
浙江省	浙江省	浙江省肿瘤防治办公室	程向东 俞 敏 杜灵彬 李辉章 陈瑶瑶 裘燕飞 钟节鸣 龚巍巍 周慧娟 朱 陈 王悠清 王 乐 陈雯冰 陈 刚
	杭州市	杭州市疾病预防控制中心	徐 珏 姜彩霞 姜 鹏 任艳军 张 艳 刘 冰 秦 康
	宁波市鄞州区	宁波市鄞州区疾病预防控制中心	林鸿波 沈 鹏 陈 奇 赵 磊
	慈溪市	慈溪市疾病预防控制中心	吴逸平 马 旭 罗 丹 刘 琼 黄振宇 罗央努 黄 文 王利君 胡 吉 岑 鑫
	温州市鹿城区	温州市鹿城区疾病预防控制中心	朱海深 谢海斌 陈 茜 陈 捷 张沛绮 徐晓旭 郑茹茹
	嘉兴市	嘉兴市疾病预防控制中心	李雪琴 陈中文 顾伟玲 谢 亮 陈文燕 金 鎏 王 林 周夏芳 金泽彬
	嘉善县	嘉善县肿瘤防治所	沈飞琼 杨金华 李其龙 吕洁萍 张小红
	海宁市	海宁市中医院	朱云峰 祝丽娟 杨 靖 封 琳 白卿长
	长兴县	长兴县疾病预防控制中心	施长苗 秦家胜 陈 蓉 臧宇凡 陈 芸 顾建萍 叶 萍
	绍兴市上虞区	绍兴市上虞区疾病预防控制中心	王家开 章 军 丁萍飞 杨晓静 赵之青 龚月江 阮建江 王少华
	永康市	永康市疾病预防控制中心	潘中伟 胡云卿 吴忠顶 胡 浩 朱洪挺 胡春生 徐玲巧 陈 璐 沈锦绣 周美儿
	开化县	开化县疾病预防控制中心	严传富 汪德兵 项彩英 吴芝兰 应武群 万红建 叶 青 王贵平 余 虹
	岱山县	岱山县疾病预防控制中心	李琼燕 虞吉寅 张彤杰 何存弘 赵剑刚 王坤炎 王志平 王建军 徐 妮 俞秀华
	仙居县	仙居县疾病预防控制中心	蔡红卫 应江伟 吴武军 周立新 王丽君 王宇多 郑 红 王敏华 陈海仙 王丹枫
	龙泉市	龙泉市疾病预防控制中心	钟伟文 梅盛华 万春松 刘卫红 潘伟文 叶水菊 尹丽梅 谢泽久 张美锦 吴国庆

续表

省(自治区、直辖市) Province (autonomous region, municipality)	肿瘤登记处 Cancer registry	登记处所在单位 Affiliation	主要工作人员 Staff
安徽省	安徽省	安徽省疾病预防控制中心	刘志荣　王华东　陈叶纪　查震球　戴　丹
	合肥市	合肥市疾病预防控制中心	孙　锋　张小鹏　张俊青　李佳佳　唐　伦　陈晓园　穆永春　屈跃斌　胡玉莹　张　欢　何丽芳
	长丰县	长丰县疾病预防控制中心	孙多壮　郑　军　陈　春　吴海燕
	肥东县	肥东县疾病预防控制中心	张全寿　徐　旭　陈海涛
	肥西县	肥西县疾病预防控制中心	胡晓先　汪　飞　魏九丹
	庐江县	庐江县疾病预防控制中心	郑诗佳　吴　骅
	巢湖市	巢湖市疾病预防控制中心	宋玉华　叶正文　王义江　刘　涛
	芜湖市	芜湖市疾病预防控制中心	朱君君　崔晓娟　陈佳瑶　盛　娟　鲍慧芬　王力炜　丁卫群　赵丽华　王秀丽　吴瑞萍　冯花平
	蚌埠市	蚌埠市疾病预防控制中心	陈　军　张威振　周国华　白　雪　陈　艳　尚晓静　苏一兰
	五河县	五河县疾病预防控制中心	夏立环　郭茂蕴　纪　琼　许美菱
	淮南市大通区	大通区疾病预防控制中心	王艳霞　张　娇　陈邦齐
	淮南市田家庵区	田家庵区卫生防疫和食品药品安全服务中心	周　蕾　李娜娜　崔　越
	淮南市谢家集区	谢家集区卫生防疫和食品药品安全服务中心	辛家魁　吕　娟
	淮南市八公山区	八公山区卫生防疫和食品药品安全服务中心	吴　婷　叶亚萍
	淮南市潘集区	潘集区卫生防疫和食品药品安全服务中心	左廷杰　孙海防　姚　媛
	凤台县	凤台县疾病预防控制中心	秦克波　郭　克　李　涛　陈志强
	马鞍山市	马鞍山市疾病预防控制中心	王　春　叶敏仕　张　燕　蔡华英　秦其荣
	当涂县	当涂县疾病预防控制中心	徐　薇　李代平　卜维霞
	濉溪县	濉溪县疾病预防控制中心	贾　林　周鹏程　杨　珂　朱　英　张贵然
	铜陵市	铜陵市疾病预防控制中心	吴　刚　钱　丹　刘　睿　汪　蕊
	铜陵市义安区	铜陵市义安区疾病预防控制中心	张　标　丁　媛　高红霞
	安庆市宜秀区	安庆市宜秀区疾病预防控制中心	郝润华　鲍克彪
	岳西县	岳西县疾病预防控制中心	范莉莉　储琼瑛　亓志强
	黄山市屯溪区	屯溪区疾病预防控制中心	叶雯雯　冯　桅
	天长市	天长市疾病预防控制中心	胡　彪　赵培甫　张　浩

省(自治区、直辖市) Province (autonomous region, municipality)	肿瘤登记处 Cancer registry	登记处所在单位 Affiliation	主要工作人员 Staff
	阜阳市颍州区	阜阳市颍州区疾病预防控制中心	张海峰　郭　青　刘俊辉　王福军　王明玉　韦冰之　韩　梅
	阜阳市颍东区	阜阳市颍东区疾病预防控制中心	马朝阳　孙　涛　郭海昊　陈　雷　徐晓晴　张静静
	太和县	太和县疾病预防控制中心	张怡楠　李诗童　张西才　王允田　谭霈源　范　鑫
	阜南县	阜南县疾病预防控制中心	杨晓波　张永红　田　侠　单文华　张家棒
	颍上县	颍上县疾病预防控制中心	王　政　吴　昊　明　超　彭姝婞
	宿州市埇桥区	埇桥区疾病预防控制中心	刘中华　刘　森　张　鹏　张圆圆　黄　磊
	灵璧县	灵璧县疾病预防控制中心	郭启高　赵　辉　汤雅丽
	寿县	寿县疾病预防控制中心	杨茂敏　蔡传毓　徐海军　黄　奎　霍圣菊　唐晶晶　周　颖　王正友　周玉雪　陶俊婷
	霍邱县	霍邱县疾病预防控制中心	吴礼娟　周明琴
	金寨县	金寨县疾病预防控制中心	俞　亮　廖家胜　张礼兵　王玉文　童　亮
	蒙城县	蒙城县疾病预防控制中心	刘珊珊　刘　翔　李银梅　张爱东
	东至县	东至县疾病预防控制中心	景燕平　张　瑶　吴泽宁
	泾县	泾县疾病预防控制中心	刘安阜　吴　鹏　程莉莉　周　伟　杨露露　马雄梅
	宁国市	宁国市疾病预防控制中心	胡倩华　付　超　唐　雯　朱韦辰
福建省	福建省	福建省肿瘤医院	周　衍　马晶昱　相智声
	福清市	福清市疾病预防控制中心	何道逢　钟女娟　翁瑜瑶　王小阳
	福州市长乐区	福州市长乐区肿瘤防治研究所	陈建顺　陈礼慈　陈　英　陈心聪　陈聪明　张祖霞
	厦门市	厦门市疾病预防控制中心	伍啸青　许连升　林艺兰　陈月珍　连真忠　陈　沁　张卓平　陈丽燕　张琼花　易艺鹏　谭林华　谢丽珊
	厦门市同安区	厦门市同安区疾病预防控制中心	陈仁忠　陈上清　陈珊瑚
	厦门市翔安区	厦门市翔安区疾病预防控制中心	柯金练　林雅秀
	莆田市涵江区	莆田市涵江区疾病预防控制中心	林玉成　方晓滨
	永安市	永安市疾病预防控制中心	范　光　李杭生　李丽丽
	惠安县	惠安县疾病预防控制中心	刘庆烟　张冬雪
	漳州市长泰区	漳州市长泰区疾病预防控制中心	郑冬柏　张碧花

续表

省(自治区、直辖市) Province (autonomous region, municipality)	肿瘤登记处 Cancer registry	登记处所在单位 Affiliation	主要工作人员 Staff
	建瓯市	建瓯市疾病预防控制中心	官文婷　裴振义　徐肖健
	龙岩市新罗区	龙岩市新罗区疾病预防控制中心	廖凌玲
	龙岩市永定区	龙岩市永定区疾病预防控制中心	黄远田　张海丽
江西省	江西省	江西省疾病预防控制中心	刘　杰　颜　玮　陈小娜
	南昌市青云谱区	青云谱区疾病预防控制中心	章文华　李培松　邓云兰
	南昌市青山湖区	青山湖区疾病预防控制中心	黄　静　杨盈华　蔡丹桃　陈昔梅
	南昌市新建区	新建区疾病预防控制中心	万　信　熊　炜　周孔香　陶永军
	芦溪县	芦溪县疾病预防控制中心	张　莉　张庆红　刘裕坤　李益球
	九江市浔阳区	浔阳区疾病预防控制中心	涂波涌　郑　坤　田绍进　邓如蕙
	武宁县	武宁县疾病预防控制中心	潘盛林　邹德政　张赣湘　熊彩云　段红政
	新余市渝水区	渝水区疾病预防控制中心	周　林　杨　竹　晏琳春　何志勇　宋　艳　毛　麒
	余江县	余江县疾病预防控制中心	曾串莲　陈紫云　危安安
	赣州市章贡区	章贡区疾病预防控制中心	廖　顺　苏德云　任学纳
	赣州市赣县区	赣县区疾病预防控制中心	罗文云　黄文姬
	信丰县	信丰县疾病预防控制中心	王昱云　何光伟
	大余县	大余县疾病预防控制中心	黄飞平　张祥金
	上犹县	上犹县疾病预防控制中心	田玉平　李舒敏
	崇义县	崇义县疾病预防控制中心	冯云洪　肖耳目　卢致强
	龙南县	龙南县疾病预防控制中心	赖永赣　彭旻微　曾志斌
	于都县	于都县疾病预防控制中心	刘冬秀　陈　军
	吉安市吉州区	吉安市吉州区疾病预防控制中心	张艳玲　刘　琦
	峡江县	峡江县疾病预防控制中心	陈志虹　袁怿飞　陈九英
	安福县	安福县疾病预防控制中心	王　剑　胡水斌　王钟舟　刘忠明　王玉婷
	万载县	万载县疾病预防控制中心	汤丽珍　卢　萍　郭巧红
	上高县	上高县疾病预防控制中心	叶江西　赵卫东　陶武明　左　程　刘梓英　游　浩
	靖安县	靖安县疾病预防控制中心	赵朝强　舒小裕　刘志英
	乐安县	乐安县疾病预防控制中心	戴招文
	宜黄县	宜黄县疾病预防控制中心	徐媛锋
	抚州市东乡区	抚州市东乡区疾病预防控制中心	陈　霞　艾欢欢
	上饶市信州区	上饶市信州区疾病预防控制中心	叶栩艺　叶梦颖　陈婉婷
	上饶市广丰区	上饶市广丰区疾病预防控制中心	胡翠芳　姚信飞　姚佳丽　严爱丽

省(自治区、直辖市) Province (autonomous region, municipality)	肿瘤登记处 Cancer registry	登记处所在单位 Affiliation	主要工作人员 Staff
	铅山县	铅山县疾病预防控制中心	黄永进　李振雄　暨丽敏　吴永丽
	横峰县	横峰县疾病预防控制中心	程立平　涂永海　毛术霞　杨　帆
	弋阳县	弋阳县疾病预防控制中心	曾雄文　林水旺　胡素华　方荣霞
	余干县	余干县疾病预防控制中心	徐建强　汤彩兰　付美玲　段　叠
	万年县	万年县疾病预防控制中心	盛根英　应　萍
	婺源县	婺源县疾病预防控制中心	叶鹏华
	德兴市	德兴市疾病预防控制中心	李彬明　许晓丹
山东省	山东省	山东省疾病预防控制中心	郭晓雷　付振涛　姜　帆
	济南市	济南市疾病预防控制中心	宫舒萍　张先慧　周　林　刘　冰　姜　超　王玉恒　李瑛鑫　李荣华　丁春明
	济南市章丘区	济南市章丘区疾病预防控制中心	刘庆皆　辛　佳　颛孙宁宁
	济南市莱芜区	济南市莱芜区疾病预防控制中心	丁丽平　常　安
	青岛市	青岛市疾病预防控制中心	张增智　宁　锋　王　康　郑晓艳
	青岛市黄岛区	青岛市黄岛区疾病预防控制中心	廖　倩　张金太
	淄博市临淄区	淄博市临淄区疾病预防控制中心	卢　斌　韦　洁　张城倩
	沂源县	沂源县疾病预防控制中心	李东芝　孙　璞　陈义菊　王　慧
	滕州市	滕州市疾病预防控制中心	徐玉銮　于雪静　李玉春　龚　理
	广饶县	广饶县疾病预防控制中心	徐海霞
	烟台市	烟台市疾病预防控制中心	于绍轶　刘海韵　曲淑娜
	烟台市芝罘区	烟台市芝罘区疾病预防控制中心	赵　冲
	烟台市福山区	烟台市福山区疾病预防控制中心	孙　昕
	烟台市莱山区	烟台市莱山区疾病预防控制中心	赵万里
	烟台市牟平区	烟台市牟平区疾病预防控制中心	李东洪
	烟台市开发区	烟台市开发区疾病预防控制中心	厉　程
	招远市	招远市疾病预防控制中心	翟玉庭　宁巍巍　李　玮
	临朐县	临朐县疾病预防控制中心	郭　超　刘卫东　张兰福　井　斌
	高密市	高密市疾病预防控制中心	黄一峰　冷冠群　马瑞花　谢　珍　宋　娟　刘　晓
	济宁市任城区	济宁市任城区疾病预防控制中心	郗帅帅　段世彬　唐　琪

省(自治区、直辖市) Province (autonomous region, municipality)	肿瘤登记处 Cancer registry	登记处所在单位 Affiliation	主要工作人员 Staff
	汶上县	汶上县疾病预防控制中心	李　岩　张　燕
	梁山县	梁山县疾病预防控制中心	张建鲁　冯昌红　谢书丹　王春秀　孔甜甜
	曲阜市	曲阜市疾病预防控制中心	孔　超　侯爱平　颜　俊　孔　晖　王　蕊　乔　乔
	邹城市	邹城市疾病预防控制中心	骆秀美　张廷番　杨建宁　刘亚琪　王　薇　李　娜
	宁阳县	宁阳县疾病预防控制中心	刘婷婷　马学成　董芙蓉　张丽杰
	肥城市	肥城市人民医院	李琰琰　尹晓燕　姜　敏　张婷婷　王　青　郑春娟
	乳山市	乳山市疾病预防控制中心	邹跃威　李立科　张玉佳　李小菲
	日照市东港区	日照市东港区疾病预防控制中心	尚明风　韩志军
	沂南县	山东省沂南县疾病预防控制中心	华国梁　王家倩
	沂水县	沂水县疾病预防控制中心	王维霞　杨登强　马襲玲　伏祥浩　张江宝　王翠翠
	莒南县	莒南县疾病预防控制中心	文章军　张斌磊　李学刚　邓　花
	德州市德城区	德州市德城区疾病预防控制中心	屠永梓　马莉莉　安德峰
	高唐县	高唐县疾病预防控制中心	刘淑梅　王秀珍　尹　红　杨亮亮　穆守常
	滨州市滨城区	滨州市滨城区疾病预防控制中心	范美霞　赵贝贝　付立平
	菏泽市牡丹区	菏泽市牡丹区疾病预防控制中心	秦　舒　国　锦　仇翠梅　刘洋洋
	单县	山东省单县疾病预防控制中心	赵海洲　李　锦　赵　娥
	巨野县	巨野县疾病预防控制中心	高杨波　张　晋
河南省	河南省	河南省肿瘤医院	张韶凯　陈　琼　刘曙正　孙喜斌　郭兰伟　徐慧芳　郑黎阳　刘　茵
	郑州市	郑州市疾病预防控制中心	李建彬　宋彩娟　郭向娇　武恩平
	巩义市	巩义市疾病预防控制中心	蒋蔚林　王燕青　张文君
	开封市祥符区	开封市祥符区疾病预防控制中心	马　师　李慎榜　田艳玲　朱方敏
	洛阳市	洛阳市疾病预防控制中心	闫云燕　常　颖　李爱红　马　凯　邢建乐　刘培培　马昊翔　魏冰燕　石晓红　陈亚楠　齐虹飞　刘青青　张菲菲　陈家琦　李　博
	孟津县	孟津县疾病预防控制中心	许瑞瑞　张琰琰
	新安县	新安县疾病预防控制中心	付文莉　翟亚楠　李　辉

省(自治区、直辖市) Province (autonomous region, municipality)	肿瘤登记处 Cancer registry	登记处所在单位 Affiliation	主要工作人员 Staff
	栾川县	栾川县疾病预防控制中心	刘爱坡　孙亚琦　周园园　刘杏杏
	嵩县	嵩县疾病预防控制中心	杨欣欣　乔　幸　石梦瑶　杨静媛　姜开霞　梁秋娟
	汝阳县	汝阳县疾病预防控制中心	李白鸟　耿振强
	宜阳县	宜阳县疾病预防控制中心	楚玉梅　李若男　陈　培
	洛宁县	洛宁县疾病预防控制中心	段乐永　刘龙安
	伊川县	伊川县疾病预防控制中心	王蜓蜓　董　芳　刘　峰
	偃师市	偃师市疾病预防控制中心	秦延锦
	平顶山市	平顶山市疾病预防控制中心	吕锐利　宋　波　颜欣颖　张泽华　许艺苑　彭　浩　李智伟　郑红云　仲晓伟　温红旭
	鲁山县	鲁山县疾病预防控制中心	王一博　郭启民　田广恩　许姗姗
	郏县	郏县疾病预防控制中心	孙　颖　王晓艳　昝　哲　宁海燕　董人阁
	舞钢市	舞钢市疾病预防控制中心	刘青兰　刘亚红　尹馨可　段慧娟
	安阳市	安阳市肿瘤医院	张金文　王能超　方　岩　张媛媛　闫焕勤　张晓星　秦永超
	林州市	林州市肿瘤医院	郭贵周　付方现　王振海　李变云　于晓东　侯　凯　王　丽　刘　畅
	鹤壁市	鹤壁市人民医院	钞利娜　王冰冰　王梦媛　胡凤琴　裴树英　任红勤　郭雪琴
	新乡市	新乡市中心医院	朱智玲　曹河璐
	辉县市	辉县市疾病预防控制中心	孙花荣　赵小聪　李　颖
	焦作市	焦作市疾病预防控制中心	孟春辉　田　珍　路娜娜　韩晓宁　高丽利　周琳菲
	孟州市	孟州市疾病预防控制中心	武晓华　潘小燕
	濮阳市华龙区	濮阳市华龙区疾病预防控制中心	王培贤　齐庆荣　胡利娟
	范县	范县疾病预防控制中心	田军艳　邢秀娟　薛　辉　王静芳　周瑞敏
	濮阳县	濮阳县疾病预防控制中心	郭秋献　穆晓红　刘　军
	禹州市	禹州市疾病预防控制中心	王全新　郭　影　李　蔚　杨宗慧　张亚楠
	漯河市	漯河市疾病预防控制中心	代　莹　孙路平　孟　蕾　胡　昕　代君君
	漯河市郾城区	漯河市郾城区疾病预防控制中心	李爱会　袁兵翔　庞　静　常帅奇　何怡聪　邓　婕　张　楠
	舞阳县	舞阳县疾病预防控制中心	何　洁　马永晓　周小佳　谷来君　张艳丽　杨艳芳
	临颍县	临颍县疾病预防控制中心	吴　真　罗　婷　秦苏丹　马玉智
	三门峡市湖滨区	湖滨区疾病预防控制中心	李粉妮　刘润娣　罗　丹

省(自治区、直辖市) Province (autonomous region, municipality)	肿瘤登记处 Cancer registry	登记处所在单位 Affiliation	主要工作人员 Staff
	南阳市卧龙区	南阳市卧龙区疾病预防控制中心	刘　凯　周　静　张　爽
	南召县	南召县疾病预防控制中心	靳万春　王青勤　陈立明　朱广博　张　营　宋　峰　樊　璞
	方城县	方城县疾病预防控制中心	马建民　马璟颖　李　谱　仝成杰　倪林静　张禄军
	内乡县	内乡县疾病预防控制中心	李亚波　金　花　代　阳
	睢县	睢县疾病预防控制中心	袁　帅　刘　艳
	虞城县	虞城县疾病预防控制中心	张亚威　冯金洪　马　宁　毕兴华　刘　威　江　培
	信阳市浉河区	信阳市浉河区疾病预防控制中心	兰宏旺　楚尚兰　耿祎祎　周　娣　李　刚
	罗山县	罗山县疾病预防控制中心	江　坤　徐蔚静　王明阳
	固始县	固始县疾病预防控制中心	张　柯　沈　玉
	沈丘县	沈丘县疾病预防控制中心	徐　玲　李庆文　郭丽花　李旭东　孙梦洋
	郸城县	郸城县疾病预防控制中心	张吉志　孙　忠　郭德银　陈　静　马　慧　李慧珍
	太康县	太康县疾病预防控制中心	董　洪　魏国成　李　昂
	西平县	西平县疾病预防控制中心	毛小辉　邵天堂　王中梅　赵春玲　刘彩霞
	济源市	济源市疾病预防控制中心	马璐瑶　刘　磊　黄艳芳　郑飞飞　张雷锋　郑莹茹
	漯河市源汇区	漯河市源汇区疾病预防控制中心	张　祥　王宏博　牛艳丽　叶　静
	漯河市召陵区	漯河市召陵区疾病预防控制中心	王军奇　陶　哲　樊永立　鞠晨云
湖北省	湖北省	湖北省肿瘤医院	庹吉妤　姚　霜　张　敏　秦　宇　孟繁地　夏雅芬
	武汉市	武汉市疾病预防控制中心	杨念念　严亚琼　金琦曼　代　娟　赵原原　张晓霞　郭　燕
	大冶市	大冶市疾病预防控制中心	徐　鹏　黄泽华　徐新建　陈旭东　曹宏利　曹群芳　袁雪冰　冯　辉
	十堰市郧阳区	十堰市郧阳区疾病预防控制中心	柯　华　左顺彦　曹　琳　贺　锐
	宜昌市	宜昌市疾病预防控制中心	胡　池　杨佳娟　刘　军　张　培　朱　婕　吴　婵　邓亚玲
	五峰土家族自治县	五峰土家族自治县疾病预防控制中心	熊　斌　邹晓丹　王仁兴

省(自治区、直辖市) Province (autonomous region, municipality)	肿瘤登记处 Cancer registry	登记处所在单位 Affiliation	主要工作人员 Staff
	襄阳市	襄阳市疾病预防控制中心	陈小慧 龚文胜 鲲 鹏 刘 杰
	宜城市	宜城市疾病预防控制中心	杨 波 龚新洪 曾卓璇 胡院芳 张家乐
	京山县	京山县疾病预防控制中心	李 宏 容艳红 杨 丹
	钟祥市	钟祥市疾病预防控制中心	赵 丽 霍军荣 廖金凤 高雅玲
	云梦县	云梦县疾病预防控制中心	周 浩 李纯波 潘雨晴 徐敏莉
	荆州市	荆州市疾病预防控制中心	毛安禄 孙 春 江 鸿 雷若倩 颜 杰
	公安县	公安县疾病预防控制中心	洪 杰 申立琼 文良军 龚 春 胡长贵 张 丹
	洪湖市	洪湖市疾病预防控制中心	廖 涛 向代成 徐海涛 刘登洪
	麻城市	麻城市疾病预防控制中心	柳以泽 丁 成 徐胜平 项维红 库守能 王金荣
	嘉鱼县	嘉鱼县疾病预防控制中心	刘晓玲 刘 庆 黄忠文 范锡芳 陈圆圆 曾 晶 肖德顺 杜清华 李小红 李 燕 唐 文 姚智敏 殷 姗 魏 雯
	通城县	通城县疾病预防控制中心	刘加军 杨 劲 熊新征 熊子鹏
	恩施市	恩施市疾病预防控制中心	王 斌 胡燕琳 刘迪军 廖荣芳
	天门市	天门市疾病预防控制中心	刘 积 罗 芬 王义华 何明辉 倪亚敏 李 锐 方 亮 邹红艳 彭菊萍 董君华 黄红艳 胡 嵘 胡珍贵 郭 芳
湖南省	湖南省	湖南省肿瘤防治研究办公室	肖亚洲 王 静 颜仕鹏 廖先珍 许可葵 邹艳花 石朝晖 肖海帆 曹世钰 李 灿 李 娜 王石玉 郭 佳
	长沙市芙蓉区	长沙市芙蓉区疾病预防控制中心	张运秋 胡辉伍 杨 丽 罗霜艳 朱 丽
	长沙市天心区	长沙市天心区疾病预防控制中心	许超伦 兰泽龙 王红江
	长沙市岳麓区	长沙市岳麓区疾病预防控制中心	苏威武 陈继怀 杨思进
	长沙市开福区	长沙市开福区疾病预防控制中心	林 玲 陈腊梅 刘 阳 刘 玲
	长沙市雨花区	长沙市雨花区疾病预防控制中心	周建湘 何 韬 黄 芬 胡 蓉 邓谦成 段利霞 廖丽艳
	长沙市望城区	长沙市望城区疾病预防控制中心	程新和 王华良 赵劲良 熊 浩 邹思伟 胡利英
	长沙县	长沙县疾病预防控制中心	罗辉琴 黄 云 彭 敏 刘 丹 刘遂怡 黄雅兰
	浏阳市	浏阳市疾病预防控制中心	许 欣 陈建伟 李 跳 龙花君 王 群 谭诗花 李光辉

省(自治区、直辖市) Province (autonomous region, municipality)	肿瘤登记处 Cancer registry	登记处所在单位 Affiliation	主要工作人员 Staff
	株洲市芦淞区	株洲市芦淞区疾病预防控制中心	何　礼　唐　晶　卞晓嘉　刘慧颖　鲍　芳
	株洲市石峰区	株洲市石峰区疾病预防控制中心	袁　湘　刘　杰　黄　平　刘　宏　彭玉梅　袁　敏　齐佳锐
	攸县	攸县疾病预防控制中心	符三乃　欧阳四新　刘孳雄　杨华艳
	湘潭市雨湖区	湘潭市雨湖区疾病预防控制中心	邓莉芳　杨玉环　马超颖　马子涵　蔡文迪
	衡东县	衡东县疾病预防控制中心	尹　炜　单健生　刘早红　肖静娴　李俊华　刘银月　周　玲　丁　莉
	常宁市	常宁市疾病预防控制中心	曹诗鹏　郭秀连　欧　琦　滕德伟　吴良元　郭　兰
	邵东县	邵东县疾病预防控制中心	曾　平　田　丽　陈文伟　谢　玉　金海燕　谢清玲　谭辉路　刘冬梅
	新宁县	新宁县疾病预防控制中心	邓海名　周前富　陈　富　刘倩文
	岳阳市岳阳楼区	岳阳市岳阳楼区疾病预防控制中心	陈艳芳　黄　平　罗江洪　罗　莎　李　盛　鲁小霞　宋　婷
	常德市武陵区	常德市武陵区疾病预防控制中心	管元平　涂林立　张志刚　彭学文　唐志敏　朱晓辉　周宏惠
	慈利县	慈利县疾病预防控制中心	朱从喜　向　英　吴　双　陈华云　刘　波　寇渝东
	益阳市资阳区	益阳市资阳区疾病预防控制中心	龚建华　王迪军　鲁　容　陈　晶　王玲玲　范朝彪　张丽情
	桃江县	桃江县人民医院	刘　军　廖亚男　薛媚娟　邹　平　黄　德　邹朝霞　郭　纯　谢　真
	临武县	临武县疾病预防控制中心	周贤文　李伟生　李国斌　谭林林　刘　冰　曹玲芳
	资兴市	资兴市疾病预防控制中心	徐贤雄　李雄豹　黎利文　夏云磊　王英籍
	道县	道县疾病预防控制中心	肖拥军　胡建湘　郑　平　何林秀　何英俊　胡雨华　刘海萍　蒋忠葵　许洪平
	宁远县	宁远县疾病预防控制中心	李万忠　李万清　欧阳小芳　陈颖香　李　玮
	新田县	新田县疾病预防控制中心	欧阳乐　谢众麟　黄　锋　何忠勇　段良祥　刘君红　刘　波
	麻阳苗族自治县	麻阳苗族自治县疾病预防控制中心	陈　琳　赵　辉　陈启佳　张春玉　滕　瑶
	洪江市	洪江市疾病预防控制中心	向湘林　易思连　寻英姿　杨小琴　向丽琼　林嘉兴
	冷水江市	冷水江市疾病预防控制中心	方吉贤　宾远忠　张彬彬　罗三峰　杨　娟

省(自治区、直辖市) Province (autonomous region, municipality)	肿瘤登记处 Cancer registry	登记处所在单位 Affiliation	主要工作人员 Staff
	涟源市	涟源市疾病预防控制中心	文申根　李秀兰　周红大　龙爱梅　黄　靖　张晓勇　肖艳慎　李　清
广东省	广东省	广东省疾病预防控制中心	林立丰　夏　亮　孟瑞琳　王　晔　许晓君　许燕君　廖　羽
	广州市	广州市疾病预防控制中心	李　科　许　欢　王穗湘　秦鹏哲　梁伯衡　陈远源　董　航
	广州市郊区	广州市疾病预防控制中心	许　欢　李　科　王穗湘　秦鹏哲　梁伯衡　陈远源　董　航
	佛山市	佛山市疾病预防控制中心	古嘉诚　孙宝志　隋丹丹
	佛山市顺德区	佛山市顺德区慢性病防治中心	杨俊杰　罗洁莹　王谦可　陈　榕　吴　焜
	佛山市南海区	佛山市南海区疾病预防控制中心	谢威龙　黄杰周　谢冬怡
	江门市	江门市疾病预防控制中心	莫兆波　于雪芳
	梅州市梅江区	梅州市疾病预防控制中心	古彩红　刘雅姬　胡艳红　林文渊
	梅州市梅县区	梅州市梅县区疾病预防控制中心	杨　慧　李加宁
	东莞市	东莞市疾病预防控制中心	陈妙嫦　钟洁莹　姚旭芳　魏建坤　黄雅卿
	南雄市	南雄市疾病预防控制中心	张艳艳　邬香华
	揭西县	揭西县疾病预防控制中心	贝晶利
	惠州市惠阳区	惠州市惠阳区疾病预防控制中心	黄惠玲　陈　萍
	中山市	中山市人民医院(中山市肿瘤研究所)	魏矿荣　梁智恒　李柱明
	深圳市	深圳市慢性病防治中心	彭　绩　赵志广　雷　林　刘芳江
	阳山县	阳山县疾病预防控制中心	毛智趣　丘银霞　梁时力　黄永杰
	罗定市	罗定市疾病预防控制中心	陈红艳　张乔珍　梁惠玲
	阳江市阳东区	阳江市阳东区疾病预防控制中心	谭家伟　关　设　李海凤　雷玉燕
	四会市	四会市惠民平价门诊部(四会市肿瘤研究所)	卢玉强　姚继洲　李晓翌　乡一萍　丁惠玲
	珠海市	珠海市慢性病防治中心	郭红革　滕勇勇　陈美婷　谢水仙
	肇庆市	肇庆市疾病预防控制中心	方艺娟　陆素颖　冼国佳　梁大艳
广西壮族自治区	广西壮族自治区	广西医科大学附属肿瘤医院	李秋林　余家华　余红平　葛莲英　曹　骥　容敏华　周子寒
	南宁市兴宁区	南宁市兴宁区疾病预防控制中心	梁翠敏　欧阳丽华　黄礼庆

续表

省(自治区、直辖市) Province (autonomous region, municipality)	肿瘤登记处 Cancer registry	登记处所在单位 Affiliation	主要工作人员 Staff
	南宁市青秀区	青秀区疾病预防控制中心	李　颖　黄绍旎　卢志玲　黄中学
	南宁市江南区	南宁市江南区疾病预防控制中心	戴　姮　卢　珠　曾　俊
	南宁市经开区	南宁市经开区疾病预防控制中心	覃燕红
	南宁市西乡塘区	南宁市西乡塘区疾病预防控制中心	苏升灿　唐盛志　韦　鹏　何雨澄
	南宁市良庆区	南宁市良庆区疾病预防控制中心	唐英花
	南宁市东盟经济开发区	广西东盟经济技术开发区疾病预防控制中心	宁　栈
	隆安县	隆安县疾病预防控制中心	陈珍莲　黄建云　方孔雄
	宾阳县	宾阳县疾病预防控制中心	陈伟强　甘晓琴　韦柳青　李秀霞　陈源珍　龚冰冰　莫少梅　张　华
	柳州市	柳州市疾病预防控制中心	覃忠书　蓝　剑　王晓伟　孟繁文　覃宇禄　陈宁钰　刘　芸　欧　蕾　朱庭萍　谭晓萍
	桂林市	桂林市疾病预防控制中心	潘定权　蒋富生　汤　杰　石　瑀
	梧州市	梧州市红十字会医院	郑裕明　汤伟文　苏韶华　谢红英　黄金菊　苏阳红　陈骐炜
	苍梧县	苍梧县疾病预防控制中心	李汉福　杨敏生　谭夏敏　麦新苗　李北金　苏石汉　林　冰　余思洁
	北海市	北海市疾病预防控制中心	梁耀洁　谢　平
	合浦县	合浦县疾病预防控制中心	苏福康　曹　松　张　强　秦晓丽　罗世琼　陈鑫祖　谢贤缤
	钦州市钦南区	钦州市钦南区疾病预防控制中心	陆玉培　黄红英
	贵港市港北区	贵港市港北区疾病预防控制中心	韦坚峥
	贵港市港南区	贵港市港南区疾病预防控制中心	莫桂琼　谭金贤　黎兆华
	贵港市覃塘区	贵港市覃塘区疾病预防控制中心	熊　维
	平南县	平南县疾病预防控制中心	冯　翠
	玉林市	玉林市疾病预防控制中心	陈立锐　周阳洋　吴定康　黄　胜
	陆川县	陆川县疾病预防控制中心	黄文宁
	北流市	北流市疾病预防控制中心	唐美玲　陈金武　李鸿玲　黎　丹　陈　雪　黄　胜

省(自治区、直辖市) Province (autonomous region, municipality)	肿瘤登记处 Cancer registry	登记处所在单位 Affiliation	主要工作人员 Staff
	百色市右江区	百色市右江区疾病预防控制中心	吴美秀
	田阳县	田阳县疾病预防控制中心	李洁玲　黄志刚　何少松
	罗城仫佬族自治县	罗城仫佬族自治县疾病预防控制中心	韦政兴　梁玉春　卢永钧　罗黎霞　韦　愿
	合山市	合山市疾病预防控制中心	黄海浪
	扶绥县	扶绥县人民医院	李海华　梁威丽　李云西　韦忠亮　黄志斌　陶哲艺
海南省	海南省	海南省肿瘤防治中心	董　华　范康琼　华　婧　王定彬
	三亚市	三亚市疾病预防控制中心	陈莲芬　黄炯媚　潘　超
	五指山市	五指山市疾病预防控制中心	符美艳　卢耿慧
	琼海市	琼海市疾病预防控制中心	符芳敏　颜李丽
	定安县	定安县疾病预防控制中心	李建斌　黎才刚　郭芳华
	昌江黎族自治县	昌江黎族自治县疾病预防控制中心	符为巨　王灵珍　钟玲慧
	陵水黎族自治县	陵水黎族自治县疾病预防控制中心	许声文　林仕栋
重庆市	重庆市	重庆市疾病预防控制中心	吕晓燕　丁贤彬
	重庆市万州区	重庆市万州区疾病预防控制中心	彭　瑾　吴　波　唐　亮
	重庆市涪陵区	重庆市涪陵区疾病预防控制中心	周义芬　陈晓明　王杨凤　王　琪
	重庆市渝中区	重庆市渝中区疾病预防控制中心	周　琦　凌瑜双
	重庆市大渡口区	重庆市大渡口区疾病预防控制中心	赵　璨　刘勇言
	重庆市江北区	重庆市江北区疾病预防控制中心	郭　梅　刘　静
	重庆市沙坪坝区	重庆市沙坪坝区疾病预防控制中心	邓丽君　支　倩　蒙　怡
	重庆市九龙坡区	重庆市九龙坡区疾病预防控制中心	汤　成　贺　明　陶　然　肖　伦
	重庆市南岸区	重庆市南岸区疾病预防控制中心	何英淑　黄治兰　廖晓澄
	重庆市北碚区	重庆市北碚区疾病预防控制中心	李大兵　邓小霞

续表

省(自治区、直辖市) Province (autonomous region, municipality)	肿瘤登记处 Cancer registry	登记处所在单位 Affiliation	主要工作人员 Staff
	重庆市綦江区	重庆市綦江区疾病预防控制中心	罗春亮　周梦雪
	重庆市大足区	重庆市大足区疾病预防控制中心	李万华　任香勇　杨　颖
	重庆市渝北区	重庆市渝北区疾病预防控制中心	郭昌融　张晓慧
	重庆市巴南区	重庆市巴南区疾病预防控制中心	陶小红　刘成果
	重庆市黔江区	重庆市黔江区疾病预防控制中心	吴　畅　吴彩霞　李　卫　王　敏
	重庆市长寿区	重庆市长寿区疾病预防控制中心	马周俊　邓　静
	重庆市江津区	重庆市江津区疾病预防控制中心	杨　媚　孟秋雨　李西同
	重庆市合川区	重庆市合川区疾病预防控制中心	贺　玲　王绍梅
	重庆市永川区	重庆市永川区疾病预防控制中心	吴　欢　程莉莎　刘　琳
	重庆市南川区	重庆市南川区疾病预防控制中心	钟　静
	重庆市万盛经开区	重庆市万盛经开区疾病预防控制中心	杨　琴　田　哲
	重庆市潼南区	重庆市潼南区疾病预防控制中心	龙　凤　陈雪莲　郝真强
	重庆市铜梁区	重庆市铜梁区疾病预防控制中心	周昇杰
	重庆市荣昌区	重庆市荣昌区疾病预防控制中心	舒　强　于均梅　熊华利
	重庆市璧山区	重庆市璧山区疾病预防控制中心	陈　静　张　瑜
	重庆市梁平区	重庆市梁平区疾病预防控制中心	游茂林　邱虹蛟
	丰都县	丰都县疾病预防控制中心	熊　薇　曾正英　刘　琳
	垫江县	垫江县疾病预防控制中心	杨世亚　谭　格
	重庆市武隆区	重庆市武隆区疾病预防控制中心	万　泉　刘浩然　李婷婷
	忠县	忠县疾病预防控制中心	熊晓世　袁　英　方　君

省（自治区、直辖市） Province （autonomous region，municipality）	肿瘤登记处 Cancer registry	登记处所在单位 Affiliation	主要工作人员 Staff
	重庆市开州区	重庆市开州区疾病预防控制中心	肖幸平　崔喜闻
	云阳县	云阳县疾病预防控制中心	张　星　张　林　王　芳
	奉节县	奉节县疾病预防控制中心	向　嫱　张克燕　罗　宇　姜孝凤
	巫山县	巫山县疾病预防控制中心	何成丹　曾　蓉　梁　辉
	巫溪县	巫溪县疾病预防控制中心	吕文宾　王发辉　任兴荣
	石柱土家族自治县	重庆市石柱土家族自治县疾病预防控制中心	汤剑峰
	秀山土家族苗族自治县	秀山土家族苗族自治县疾病预防控制中心	郭　敏
	酉阳土家族苗族自治县	酉阳土家族苗族自治县疾病预防控制中心	冉悦函
	彭水苗族土家族自治县	彭水苗族土家族自治县疾病预防控制中心	陈　节　郭　超　杨　璇　胡元红
四川省	四川省	四川省疾病预防控制中心	成姝雯　邓　颖　胥馨尹　董　婷　曾　晶　张　新　乔　良　刘潇霞
	成都市青羊区	成都市青羊区疾病预防控制中心	韩湘意　彭长燕　蔡　鹏　刘　嘉
	成都市成华区	成都市成华区疾病预防控制中心	胡　莹　许　凌　王　超　周　静　赵子君
	成都市龙泉驿区	成都市龙泉驿区疾病预防控制中心	卢清平　江　柯　张群英　阮红海
	成都市新都区	成都市新都区疾病预防控制中心	文婧唯　焦　娇　刘　芳　赵子贺　刘　燕
	金堂县	金堂县疾病预防控制中心	李林容　叶立力
	成都市双流区	成都市双流区疾病预防控制中心	王照华　胡　容　黄先志　唐　爽　裴宗琴
	成都市天府新区	成都市天府新区疾病预防控制中心	袁晓宇　罗　刚　袁　伟　姚菲菲　罗　杰
	成都市郫都区	成都市郫都区疾病预防控制中心	林超兰　江　秀　黄小芳　余　林
	成都市新津区	成都市新津区疾病预防控制中心	刘凤容　杨　杰　苟念秋
	彭州市	彭州市疾病预防控制中心	蒋　微　罗国金　李建国　陈小芳　刘佳秋　孙　强　王建娜
	自贡市自流井区	自贡市自流井区疾病预防控制中心	熊端萍　冯小伟　李　刚　刘筱颖　商　静

续表

省(自治区、直辖市) Province (autonomous region, municipality)	肿瘤登记处 Cancer registry	登记处所在单位 Affiliation	主要工作人员 Staff
	自贡市贡井区	自贡市贡井区疾病预防控制中心	邱玉琼　江　超　毛喜艳
	自贡市大安区	自贡市大安区疾病预防控制中心	徐　爽　倪　嘉　张小林　李蕾思
	自贡市沿滩区	自贡市沿滩区疾病预防控制中心	陈　燕　郑尚红
	荣县	荣县疾病预防控制中心	陈　莉　刘　莉　夏和珍　胡　杰　杨　玲
	富顺县	富顺县疾病预防控制中心	刘兴莉　黄帮雨　关晓旭　徐小丽　吴　帆
	攀枝花市东区	攀枝花市东区疾病预防控制中心	陈　莹　周川楠　徐静亚　张　琳　李　燕
	攀枝花市西区	攀枝花市西区疾病预防控制中心	贺绍琼　李　英　关绍婷
	攀枝花市仁和区	攀枝花市仁和区疾病预防控制中心	毛　鹏　赫永新　汪　杰　周玉萍
	米易县	米易县疾病预防控制中心	甘　泉　曾文海　罗　欢　廖长春　曹　珊　董家君　刘天慧
	盐边县	盐边县疾病预防控制中心	程　平　任宗良
	泸州市江阳区	泸州市江阳区疾病预防控制中心	邵　红　李　奕　杨廷婷　李娅凌　林叶清
	泸州市纳溪区	泸州市纳溪区疾病预防控制中心	林　利　虞旭东　曾世林
	泸州市龙马潭区	泸州市龙马潭区疾病预防控制中心	唐　伟　韦汉淬　雷启云　李春艳　曾　瑜
	泸县	泸县疾病预防控制中心	谢　婧　余　军　熊　君　汪正刚　陈平平
	合江县	合江县疾病预防控制中心	胡　东　王　蓉　黎　溢　邓艳艳　刘明海
	叙永县	叙永县疾病预防控制中心	郭庆洁　魏策进　黄　嵩　罗　刚　李玉开
	古蔺县	古蔺县疾病预防控制中心	邓　波　文　兵　姜春霞　冯华强　龙巧林
	德阳市旌阳区	德阳市旌阳区疾病预防控制中心	叶先太　苏小波　于　进　陈　思　周小华
	中江县	中江县疾病预防控制中心	邹　红　蒋文斌　邓绍清　秦国胜　谢　伟　邓　庆
	德阳市罗江区	德阳市罗江区疾病预防控制中心	管小琴　彭　茹　刘怀淑
	广汉市	广汉市疾病预防控制中心	肖昌华　刘丹丹　王　玲　龙小刚　何　柳
	什邡市	什邡市疾病预防控制中心	蒋　丽　郑小军　钟雪飞　肖家慧　邢婷婷
	绵竹市	绵竹市疾病预防控制中心	张　桃　周道兴　周　平　何启明　周义健　廖伯勇

省（自治区、直辖市） Province (autonomous region, municipality)	肿瘤登记处 Cancer registry	登记处所在单位 Affiliation	主要工作人员 Staff
	绵阳市涪城区	绵阳市涪城区疾病预防控制中心	李　洁　王蒙杰　周晓凤
	绵阳市游仙区	绵阳市游仙区疾病预防控制中心	安水玲　王　慧
	绵阳市安州区	绵阳市安州区疾病预防控制中心	季洪兵　许　强　李艳梅　周海英　滕　樛
	三台县	三台县疾病预防控制中心	黄　丽　周　欢
	盐亭县	盐亭县肿瘤防治研究所（肿瘤医院）	李　军　李　林　黄　政
	梓潼县	梓潼县疾病预防控制中心	帖映伟　赵金华
	北川羌族自治县	北川羌族自治县疾病预防控制中心	蒋素红　韩　丽
	平武县	平武县疾病预防控制中心	严松林　焦　剑　罗　健　刘严娇　黄莉蓉
	江油市	江油市疾病预防控制中心	夏丽莉　竹晓琴　王定邦　李　宁　李春梅　薛　莉
	广元市	广元市疾病预防控制中心	侯　敏　胡晓波
	广元市利州区	广元市利州区疾病预防控制中心	张小玲　王　平　谢晓莉
	广元市昭化区	广元市昭化区疾病预防控制中心	曹　智　漆志军　李小建
	广元市朝天区	广元市朝天区疾病预防控制中心	何　磊　解明成　张玉芬
	旺苍县	旺苍县疾病预防控制中心	陈晓红　米家君　贾正常
	青川县	青川县疾病预防控制中心	张淑兰　袁正华　袁伟贤　柳青蓉　王桂花
	剑阁县	剑阁县疾病预防控制中心	田　辉　吴　婷　赵　彬
	苍溪县	苍溪县疾病预防控制中心	张　娟　吴德明　何　楠　朱友德
	遂宁市船山区	遂宁市船山区疾病预防控制中心	王　婧　刘　淼
	遂宁市安居区	遂宁市安居区疾病预防控制中心	李　谦　吴　高　冯裕如　陈胜春
	蓬溪县	蓬溪县疾病预防控制中心	邱　林　杨建红　梁　波　陈　恒
	射洪县	射洪县疾病预防控制中心	石晓柳　刘　扬　杜思豪
	大英县	大英县疾病预防控制中心	夏　冰　唐　霞　韦　伊
	内江市市中区	内江市市中区疾病预防控制中心	董永年　唐纯丽　尤　霄　达　希　刘小波
	内江市东兴区	内江市东兴区疾病预防控制中心	黄　艳　冷江涛

续表

省(自治区、直辖市) Province (autonomous region, municipality)	肿瘤登记处 Cancer registry	登记处所在单位 Affiliation	主要工作人员 Staff
	威远县	威远县疾病预防控制中心	陈秀兰　陈　娜　杨卉玲
	资中县	资中县疾病预防控制中心	崔红刚　钟　鸣　李　静　陈　璐　孙于茹
	隆昌市	隆昌市疾病预防控制中心	罗　睿　高雪娅　代　敬
	乐山市市中区	乐山市市中区疾病预防控制中心	赵彬茜　钟　钰　岑晓喻　冯　亮
	乐山市沙湾区	乐山市沙湾区疾病预防控制中心	朱　攀　张春霞　苟　伟
	乐山市五通桥区	乐山市五通桥区疾病预防控制中心	侯　亮
	乐山市金口河区	乐山市金口河区疾病预防控制中心	吕伟华　刘海燕　江旭婷
	犍为县	犍为县疾病预防控制中心	谯　宇　余美帆　童　宇
	井研县	井研县疾病预防控制中心	税智群　李泳梅　何　芳　吕中林
	夹江县	夹江县疾病预防控制中心	晏　荧　龙建坤　干晓辉
	沐川县	沐川县疾病预防控制中心	周玉萍　郑　玲
	峨边彝族自治县	峨边县疾病预防控制中心	黄代骥　李忠林
	马边彝族自治县	马边彝族自治县疾病预防控制中心	立机妹美
	峨眉山市	峨眉山市疾病预防控制中心	吴　洁　伍毕英　吴凌燕　周　敏　费　琳
	南充市顺庆区	南充市顺庆区疾病预防控制中心	杨　欢　徐　捷　梁　熙　肖　强
	南充市高坪区	南充市高坪区人民医院	邢　丽　岳小林　廖　波
	南充市嘉陵区	南充市嘉陵区疾病预防控制中心	黄　维　祝　倩　彭小倩
	南部县	南部县疾病预防控制中心	陈　进　杨晓萍　张燕军
	营山县	营山县疾病预防控制中心	苟军平　彭　勇
	蓬安县	蓬安县疾病预防控制中心	林　波　罗　容　蒲泓兵
	仪陇县	仪陇县疾病预防控制中心	曹　成　曹秋菊　何　倩　吴相遇　刘　燕
	西充县	西充县疾病预防控制中心	赵　辉　孙青青
	阆中市	阆中市疾病预防控制中心	游宁静　任　焱　刘　刚　许　华
	眉山市东坡区	眉山市东坡区疾病预防控制中心	陈兰芬
	眉山市彭山区	眉山市彭山区疾病预防控制中心	周建容　潘　耀　余志祥
	仁寿县	仁寿县疾病预防控制中心	宋良文　瞿遥来　黄佳玲　宁　芳　杨　红

省(自治区、直辖市) Province (autonomous region, municipality)	肿瘤登记处 Cancer registry	登记处所在单位 Affiliation	主要工作人员 Staff
	洪雅县	洪雅县疾病预防控制中心	赖　兵　吴　莹　杨利琴
	丹棱县	丹棱县疾病预防控制中心	罗　源　梁学祥
	青神县	青神县疾病预防控制中心	徐　琴　张　邻　黄彬鑫
	宜宾市翠屏区	宜宾市翠屏区疾病预防控制中心	马坤容　刘如葵　戴自强　陈志富　应元玲　黄昌学　朱德琴
	宜宾市叙州区	宜宾市叙州区疾病预防控制中心	陈小芳　周　刘
	江安县	江安县疾病预防控制中心	王　芳　李　军　李必容　杨　晴　程　彦
	长宁县	长宁县疾病预防控制中心	王　宇
	高县	高县疾病预防控制中心	黄小清　任　燃
	筠连县	筠连县疾病预防控制中心	张　迪
	屏山县	屏山县疾病预防控制中心	程　伟　徐江红
	广安市广安区	广安市广安区疾病预防控制中心	李国辉　杜承彬　李荣川
	广安市前锋区	广安市前锋区疾病预防控制中心	王　维　黄春凤　叶正明　李　川
	岳池县	岳池县疾病预防控制中心	邓　平　聂　勇
	武胜县	武胜县疾病预防控制中心	王文婷　张泽军　张建东　米惠琼　王惊秋
	邻水县	邻水县疾病预防控制中心	廖冬娟　刘　健　钟晓辉
	华蓥市	华蓥市疾病预防控制中心	何　阳　李建川　韩小月
	达州市达川区	达州市达川区疾病预防控制中心	段凯岚　罗　玲　周　莉　熊舒书
	宣汉县	宣汉县疾病预防控制中心	赵鹏飞　李　波　桂国尧　张冬梅
	开江县	开江县疾病预防控制中心	卢有见　舒进川　陈　红
	大竹县	大竹县疾病预防控制中心	袁东娅　王大骞　叶明兰　赵　红　艳师小林
	渠县	渠县疾病预防控制中心	李　平　王秀瑛
	万源市	万源市疾病预防控制中心	何　莉　黄明锋　徐　洁
	雅安市雨城区	雅安市雨城区疾病预防控制中心	王登琪　吴　波　朱春明　李雅苹　刘　杰　范　娟
	雅安市名山区	雅安市名山区疾病预防控制中心	王修华　胡启源
	荥经县	荥经县疾病预防控制中心	李明远
	汉源县	汉源县疾病预防控制中心	廖卓航　王　新　杜　涓　辜　豪
	石棉县	石棉县疾病预防控制中心	李桂芬　王　琴　廖艳萍

续表

省(自治区、直辖市) Province (autonomous region, municipality)	肿瘤登记处 Cancer registry	登记处所在单位 Affiliation	主要工作人员 Staff
	天全县	天全县疾病预防控制中心	高鸿敏
	芦山县	芦山县疾病预防控制中心	李唐芳 王 鸿 熊 欣
	宝兴县	宝兴县疾病预防控制中心	徐新红 姜 亚
	巴中市巴州区	巴中市巴州区疾病预防控制中心	叶南宁 李俊杰
	巴中市恩阳区	巴中市恩阳区疾病预防控制中心	罗 斌 张 翼 谢明芳 谯 健
	通江县	通江县疾病预防控制中心	刘德泉 赵廷明 张 劲 陈 静 谢东柏 岳秀凤 王 丽 李 骁 王清华 何开莉 李 鑫 徐 畅 杨 清
	南江县	南江县疾病预防控制中心	赵正强 郭春燕 王光秀 谢 蓉 刘 兰
	平昌县	平昌县疾病预防控制中心	邹晓兰 谢 凯 涂亚平 李健生 何 勇 钟 鑫 杨晓莉
	资阳市雁江区	资阳市雁江区疾病预防控制中心	李仕海 王红艳 李成维
	安岳县	安岳县疾病预防控制中心	杨 建 谢益琼 江 霁 唐承美
	乐至县	乐至县疾病预防控制中心	吴志敏 李 光 雷方君
	马尔康县	马尔康县疾病预防控制中心	陈跃文 任跃文 马武胜
	汶川县	汶川县疾病预防控制中心	余小芳 张 胜 姚 云 张诗卓
	理县	理县疾病预防控制中心	余石花 班玉萍 杨敏菲 晏名辉
	茂县	茂县疾病预防控制中心	黄德亮 夏 明 文德强 付 琴
	松潘县	松潘县疾病预防控制中心	马静瑶 罗金磋 如妹磋
	金川县	金川县疾病预防控制中心	马华美 熊 云
	小金县	小金县疾病预防控制中心	张测铭 王术琼
	黑水县	黑水县疾病预防控制中心	江友林
	若尔盖县	若尔盖县疾病预防控制中心	欧志婷 邓 斌
	红原县	红原县疾病预防控制中心	尕尔姆
贵州省	贵州省	贵州省疾病预防控制中心	刘 涛 李 凌 周 婕
	贵阳市花溪区	贵阳市花溪区疾病预防控制中心	刘 靖
	开阳县	开阳县疾病预防控制中心	颜克梅
	息烽县	息烽县疾病预防控制中心	吴 会
	清镇市	清镇市疾病预防控制中心	付 敏
	六盘水钟山区	六盘水市钟山区疾病预防控制中心	朱 娟

省(自治区、直辖市) Province (autonomous region, municipality)	肿瘤登记处 Cancer registry	登记处所在单位 Affiliation	主要工作人员 Staff
	六盘水市六枝特区	六盘水市六枝特区疾病预防控制中心	张徐巾
	水城县	六盘水市水城县疾病预防控制中心	刘作英
	盘州市	六盘水市盘州市疾病预防控制中心	章有建
	遵义市红花岗区	遵义市红花岗区疾病预防控制中心	陈艳娟
	遵义市汇川区	遵义市汇川区疾病预防控制中心	杨　敏
	习水县	习水县疾病预防控制中心	杨存焜
	赤水市	赤水市疾病预防控制中心	邓金勇
	安顺市西秀区	安顺市西秀区疾病预防控制中心	鲁玲亚
	镇宁布依族苗族自治县	镇宁布依族苗族自治县疾病预防控制中心	杨　琳
	毕节市七星关区	毕节市七星关区疾病预防控制中心	李　琴
	金沙县	金沙县疾病预防控制中心	王天赐
	铜仁市碧江区	铜仁市碧江区疾病预防控制中心	杨江艳
	玉屏侗族自治县	玉屏侗族自治县疾病预防控制中心	陆承凯
	思南县	思南县疾病预防控制中心	王伟忠
	普安县	黔西南州普安县疾病预防控制中心	顾凤莉
	册亨县	黔西南州册亨县疾病预防控制中心	覃明江
	黄平县	黔东南州黄平县疾病预防控制中心	杨　玲
	镇远县	黔东南州镇远县疾病预防控制中心	顾先桃
	榕江县	黔东南州榕江县疾病预防控制中心	吴永莲
	雷山县	黔东南州雷山县疾病预防控制中心	毛　海
	麻江县	黔东南州麻江县疾病预防控制中心	吴晓云

省(自治区、直辖市) Province (autonomous region, municipality)	肿瘤登记处 Cancer registry	登记处所在单位 Affiliation	主要工作人员 Staff
	都匀市	黔南州都匀市疾病预防控制中心	李国叶
	福泉市	黔南州福泉市疾病预防控制中心	唐秋红
	荔波县	黔南州荔波县疾病预防控制中心	周雪梅
	独山县	黔南州独山县疾病预防控制中心	马清兰
	龙里县	黔南州龙里县疾病预防控制中心	杜月清
云南省	云南省	云南省疾病预防控制中心	文洪梅　陈　杨　石青萍
	昆明市	昆明市疾病预防控制中心	李　吉　杨　昭
	昆明市五华区	昆明市五华区疾病预防控制中心	周　丽　刘　畅　许秋婧　曾成琴　高柏强　王紫玉
	昆明市盘龙区	昆明市盘龙区疾病预防控制中心	何丽明　王睿翊　马琳玲　何开浚
	昆明市官渡区	昆明市官渡区疾病预防控制中心	张　龙　詹　恒　王晓珺　张慧萍　王　丽　段培华　佘旭敏
	昆明市西山区	昆明市西山区疾病预防控制中心	李　杰　周欣霞　龚　林　李赛云　李子美　张艺嘉　袁寂州　李绍叶
	昆明市东川区	昆明市东川区疾病预防控制中心	赵亚楠　韩贵卫
	昆明市晋宁区	昆明市晋宁区疾病预防控制中心	张美莲　李明珠
	昆明市呈贡区	昆明市呈贡区疾病预防控制中心	张永丽
	富民县	富民县疾病预防控制中心	李俊兴
	嵩明县	嵩明县疾病预防控制中心	郭树岚　保　尚
	禄劝县	禄劝县疾病预防控制中心	钟玉美　王　鑫　潘庆葵　杨祖宏　李泽蕊　耿天顺　李锡军
	安宁市	安宁市疾病预防控制中心	杨保学　赵会联
	曲靖市	曲靖市疾病预防控制中心	李继华　李　云　牛文倩
	曲靖市麒麟区	曲靖市麒麟区疾病预防控制中心	雷芸华　关秋艳　施红娟　丁鹏俊　吴林凤
	曲靖市沾益区	曲靖市沾益区疾病预防控制中心	雷宝琼　付　进
	马龙县	马龙县疾病预防控制中心	王慈蓉　万正文
	陆良县	陆良县疾病预防控制中心	钱康林　朱　姗
	富源县	富源县疾病预防控制中心	王　云

省(自治区、直辖市) Province (autonomous region, municipality)	肿瘤登记处 Cancer registry	登记处所在单位 Affiliation	主要工作人员 Staff
	宣威市	宣威市疾病预防控制中心	宁伯福
	玉溪市	玉溪市疾病预防控制中心	李六九 马真飞 李 吉
	玉溪市红塔区	玉溪市红塔区疾病预防控制中心	瞿 媛 杜春华 张 莉 刘 蕊 林 蕾 陶 然 邹 容 白光宝 管 颖 赵明洪 孟源珂
	玉溪市江川区	玉溪市江川区疾病预防控制中心	史伊冉 陈艺丹 赵媛丽
	澄江县	澄江县疾病预防控制中心	马重义 周红云 董志鹏
	通海县	通海县疾病预防控制中心	高瑞芳 李德雄 杨春琼 李 艳
	华宁县	华宁县疾病预防控制中心	施云丽 王志鹏 杨 蓉 杨忠卫
	易门县	易门县疾病预防控制中心	樊学琼 吕 宏 许 葵 阮 伟 王冬梅
	峨山彝族自治县	峨山彝族自治县疾病预防控制中心	李晓燕
	新平彝族傣族自治县	新平彝族傣族自治县疾病预防控制中心	殷文学
	元江哈尼族彝族傣族自治县	元江哈尼族彝族傣族自治县疾病预防控制中心	张坤平 杨太专 卫 芳 杨忠强 杨生宝 陆拾妹
	保山市	保山市疾病预防控制中心	徐仙会 李明松 邓 丽 褚钊颖
	保山市隆阳区	保山市隆阳区疾病预防控制中心	杨璐竹 杨善华 董全玉 杨保国 陈 浩 王 伟
	施甸县	施甸县疾病预防控制中心	吴新会 朱海燕 杨丝丝 杨继虎 杨进水
	腾冲市	腾冲市疾病预防控制中心	刘晓丽 李亚丹 杨艳芳 封占益 段立敏 李相妹
	龙陵县	龙陵县疾病预防控制中心	杨福娣 寸勐震 李菊云 王云春
	昌宁县	昌宁县疾病预防控制中心	曾映竹 杨绍杰 宋金阳 黄丽琼
	昭通市	昭通市疾病预防控制中心	马东琼
	昭通市昭阳区	昭通市昭阳区疾病预防控制中心	刘 卫 刘红英 陈 会
	巧家县	巧家县疾病预防控制中心	王开芳
	绥江县	绥江县疾病预防控制中心	刘晓静
	水富县	水富县疾病预防控制中心	朱晓蕾
	丽江市	丽江市疾病预防控制中心	杨丽梅 冉钦玉 段 珏 李光聪 杨永寿 王恭汉
	丽江市古城区	丽江市古城区疾病预防控制中心	和臣慧 王艳红 崔舒静
	玉龙纳西族自治县	玉龙纳西族自治县疾病预防控制中心	杨翠香 杨 俊 和致祥
	华坪县	华坪县疾病预防控制中心	王正英 黄同琼 卢国春
	普洱市	普洱市疾病预防控制中心	周锦涛 唐 颖 段义军
	景东彝族自治县	景东彝族自治县疾病预防控制中心	祝章美 龚 晨 陶 梅 周晓波

续表

省(自治区、直辖市) Province (autonomous region, municipality)	肿瘤登记处 Cancer registry	登记处所在单位 Affiliation	主要工作人员 Staff
	景谷傣族彝族自治县	景谷傣族彝族自治县疾病预防控制中心	周新玉　王丽娇　李　健
	镇沅彝族哈尼族拉祜族自治县	镇沅彝族哈尼族拉祜族自治县疾病预防控制中心	自家梅　罗开萍　吴容容
	江城哈尼族彝族自治县	江城哈尼族彝族自治县疾病预防控制中心	鲍月月　刘红兵　罗　路
	临沧市	临沧市疾病预防控制中心	李秋圆　曹建英　胡　红
	临沧临翔区	临翔区疾病预防控制中心	罗忠芳　王新梅　董秀玲　施正仙　李天玺
	镇康县	镇康县疾病预防控制中心	杨　凤　刘志梅
	沧源佤族自治县	沧源佤族自治县疾病预防控制中心	赵福芳　李　瑶　李　波
	楚雄彝族自治州	楚雄彝族自治州疾病预防控制中心	赵会勇
	楚雄市	楚雄市疾病预防控制中心	刘家早　仇剑芝
	双柏县	双柏县疾病预防控制中心	张雅薇
	牟定县	牟定县疾病预防控制中心	何　磊　杨　芳
	南华县	南华县疾病预防控制中心	吕美英　费建琼
	姚安县	姚安县疾病预防控制中心	苏菊芬　刘洪文
	大姚县	大姚县疾病预防控制中心	班琼珍　赵宗和
	永仁县	永仁县疾病预防控制中心	肖甫仁　孙丽华
	元谋县	元谋县疾病预防控制中心	仲丽红
	武定县	武定县疾病预防控制中心	赵学敏
	禄丰县	禄丰县疾病预防控制中心	刘雪丽　毕志梅
	红河哈尼族彝族自治州	红河州第三人民医院	潘龙海　后　群
	个旧市	个旧市肿瘤防治工作领导小组办公室	王建宁
	开远市	开远市疾病预防控制中心	杜晓芳　顾春芳　陈亚苏　闫友芸
	蒙自县	蒙自市疾病预防控制中心	杨　涛
	弥勒市	弥勒市疾病预防控制中心	徐建华　杨晓静
	屏边苗族自治县	屏边苗族自治县疾病预防控制中心	吴　娅
	建水县	建水县疾病预防控制中心	周艳梅　张艳芳　刘　怡　白玉仙　白　琼
	石屏县	石屏县疾病预防控制中心	王昌钰　高　霞
	泸西县	泸西县疾病预防控制中心	戴　丽　王秋婷
	河口瑶族自治县	河口瑶族自治县疾病预防控制中心	王海波　刘　源　姚　倩

续表

省(自治区、直辖市) Province (autonomous region, municipality)	肿瘤登记处 Cancer registry	登记处所在单位 Affiliation	主要工作人员 Staff
	文山壮族苗族自治州	文山壮族苗族自治州疾病预防控制中心	程　艳
	砚山县	砚山县疾病预防控制中心	祁红芬
	西畴县	西畴县疾病预防控制中心	袁　丽
	丘北县	丘北县疾病预防控制中心	杨燕琼
	富宁县	富宁县疾病预防控制中心	何利华
	西双版纳傣族自治州	西双版纳傣族自治州疾病预防控制中心	陈　萍　范芸苑
	景洪市	景洪市疾病预防控制中心	石保英　杨舒寒
	大理市	大理市疾病预防控制中心	何俊涵　杨　清　张　莹　杜雅素　魏朝晖　赵庆平
	祥云县	祥云县疾病预防控制中心	周亚娟　张建荣　丁雪琴
	弥渡县	弥渡县疾病预防控制中心	孙海欧　姚绍梅　张美华
	永平县	永平县疾病预防控制中心	马迎春　李亚芳
	鹤庆县	鹤庆县疾病预防控制中心	洪　梅　吴玉蓉　董　垚
	德宏傣族景颇族自治州	德宏傣族景颇族自治州疾病预防控制中心	李家才　高右东
	梁河县	梁河县疾病预防控制中心	李素一　方永兴
	盈江县	盈江县疾病预防控制中心	刘永艳　杨　洁　毕　锐
	怒江傈僳族自治州	怒江傈僳族自治州疾病预防控制中心	杨卫美
	兰坪白族普米族自治县	兰坪白族普米族自治县疾病预防控制中心	李晓燕　和绍梅　杨红玉
西藏自治区	西藏自治区	西藏自治区疾病预防控制中心	扎西宗吉　于　跃
	拉萨市城关区	拉萨市疾病预防控制中心	袁　静　杨永艳
	林芝市巴宜区	林芝市疾病预防控制中心	王　英
	山南市乃东区	山南市乃东区疾病预防控制中心	益西热强　刘月英
陕西省	陕西省	陕西省疾病预防控制中心	刘　峰　程永兵　邱　琳　王艳平
	西安市碑林区	西安市碑林区疾病预防控制中心	范　颖　周　鼎　李福强　朱　倩　郑君茹
	西安市莲湖区	西安市莲湖区疾病预防控制中心	李　凡　孙婷婷
	西安市未央区	西安市未央区疾病预防控制中心	李　倩　杨　梦
	西安市雁塔区	西安市雁塔区疾病预防控制中心	王　宁　薛静怡

续表

省(自治区、直辖市) Province (autonomous region, municipality)	肿瘤登记处 Cancer registry	登记处所在单位 Affiliation	主要工作人员 Staff
	西安市高陵区	西安市高陵区疾病预防控制中心	黄维娜　汪　洋
	西安市鄠邑区	西安市鄠邑区疾病预防控制中心慢病科	张　莹　丁　珍
	铜川市王益区	铜川市王益区疾病预防控制中心	赵旭东
	铜川市耀州区	铜川市耀州区疾病预防控制中心	陈雯雯
	宝鸡市金台区	宝鸡市金台区疾病预防控制中心	李　倩
	宝鸡市陈仓区	宝鸡市陈仓区疾病预防控制中心	王新梅
	凤翔县	凤翔县疾病预防控制中心	周晓梅
	岐山县	岐山县疾病预防控制中心	袁小红
	眉县	眉县疾病预防控制中心	赵　云
	陇县	陇县疾病预防控制中心	郭小兰
	千阳县	千阳县疾病预防控制中心	茹夏丽　赵　倩　尚　博
	麟游县	麟游县疾病预防控制中心	马方伟
	泾阳县	泾阳县疾病预防控制中心	闫阿妮
	渭南市临渭区	渭南市临渭区疾病预防控制中心	权巧玲
	渭南市华州区	渭南市华州区疾病预防控制中心	张亚莹
	潼关县	潼关县疾病预防控制中心	亢　静
	大荔县	大荔县疾病预防控制中心	陈艳萍　高卫丽
	合阳县	合阳县疾病预防控制中心	雷艳玲　梁忠义
	澄城县	澄城县疾病预防控制中心	王　鹏　雷晓利　楚　莹
	蒲城县	蒲城县疾病预防控制中心	赵　莹
	富平县	富平县疾病预防控制中心	苏木兰　简　琳
	华阴市	华阴市疾病预防控制中心	张济德　郝青青
	延安市宝塔区	延安市宝塔区疾病预防控制中心	刘　鑫　贺军宏　尹明萍　孙　婧
	富县	富县疾病预防控制中心	冯　超　王忠学　吕亚军　罗英利
	黄陵县	黄陵县疾病预防控制中心	雷云云　王　曼　杨明霞
	汉中市汉台区	汉中市汉台区疾病预防控制中心	杨宝亮　刘轩岐
	城固县	城固县疾病预防控制中心	尹　勇　高智平　李　罡
	宁强县	宁强县疾病预防控制中心	向凤义

省(自治区、直辖市) Province (autonomous region, municipality)	肿瘤登记处 Cancer registry	登记处所在单位 Affiliation	主要工作人员 Staff
	绥德县	绥德县疾病预防控制中心	刘　成
	安康市汉滨区	安康市汉滨区疾病预防控制中心	单林涛　刘卫军　王大锋　柯　娴
	汉阴县	汉阴县疾病预防控制中心	王　鹏
	石泉县	石泉县疾病预防控制中心	冯如月　陈梨花
	宁陕县	宁陕县疾病预防控制中心	代　鹏　易秉涛
	紫阳县	紫阳县疾病预防控制中心	许金华　陈　涛
	镇坪县	镇坪县疾病预防控制中心	杜誉淇
	旬阳县	旬阳县疾病预防控制中心	沈　龙　杜小菊
	商洛市商州区	商洛市商州区疾病预防控制中心	王天军　张　琪
	镇安县	镇安县疾病预防控制中心	刘家政　王　雯
甘肃省	甘肃省	甘肃省肿瘤医院/甘肃省癌症中心	刘玉琴　丁高恒
	兰州市	兰州市疾病预防控制中心	史危安　陆署元
	兰州市城关区	兰州市城关区疾病预防控制中心	杨海峰　韩　霞　杨　菁
	兰州市七里河区	兰州市七里河区疾病预防控制中心	陶　涛　王志龙
	兰州市西固区	兰州市西固区疾病预防控制中心	苟丽萍　徐　梅　徐　洁
	兰州市安宁区	兰州市安宁区疾病预防控制中心	何秀芬　殷　行
	兰州市红古区	兰州市红古区疾病预防控制中心	齐国怀　张　青
	白银市	白银市疾病预防控制中心	马骥雄　鲁朝霞
	白银市白银区	白银市白银区疾病预防控制中心	李顺翠　张小琴
	白银市平川区	白银市平川区疾病预防控制中心	李　霞　胡晓俊
	靖远县	靖远县疾病预防控制中心	高跟霞　欧志秀
	会宁县	会宁县疾病预防控制中心	程永莲　党丽琴
	景泰县	景泰县疾病预防控制中心	梁志龙　周福新　王生芸
	天水市	天水市疾病预防控制中心	张　庆　杨　婧
	天水市秦州区	天水市秦州区疾病预防控制中心	马　明　安珊珊
	天水市麦积区	天水市麦积区疾病预防控制中心	杨　慧　王　芳
	武威市	甘肃省武威肿瘤医院	叶延程　胡军国　高彩云

省(自治区、直辖市) Province (autonomous region, municipality)	肿瘤登记处 Cancer registry	登记处所在单位 Affiliation	主要工作人员 Staff
	武威市凉州区	武威市凉州区疾病预防控制中心	刘海峰　李玉霞
	民勤县	民勤县疾病预防控制中心	姜玉平
	古浪县	古浪县疾病预防控制中心	严艳玲　高娟娟
	天祝藏族自治县	天祝藏族自治县疾病预防控制中心	石福娟　王生玲
	张掖市	张掖市疾病预防控制中心	银万栋　王　清
	张掖市甘州区	甘州区疾病预防控制中心	王金金　陈国辉
	高台县	高台县疾病预防控制中心	黄充盈　闫述凯
	静宁县	静宁县疾病预防控制中心	闫润芳　杨　娟　师　慧
	敦煌市	敦煌市疾病预防控制中心	淳志明　殷海燕　杜文倩
	庆城县	庆城县疾病预防控制中心	慕杰民　项霞霞
	临洮县	临洮县疾病预防控制中心	汪生虎　康玉霞
	临潭县	临潭县疾病预防控制中心	姚文林　祁少华
青海省	青海省	青海省疾病预防控制中心	周素霞
	西宁市	西宁市疾病预防控制中心	汤海霞
	西宁市	城中区疾病预防控制中心	年晓亮
	西宁市	城东区疾病预防控制中心	马　萍　马丽娟
	西宁市	城西区疾病预防控制中心	张丁鑫乐
	西宁市	城北区疾病预防控制中心	郝广洪
	大通回族土族自治县	大通回族土族自治县疾病预防控制中心	张　莹　罗　燕
	湟中县	湟中县疾病预防控制中心	汪有库
	海东市	海东市疾病预防控制中心	魏　青
	海东市乐都区	青海省海东市乐都区疾病预防控制中心	谢淑雯
	民和回族土族自治县	民和回族土族自治县疾病预防控制中心	张学强
	互助土族自治县	互助土族自治县疾病预防控制中心	王小庆
	循化撒拉族自治县	循化撒拉族自治县疾病预防控制中心	陕国清
	海南藏族自治州	海南藏族自治州疾病预防控制中心	拉毛才让
	海南藏族自治州	共和县疾病预防控制中心	齐迎兰
	海南藏族自治州	同德县疾病预防控制中心	朱祖祯　拉先太
	海南藏族自治州	贵德县疾病预防控制中心	贺永庆
	海南藏族自治州	兴海县疾病预防控制中心	张　琼

续表

省(自治区、直辖市) Province (autonomous region, municipality)	肿瘤登记处 Cancer registry	登记处所在单位 Affiliation	主要工作人员 Staff
	海南藏族自治州	贵南县疾病预防控制中心	石君红
宁夏回族自治区	宁夏回族自治区	宁夏疾病预防控制中心	马　芳　杨　艺　魏　嵘
	银川市兴庆区	兴庆区疾病预防控制中心	王洪丽　王　晶　侯静娅
	银川市西夏区	西夏区疾病预防控制中心	张　婷　仇婷婷
	银川市金凤区	金凤区疾病预防控制中心	保红莉　王海霞
	贺兰县	贺兰县疾病预防控制中心	盛春宁　陈海荣　姜旭红　董　威　陈　娥　马美娜
	石嘴山市大武口区	石嘴山市疾病预防控制中心	马　洁　张平稳　任海丽　刘　英　吴永军　张　悦
	石嘴山市惠农区	石嘴山市惠农区疾病预防控制中心	叶　璐　李冬梅　冯　羽
	平罗县	平罗县疾病预防控制中心	刘凤香
	青铜峡市	青铜峡市疾病预防控制中心	哈艳茹　赵仲刚　马　丽
	固原市原州区	固原市原州区疾病预防控制中心	南　艳
	中卫市沙坡头区	中卫市疾病预防控制中心	姚永红
	中宁县	中宁县疾病预防控制中心	赵寿桃
新疆维吾尔自治区	新疆维吾尔自治区	新疆维吾尔自治区疾病预防控制中心	董　言　张　荣　者　炜　王雯雷　张　俊　方　萍
	乌鲁木齐市天山区	乌鲁木齐市天山区疾病预防控制中心	郭颖贞　张招辉
	乌鲁木齐市米东区	乌鲁木齐市米东区疾病预防控制中心	刘　馨　马　芳
	克拉玛依市	克拉玛依市疾病预防控制中心	陈志萍　陈雪莹
	新源县	新源县疾病预防控制中心	田鹏昊　杨贺霞
	库尔勒市	库尔勒市疾病预防控制中心	木克热木・于努斯
	和田市	和田市疾病预防控制中心	阿曼古丽・阿迪力
	和田县	和田县疾病预防控制中心	古丽洁米娜・阿不杜喀迪尔
新疆生产建设兵团	新疆生产建设兵团	兵团疾病预防控制中心	申嘉丛　李凡卡　张宏伟　敬　雯
	第二师	第二师疾病预防控制中心	文　静　周喜元　丁宏达　闫　澈
	第七师	第七师疾病预防控制中心	周　倩　杨海东　龚　耀　刘长龙
	石河子市	石河子大学	李　锋　崔晓宾　李述刚　胡云华　刘春霞　刘成刚　陈　瑜　王　蓉　牛　强　闫贻忠　卢香云